Rhinoplasty:
A Multispecialty Approach

Editor

BABAK AZIZZADEH

CLINICS IN
PLASTIC SURGERY

www.plasticsurgery.theclinics.com

Section Editors
DANIEL BECKER
RONALD P. GRUBER

January 2016 • Volume 43 • Number 1

ELSEVIER

1600 John F. Kennedy Boulevard • Suite 1800 • Philadelphia, Pennsylvania, 19103-2899

http://www.theclinics.com

CLINICS IN PLASTIC SURGERY Volume 43, Number 1
January 2016 ISSN 0094-1298, ISBN-13: 978-0-323-41464-7

Editor: Jessica McCool
Developmental Editor: Donald Mumford

Clinics in Plastic Surgery (ISSN 0094-1298) is published quarterly by Elsevier Inc., 360 Park Avenue South, New York, NY 10010-1710. Months of issue are January, April, July, and October. Business and Editorial Offices: 1600 John F. Kennedy Blvd., Suite 1800, Philadelphia, PA 19103-2899. Periodicals postage paid at New York, NY and additional mailing offices. Subscription prices are $490.00 per year for US individuals, $793.00 per year for US institutions, $100.00 per year for US students and residents, $555.00 per year for Canadian individuals, $944.00 per year for Canadian institutions, $630.00 per year for international individuals, $944.00 per year for international institutions, and $305.00 per year for Canadian and foreign students/residents. To receive student/resident rate, orders must be accompanied by name of affiliated institution, date of term, and the *signature* of program/residency coordinator on institution letterhead. Orders will be billed at individual rate until proof of status is received. Foreign air speed delivery is included in all *Clinics* subscription prices. All prices are subject to change without notice. **POSTMASTER:** Send address changes to *Clinics in Plastic Surgery,* Elsevier Health Sciences Division, Subscription Customer Service, 3251 Riverport Lane, Maryland Heights, MO 63043. **Customer Service: 1-800-654-2452 (US and Canada). From outside of the United States and Canada, call 314-447-8871. Fax: 314-447-8029. E-mail: JournalsCustomerService-usa@elsevier.com (for print support); JournalsOnlineSupport-usa@ elsevier.com (for online support).**

Reprints. For copies of 100 or more of articles in this publication, please contact the Commercial Reprints Department, Elsevier Inc., 360 Park Avenue South, New York, New York 10010-1710. Tel.: +1-212-633-3874; Fax: +1-212-633-3820; E-mail: reprints@elsevier.com.

Clinics in Plastic Surgery is covered in *Current Contents, EMBASE/Excerpta Medica, Science Citation Index, MEDLINE/ PubMed (Index Medicus), ASCA, and ISI/BIOMED.*

Contributors

EDITOR

BABAK AZIZZADEH, MD, FACS
Associate Clinical Professor, Department of
Head and Neck Surgery, David Geffen School
of Medicine at UCLA, Los Angeles, California;
Center for Advanced Facial Plastic Surgery,
Beverly Hills, California

SECTION EDITORS

DANIEL G. BECKER, MD, FACS
Clinical Professor, Division of Facial Plastic and
Reconstructive Surgery, Department of
Otolaryngology-Head and Neck Surgery,
University of Pennsylvania Medical Center,
Philadelphia, Pennsylvania; Clinical Associate
Professor, Department of Otolaryngology-
Head and Neck Surgery, University of Virginia
Medical Center, Charlottesville, Virginia

RONALD P. GRUBER, MD
Clinical Associate Professor, Division of Plastic
and Reconstructive Surgery, University of
California, San Francisco, Oakland, California;
Adjunct Clinical Associate Professor of
Surgery, School of Medicine, Stanford
University, Stanford, California

AUTHORS

JAMIL AHMAD, MD, FRCSC
Director of Research and Education, The
Plastic Surgery Clinic, Mississauga, Ontario,
Canada; Assistant Professor, Division of
Plastic and Reconstructive Surgery,
Department of Surgery, University of Toronto,
Toronto, Ontario, Canada

AMIR ALLAK, MD, MBA
Department of Otolaryngology–Head and Neck
Surgery, University of Virginia, Charlottesville,
Virginia

FAZIL APAYDIN, MD
Professor, Department of Otolaryngology, Ege
University Medical Faculty, Bornova, İzmir,
Turkey

BABAK AZIZZADEH, MD, FACS
Associate Clinical Professor, Department of
Head and Neck Surgery, David Geffen School
of Medicine at UCLA, Los Angeles, California;
Center for Advanced Facial Plastic Surgery,
Beverly Hills, California

DANIEL G. BECKER, MD, FACS
Clinical Professor, Division of Facial Plastic and
Reconstructive Surgery, Department of
Otolaryngology-Head and Neck Surgery,
University of Pennsylvania Medical Center,
Philadelphia, Pennsylvania; Clinical Associate
Professor, Department of Otolaryngology-
Head and Neck Surgery, University of Virginia
Medical Center, Charlottesville, Virginia

R. LAURENCE BERKOWITZ, MD
Diplomate, American Board of Plastic Surgery;
Aesthetic and Reconstructive Plastic Surgery,
Campbell, California

ASHLEY CAFFERTY, BA
Post-Baccalaureate PreMedical Program,
Thomas Jefferson University, Philadelphia,
Pennsylvania

BARıŞ ÇAKıR, MD
Plastic Surgeon, Private Practice, Terrace
Fulya, Istanbul, Turkey

NAZIM CERKES, MD
Private Practice, Istanbul, Turkey

GERALD J. CHO, MD
Division of Plastic and Reconstructive Surgery,
University of California, San Francisco,
San Francisco, California

ROXANA COBO, MD
Chief, Department of Otolaryngology, Centro
Médico Imbanaco, Cali, Colombia

CHRISTOPHER SPENCER COCHRAN, MD
Clinical Assistant Professor,
Department of Otolaryngology-Head
and Neck Surgery, University of Texas
Southwestern Medical Center at Dallas,
Dallas, Texas

JEFFREY D. CONE Jr, MD
Wellspring Plastic Surgery, Austin, Texas

ROLLIN K. DANIEL, MD
Clinical Professor, Aesthetic Plastic Surgery
Institute, University of California Irvine, Irvine,
California

KARAN DHIR, MD
Assistant Clinical Professor, Department of
Head and Neck Surgery, Harbor-UCLA
Medical Center, Beverly Hills, California

FRED G. FEDOK, MD, FACS
Adjunct Professor, Department of Surgery,
University of South Alabama Medical Center,
Mobile, Alabama; Professor, Facial Plastic and
Reconstructive Surgery, Otolaryngology/Head
and Neck Surgery, Hershey Medical Center,
Pennsylvania State University, Hershey,
Pennsylvania

OREN FRIEDMAN, MD
Director, Facial Plastic Surgery; Associate
Professor, Department of
Otorhinolaryngology–Head and Neck Surgery,
University of Pennsylvania, Philadelphia,
Pennsylvania

REBECCA M. GARZA, MD
Division of Plastic and Reconstructive Surgery,
Stanford University, Stanford, California

ASHKAN GHAVAMI, MD
Assistant Clinical Professor, Department of
Plastic and Reconstructive Surgery, David
Geffen School of Medicine, University of
California, Los Angeles, Beverly Hills, California

ANKONA GHOSH, MD
Department of Otorhinolaryngology–Head and
Neck Surgery, University of Pennsylvania,
Philadelphia, Pennsylvania

RONALD P. GRUBER, MD
Clinical Associate Professor, Division of Plastic
and Reconstructive Surgery, University of
California, San Francisco, Oakland, California;
Adjunct Clinical Associate Professor of
Surgery, School of Medicine, Stanford
University, Stanford, California

BAHMAN GUYURON, MD
Zeeba Clinic, Lyndhurst, Ohio; Emeritus
Professor, Case Western Reserve University,
Cleveland, Ohio

P. CRAIG HOBAR, MD
Director of International Development
of Cleft and Craniofacial Surgery,
Medical City Children's Hospital, Dallas,
Texas

HONG RYUL JIN, MD, PhD
Department of Otorhinolaryngology-Head and
Neck Surgery, Boramae Medical Center, Seoul
National University College of Medicine, Seoul,
Republic of Korea

MYRIAM LOYO, MD
Assistant Professor, Division of Facial Plastic
and Reconstructive Surgery, Department of
Otolaryngology-Head and Neck Surgery,
Oregon Health and Science University,
Portland, Oregon

IAN R. MacARTHUR, MD, FRCSC
Craniofacial Surgery Fellow, Plastic and
Reconstructive Surgery, Nicklaus Children's
Hospital, Miami, Florida

DIRK JAN MENGER, MD, PhD
Department of ENT/FPRS, University Medical
Center Utrecht, Utrecht, The Netherlands

HYOUNG JIN MOON, MD
President of Dr Moon's Aesthetic Plastic
Surgery Clinic, Seoul, Republic of Korea

PAUL S. NASSIF, MD, FACS
Department of Otolaryngology, Head and
Neck Surgery, Keck School of Medicine,
University of Southern California, Los Angeles,
California

NIRMAL R. NATHAN, MD
Craniofacial Surgery Fellow, Plastic and
Reconstructive Surgery, Nicklaus Children's
Hospital, Miami, Florida

ALI RıZA ÖREROĞLU, MD
Assistant Professor of Plastic Surgery,
Acıbadem Fulya Hospital, Istanbul, Turkey

STEPHEN S. PARK, MD
Vice Chairman and Professor, Department of
Otolaryngology–Head and Neck Surgery,
University of Virginia, Charlottesville, Virginia

GRACE LEE PENG, MD
Department of Otolaryngology, Head and
Neck Surgery, Keck School of Medicine,
University of Southern California, Los Angeles,
California

MICHAEL REILLY, MD
Associate Professor, Department of
Otolaryngology—Head and Neck Surgery,
Georgetown University Medical Center,
Washington, DC

ROD J. ROHRICH, MD, FACS
Professor and Founding Chairman,
Department of Plastic Surgery, University of
Texas Southwestern Medical Center at Dallas,
Dallas, Texas

ALI SAJJADIAN, MD, FACS
Department of Plastic Surgery, Hoag Hospital,
Newport Beach, California

GUSTAVO A. SUÁREZ, MD
Department of Otolaryngology - Head and
Neck Surgery, Bellvitge University Hospital,
Barcelona, Spain

JONATHAN M. SYKES, MD
Professor and Director, Facial Plastic Surgery,
Division of Facial Plastic and Reconstructive
Surgery, Department of Otolaryngology,
University of California Davis, Sacramento,
California

NEIL TANNA, MD, MBA
Associate Professor of Surgery, Division of
Plastic and Reconstructive Surgery, North
Shore – LIJ Health System, Lake Success,
New York

ABEL-JAN TASMAN, MD
Rhinology and Facial Plastic Surgery,
Department of Otolaryngology-Head and Neck
Surgery, Cantonal Hospital, St. Gallen,
Switzerland

JOHN F. TEICHGRAEBER, MD
Professor of Surgery, Division of Plastic and
Reconstructive Surgery, University of Texas
Health Science Center at Houston, Houston,
Texas

ALI TOTONCHI, MD
Plastic Surgery Division, MetroHealth
Medical Center; Assistant Professor, Case
Western Reserve University, Cleveland,
Ohio

DEV VIBHAKAR, DO
Adult Craniofacial Reconstructive and
Aesthetic Fellow, Division of Plastic and
Reconstructive Surgery, Massachusetts
General Hospital, Harvard Medical School,
Boston, Massachusetts

TOM D. WANG, MD
Professor and Chief, Division of Facial Plastic
and Reconstructive Surgery, Department of
Otolaryngology-Head and Neck Surgery,
Oregon Health and Science University,
Portland, Oregon

**STEPHEN ANTHONY WOLFE, MD, FACS,
FAAP**
Chief of Plastic and Reconstructive
Surgery, Nicklaus Children's Hospital,
Miami, Florida

TAE-BIN WON, MD, PhD
Department of Otorhinolaryngology-Head and
Neck Surgery, Seoul National University
Hospital, Seoul, Republic of Korea

MICHAEL J. YAREMCHUK, MD
Program Director, Harvard Plastic Surgery
Training Program, Chief of Craniofacial
Surgery, Division of Plastic and Reconstructive
Surgery, Massachusetts General Hospital,
Clinical Professor of Surgery, Part-Time,
Harvard Medical School, Boston,
Massachusetts

Contents

Surface aesthetics of an attractive nose result from certain lines, shadows, and highlights with specific proportions and breakpoints. Analysis emphasizes geometric polygons as aesthetic subunits. Evaluation of the complete nasal surface aesthetics is achieved using geometric polygons to define the existing deformity and aesthetic goals. The relationship between the dome triangles, interdomal triangle, facet polygons, and infralobular polygon are integrated to form the "diamond shape" light reflection on the nasal tip. The principles of geometric polygons allow the surgeon to analyze the deformities of the nose, define an operative plan to achieve specific goals, and select the appropriate operative technique.

Most surgeons recognize the broad utility of both endonasal and external rhinoplasty approaches. Most understand that there are situations when a given approach offers advantages and may be considered preferable. In this article, the anatomy, incisions, and approaches that are available to the surgeon are reviewed. General indications are discussed for the external and endonasal approaches. The pros and cons of each approach are discussed, and further thoughts on the decision-making process are provided.

The key to a successful septorhinoplasty includes an understanding of nasal anatomy and physiology. This allows the surgeon the ability to properly address both form and function during the operation. History and physical examination are paramount in diagnosing and subsequently treating the epicenter of obstruction, which is commonly found among the internal and external nasal valve, the septum, or the turbinates. Treatment of each of these areas is nuanced and multiple approaches are discussed to provide an understanding of the current surgical techniques that allow for excellent functional and cosmetic rhinoplasty results.

The management and diagnosis of nasal airway obstruction requires an understanding of the form and function of the nose. Nasal airway obstruction can be structural, physiologic, or a combination of both. Anatomic causes of airway obstruction include septal deviation, internal nasal valve narrowing, external nasal valve collapse, and inferior turbinate hypertrophy. Thus, the management of nasal air obstruction must be selective and carefully considered. The goal of surgery is to address the deformity and not just enlarge the nasal cavity.

This article discusses the technique for planning, executing, and troubleshooting dorsal hump reduction for the cosmetic rhinoplasty patient. Details of the discussion include the necessary elements of the preoperative consultation with the patient, the specific instruments used to effectively and reproducibly create osteotomies, the anatomic and patient variables that require special attention, and the necessary measures to guard against potential complications.

Rhinoplasty is not so much an art, but rather an architectural undertaking: a methodical approach to reconfiguring the nasal components to give a proportionate nose that both pleases the eye and satisfies functional requirements. The dorsum and dorsal aesthetic lines are some of the most important components of the nose in terms of aesthetics and function. The middle vault is the critical portion of the nose that will guide the management of the bony vault and the tip. The role of the spreader flap and its extension into the bony vault is stressed to re-create the barrel vaultlike nasal architecture.

Controlling the shape of the nasal bones has long been a frustrating problem. Conventional osteotomies are associated with bleeding, loss of reduction, inability to achieve the desired alignment, improperly placed osteotomy sites, and spicule formation. A nonpowered osteotomy method empirically provided the safest and most controlled technique to achieve the desired anatomic result. The nasal bones should be thought of as 2 thin nasal plates that can be released from their medial and lateral attachments to become mobile units that can affect the dorsal width and bony base independently. There is a learning curve to osteotomies.

The middle nasal vault is a sensitive region of the nose from both an esthetic and a functional perspective. It is critical for the rhinoplasty surgeon to properly evaluate and identify abnormalities of the middle vault when considering patients for primary or secondary surgery. This article addresses the surgical management of the cosmetic deformities and functional deficits of the middle vault and provides guidance for avoiding complications in this structurally critical region of the nose.

(▶) Videos of the steps in the correction of the twisted nose accompany this article

The twisted nose is a challenging procedure in rhinoplasty. The goal of surgery is to realign the nasal skeleton to create symmetry in the face and restore nasal patency. Key in the surgical procedure is that all structures of the nasal skeleton be dissected free, mobilized, repositioned, and stabilized. Important surgical steps are intermediate osteotomies on the contralateral side of the deviation for the upper nasal third; for the mid nasal third, a unilateral spreader graft or splint on the non-deviated side, and for the lower nasal third, fixation of the caudal septum to the anterior nasal spine.

Correction of a crooked nose is one of the most common requests from patients presenting for rhinoplasty. Both esthetic and functional issues are typically present in patients with this deformity. Rhinoplasty for the crooked nose is particularly challenging because multiple nasal structures, both external and internal, are commonly involved. A major septal deformity is almost always a component of severely deviated noses. The crooked nose results from extrinsic and intrinsic forces that produce distortion of the nasal structures and nasal deviation. The open approach is particularly useful and is the focus of this article.

This article presents a contemporary overview of tip suturing and tip structural grafting techniques used to refine the wide nasal tip. Previous reductive techniques have proved to produce unnatural results over time. It is imperative to correctly evaluate the nose and assess all possible pitfalls during the preoperative period before outlining a surgical plan. Intraoperatively, an algorithmic approach helps obtain a reproducible and refined yet properly narrowed domal tip region with graceful contours that extend laterally to the alar lobule with proper shadowing.

The alar rim plays an important role in nasal harmony. Alar rim flaws are common following the initial rhinoplasty. Classification of the deformities helps with diagnosis and successful surgical correction. Diagnosis of the deformity requires careful observation of the computerized or life-sized photographs. Techniques for treatment of these deformities can easily be learned with attention to detail.

 Videos of strengthening of a deficient nasal tip; correction of cephalic malposition; elongation of short alar cartilages; and bending technique for lateral crura and dome reconstruction using rib cartilage accompany this article

Nasal tip deficiency can be congenital or secondary to previous nasal surgeries. Underdeveloped medial crura usually present with underprojected tip and lack of tip definition. Weakness or malposition of lateral crura causes alar rim retraction and lateral nasal wall weakness. Structural grafting of alar cartilages strengthens the tip framework, reinforces the disrupted support mechanisms, and controls the position of the nasal tip. In secondary cases, anatomic reconstruction of the weakened or interrupted alar cartilages and reconstitution of a stable nasal tip tripod must be the goal for a predictable outcome.

Satisfactory and consistent long-term results in primary and secondary rhinoplasty rely on adequately resupporting or reconstructing the nasal osseocartilagenous framework. Autogenous rib cartilage has been our graft material of choice for major nasal reconstruction when sufficient septal cartilage is not available. The rib provides the most abundant source of cartilage for graft fabrication and is the most reliable when structural support is needed.

Cartilage grafts are regularly used in rhinoplasty. Septal and auricular donor sites are commonly used. Many situations compel the surgeon to use other alternative donor sites, including revision rhinoplasty and trauma. Many patients have a small amount of native septal cartilage and are unable to provide adequate septal cartilage to be used for frequently performed rhinoplasty maneuvers. The rib cage provides an enormous reserve of costal cartilage that can be carved into a variety of necessary grafts. A description of the technique of harvesting costal cartilage, a review of complications and management, and illustrative cases are included as examples.

This article presents an overview of the cleft lip nasal deformity and its treatment. The complex pathologic changes to normal nasal anatomy are described, and treatment strategies for both unilateral and bilateral cleft lip patients are presented. The surgical technique for management of the cleft lip nasal deformity is discussed as it pertains to both primary and secondary correction.

All patients with a cleft lip deformity have an associated nasal deformity that varies in degree of severity. A three-dimensional understanding of the anatomy of the cleft nose aids surgeons in selecting the proper technique for repair. Analysis and performance of orthognathic surgery should be done before nasal surgery to optimize the overall result. Goals of the secondary rhinoplasty include relief of nasal obstruction, creation of symmetry and definition of the nasal base and tip, and management of nasal scarring and webbing. Septal reconstruction in the cleft nose is a key maneuver in cleft rhinoplasty.

 Videos of placement of intercrural and septoclumellar sutures accompany this article

Rhinoplasty is the main facial plastic procedure performed in Latin America. Mestizo or Latino patients tend to have noses with thick skin, bulbous tips with poor projection, and flimsy osteocartilaginous underlying frameworks. A technique is presented in which structural grafts are used to strengthen support structures of the nose. A gradual approach is used to obtain tip definition, rotation, and projection using sutures and grafts. Simple techniques are used initially, progressing to more aggressive and less predictable ones in patients who require greater changes. The result should be noses that look more refined, with greater definition, but without looking bigger.

concurrent augmentation or reduction mentoplasty. Alloplastic chin implants and sliding genioplasty represent the main accepted methods of chin augmentation. Although both procedures may be used for retrognathia or microgenia, the sliding genioplasty may also be used in chin asymmetry, prognathia, and vertical height discrepancies. This article outlines the methods to analyze the chin, and discusses the treatment options available for correction of chin deformities as an adjunct to rhinoplasty.

Use of Fillers in Rhinoplasty

Hyoung Jin Moon

Surgical rhinoplasty is the one of the most common cosmetic procedures in Asians. But there are limitations, such as down time, high cost, and a steep learning curve. Most complications are implant related. A safer and less invasive procedure is rhinoplasty using fillers. Good knowledge of the nasal anatomy is essential for rhinoplasty using fillers. Knowledge of nerves, blood supply, and injection plane allows avoiding complications. There are several planes in the nose. The deep fatty layer is recommended for injection, because it is wide and loose and there are less important neurovascular structures. Botulinum toxin also can be used for noninvasive rhinoplasty.

Index

CLINICS IN PLASTIC SURGERY

FORTHCOMING ISSUES

April 2016
Complications in Breast Reduction
Dennis C. Hammond, *Editor*

July 2016
Minimally Invasive Plastic Surgery for the Aging Face
Kenneth Rothaus, *Editor*

October 2016
Free Tissue Transfer to Head and Neck: Lessons Learned from Unfavorable Results
Fu-Chan Wei and Nidal Farhan AL Deek, *Editors*

RECENT ISSUES

October 2015
Breast Augmentation
Bradley P. Bengtson, *Editor*

July 2015
Fat Grafting: Current Concept, Clinical Application, and Regenerative Potential, Part 2
Lee L.Q. Pu, Kotaro Yoshimura, and Sydney R. Coleman, *Editors*

April 2015
Fat Grafting: Current Concept, Clinical Application, and Regenerative Potential, Part 1
Lee L.Q. Pu, Kotaro Yoshimura, and Sydney R. Coleman, *Editors*

ISSUE OF RELATED INTEREST

Facial Plastic Surgery Clinics of North America
Editor: Richard E. Davis
Rhinoplasty: Contemporary Innovations
February 2015. Volume 23, Issue 1
Available at: http://www.facialplastic.theclinics.com/

THE CLINICS ARE AVAILABLE ONLINE!
Access your subscription at:
www.theclinics.com

Preface
Rhinoplasty: Education Through Multispecialty Collaboration

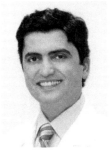

Babak Azizzadeh, MD, FACS

Editor

It is a great honor to be part of this special issue of *Clinics in Plastic Surgery* dedicated to multispecialty rhinoplasty. I embarked several years ago in partnership with *Clinics in Plastic Surgery* to develop publications that bring together viewpoints of different core specialists in order to provide the most up-to-date and advanced educational forum. The first two issues focused on eyelid, brow, and midface rejuvenation. This issue is solely dedicated to rhinoplasty and nasal surgery. Rhinoplasty has long been considered one of the most challenging operations in esthetic and reconstructive surgery. Although plastic surgeons and facial plastic surgeons have for decades worked alongside one another in teaching and practicing this beautiful surgery, very few publications have put forth techniques by experts in both specialties. This unfortunate fact has truly affected multispecialty education and collaboration. We hope that these series of journals will be the beginning of many more collaborative efforts by experts from various different specialties.

The guest editors, Drs Daniel Becker and Ronald Gruber, are among the most prolific rhinoplasty surgeons and educators in their respective fields of facial plastic surgery and plastic surgery.

They have done a remarkable job of putting together a rhinoplasty compendium that will serve both the novice and the experienced surgeon alike. I owe them a debt of gratitude that is beyond words. This project could not have been completed without the tireless effort of the editors at Elsevier, specifically Donald Mumford, Jessica McCool, and Mahalakshmi Narayanan. Finally, I would like to thank my wonderful family for supporting not just this effort but countless other projects. Their selfless sacrifice will never be forgotten.

Babak Azizzadeh, MD, FACS
Center for Advanced Facial Plastic Surgery
9401 Wilshire Boulevard, Suite 650
Beverly Hills, CA 90212, USA

Department of Head and Neck Surgery
David Geffen School of Medicine at UCLA
Los Angeles, CA, USA

E-mail address:
drazizzadeh@gmail.com
Website: http://www.facialplastics.info (B. Azizzadeh)

Surface Aesthetics and Analysis

Barış Çakır, MD[a],*, Ali Rıza Öreroğlu, MD[b], Rollin K. Daniel, MD[c]

KEYWORDS

- Rhinoplasty • Nasal surface aesthetics • Nasal aesthetic polygons • Lateral crus resting angle

KEY POINTS

- Surface aesthetics of an attractive nose are the result of certain lines, shadows, and highlights with specific proportions and breakpoints.
- Evaluation of the complete nasal surface aesthetics is achieved using the concept of geometric polygons to define the existing deformity and the aesthetic goals.
- The concept of a lateral crus resting angle in the ideal nose is defined.
- The relationship between dome triangles, interdomal triangle, facet polygons, and infralobular polygon is integrated to form the "diamond shape" light reflection on the nasal tip.
- The principles of geometric polygons allow the surgeon to analyze deformities, define an operative plan to achieve specific goals, and select the appropriate operative technique.

The primary objective of rhinoplasty surgery is to create an attractive functional nose without any surgical stigmata. However, this goal can only be achieved if the surgeon understands the direct linkage between surface aesthetics, underlying anatomic structures, and functional factors. The appearance of an attractive nose is created by certain lines, shadows, and highlights covering the nasal dorsum, tip, and base. During rhinoplasty surgery, these surface aesthetics with their proportions and breakpoints must be maintained, emphasized, and created. Analysis of the nasal anatomy through the surface aesthetic concepts enables proper identification of the underlying anatomic structures contributing to the shape and hence proper planning of surgery (**Fig. 1**). The following aesthetic concepts enable the rhinoplasty surgeon to analyze the underlying nasal anatomy and the reflections on the surface, and to plan and perform the rhinoplasty procedure with respect to the surface aesthetics of the nose.

NASAL ANALYSIS: LEARN TO SKETCH THE NOSE

You cannot perform a good surgery unless you can draw the organ precisely. Design increases awareness. You cannot solve a problem that you cannot see. Design allows you to analyze a good nose and imitate it well. Draw the nose contours; create the shades. Draw the edges of the cartilages.

Sketch from the Front

The nose tip is composed of 3 circles. The middle circle includes more cartilage than the circles on the sides. There is a 3:2 ratio for these circles. Investigate the boundaries where the nose

Financial Disclosure and Products: No financial aid or funding has been received from any institution for preparation of this paper by any of the authors. Dr B. Çakır: (1) Springer Publications; (2) Medicon Instruments. Dr R.K. Daniel: (1) Springer Publications; (2) Medicon Instruments.
[a] Private Practice, Terrace Fulya, Hakkı Yeten Cad., No: 11, Center: 1, Apt: 5 Şişli, Istanbul 34349, Turkey;
[b] Acıbadem Fulya Hospital, Yeşilçimen Sok. No: 23 Dikilitaş Mah. Hakkı Yeten Cad., Beşiktaş, Istanbul 34349, Turkey; [c] Aesthetic Plastic Surgery Institute, University of California Irvine, Irvine, CA 92697, USA
* Corresponding author.
E-mail address: op.dr.bariscakir@gmail.com

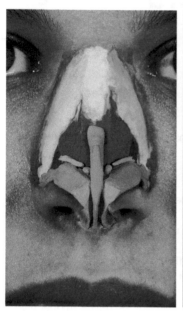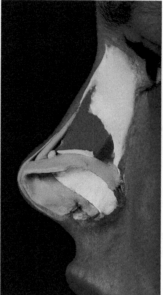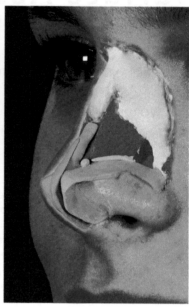

Fig. 1. Clay model superposition of the nasal anatomy. Yellow, bony vault; red, upper lateral cartilages; blue, lower lateral cartilages; green, Pitanguy's midline ligament and scroll ligaments.

touches the face. Also draw the lateral aesthetic lines. Investigate the relation between lateral aesthetic lines and dorsum aesthetic lines, the beginning and ending points. Look at your friend's nose during the drawing. You will start to see details that you never recognized before. This will increase your awareness. Draw the "nostril sill" and understand its anatomy well. See the close relation between the nostril sill and the footplate. Investigate the endpoint of the nostril sill. If the scar of the alar surgery conforms to the nostril sill anatomy, then the human eye cannot recognize the scar. Investigate the fusiform structure constituted by the nasal dorsum. You can understand the dorsal aesthetic lines better. Shadowing is a further step. Investigate the relation between dorsal aesthetic lines and shadows. Adding some light to the dorsal aesthetic lines will make your drawing more realistic (**Fig. 2**).

Sketch from the Side

Determine the length and height of the nose. Determine the nasolabial angle. We will use the same circles again. The 3:2 ratio is the same as from the front. The line that passes tangent to the bottom edge of the circles gives us the nasolabial angle. The lateral view of the nostrils is also very important. Examine the nostril peak point and the C point relation. Examine the columellar and lobule ratio. You can copy from beautiful noses in these drawings. It is easier to make drawings from beautiful nose photos (**Fig. 3**).

Sketch from Above and Below

It is also important to draw the nose from top and bottom. If you make drawings from all angles by using the same cubic forms, your brain will take the photo of the cartilages and make a 3-dimensional model of it (**Fig. 4**).

AESTHETIC NASAL POLYGONS

The nose can be analyzed as aesthetic units using the concept of geometric polygons.[1] A polygon is defined as a plane figure with at least 3 straight sides and angles. Evaluation of the nasal surface using polygons allows identification of shadows and highlights that are linked to the underlying anatomic structures that can be modified surgically. Thus, the goal of surgery is to modify, rearrange, and/or reconstruct the nasal infrastructure, thereby creating nasal surface polygons that are symmetric and aesthetically pleasing.

From the glabella downward, we can define the glabella polygon, dorsal bone polygon, dorsal cartilage triangle, lateral bone polygons, upper lateral polygons, dome triangles, lateral crus polygons, interdomal triangle, facet polygons, infralobular polygon, columellar polygon, and footplate polygons (**Fig. 5**). The intersection and juxtaposition of the polygons define the "lines" and "points" that rhinoplasty surgeons use to analyze the nose. Although somewhat tedious to define, these polygons are easily sketched on standard nasal photographs and quickly mastered for operative planning.[1]

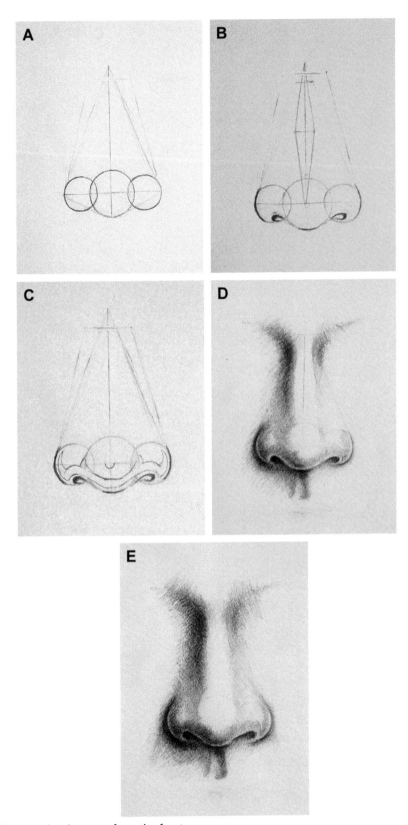

Fig. 2. (*A–E*) Steps to sketch a nose from the front.

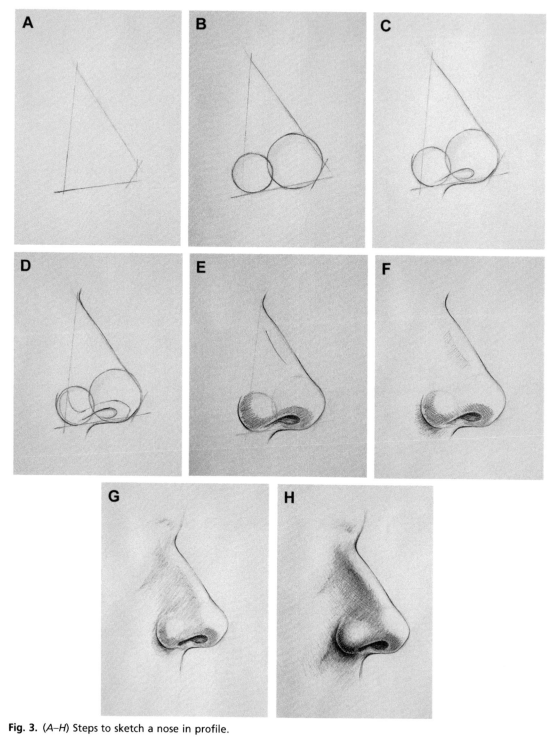

Fig. 3. (*A–H*) Steps to sketch a nose in profile.

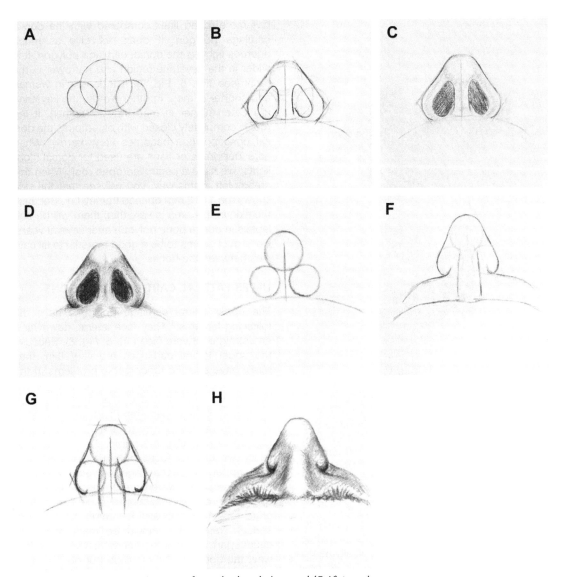

Fig. 4. (*A–D*) Steps to sketch a nose from the basal view and (*E–H*) top view.

THE NON-MOBILE UPPER NOSE

These polygons are mass polygons. They are created from cartilage and bone.

1. Glabellar polygon
2. Dorsal bone polygon
3. Dorsal cartilage polygon
4. Lateral bone polygons
5. Upper lateral cartilage polygons

THE MOBILE TIP AREA
Mass Polygons

1. Dome triangles
2. Lateral crus polygons

Gap Polygons (Cannot Be Seen When the Skin Is Raised)

1. Interdomal polygon
2. Facet polygon
3. Columellar polygon
4. "Footplate" polygon (we do not raise the skin in this region)

DORSAL CARTILAGE POLYGON

The dorsal cartilage polygon is the area from the tip until the keystone region.[1] It can be seen clearly as a section looking anterior in thin-skinned patients (see **Fig. 5**; **Fig. 6**). In the cartilage anatomy, there is a groove from the center of the cartilage

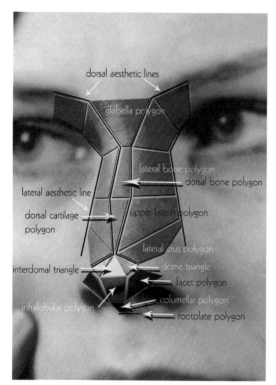

Fig. 5. The nasal surface aesthetics can be analyzed in terms of geometric polygons including the glabella polygon, dorsal bone polygon, dorsal cartilage triangle, lateral bone polygons, upper lateral polygons, dome triangles, lateral crus polygons, interdomal triangle, facet polygons, infralobular polygon, columellar polygon, and footplate polygons.

top point until the keystone. This groove is 1 to 2 mm deep and filled by the dorsal perichondrium. The Pitanguy ligament is on top of this perichondrium.[2] The Pitanguy ligament was initially named the "dermocartilaginous ligament." Pitanguy stated that this ligament begins from the supratip dermis, passes through the area between the dome and the septal angle, and is finally attached to the medial crura. In terms of surgical importance, he has stated: "cut this ligament for nose rotation, if the ligament is too much then resect."[3]

If you are making a subperichondrial dissection, forming this groove wherein the tissues above fit will strengthens dorsal highlights.[2] Because of this, the dorsal cartilage polygon is longer. As the dorsal cartilages approach the nasal tip, the thickness of the Pitanguy tissue increases. The dorsal cartilages end as it forms the septal angle after entering between the lateral crura.

DORSAL BONE POLYGON

The dorsal bone polygon is the area between the keystone and radix.[1] The dorsum bone polygon has more round lines compared with the dorsal cartilage polygon. It does not give as much rigorous light as the dorsal cartilage polygon. It is wider in the keystone region and narrower in the radix (see **Fig. 5**; **Fig. 7**). It is longer in women and shorter in men. In other words, the keystone is located higher in men than in women. If the roof is completely closed with osteotomy, the dorsal bone polygon becomes very narrow. When spreader grafts or flaps are used for dorsal highlights, we have a controlled open roof. When this area is left in this way, you will see that the skin shows the 1 to 2 mm opened framework. Because the skin in this area is very thin, there will be collapses in dorsal bone polygon after several years. Bone dust seems to be a good material to fill cavities between the bones.

UPPER LATERAL CARTILAGE POLYGONS

The upper lateral cartilage polygons have the following features.[1] They face lateral, downward, and straight forward (see **Fig. 5**; **Fig. 8**). Because the upper lateral cartilages are very thin, they rarely have specific topographic problems. If the dorsum cartilage polygon is shaped correctly, this section will not cause a problem. Because the height of the upper lateral cartilage is greater, we perform a resection from the upper lateral cartilage while removing the hump. The problem on which we did not focus much is the case of a long upper lateral cartilage polygon. In noses with a droopy tip, we ensure the nose tip rotation by septum caudal resection and cephalic lateral crura resections (usually 1–4 mm). If this is not enough, resections should be made from the caudal part of the upper lateral cartilages. In this way, the upper lateral cartilage polygons can be shortened.

LATERAL BONE POLYGONS

The nasal bones form the lateral bone polygons.[1] They face lateral, upward, and straight forward. They are generally convex and often asymmetry can be observed (see **Fig. 5**; **Fig. 9**). We can mobilize the bones like flaps. However, topographic problems of the bone can result in asymmetry. You can correct these asymmetries with a rasp after a wide dissection.

DORSAL AESTHETIC LINES

Classically, the nose is shown in frontal view with two divergent concave lines that extend from the supraorbital rim through the radix area and then continue as paired lines to the nasal tip.[4] However, these traditional dorsal aesthetic lines are slightly

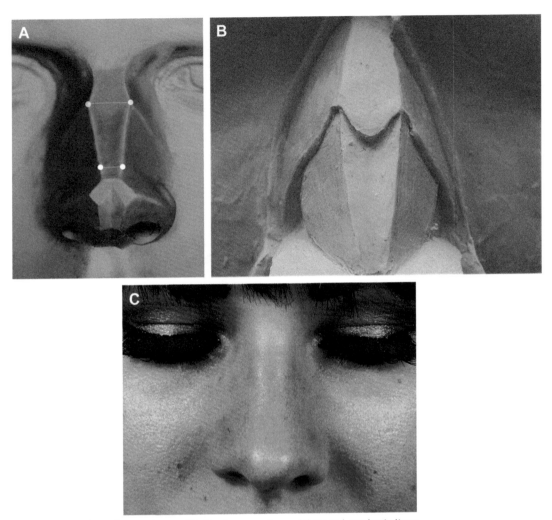

Fig. 6. (*A*) Dorsal cartilage polygon. (*B*) Keystone anatomy. (*C*) Dorsal aesthetic lines.

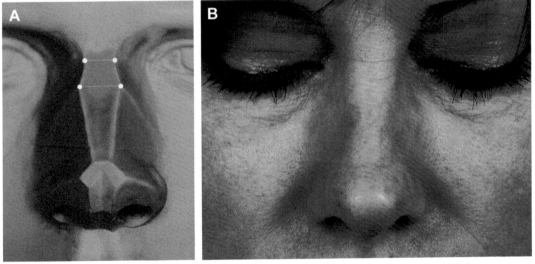

Fig. 7. (*A*) Dorsal bone polygon on the cubic clay model. (*B*) Dorsal bone polygon on a beautiful nose.

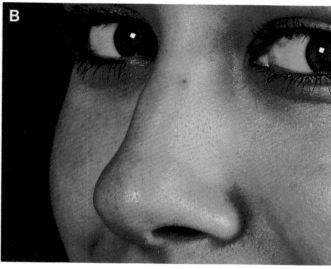

Fig. 8. (*A*) Lateral cartilage polygon. (*B*) Lateral cartilage polygon on a beautiful nose.

different when viewed through the nasal polygon aesthetic unit concept. As seen in **Fig. 5**, the dorsal aesthetic lines should have a fusiform pattern starting at the brows with the nasal radix area being narrow, the keystone area wider, and the supratip region narrow again before ultimately diverging at the tip. This fusiform pattern is important for creating a natural-looking aesthetic dorsum (**Fig. 10**). The dorsal aesthetic lines are formed when the skin softens the lines that join the glabellar, the dorsal bone, the dorsal cartilage and the lateral edges of the dome polygons (see **Fig. 5**).

LATERAL AESTHETIC LINES

These lines are created by combining the lateral edges of the lateral bone polygons, the upper lateral polygons, and partially by the lateral crura polygons (see **Fig. 5**). The importance of the lateral aesthetic lines is to emphasize the triangularity of the nose and to offset the nose from the cheek.[1] The lateral aesthetic lines are as important as the dorsal subunit, but not as complex. The nasal base on both sides should also produce a highlight creating two convergent convex lines extending from the supratarsal folds toward the nasal alae, with the narrowest point being at the medial canthus.

THE NOSTRIL CREASE

The nostril crease begins superficially in the medial with the nostril sill. It deepens towards the inferolateral and then becomes more shallow towards the superolateral. Where it joins the nasolabial fold at the line between 10 and 2 o'clock, it loses its linear character and turns into a groove. If surgery on the nostril base is performed higher than at the line between 3 and 9 o'clock, then the scar becomes more obvious. The nostril crease forms a dimple at the highest point and then turns downwards again, terminating in the free edge of the nostril (**Fig. 11**). This is why one should stay below the 3 to 9 o'clock area in nostril surgery. Incisions extending superiorly are more visible.

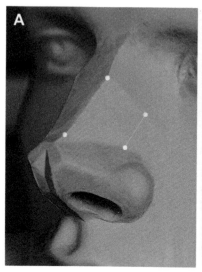

Fig. 9. Lateral bone polygon.

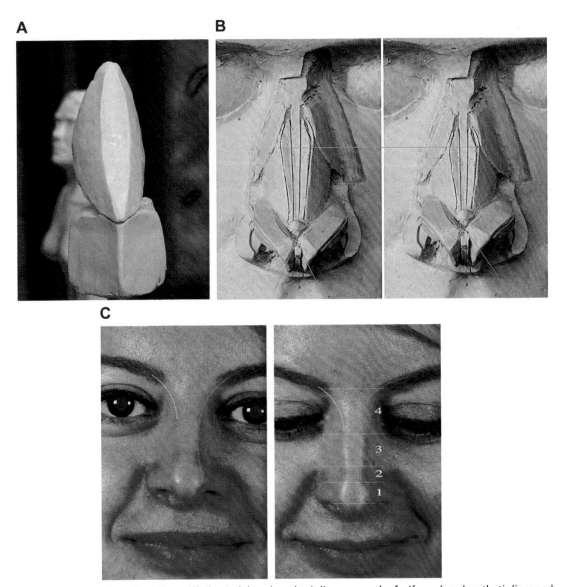

Fig. 10. (*A, B*) Dorsal aesthetic lines. (*C*) Classical dorsal aesthetic lines versus the fusiform dorsal aesthetic lines and the dorsalaesthetic lines' light intensity (1–3 sharp light, 2–4 soft light, sharp edge is required in the keystone area).

THE NASAL TIP

Sheen and Sheen[5] described the ideal tip shape as two equilateral geodesic triangles with a common base formed by a line connecting the two domes. They note that the highest projecting point of the tip should lie along the apogee of the curved line that connects both domes. They define the intercrural distance as the distance between the domes, which also represents the common base of the two geodesic triangles. Daniel[6] notes an angle of dome definition at the domal junction line with the most aesthetically pleasing tips having a convex domal segment and concave lateral crus. In contrast, our concept of tip surface

aesthetics is composed of 2 dome triangles, an interdomal triangle, a pair of facet polygons, and an infralobular polygon (see **Fig. 5**).

DOME TRIANGLES AND THE INTERDOMAL TRIANGLE

The dome triangles are a pair of isosceles triangles, in between the superior tip (Ts), inferior tip (Ti), and medial rim (Rm) points, each having their bases in contact with the facet polygons.[1] The interdomal triangle, on the other hand, is the triangle between the dome triangles created by Ts and the bilateral Ti points. Ideally, the base of the dome triangle should be 0.7 times the length of the two

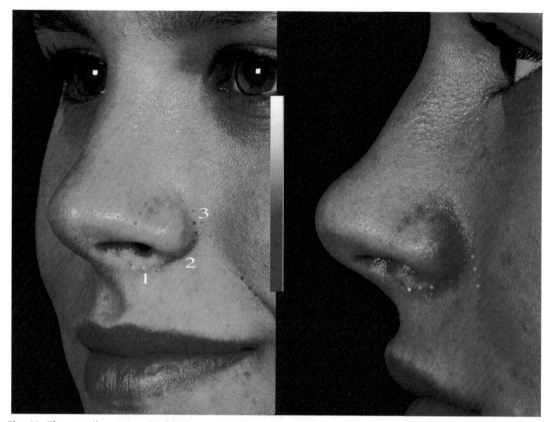

Fig. 11. The nostril crease zone. (1) The nostril sill creates a soft line. (2) The crease deepens in zone 2. (3) The nostril crease joins the nasoloabial fold at 2–10 o'clock and first forms a groove, then a crease. Insicions in zone 1–2 are less visible than in zone 3.

sides. The base of the triangle should never be narrowed. Any attempt to narrow the caudal base will result in widening the infralobular polygon, which results in the medialization of the caudal edges of the lateral crura and an unwanted notching effect on the nostrils (see **Fig. 5**; **Fig. 12**).

The line between the Rm points is the widest area of the tip point. Closing the dome and interdomal triangles with sutures creates a pointed tip deformity. The medial edge of each dome triangle corresponds to the lateral edge of the interdomal triangle (see **Figs. 5** and **12**).

In men, the tip is narrower, while it is wider in women. The superior angle of the interdomal triangle, corresponding to the angle formed by the two dome triangles, is also an important structural detail, with an ideal value of 80° in males and 100° in females (see **Fig. 12**).

TIP-DEFINING POINTS

The oblique and lateral views of the nose reveal important breaking points at the tip, which have been defined previously in the literature under various nomenclature.[7] Our approach to the tip

surface structural anatomy requires the definition of specific points, namely the Ts, Ti, Rm and lateral rim points for precise description of the tip polygons[1,8] (see **Fig. 12**).

The Ts point corresponds to the combined vertices of the dome triangles, as described elsewhere in this article. The Ti points correspond to the inferomedial corners of the dome triangles, hence the two inferolateral vertices of the interdomal triangle. These points should ideally be positioned in the same vertical plane in the lateral profile view, to create an aesthetically pleasing tip shape.

The Rm points represent the medial ends of the lateral crura caudal border, whereas the lateral rim points (R1) correspond to the lateral ends of the lateral crura at the caudal border (see **Fig. 12**). These landmarks and breakpoints help to define and evaluate the tip polygons, thus facilitating analysis of the nasal surface aesthetics.

WHAT IS THE FACET?

Facets are the multiedged flat areas that surround the 3-dimensional objects and provide the easiest method for making sculptures. You create the

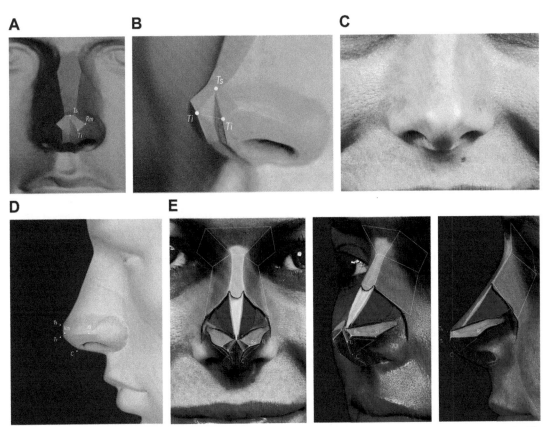

Fig. 12. (A) The tip surface structural anatomy: Rl, lateral rim; Rm, medial rim; Ti, inferior tip; Ts, superior tip. The Ts point corresponds to the combined vertices of the dome triangles. The Ti points correspond to the inferomedial corners of the dome triangles, hence the two inferolateral vertices of the interdomal triangle. The Rm points represent the medial ends of the lateral crura caudal border, and the Rl points correspond to the lateral ends of the lateral crura at the caudal border. (B) Tip polygons on a cubic clay model in oblique view. (C) A thin-skinned beautiful nose has clear polygon anatomy. (D) The lateral view of the cubic clay model shows two tip breaking points which are at the same vertical level: C point, Columella break point. (E) Polygon illustration of a beautiful a nose in front, oblique and lateral views.

same sections that are on the object within the sculpting clay. The size of the sections, their angles, and the ratio between them are important. Organic models have mixed round edges. Imagining organic models as angled and seeing their sections in this way, together with analyzing them as cubic forms, is one of the basic rules for design knowledge.

FACET POLYGONS

The facet polygon in the nasal tip is a critical surface structure that should be respected in tip rhinoplasty.[1,8] It is the polygon between Ti, Rm, lateral rim, and C points. It looks downward and lateral 45° (see **Fig. 5**; **Fig. 13**). In the front view, the height of the dome triangle and the height of the facet should be similar.

One of the essential objections is this region. This area is not a triangle. There is a 2- to 3-mm

edge between the Ti and Rm points (see **Fig. 13**). The facet polygon is not a space that has to be filled. It can be seen clearly in beautiful noses. A thin-skinned nose without the facet polygon clearly shows that it has been operated on. It has an anatomy like a tent.

LATERAL CRUS POLYGONS

The lateral crus polygon is a mass polygon made up from the body of the lateral crus.[1,8] The caudal edge of the lateral crus is in front of the cephalic edge. This position produces a clear facet polygon and a "scroll" line in the skin (see **Fig. 5**; **Fig. 14**).

RESTING ANGLE

Correcting the resting angle of the lateral crura is vital for the surface aesthetics of the tip. The notion of cephalic malpositioning is, for example, an important concept that can be analyzed through

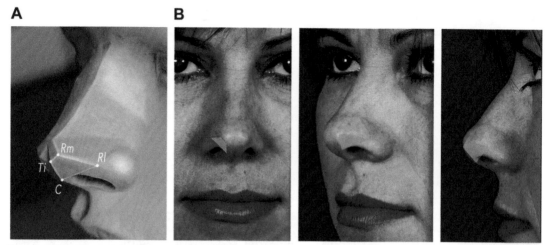

Fig. 13. (*A*) Vertices of the facet polygon. C, columella break point; Rl, lateral rim; Rm, medial rim; Ti, inferior tip. (*B*) Facet polygon on a beautiful nose.

surface aesthetics. A high nostril crease can, for example, define a true cephalically malpositioned nose. The scroll line is high, the resting angle is wrong, the lateral crura are convex, and the facet polygons are narrow.

This is the angle between the surface of the lateral crus and the upper lateral cartilage surface.[1,8] It should be around 100° (see **Fig. 14**). Surgical techniques that ruin the nose tip also ruin the lateral crus resting angle. If this angle is regular, then the need for a rim graft dramatically decreases. As the resting angle broadens, the nose starts to become pinched. If the resting angle is 100°, the facet polygon appears pleasing to the eye.[9]

A resting angle of 100° or less creates a well-defined scroll groove. Lateral crura with an abnormal resting angle result in loss of the scroll groove and excessive fullness in the supratip region, and make the nose look as though the lower lateral cartilages were cephalically malpositioned, described as a pseudocephalic malposition of the lateral crura.[1] A resting angle of 180° or more results in the medialization of the lateral crus cephalic border when compared with the upper lateral cartilage, hence creating a "pinch nose" appearance (**Fig. 15**).

SCROLL LINE

The scroll line is the area where the upper lateral cartilage and the lateral crus meet, forming a groove that is visible in the skin.[1] It is a groove

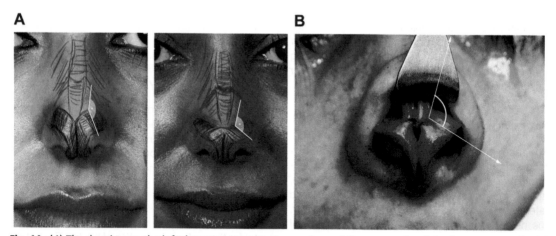

Fig. 14. (*A*) The drawing on the left shows a wrong resting angle, and the one on the right the correct angle. (*B*) The resting angle is the angle between the upper lateral and lateral crura, and this figure shows a resting angle corrected with a cephalic dome suture in the open approach.

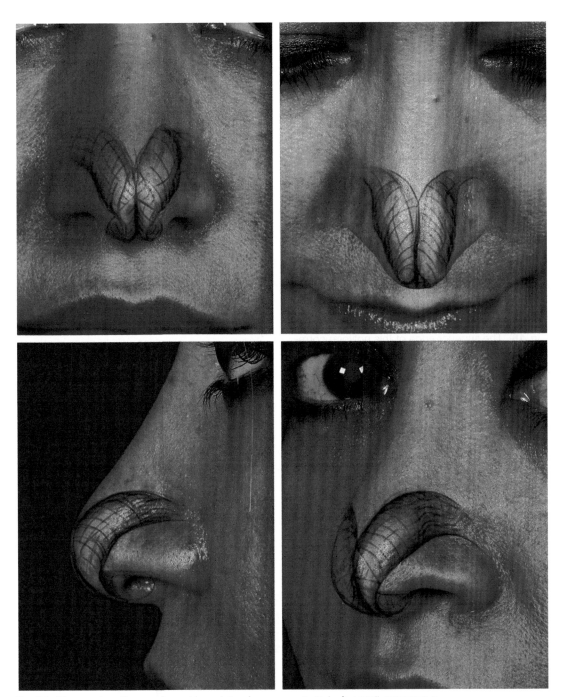

Fig. 15. Abnormal resting angle and long lateral crura create "pinch nose" appearance.

indicating the transition from the upper lateral polygon to the lateral crus polygon (see **Fig. 5**). The scroll junction between the upper lateral cartilage and the lateral crus marks the transition from the static nasal body to the dynamic moving nasal tip.[10] The groove over the scroll area should meet in the center to create a supratip breakpoint, especially in the female profile.

If we do not form this line, the nose becomes round. If the lateral supratip skin does not fit completely over the cartilage skeleton after rhinoplasty surgery, the dead space fills with fibrosis and the scroll line becomes indistinct. For a beautiful scroll line, a correct resting angle is essential because it is formed by the pit where the upper lateral cartilage and lateral crus connect.

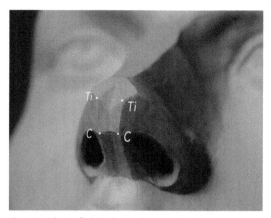

Fig. 16. The infralobular polygon. C, columella break point; Ti, inferior tip.

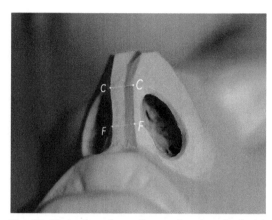

Fig. 17. The columellar polygon. C, columella break point; F, footplate point.

INFRALOBULAR POLYGON

The infralobular polygon is formed in between the interdomal triangle and the columellar polygon (**Fig. 16**). The superior edge of this polygon corresponds with the interconnection of the Ti points. The base of the infralobular polygon is at the columella breakpoint, represented by the interconnecting line between the C points (see **Figs. 5** and **16**), which is ideally placed at the apical edge of the nostrils. If the columellar point is posterior to the nostril apex level, the nostrils are more exposed in the frontal view. The infralobular polygon has a relatively wider superior edge in females and a narrower one in males.[1,8]

The infralobular polygon looks down at a 45° angle. It is a space polygon. The superficial part of the superficial muscular aponeurotic system (SMAS) fills this space and makes it a plane. A "strut" graft is also located within this polygon. If the strut graft is placed near the caudal edge of the medial crus, the infralobule polygon will seem to be round. The infralobule polygon is constituted by the weakest part of the lower lateral cartilage, which is named the middle crus. After dissection, this part weakens and contour grafts may be needed to strengthen it.

COLUMELLAR POLYGON

The columellar polygon is a space polygon between the C points and the footplate polygon (see **Fig. 5**; **Fig. 17**). The columellar polygon looks downwards. The space between the caudal edges of the medial crus should be protected. A common error is the extreme grafting of this region or setting the caudal edges too close to each other. Extreme grafting expands the columellar polygon. Suturing the caudal edges narrows the columellar polygon. However, in a

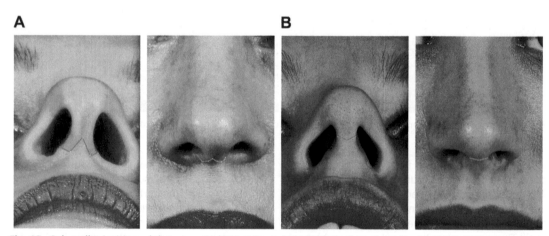

Fig. 18. Columellar incisions. (*A*) An inverted-V incision is less visible in the columellar base. (*B*) A V incision is less visible in the midcolumellar region. The V incision has shorter mucosa flaps than the inverted-V incision; therefore, elevation and wound adaptation is easy.

normal and beautiful nose, the columellar polygon can be seen clearly. A little space seems to be natural and will not disturb the patient. The medial crura turn laterally and upward to form the footplates. If the columellar polygon is short, then it is possible to lengthen the columellar polygon by suturing the footplates to each other.[1,8]

When the tip surgery is finished, the superficial SMAS and perichondrium may cause bulging on perform for the bulging on the columellar polygon or make small flaps and turn them into the space in the infralobular polygon.

The columellar polygon is located in between the infralobular polygon and the footplate polygon. It begins at the columellar breakpoint and continues down until the divergence of the medial crura.

Another concept that should be taken into account especially in open rhinoplasty surgery consists of the columellar incision. Although a V incision is less visible in the midcolumellar region, an inverted V incision will be less visible in the columellar base (**Fig. 18**).

FOOTPLATE POLYGONS

The footplate polygons begin at the divergence point of the medial crura footplates and end just above the lip junction. These two polygons reflect the underlying division of the medial crura into a columellar segment and a footplate segment.[6,10] They look sidewards and downward (**Fig. 19**). The footplate polygon, columellar polygon, and lip may not be separated from each other clearly.

It can be fleshier in women and not uncommon to make sharp angles with the lip in men. In tension noses, the excess part of the caudal posterior of the septum goes between the footplates and expands this polygon. In patients with short columellar polygons, it is possible to make the columellar polygon longer by suturing the footplates.

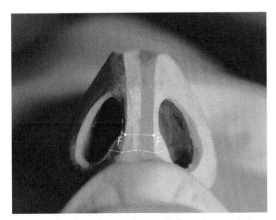

Fig. 19. The footplate polygon. F, footplate point.

The footplate polygon may be wide enough to obstruct breathing. In surgery this region should be usually constricted.

SUMMARY

Nasal aesthetics can be defined in terms of polygons and triangles with a new emphasis on the lateral crus spatial position and a proper lateral crus resting angle. For example, the critical "tip diamond" is created by the interrelationship between the dome triangles, the interdomal triangle, the facet polygons, and the infralobule polygon. This type of analysis has led to new surgical techniques. The cephalic dome suture is used to create the desired tip by emphasizing the dome triangles, the infralobule polygon and the interdomal triangle aesthetic subunits. The Libra graft is used to create a natural fusiform dorsum with reconstruction of the dorsal bone polygons and the dorsal cartilage triangle. Use of these techniques enables manipulation of the surface aesthetic polygons, facilitating the reconstruction of proportions and aesthetic subunits associated with an attractive nose. Cubic form analyses based on nasal polygons can serve as a guide for surgeons to manage surgical techniques.

REFERENCES

1. Çakır B, Doğan T, Öreroğlu AR, et al. Rhinoplasty: surface aesthetics and surgical techniques. Aesthet Surg J 2013;33(3):363–75.

2. Çakır B, Öreroğlu AR, Doğan T, et al. A complete subperichondrial dissection technique for rhinoplasty with management of the nasal ligaments. Aesthet Surg J 2012;32(5):564–74.

3. Pitanguy I. Surgical importance of a dermocartilaginous ligament in bulbous noses. Plast Reconstr Surg 1965;36:247–53.

4. Toriumi DM. New concepts in nasal tip contouring. Arch Facial Plast Surg 2006;8(3):156–85.

5. Sheen JH, Sheen AP. Aesthetic rhinoplasty. 2nd edition. St Louis (MO): CV Mosby; 1987.

6. Daniel RK. The nasal tip: anatomy and aesthetics. Plast Reconstr Surg 1992;89:216–24.

7. Daniel RK. Tip refinement grafts: the designer tip. Aesthet Surg J 2009;29(6):528–37.

8. Çakır B, Öreroğlu AR, Daniel RK. Surface aesthetics in tip rhinoplasty: step-by-step surgery. Aesthet Surg J 2014;34(6):941–55.

9. Toriumi DM, Checcone MA. New concepts in nasal tip contouring. Facial Plast Surg Clin North Am 2009;17(1):55–90.

10. Daniel RK, Letourneau A. Rhinoplasty: nasal anatomy. Ann Plast Surg 1988;20(1):5–13.

Open and Closed Rhinoplasty

Ashley Cafferty, BA[a], Daniel G. Becker, MD[b,c],*

KEYWORDS

- Rhinoplasty • Transcartilaginous • Intercartilaginous • Marginal • Transcolumellar

KEY POINTS

- Most surgeons now recognize the broad utility of both endonasal and external rhinoplasty approaches. In this chapter the pros and cons are discussed and further thoughts on the decision-making process are provided.
- Based on an analysis of the individual patient's anatomy, appropriate incisions, approaches and tip-sculpting techniques may be selected.
- Much can be gained from considering the experiences of surgeons who have had the opportunity to see the consequences over time. The important philosophic concept is not open or closed, but instead, the emphasis on anatomical diagnosis and preservation of structural support.
- There is no ideal approach. Each surgeon will develop a unique approach based on the concepts outlined and based on the techniques and experiences he or she has developed in the course of an eclectic training.

INTRODUCTION

In the modern era of rhinoplasty, the introduction of external rhinoplasty was greeted by enthusiastic advocates and also met with spirited opposition. Over time, however, the tenor of this debate has become more ecumenical. Most surgeons now recognize the broad utility of both endonasal and external approaches. Most understand that there are situations when a given approach offers advantages and may be considered preferable. Most also agree that there is a large "gray area," where either the endonasal or the external approach would be appropriate, and the choice may be considered a toss-up. Most surgeons readily acknowledge that surgeon comfort with a procedure is an appropriately important factor.

In this article the anatomy, incisions, and approaches that are available to the surgeon are reviewed. General indications are discussed for the external and endonasal approaches. The pros and cons of each approach are discussed, and further thoughts on the decision-making process are provided.

ANATOMY, INCISIONS, AND APPROACHES
Nasal Anatomy

Although the anatomy of the nose has been fundamentally understood for many years, only relatively recently has there been an increased understanding of the long-term effects of surgical changes on the function and appearance of the nose. A detailed understanding of nasal anatomy is critical for successful rhinoplasty. Accurate assessment of the anatomic variations presented by a patient allows the surgeon to develop a rational and realistic surgical plan. Furthermore, recognizing variant or aberrant anatomy is critical to preventing functional compromise or untoward esthetic results. This section presents a limited diagrammatic overview of nasal anatomy (**Figs. 1–4**). More

[a] Post-Baccalaureate PreMedical Program, Thomas Jefferson University, Philadelphia, PA, USA; [b] Division of Facial Plastic & Reconstructive Surgery, Department of Otolaryngology-Head and Neck Surgery, University of Pennsylvania Medical Center, Philadelphia, PA, USA; [c] Department of Otolaryngology-Head and Neck Surgery, University of Virginia Medical Center, Charlottesville, VA, USA
* Becker Nose and Sinus Center, LLC, 570 Egg Harbor Drive, Suite B-2, Sewell, NJ 08080.
E-mail address: beckermailbox@aol.com

Clin Plastic Surg 43 (2016) 17–27
http://dx.doi.org/10.1016/j.cps.2015.09.002
0094-1298/16/$ – see front matter © 2016 Elsevier Inc. All rights reserved.

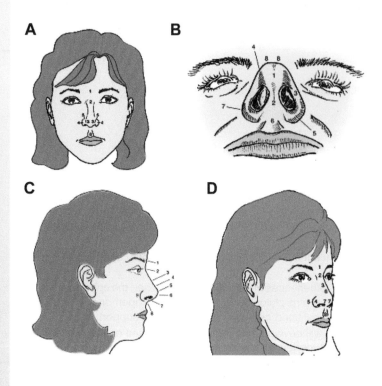

Fig. 1. Surface anatomy. (*A*) Frontal. 1. Glabella; 2. Nasion; 3. Tip-defining points; 4. Alar-sidewall; 5. Supra-alar crease; 6. Philtrum. (*B*) Base. 1. Infratip lobule; 2. Columella; 3. Alar sidewall; 4. Facet, or soft tissue triangle; 5. Nostril sill; 6. Columella-labial angle or junction; 7. Alar-facial groove or junction; 8. Tip defining points. (*C*) Lateral. 1. Glabella; 2. Nasion, nasofrontal angle; 3. Rhinion (osseocartilaginous junction); 4. Supratip; 5. Tip-defining points; 6. Infratip lobule; 7. Columella; 8. Columella-labial angle or junction; 9. Alar-facial groove or junction. (*D*) Oblique. 1. Glabella; 2. Nasion, nasofrontal angle; 3. Rhinion; 4. Alar sidewall; 5. Alar-facial groove or junction; 6. Supratip; 7. Tip-defining point; 8. Philtrum.

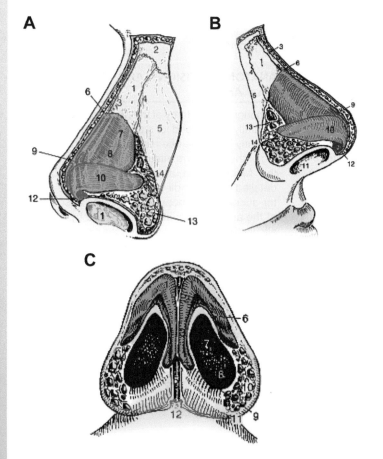

Fig. 2. Bony-cartilaginous anatomy. (*A*) Oblique. 1. Nasal bone; 2. Nasion (nasofrontal suture line); 3. Internasal suture line; 4. Nasomaxillary suture line; 5. Ascending process of maxilla; 6. Rhinion (osseocartilaginous junction); 7. Upper lateral cartilage; 8. Caudal edge of upper lateral cartilage; 9. Anterior septal angle; 10. Lower lateral cartilage–lateral crus; 11. Medial crural footplate; 12. Intermediate crus; 13. Sesamoid cartilage; 14. Pyriform aperture. (*B*) Lateral. 1. Nasal bone; 2. Nasion (nasofrontal suture line); 3. Internasal suture line; 4. Nasomaxillary suture line; 5. Ascending process of maxilla; 6. Rhinion (osseocartilaginous junction); 7. Upper lateral cartilage; 8. Caudal edge of upper lateral cartilage; 9. Anterior septal angle; 10. Lower lateral cartilage lateral crus; 11. Medial crural footplate; 12. Intermediate crus; 13. Sesamoid cartilage; 14. Pyriform aperture. (*C*) Base. 1. Tip-defining point; 2. Intermediate crus; 3. Medial crus; 4. Medial crural footplate; 5. Caudal septum; 6. Lateral crus; 7. Naris; 8. Nostril floor; 9. Nostril sill; 10. Alar lobule; 11. Alar-facial groove or junction; 12. Nasal spine.

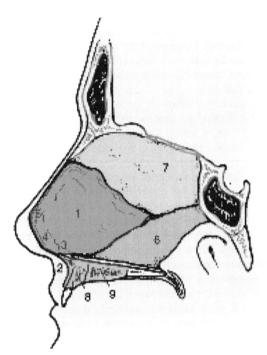

Fig. 3. Septum. 1. Quadrangular cartilage; 2. Nasal spine; 3. Posterior septal angle; 4. Middle septal angle; 5. Anterior septal angle; 6. Vomer; 7. Perpendicular plate of ethmoid bone; 8. Maxillary crest maxillary component; 9. Maxillary crest–palatine component.

detailed study of nasal and facial anatomy is recommended.[1–3]

Incisions and approaches

Incisions are methods of gaining access to the bony and cartilaginous structures of the nose and include transcartilaginous, intercartilaginous, marginal, and transcolumellar incisions. Approaches provide surgical exposure of the nasal structures such as the nasal tip and dorsum. The main rhinoplasty approaches include cartilage-splitting (transcartilaginous incision), retrograde (intercartilaginous incision with retrograde dissection), delivery approach (intercartilaginous + marginal incisions), and external (transcolumellar and marginal incisions) (**Box 1**). Based on an analysis of the individual patient's anatomy, appropriate incisions, approaches, and tip-sculpturing techniques may be selected (**Fig. 5**).[3–5]

Regardless of the incisions and approaches selected, the surgical dissection must be performed in the proper areolar tissue planes to minimize tissue damage and scarring, maintain hemostasis, and maximize redraping of the skin–soft tissue envelope. Dissection in proper tissue planes will help preserve vascular structures of the flap, insure flap viability, and minimize bleeding, postoperative edema, and scarring.[2]

Indications for endonasal versus external

An operative algorithm often provides a helpful starting point in selecting the incisions, approaches, and techniques used in nasal tip surgery (**Fig. 6**). In every case, the patient's anatomy directs the selection of appropriate technique. As the anatomic deformity becomes more abnormal, a graduated, stepwise approach is taken. However, other factors, such as the need for spreader grafts, complex nasal deviation, surgeon preference, and other factors may also appropriately affect the ultimate selection of approach.[5]

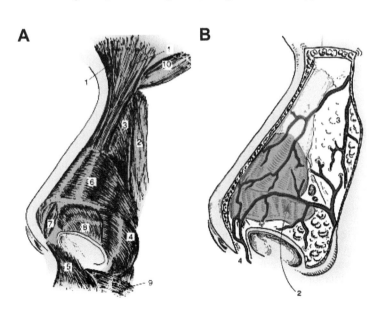

A   B

Fig. 4. Nasal musculature and blood vessels. The surgeon must fully recognize the importance of this plane and must carefully avoid operating in the incorrect tissue planes, which can result in violation of the muscle and blood vessels and subsequent abnormal scarring. (A) Musculature. A: Elevator muscles. 1. Procerus; 2. Levator labii alaequae nasi; 3. Anomalous nasi. B: Depressor muscles. 4. Alar nasalis; 5. Depressor septi nasi. C: Compressor muscles. 6. Transverse nasalis; 7. Compressor narium minor. D: Minor dilator muscles. 8. Dilator naris anterior. E: Other. 9. Orbicularis oris; 10. Corrugator. (B): Vasculature. 1. Dorsal nasal artery; 2. Lateral nasal artery; 3. Angular vessels; 4. Columellar artery.

Box 1

Tip support mechanisms, incisions, and approaches

Major tip support mechanisms

1. Size, shape, and strength of lower lateral cartilages
2. Medial crural footplate attachment to caudal septum
3. Attachment of caudal border of upper lateral cartilages to cephalic border of lower lateral cartilages
   (Nasal septum is also considered a major support mechanism of the nose.)

Minor tip support mechanisms

1. Ligamentous sling spanning the domes of the lower lateral cartilages (ie interdomal ligament)
2. Cartilaginous dorsal septum
3. Sesamoid complex of lower lateral cartilages
4. Attachment of lower lateral cartilages to overlying skin-soft tissue envelope
5. Nasal spine
6. Membranous septum

Incisions: methods of gaining access

Intercartilaginous

Transcartilaginous

Marginal (NOT to be confused with rim incision)

Transcolumellar

Approaches: provide surgical exposure

Cartilage-splitting

Retrograde

Delivery: Marginal + intercartilaginous incision

External approach: marginal + trans-columellar incision

Sculpting techniques: surgical modifications

Complete strip: that is, cephalic resection, or volume reduction of lateral crura

Incomplete strip (dome division)

Transdomal/domal sutures

Augmentation grafting

Tip graft

Other

---

undertaken (**Fig. 7**). Advantages of less invasive approaches include less dissection, less edema, less healing. However, less invasive approaches provide by their very nature less exposure, which in some cases may be a disadvantage.

Indications for external rhinoplasty approach[3,6–14] (**Box 2**) generally include asymmetric nasal tip, crooked nose deformity (lower two-thirds of nose), saddle nose deformity, cleft-lip nasal deformity, secondary rhinoplasty requiring complex structural grafting, and septal perforation repair. Other indications may include complex nasal tip deformity, middle nasal vault deformity, and selected nasal tumors. Some surgeons prefer the open approach for less complex nasal tip deformities due to the precision that they think it offers them when compared with the endonasal approach.

Advantages of the external approach include the maximal surgical exposure, allowing the surgeon a more accurate anatomic diagnosis. The external approach also provides the opportunity for precise tissue manipulation, suturing, and grafting. Disadvantages include the transcolumellar incision, wide field dissection resulting in loss of support, and increased nasal tip edema.

Regardless of approach, one must be mindful of the need to maintain appropriate structural support. When the approach is disruptive of tip support, countermeasures, such as the placement of a columellar strut, are warranted. When the support to the upper lateral cartilages has been disrupted, spreader grafts may be appropriate.

External and endonasal approaches to the upper third

The bony pyramid can be reliably reduced, repositioned, or augmented through a closed approach. However, Larrabee[15] reports that open rhinoplasty may allow a more precise refinement of its contour and lower incidence of profile irregularities.

He points out that although there is a tendency to treat the bony pyramid in an essentially closed fashion when using the open approach, the benefits of increased exposure to the dorsum with the open rhinoplasty approach should be exploited whenever possible.

In the author's experience, a closed approach has been reliable for addressing most bony profile problems. However, when the author performs an open rhinoplasty, at times he will undertake hump reduction under direct visualization. When using an osteotome, he typically uses a 12-mm non-guarded osteotome. (Wider osteotomes can create an injury to the skin–soft tissue envelope.) When rasping during open rhinoplasty, he uses a powered rasp under direct visualization.[16]

The endonasal approach may be generally preferred for patients requiring conservative profile reduction, conservative tip modification, selected revision rhinoplasty patients, and other situations in which conservative changes are being

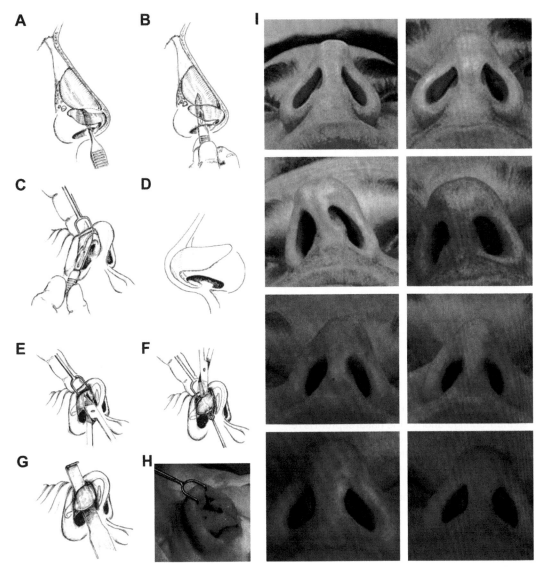

Fig. 5. Incisions and endonasal approaches. (*A*) Transcartilaginous incision and approach. (*B*) Intercartilaginous incision and approach. (*C, D*) Marginal incision. (*E–G*) Delivery approach combines marginal and intercartilaginous incisions. (*H*) The open rhinoplasty approach combines marginal and columellar incisions. (*I*) Before and after external rhinoplasty. Tension-free closure improves final scar appearance.

External and endonasal approaches to the middle nasal vault

The determination of the need for spreader grafts or spreader flaps may play a significant role in determining whether the open approach will be used, even when the tip could be satisfactorily addressed by endonasal approaches. Modern rhinoplasty techniques increasingly emphasize preservation of cartilaginous and bony substructure. Preservation of cartilaginous and bony substructure is of particular importance in the middle nasal vault, because preservation of support for the upper lateral cartilages helps to avoid collapse of the middle vault and the associated internal nasal valve. Middle vault and nasal valve collapse can cause overnarrowing of the middle third of the nose, with the inverted V deformity and nasal obstruction. When support and contour of the middle vault require reconstitution, spreader grafts or spreader flaps can be used.

Use of spreader grafts and spreader flaps in primary rhinoplasty is becoming much more common.[10,17,18] They can be effective in maintaining the contour of the middle vaults after hump reduction. Although it may be technically easier to place spreader grafts and spreader flaps via an external approach, they can also be placed via the endonasal approach.[6,9,10,19,20]

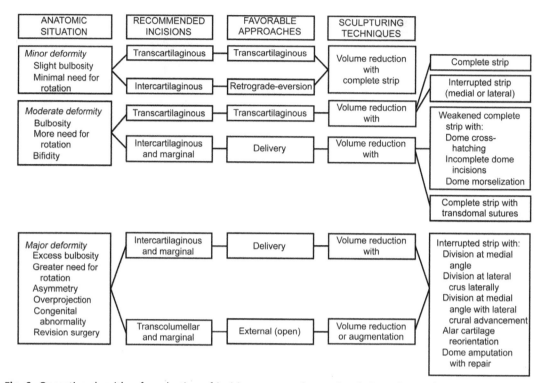

ANATOMIC SITUATION	RECOMMENDED INCISIONS	FAVORABLE APPROACHES	SCULPTURING TECHNIQUES	
Minor deformity Slight bulbosity Minimal need for rotation	Transcartilaginous	Transcartilaginous	Volume reduction with complete strip	Complete strip
	Intercartilaginous	Retrograde-eversion		Interrupted strip (medial or lateral)
Moderate deformity Bulbosity More need for rotation Bifidity	Transcartilaginous	Transcartilaginous	Volume reduction with	Weakened complete strip with: Dome cross-hatching Incomplete dome incisions Dome morselization
	Intercartilaginous and marginal	Delivery	Volume reduction with	
				Complete strip with transdomal sutures
Major deformity Excess bulbosity Greater need for rotation Asymmetry Overprojection Congenital abnormality Revision surgery	Intercartilaginous and marginal	Delivery	Volume reduction with	Interrupted strip with: Division at medial angle Division at lateral crus laterally Division at medial angle with lateral crural advancement Alar cartilage reorientation Dome amputation with repair
	Transcolumellar and marginal	External (open)	Volume reduction or augmentation	

Fig. 6. Operative algorithm for selection of incisions, approaches and techniques in nasal tip surgery.

Narrowing of the middle nasal vault that occurs when the T configuration of the nasal septum is resected with dorsal hump removal may be problematic in the high-risk patient.[10] Spreader grafts and flaps act as a spacer between the upper lateral cartilage and septum, preventing excessive narrowing in the high-risk patient or correcting an overnarrow middle vault when it exists.

As described by Sheen,[19] unilateral or bilateral submucoperichondrial tunnels may be prepared by elevating the mucoperichondrium bridging the upper lateral cartilages to the septum. The space between the upper lateral cartilage and septum can be filled by a cartilage strip insinuated and secured by suture-fixation into the pocket, thereby lateralizing the upper lateral cartilage or cartilages, improving the airway, and effectively maintaining or widening the width of the middle nasal vault. Spreader grafts are well-addressed and well-illustrated in other articles in this issue.

Spreader grafts and spreader flaps may be comfortably carried out through both external and endonasal techniques. In more complex reconstructions, particularly complicated by multiple abnormalities, an external rhinoplasty approach may facilitate accurate dissection and graft suture fixation. Some surgeons find that the external approach is simply a technically easier method to undertake spreader graft or spreader flap placement.

It should be noted that the use of the external rhinoplasty approach may lead to a greater need for spreader grafts or spreader flaps to preserve the nasal valve and middle nasal width, which may be put at risk due to the loss of support to the upper lateral cartilages caused by more extensive skin undermining.

Identifying the high-risk patient during initial preoperative analysis is essential to the prevention of excessive narrowing of the middle nasal vault with internal nasal valve collapse.[10] Sheen[19] identified an anatomic variant that he labeled the narrow nose syndrome. Short nasal bones, long weak upper lateral cartilages, thin skin, and a narrow projecting nose predispose to middle vault collapse.[9,10] As described by Toriumi,[10] commonly performed surgical maneuvers can result in loss of support to the middle vault. A large en-bloc hump removal should be avoided, as the T-shaped support of the nasal septum is eliminated and the intranasal mucosa (which provides important support to the upper lateral cartilage) is at risk of injury. Cephalic trim (volume reduction) of the lateral crura disrupts the scroll recurvature and frees the caudal margin of the upper lateral cartilage. Lateral osteotomies may further medialize the upper lateral cartilages. The upper lateral cartilages can fall toward the narrowed dorsal septal edge, producing middle vault and internal valvular collapse.[10] Collapse of the middle vault

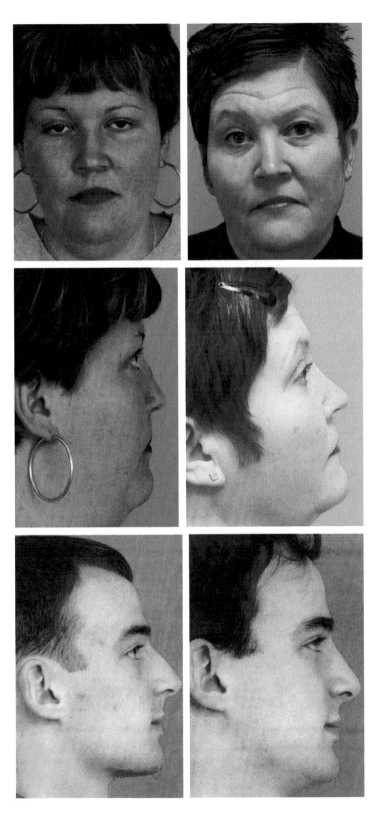

Fig. 7. In a patient in whom relatively conservative changes are being undertaken, the endonasal approach may be advantageous, as in these patients seeking only conservative profile reduction. First patient's photos are 15 years postoperatively; the second patient's photos are 1 year postoperatively.

may highlight the caudal edges of the nasal bones to produce the characteristic inverted V deformity.[10,19]

In most patients, the combination of these maneuvers will not result in a problem; however, in high-risk patients, this combination of maneuvers may contribute to excessive narrowing of the middle vault with internal valve collapse.

Experience is required to develop reliable surgical judgment regarding the appropriate use of spreader grafts and spreader flaps. After spreader grafts or spreader flaps are secured in position internally or via the open approach, the middle vault may appear slightly wide. Over time, this area of the nose tends to narrow as edema

resolves and scar contracture pulls the upper lateral cartilages medially.[10]

External and endonasal approaches to the nasal tip

Traditional tip rhinoplasty techniques, such as cephalic trim and dome binding sutures, have been well described for both external and endonasal rhinoplasty. Complex nasal tip procedures, such as lateral crural strut grafts, lateral or intermediate crural overlay techniques, and "tongue-in-groove" retrodisplacement of the medial crura onto the caudal septum, may also be performed via either approach. For some of these nasal tip techniques, the individual surgeon may find the exposure afforded by the open approach to be preferable **(Fig. 8)**.[21–24]

External and endonasal approaches to revision rhinoplasty

In revision surgery, once the nose is open, any supportive relationships that exist between the scar tissue and underlying structure is lost, and cartilage grafting may be required to support and contour the skin–soft tissue envelope that will now undergo renewed scar contracture and healing. If not, healing and scar contracture may leave a worse deficit than before. Therefore, in revision cases with relatively mild deformities or those

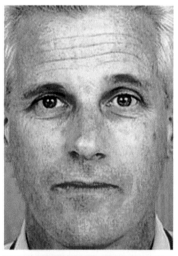
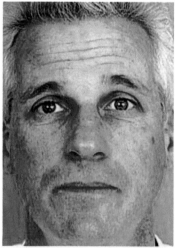
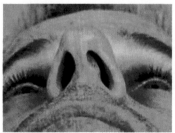
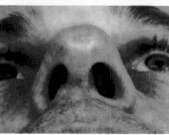

Fig. 8. This patient had a significant caudal septal deviation and severe concavity of the right lateral crus. Correction of the tip deformity required excision and "flipping" of the right lateral crus. Although this can be performed using an external or a delivery approach, the surgeon found that the exposure afforded by the external approach was preferable.

that can be corrected with precise pocket grafting, a closed approach is preferred. Spreader grafts, batten grafts, and onlay grafts are examples of maneuvers that can be well-placed via precise pocket, endonasal techniques (**Fig. 9**).[25] Although endonasal surgery could be an option for a significant percentage of revision cases, an open approach may be unavoidable in complex revision cases.

Endonasal and external approaches to the deviated caudal septum

For severe caudal septal deviation, the open approach may provide a more facile and efficacious approach, when swinging door, doorstop, and other similar maneuvers have failed.[11,26] Although many techniques to address a severe caudal deviation can be done open or closed, the pros and cons of each technique must be compared to determine the best approach. To some extent, this is ultimately a personal judgment, guided by critical self-evaluation.

Philosophic considerations—a graduated approach: the big picture

When considering the decision-making around the choice of approach, much can be gained by considering the experiences of surgeons who have had the opportunity to see the consequences over time. The important philosophic concept is not open or closed, but instead, the emphasis on anatomic diagnosis and preservation of supportive structures.

A central tenet of rhinoplasty decision-making has been the concept of a graduated approach. This concept is based on the idea that achieving the desired goals with the least amount of surgical dissection provides the best chance of success. However, the critical issue here is how much

exposure is needed for reliable execution of any specific technical maneuver.

Adamson[27] has astutely observed that there is no ideal approach; each surgeon will develop a unique approach based on the concepts outlined and the techniques and experiences he or she has developed in the course of an eclectic training. The skillful surgeon can make astute intraoperative anatomic diagnosis via the endonasal or external approach. Notwithstanding this, an important factor that can compromise results is the potential difficulty in diagnosis of various deformities and abnormalities using the endonasal approach. Another factor is the manual difficulty in correcting such deformities once diagnosed, especially effecting such maneuvers as vertical cartilage division, graft placement, and suturing techniques. Those trained in the closed approach will still tend to perform most of their rhinoplasties in this fashion, reserving the open approach for more difficult noses. This assessment will vary from surgeon to surgeon (**Fig. 10**).

Perkins[28] describes an evolution in his personal philosophy that reflects some of the issues involved in the decision-making process and provides valuable insight into the evolution in the decision-making that has occurred over the last 15 to 20 years. Although the concept of a graduated approach to achieve a pleasing esthetic result has been foremost in his personal philosophy, the evolving need to achieve more refined results and prevent late complications has resulted in his increased use of the open approach, which allows the opportunity to use certain grafting techniques. Perkins continues to strongly advocate the philosophy that the approach selected should provide the least intervention in the shortest time to achieve a satisfactory result and satisfy the patient's goals. However, his choice of approach has changed due to late

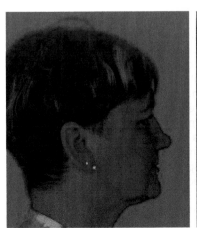 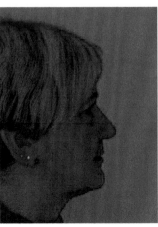

Fig. 9. This patient required a triple layer ear cartilage onlay graft to address her saddle nose abnormality. This graft was well-placed via a precise pocket, endonasal approach.

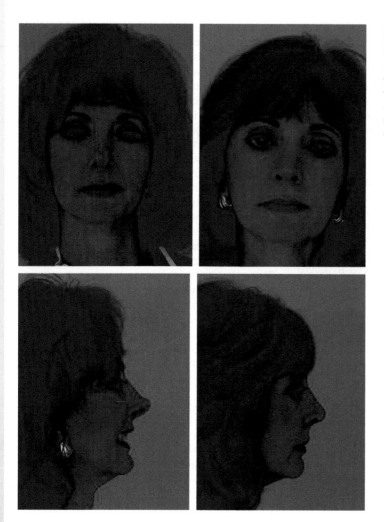

Fig. 10. Although some surgeons would choose to address this revision rhinoplasty via a closed approach, the author thought that, in his hands, the exposure obtained from the external approach offered the best opportunity for successful correction of the tip deformity.

complications that he has seen occur. The 2 areas that he found most commonly cause late complications in rhinoplasty are the midnasal pyramid and lateral alar sidewalls. He reports that it is paramount to provide a structural foundation for the middle vault (ie, spreader grafts). Although issues such as these can be addressed using the endonasal approach, it is sometimes far easier to place structural grafts via the external approach. Also, when marked reduction of over-projection is required, it is often easier to use the external columellar approach.

Although one often thinks of "open versus closed rhinoplasty," this text has instead focused on "open and closed rhinoplasty." Although this may seem like a semantic point, the surgeon should understand the advantages offered by every surgical approach. The concepts of minimizing dissection, born from endonasal techniques, also apply to external rhinoplasty. Every surgeon should be able to "think like an endonasal surgeon"; that is, to understand the advantages of limiting the surgical dissection. However, one should also be able to recognize when the additional exposure offered by the external approach may be useful and even necessary. When the external approach is undertaken, the surgeon must understand the commitment that has been made to additional support maneuvers.

There is no single answer when one considers open versus closed rhinoplasty. In each patient, diligent attention must be paid to the patient's goals and anatomy. The wise surgeon includes external and endonasal rhinoplasty as choices in his or her armamentarium and understands the critical issues of maintaining or adding structural support for improving long-term outcomes. The choice for a specific patient will ultimately depend on the surgeon's personal opinion as to which approach, in their hands, will provide the best chance of long-term success with the least amount of surgical dissection.

REFERENCES

1. Tardy ME, Brown R. Surgical anatomy of the nose. New York: Raven Press; 1990.
2. Toriumi DM, Mueller RA, Grosch T, et al. Vascular anatomy of the nose and the external rhinoplasty approach. Arch Otolaryngol Head Neck Surg 1996;122:24–34.
3. Toriumi DM, Becker DG. Rhinoplasty dissection manual. Philadelphia: Lippincott, Williams and Wilkins; 1999.
4. Tardy ME, Toriumi DM. Philosophy and principles of rhinoplasty. 2nd edition. In: Cummings. Chapter 31 in otolaryngology-head & neck surgery. Philadelphia: Saunders; 2001. p. 278–4.
5. Tardy ME. Rhinoplasty: the art and the science. Philadelphia: W.B. Saunders; 1997.
6. Johnson CM Jr, Toriumi DM. Open structure rhinoplasty. Philadelphia: Saunders; 1990.
7. Adamson PA. Open rhinoplasty. In: Papel ID, Nachlas NE, editors. Facial plastic & reconstructive surgery. St Louis (MO): Mosby Year Book; 1992. p. 295–304.
8. Becker DG. Open and closed rhinoplasty. Available at: www.RhinoplastyArchive.com. Philadelphia: SCR Publishers; 2012.
9. Toriumi DM, Johnson CM. Open structure rhinoplasty—featured technical points and long-term follow-up. Facial Plast Surg Clin North Am 1993; 1(1):1–22.
10. Toriumi DM. Management of the middle nasal vault. Operat Tech Plast Reconstr Surg 1995;2(1):16–30.
11. Toriumi DM, Ries WR. Innovative surgical management of the crooked nose. Facial Plast Surg Clin North Am 1993;1(1):63–78.
12. Toriumi DM, Johnson CM. Management of the lower third of the nose—open structure rhinoplasty technique. In: Papel ID, Nachlas NE, editors. Chapter 33 in Facial plastic & reconstructive surgery. St Louis: Mosby Year Book; 1992. p. 305–3.
13. Gunter JP. The merits of the open approach in rhinoplasty. Plast Reconstr Surg 1997;99(3):863–7.
14. Thomas JR. External rhinoplasty:intact columellar approach. Laryngoscope 1990;100(2 Pt 1):206–8.
15. Larrabee WF. Open rhinoplasty and the upper third of the nose. Facial Plast Surg Clin North Am 1993; 1(1):23–38.
16. Becker DG. The powered rasp: advanced instrumentation for rhinoplasty. Arch Facial Plast Surg 2002;4(4):267–8.
17. Constantian MB, Clardy RB. The relative importance of septal and nasal valvular surgery in correcting airway obstruction in primary and secondary rhinoplasty. Plast Reconstr Surg 1996;98(1):38–54.
18. Teichgraeber JF, Wainwright DJ. The treatment of nasal valve obstruction. Plast Reconstr Surg 1994; 93(6):1174–84.
19. Sheen JH. Spreader graft: a method of reconstructing the roof of the middle nasal vault following rhinoplasty. Plast Reconstr Surg 1984;73(2):230–7.
20. Aiach G. Atlas de rhinoplastie. Paris: Masson; 1989. p. 74–85.
21. Soliemanzadeh P, Kridel RWH. Nasal tip overprojection: algorithm of surgical deprojection techniques and introduction to medial crural overlay. Arch Facial Plast Surg 2005;7:374–80.
22. Konior RJ, Kridel RWH. Controlled nasal tip positioning via the open rhinoplasty approach. Facial Plast Surg Clin North Am 1993;1(1):53–62.
23. Adamson PA. Nasal tip surgery in open rhinoplasty. Facial Plast Surg Clin North Am 1993;1(1):39–52.
24. Wise JB, Becker SS, Sparano A, et al. Intermediate crural overlay in rhinoplasty: a deprojection technique that shortens the medial leg of the tripod without lengthening the nose. Arch Facial Plast Surg 2006;8:240–4.
25. Perkins SW, Tardy ME. External columellar incisional approach to revision of the lower third of the nose. Facial Plast Surg Clin North Am 1993;1(1):79–98.
26. Pastorek NJ, Becker DG. Treating the caudal septal deflection. Arch Facial Plast Surg 2000;2:217–20.
27. Adamson PA. Nasal tip surgery in open rhinoplasty. Facial Plast Surg Clin North Am 1993;1(1):39–52.
28. Perkins SW. The evolution of the combined use of endonasal and external columellar approaches to rhinoplasty. Facial Plast Surg Clin North Am 2004; 12:35.

Surgical Treatment of Nasal Obstruction in Rhinoplasty

Ankona Ghosh, MD, Oren Friedman, MD*

KEYWORDS

- Nasal obstruction • Septal deviation • External valve • Internal valve • Turbinate • Batten graft
- Spreader graft

KEY POINTS

- Nasal obstruction is an important consideration in both functional and aesthetic septorhinoplasty.
- For a successful surgical correction of nasal obstruction, diagnosing the precise anatomic point of collapse is fundamental.
- Recognition of the nature and location of nasal valve, septal, and turbinate disorders allows adequate correction and acceptable functional results.

INTRODUCTION

Nasal obstruction is a common problem. Normal nasal breathing involves the interaction of static and dynamic forces, including the nasal septum, lateral nasal walls, and nasal mucosa. Although many patients who present for rhinoplasty evaluation have predominantly aesthetic concerns, many patients are also concerned for nasal airway obstruction. In addition, postoperative airway compromise can detract significantly from an otherwise good aesthetic surgical result. As such, preoperative analysis of the nasal airway is an imperative step in operative planning even if the patient does not necessarily raise concerns over this issue. Modern rhinoplasty techniques allow for success in both nasal aesthetics and function, improving the quality of life functionally and cosmetically as well as allowing for mutual satisfaction of patient and surgeon alike.[1] It is therefore a paramount consideration in surgical planning. When evaluating patients with nasal obstruction, the most important variable of nasal airflow is the diameter of the nasal passage. The key to a successful surgical correction of nasal obstruction is diagnosing the precise anatomic point of collapse.[2] Causes of nasal obstruction with particular relevance for rhinoplasty surgeons are discussed later.

ANATOMIC CONSIDERATION

Proper postoperative function of the inferior turbinates, septum, and nasal valves determines, to a large degree, the success of functional rhinoplasty. Although there are other anatomic aspects to consider, these structures largely contribute to the size and patency of the nasal airway. Constantian and Clardy[3] performed nasal air flow measurements on patients with postrhinoplasty nasal obstruction and found septal deviation, internal nasal valve obstruction, and external nasal valve collapse to be the primary causes.

The Nasal Valves

The nasal valve area has been the subject of numerous studies because of its functional

Disclosures: The authors have no financial disclosures.
Department of Otorhinolaryngology–Head and Neck Surgery, University of Pennsylvania, Philadelphia, PA, USA
* Corresponding author. 18th Floor, 800 Walnut Street, Philadelphia, PA 19004.
E-mail address: orenfriedman@hotmail.com

Clin Plastic Surg 43 (2016) 29–40
http://dx.doi.org/10.1016/j.cps.2015.09.007

importance. It was first described by Mink[4] in 1903, and in 1970 Bridger[5] further described this area as the flow-limiting segment of the nasal airway.[4–6] The nasal valve area represents the area bound by the septum, the caudal aspect of the upper lateral cartilages and lower lateral cartilages, the lateral nasal wall, the nasal floor, and sometimes the head of the inferior turbinate. The valves, classified as external and internal, represent the narrowest portion of the nasal airway and account for half the total nasal airway resistance. Distinguishing between the internal valve and the external nasal valve helps to direct treatment among the different regions of the nasal sidewall.

The External Nasal Valve

The external nasal valve is supported by the caudal aspect of the nasal side wall and is delineated by the nostril rim; it is referred to as the nasal inlet. It is defined medially by the medial crus of the lower lateral cartilage and inferiorly by the nasal spine and the soft tissues over the nasal floor.[7] External nasal valve collapse is described as collapse of the alar margin of the nose on moderate to deep inspiration, caused by negative pressure during inspiration under the influence of Bernoulli forces.[5] The collapse of the external nasal valve is most often seen in patients with narrow nostrils; an overprojected tip; and thin, weak sidewalls. It is often seen in patients with cephalically malpositioned lower lateral cartilage in whom the absence of cartilage support along the nostril rim leads to weakness of the sidewall. The external valve may also be narrow at rest, unrelated to dynamics of inspiration.

The Internal Nasal Valve

The internal nasal valve angle is the angle created by the junction of the caudal border of the upper lateral cartilage and the nasal septum (**Fig. 1**). The valve angle measures 10° to 15°. However, the importance of this valve rests primarily with its area. The area of the internal nasal valve is the narrowest portion of the nasal airway and therefore it is the primary determinant of nasal air flow. Cole[8] describes the 4 functional components of the internal nasal valve area as being the structural elements, which include the internal nasal valve angle and the bony pyriform aperture; and the mucovascular elements, which include the anterior head of the inferior turbinate and the erectile body of the septum. Internal nasal valve collapse is usually observed after previous reductive rhinoplasty or in patients with weakening of the supportive structures of the nose, such as the upper and lower lateral cartilages.

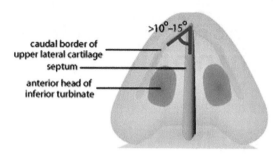

Fig. 1. Internal nasal valve area. (*From* Lam SM, Williams EF. Comprehensive facial rejuvenation. Philadelphia: LWW, 2003; with permission. Available at: http://www.lamfacialplastics.com/dallas-plastic-surgery-learning-modules/rhinoplasty-tutorial/.)

The Septum

The septum is a midline nasal structure. Posteriorly, the bony nasal septum is formed by the perpendicular plate of the ethmoid bone and the vomer. Anteriorly, the quadrangular cartilage forms the cartilaginous septum, which articulates with the upper lateral cartilages. Septal deviation off the midline can result in structural blockage of nasal air flow during inspiration or it may cause turbulent airflow. This condition can be congenital or a result of previous nasal trauma. Specifically for nasal valve surgery, the important areas of the nasal septum are the caudal aspect at the nasal vestibule (which would narrow the external valve) and the internal nasal valve area (which relates to Cottle area 2). Cottle's[9] subdivision of the nasal cavities in 5 areas, based on morphologic and rhinomanometric observations, provided a practical scheme that is still useful to understand the relationship between obstruction and anatomic considerations, thus benefiting modern understanding of functional nasal surgery. In addition, deflection of the posterior septum can result in significant narrowing of the nasal airway and should not be overlooked when evaluating for causes of nasal obstruction. Nasal septal perforations may also contribute to the sensation of nasal airway obstruction.

The Turbinates

The arteries of the nasal mucosa branch off to capillary vessels, which drain into the venous sinusoids of the erectile tissues of the mucosa. A major component of these erectile tissues contributes to the volume of the nasal mucosa; these are especially well developed at the interior part of the inferior turbinate and on the nasal septum. This expansile tissue can regulate nasal air flow because congestion of this entity can cause changes to the nasal cross-sectional area and resistance to airflow[10]; it is also a functional component of the nasal valve as described by Cole.[8] Inferior turbinate hypertrophy is a common contributor to nasal obstruction, but the inferior turbinates are also an essential functional component of the nose and should be approached cautiously.

PHYSICAL EXAMINATION

As with any preoperative planning, the history and physical examination are key to identifying the causes of nasal airway obstruction. Although most rhinoplasty planning is based on study of the standard preoperative photographic images (frontal, base, lateral, oblique), an anterior rhinoscopy with headlight allows visualization of the nasal septum and the inferior turbinate as well as any disorders associated with these structures, especially after the decongestion of nasal mucosa. Nasopharyngoscopy is often useful to further assess the disorders of the posterior septum, middle turbinate, middle meatus, nasopharynx, and all regions that are in limited view with anterior rhinoscopy. It is also extremely important, when surgery is considered, to identify all intranasal disorders, to determine the amount of cartilage available for grafting and to rule out tumors, perforations, or nasopharyngeal lesions that could contribute to the patient's symptoms. Approaching surgery with the greatest possible amount of information can help ensure the best outcome.

An inspection of the base view of the nose yields important information. On base view, special attention should be given to triangularity and symmetry for sources of nasal obstruction as well as cosmesis. The nasal base should be configured as an isosceles triangle with a gently rounded apex at the nasal tip and subtle flaring of the alar sidewalls (**Fig. 2**). The caudal septum may be seen protruding into one of the nostrils (**Fig. 3**). The base view on normal breathing and deep inspiration can reveal collapse of the alar margin of the nose, which is diagnostic of external nasal valve collapse (**Fig. 4**).

During physical examination, some patients report marked improvement in nasal obstruction when the nasal sidewall is distended with the wooden end of a cotton-tipped applicator or other device, or lateral retraction of the cheek. This maneuver, known as the Cottle maneuver, allows reliable identification of an internal nasal valve disorder and helps in identifying appropriate surgical candidates (**Fig. 5**).

Objective obstruction measures include rhinomanometry and acoustic rhinometry. Rhinomanometry is the most commonly used objective test of the nasal airway. Although there are various

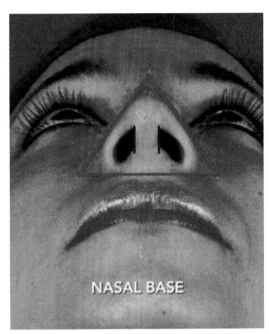

Fig. 2. Base view. (*Courtesy of* John Hilinski, MD, San Diego, CA.)

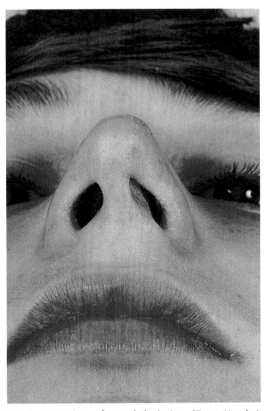

Fig. 3. Base view of septal deviation. (*From* Haack J, Papel ID. Caudal septal deviation. Otolaryngol Clin North Am 2009;42(3):427–36; with permission.)

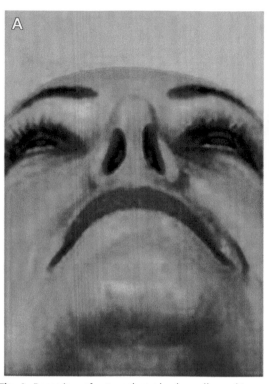

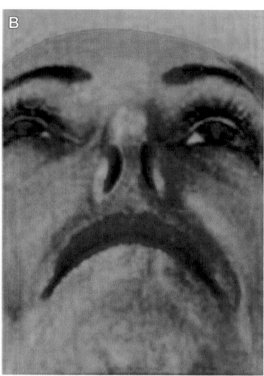

Fig. 4. Base view of external nasal valve collapse (*A*, normal breathing and *B*, inspiration). (*From* Becker D. Revision rhinoplasty. New York: Thieme; 2008; with permission.)

methods of rhinomanometry distinguished by the varying placement of the pressure sensor, anterior active rhinometry is the most commonly used in the clinical setting. The purpose of this testing is to measure airflow as a function of air pressure for each nasal cavity separately. To isolate one nasal cavity, the contralateral naris is occluded with a pressure-sensing plug, and the nasal airflow through the unoccluded cavity is quantified by a flow sensor embedded in a tight-fitting face mask.[11] Acoustic rhinometry, developed by Hilberg and colleagues[12] in 1989, measures intranasal volume, the size and location of minimal cross-sectional area, and dimensional changes using sound reflections created by a sound generator and microphone coupled to a patient's nose with a flexible silicon tube. Despite considerable interest and research, use of these objective tests is limited and rhinoplasty surgeons instead favor patient-reported subjective symptoms as well as the validated Nasal Obstruction Symptom Evaluation (NOSE) questionnaire as subjective assessments of patient breathing. Previously published research validates the practice of relying on patient subjective assessment of breathing along with the clinician's physical examination in determining nasal obstruction and surgical candidacy.[13,14]

Once the history and physical examination have revealed the potential sources of nasal obstruction, operative planning can begin.

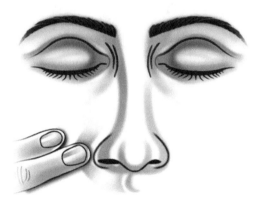

Fig. 5. Cottle maneuver. (*From* Payam V, Behnam B. Contemporary rhinoplasty techniques. In: Motamedi MHK, editor. A textbook of advanced oral and maxillofacial surgery. vol. 2. Croatia: InTech; 2015. p. 750.)

EXTERNAL NASAL VALVE

Nasal obstruction from a narrowing or collapse of the external nasal valves can occur as a consequence of congenital malposition of the lower lateral cartilages, pyriform aperture stenosis, caudal septal deviation, facial paralysis, normal aging, or complication following rhinoplasty. In most cases, the lateral crura of the lower lateral cartilages does not support the nasal ala effectively because of innate or acquired weakness, cephalic malposition, and/or protrusion of the distal part into the vestibule. Overresection of the lateral crura of the lower lateral cartilage is cited as the most common cause of external nasal valve collapse following rhinoplasty. To prevent collapse, the cross-sectional area of this segment needs to increase and the lateral component of the external nasal valve area needs to gain rigidity and strength.

Various techniques to restore the external nasal valve strength and stability have been reported, most commonly cartilage grafts such as alar rim graft, alar batten graft, and shield-tip type grafts. An alar batten graft, which is a common surgical technique, is harvested from septal cartilage or ear cartilage and provides strength and structural support to the lateral crura. This graft can be achieved during rhinoplasty through a marginal incision (**Fig. 6**) or through a limited alar-facial stab approach (**Fig. 7**).

In the marginal incision, an intranasal incision coursing along the caudal margin of the lower lateral cartilage is made. A sharp wide double hook is placed just inside the nostril margin retracting the skin. A pocket is then created with blunt scissors dissecting toward the alar-facial groove[15] and the graft is placed in this pocket. The marginal incision is then closed with interrupted 5-0 chromic sutures.

In the alar-facial stab method, described in 2010,[16] a 2-mm stab incision is made in the alar-

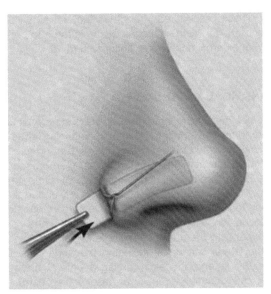

Fig. 7. Facial stab, alar rim. (*From* Deroee AF, Younes AA, Friedman O. External nasal valve collapse repair: the limited alar-facial stab approach. Laryngoscope 2011;121:475; with permission.)

facial groove. Blunt dissection through the alar fibrofatty tissue is carried superiorly to create a pocket extending to the soft tissue triangle of the alar rim. Cartilage grafts are cut to appropriate dimensions (3–4 mm by 1.5 cm long) and inserted into the pocket using Brown-Adson forceps. The external stab incision is then closed with two 5-0 chromic sutures.

Although suspension sutures are more commonly used for internal nasal valve repair, the lateral crus pull-up suture is described for isolated external nasal valve collapse. It has been described through an endonasal delivery approach to rotate the lateral crus of the lower lateral cartilage in a superolateral direction, held in place with a permanent spanning suture through the pyriform aperture. This technique is thought to supply strength and firmness to the lateral wall as a result of the continuous traction of the permanent spanning suture.[17]

Internal recurvature of the lateral crus to obstruct the nasal airway at the external nasal valve is commonly seen as a significant cause of nasal obstruction. Lateral crural strut grafts and lateral crural transposition techniques may be used to correct this problem. Structural shield tip–type grafts are often used to maintain stability of the restructured lateral nasal crura.[18] In addition, cephalic malpositioning of the lower lateral cartilages often results in poorly supported alar sidewalls. Repositioning the lower lateral cartilages in a more caudal location helps improve nasal vestibule support.[19]

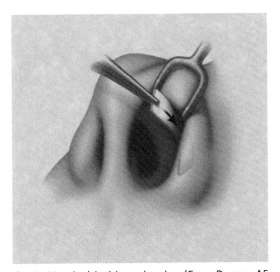

Fig. 6. Marginal incision, alar rim. (*From* Deroee AF, Younes AA, Friedman O. External nasal valve collapse repair: the limited alar-facial stab approach. Laryngoscope 2011;121:475; with permission.)

These procedures strengthen the alar sidewall and provide both static and dynamic force to prevent external nasal valve collapse (**Fig. 8**).

INTERNAL NASAL VALVE

When discussing internal nasal valve surgery, it is important to understand that maintaining structural integrity of the central pillar of the Anderson tripod (the combined medial crura, membranous septum, and caudal end of the septum) is imperative to a successful repair, such that any undertaking to perform internal nasal valve surgery should focus on strengthening the medial crura or expanding the nasal valve angle by repositioning the lateral cartilages, including the upper lateral cartilage and the alar cartilages (lateral crura). Kern[20] described causes of nasal valve obstruction according to the affected functional component of the valve, including septal disorders, mucocutaneous disorders, and upper lateral cartilage disorders. Common septal disorders are discussed later. If the relationship between the upper lateral cartilage and the septum is appropriate and there is no mucocutaneous disorder, then the lateral aspect of the valve along the nasal sidewall is addressed.

In patients presenting after previous surgery, previous resection of the cephalic border of the lower lateral cartilages or dome division may lead to structural weakness at the transition of the upper lateral cartilage and lower lateral cartilage, as well as structural weakness at the domal angle between the intermediate crus and the lateral crus. In these cases, batten grafts are a valuable mechanism in correcting these deficiencies. These grafts, consisting of curved septal cartilage or auricular cartilage, can be applied into a precise pocket at the site of maximal lateral nasal wall collapse via a limited intercartilaginous endonasal incision or via the external rhinoplasty approach.[21] The convex surface of the graft is oriented laterally to allow maximal lateralization of the collapsed portion of the lateral nasal wall and the graft may be fixated with mattress sutures to the upper lateral cartilage. One limitation of batten grafts is that they cannot correct valve obstruction associated with deformities of the middle vault and the valve angle.

The middle vault is critical for nasal breathing. The insertions of the upper lateral cartilages into the septum typically form a rounded arch that shapes the nasal valve angle at its caudal margin (**Fig. 9**). Following dorsal reduction, in which the upper lateral cartilage has been resected and

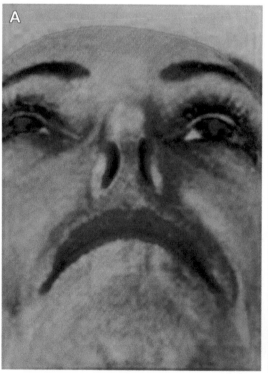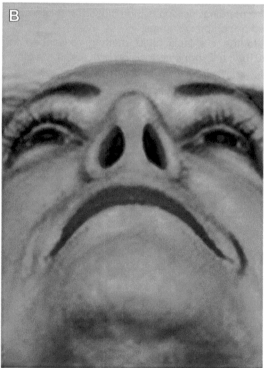

Fig. 8. (*A*) Before and (*B*) after correction of external nasal valve collapse. (*From* Becker, D. Revision rhinoplasty. New York: Thieme; 2008; with permission.)

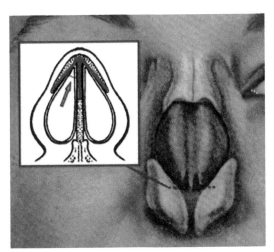

Fig. 9. Middle nasal vault. (*Courtesy of* John Hilinski, MD, San Diego, CA.)

curved auricular cartilage. The butterfly graft can be placed through an endonasal or external approach, and is placed symmetrically over the nasal dorsum. If necessary, the dorsal septum can be shaved to accommodate the thickness of the graft to avoid a polly-beak deformity. The graft is then secured with a suture to the upper lateral cartilage on each side,[24] which flares the upper lateral cartilages and widens the internal nasal valve angle (**Fig. 12**), thereby enlarging the nasal valve area. Autospreader grafts, or spreader flaps, are created by using the redundant dorsal portion of the upper lateral cartilage as the spreader graft. One advantage of this technique is that it obviates the harvesting of septal cartilage.[25]

Another method that allows excellent functional and cosmetic results is the placement of a longitudinal graft along the septum after the septum is slightly reduced in height. The upper lateral cartilages are then sutured along their entire length to the undersurface of this graft, resulting in a smooth dorsal contour and upward pull on the upper lateral cartilages.

In addition, some surgeons advocate the use of suture techniques to repair nasal valve disorders. The flaring suture across the upper lateral cartilages may be useful when used in conjunction with other techniques of valve repair.[26] Paniello[27] described the suspension suture technique, in which external sutures attached to the maxillary periosteum are used to pull out the nasal sidewalls. However, this technique requires external incisions and drilling anchor locations. These techniques can be used as alternatives to definite anatomic repair for patients who are poor candidates for rhinoplasty. There are a

separated from the dorsal septum, the natural wide and convex relationship between the upper lateral cartilage and the septum may become concave and narrowed. Therefore during rhinoplasty, separation of the upper lateral cartilages from the septum is frequently followed by spreader graft placement (fashioned from septal or auricular cartilage), to reapproximate, stabilize, and widen the nasal valve angle (**Fig. 10**). Spreader grafts can be bilateral or unilateral to correct asymmetries.[22] Another technique to reconstruct the middle vault is described by Alsarraf and Murakami[23] and involves a dorsal onlay graft sutured to the edges of the upper lateral cartilages to widen the nasal valve (**Fig. 11**). A type of onlay graft that is gaining popularity is the butterfly graft, which is composed of

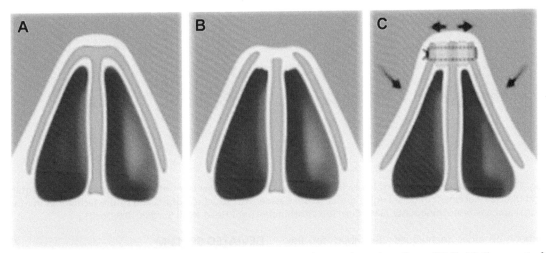

Fig. 10. Middle vault (*A*) with spreader grafts. (*B*) Separation of upper lateral cartilages (ULC). (*C*) Placement of spreader grafts between septum and ULC. (*From* Gassner HG. Structural grafts and suture techniques in functional and aesthetic rhinoplasty. GMS Curr Top Otorhinolaryngol Head Neck Surg 2010;9:Doc01.)

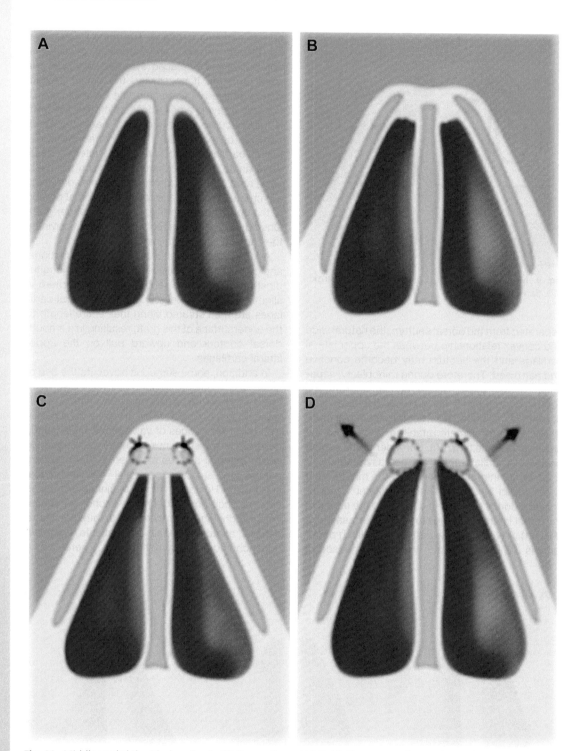

Fig. 11. Middle vault (*A*) with dorsal only. (*B*) Separation of ULC. (*C*) Placement of spreader graft between septum and ULC. (*D*) Placement of dorsal onlay grafts. (*From* Gassner HG. Structural grafts and suture techniques in functional and aesthetic rhinoplasty. GMS Curr Top Otorhinolaryngol Head Neck Surg 2010;9:Doc01.)

variety of other techniques described for the repair of internal nasal valve collapse, and interested readers are encouraged to pursue additional sources.

DEVIATED SEPTUM

Although the general techniques of septoplasty are discussed elsewhere, there are several critical

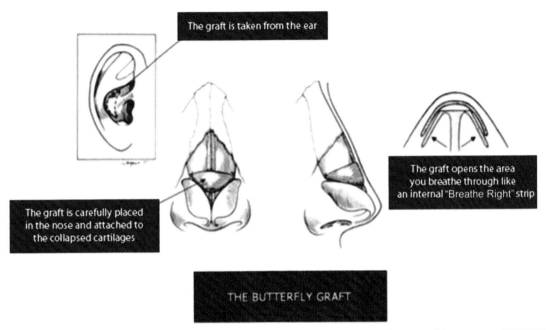

The graft is taken from the ear

The graft is carefully placed in the nose and attached to the collapsed cartilages

The graft opens the area you breathe through like an internal "Breathe Right" strip

THE BUTTERFLY GRAFT

Fig. 12. Middle vault with butterfly graft. (*From* http://noserevisionsurgeryandsurgeons.blogspot.com/2010/10/mystery-of-different-types-of-nose.html; with permission.)

aspects to consider when performing septoplasty for nasal obstruction. For posterior septal deviations and septal spurs, standard septoplasty techniques are effective. However, it is important to understand the relationship of the dorsal septum to the upper lateral cartilages and to appreciate caudal septal deviation. In the former case, marked dorsal septal deformities may require separation of the upper lateral cartilages from the septum; this disarticulation may lead to both functional and aesthetic deformities when this area becomes weak and causes blunting of the internal nasal valve angle. Spreader grafts may be required at the time of the septoplasty to straighten the dorsal septal deviation, prevent internal nasal valve collapse, and/or correct preexisting valve defects that may be present. Furthermore, spreader grafts help the aesthetic deformity caused by dorsal septal deviation, which often causes crooked nose deformity.

Caudal septal deviation should also be recognized early as a source of nasal obstruction, and one that can be challenging to correct. The goal of surgical treatment of caudal septal deformities is to reduce or eliminate the deviation while maintaining support of the nasal tip to prevent tip ptosis. Several maneuvers are at the surgeon's disposal for treating caudal septal deviation. Traditional approaches include scoring the septal cartilage on the concave side, thereby relaxing the spring of the cartilage. Another traditional

approach is the swinging-door repositioning technique described by Gubisch[28] and Peer,[29] which involves excising a wedge of cartilage along the maxillary crest to release the caudal septal attachments and allow the septum to swing to the midline. The midline position may be secured with an absorbable suture attached to the periosteum adjacent to the opposite side of the nasal spine or attached to the midline maxillary crest.

In severe cases, it may be necessary to perform a septal transplant. During this procedure, the surgeon may completely resect the anterior septum keeping a dorsal strut in place and subsequently reconstruct the caudal strut from a septal cartilage graft harvested during the septoplasty[30] or, alternatively, rib cartilage or other grafting material. This neostrut is placed within the septal space and secured to the intact dorsal strut and maxillary spine, acting as both a strut graft for nasal tip stability and as a spreader graft within the middle nasal vault (**Fig. 13**). Additional strength may be created through the use of extended spreader grafts, which help secure the newly positioned caudal septal replacement.

Another location of septal disorders less commonly seen is an elongated membranous septum resulting in tip ptosis and bilateral nasal valve obstruction. During the history and physical, the patient may indicate that pushing the nasal tip up relieves the obstruction. In addition to correcting any middle nasal vault disorders, recreation of

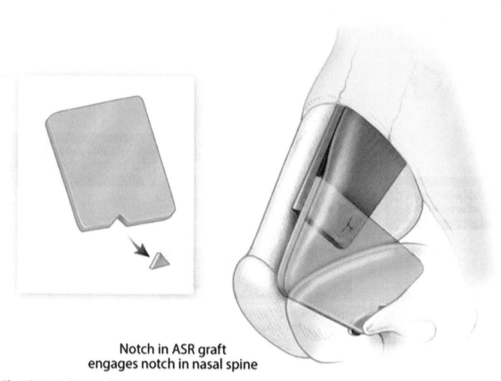

Notch in ASR graft
engages notch in nasal spine

Fig. 13. Anterior septal reconstruction (ASR). (*From* Surowitz J, Lee MK, Most SP. Anterior septal reconstruction for treatment of severe caudal septal deviation: clinical severity and outcomes. Otolaryngol Head Neck Surg 2015;153(1):27–33; with permission.)

the relationship between the columella and the caudal septum is important to correct such a deformity.

INFERIOR TURBINATE

Although turbinate hypertrophy has not been well defined and is still poorly understood, recent literature suggests that there is some merit to addressing this entity. Before attributing nasal obstruction to turbinate hypertrophy, the integrity of the nasal valve should be verified, and the straightness of the septum should be ensured. Once this is complete, turbinate hypertrophy can be considered as a contribution to nasal obstruction. Turbinate hypertrophy should be refractory to antiinflammatory medical therapies before surgical intervention is considered. Because of the physiologic function of the turbinates, we also recommend that all other disorders be addressed in correcting nasal obstruction first. If the patient continues to have an obstructive airway, the surgeon may proceed with turbinate procedure.

Various techniques of turbinate reduction have been reported in the literature. Passali and colleagues[31] showed that submucous resection with or without lateralization of the inferior turbinate via outfracture resulted in longer-lasting reduction of nasal airway resistance compared with turbinectomy, laser cautery, electrocautery, or cryotherapy. However, risk of atrophic rhinitis as a result of removal of this mucosa is substantial and should be considered in all patients who develop nasal congestion, crusting, and dryness secondary to turbinate surgery; this is known as empty nose syndrome. These symptoms occur when the humidifying function of the nasal mucosa decompensates after removal of important nasal mucosa.[32] Lateral outfracture and selective submucous resection of bone seem to be the only surgical maneuvers that allow reduction of the impact of the turbinates on nasal resistance without destruction of their physiologic function. Because the excision of turbinate tissue has been associated with major morbidity such as empty nose syndrome, the resection of healthy functionally important turbinate tissue should be approached in extreme cases only.[33] In almost all cases, correction of septal and nasal valve disorders provides patients with extremely satisfying nasal airways and turbinate reduction is rarely required.

OSTEOTOMY

An additional consideration for nasal obstruction in rhinoplasty involves complications secondary to osteotomy. Inadequate lateral osteotomies after removal of a dorsal hump may result in an open roof deformity. However, the lateral osteotomy required to correct nasal deformities while closing or preventing an open roof could lead to nasal valve obstruction. Webster and colleagues[34] showed that the risk of nasal valve obstruction could be reduced by initiating the lateral osteotomy higher on the pyriform aperture. This risk reduction is thought to be caused by preservation of a triangular piece at the edge of the pyriform aperture that prevents medial displacement of fibromuscular tissues of the ala and possibly the inferior turbinate. Thus high-low-high osteotomies are performed whenever possible in order to ensure preservation of airway patency.

Another complication of dorsal hump reduction (alluded to earlier) is the inverted V deformity, which is especially common in patients with short nasal bones. This deformity may be prevented by exact placement of spreader grafts in the manner discussed earlier. Preventative reconstruction and strengthening of the middle nasal vault with spreader grafts or other techniques in patients with short nasal bones are encouraged.

SUMMARY

The key to a successful functional septorhinoplasty includes an understanding of nasal anatomy and physiology. History and physical are paramount in diagnosing and subsequently treating an epicenter of obstruction, which is commonly found in one of the following locations: internal or external nasal valve, caudal septum, or turbinate. Treatment of each of these centers is nuanced and multiple approaches are discussed to provide an understanding of the current surgical techniques that allow adequate correction and excellent functional results.

REFERENCES

1. Salem AM, Younes A, Friedman O. Cosmetics and function: quality-of-life changes after rhinoplasty surgery. Laryngoscope 2012;122:254–9.
2. Rohrich RJ, Raniere J Jr, Ha RY. The alar contour graft: correction and prevention of alar rim deformities in rhinoplasty. Plast Reconstr Surg 2002;109:2495–505.
3. Constantian MB, Clardy RB. The relative importance of septal and nasal valvular surgery in correcting airway obstruction in primary and secondary rhinoplasty. Plast Reconstr Surg 1996;98:38–58.
4. Mink PJ. Le nez comme voi repiratorie. Presse Otolaryngol Belg 1903;5:481–96.
5. Bridger GP. Physiology of the nasal valve. Arch Otolaryngol 1970;92:543–53.
6. Haight JS, Cole P. The site and function of the nasal valve. Laryngoscope 1983;93:49–55.
7. Constantine MB. The incompetent external nasal valve: pathophysiology and treatment in primary and secondary rhinoplasty. Plast Reconstr Surg 1994;93:919–31.
8. Cole P. The four components of the nasal valve. Am J Rhinol 2003;17:107–10.
9. Cottle MH. Rhino-sphygmo-manometry and aid in physical diagnosis. Intern Rhinol 1968;6:7–26.
10. Wexler D, Braverman I, Amar M. Histology of the nasal septal swell body (septal turbinate). Otolaryngol Head Neck Surg 2006;134:596–600.
11. Masing H. Rhinomanometry, different techniques, and results. Acta Otorhinolaryngol Belg 1979;33:566–71.
12. Hilberg O, Jackson AC, Swift DL, et al. Acoustic rhinometry evaluation of nasal cavity geometry by acoustic reflection. J Appl Physiol 1989;66:295–303.
13. Chisholm E, Jallali N. Rhinoplasty and septorhinoplasty outcome evaluation. Ear Nose Throat J 2012;91:E10–4.
14. Rhee JS, Poetker DM, Smith TL, et al. Nasal valve surgery improves disease-specific quality of life. Laryngoscope 2005;115(3):437–40.
15. Guida RA. Surgical approaches to the nasal skeleton. Oper Tech Otolaryngol Head Neck Surg 1999;10:228–31.
16. Deroee AF, Younes AA, Friedman O. External nasal valve collapse repair: the limited alar-facial stab approach. Laryngoscope 2011;121:474–9.
17. Menger DJ. Lateral crus pull-up: a method for collapse of the external nasal valve. Arch Facial Plast Surg 2006;8:333–7.
18. Friedman O, Ackcam T, Cook T. Reconstructive rhinoplasty: the three-dimensional nasal tip. Arch Facial Plast Surg 2006;8:195–201.
19. Toriumi DM. New concepts in nasal tip contouring. Arch Facial Plast Surg 2006 May-Jun;8(3):156–85.
20. Kern EB. Surgery of the nasal valve. In: Sisson GA, Tardy ME Jr, editors. Plastic and reconstructive surgery of the face and neck: Proceedings of the Second International Symposium. vol. 2. New York: Grune and Stratton; 1977. p. 43–59.
21. Toriumi DM, Josen J, Weinberer M, et al. Use of alar batten grafts for correction of nasal valve collapse. Arch Otolaryngol Head Neck Surg 1997;123:802–8.

22. Sheen JH. Spreader graft: a method of reconstructing the roof of the middle nasal vault following rhinoplasty. Plast Reconstr Surg 1984;72:230.

23. Alsarraf R, Murakami CS. The saddle nose deformity. Facial Plast Surg Clin North Am 1999;7:303–10.

24. Clark JM, Cook TA. The butterfly graft in functional secondary rhinoplasty. Laryngoscope 2002;112: 1917–25.

25. Oneal RM, Berkowitz RL. Upper lateral cartilage spreader flaps in rhinoplasty. Aesthet Surg J 1998; 18(5):370–1.

26. Park SS. The flaring suture to augment the repair of the dysfunctional nasal valve. Plast Reconstr Surg 1998;101:1120–2.

27. Paniello RC. Nasal valve suspension: an effective technique for nasal valve collapse. Arch Otolaryngol Head Neck Surg 1996;122:1342–6.

28. Gubisch W. The extra-corporeal septum plasty: a technique to correct difficult nasal deformities. Plast Reconstr Surg 1995;95(4):672–82.

29. Peer L. An operation to repair lateral displacement of the lower border of septal cartilage. Arch Otolaryngol 1937;25:475–7.

30. Surowitz J, Lee MK, Most SP. Anterior septal reconstruction for treatment of severe caudal septal deviation: clinical severity and outcomes. Otolaryngol Head Neck Surg 2015;153(1):27–33.

31. Passali D, Passali FM, Damiani V, et al. Treatment of inferior turbinate hypertrophy: a randomized clinical trial. Ann Otol Rhinol Laryngol 2003;112:683–8.

32. Lindemann J, Lieacker R, Sikora T, et al. Impact of unilateral sinus surgery with resection by means of midfacial degloving on nasal air conditioning. Laryngoscope 2002;112:2062–6.

33. Chhabra N, Houser SM. The diagnosis and management of empty nose syndrome. Otolaryngol Clin North Am 2009;42:311–30.

34. Webster RC, Davidson TM, Smith RC. Curved lateral osteotomy for airway protection in rhinoplasty. Arch Otolaryngol Head Neck Surg 1977;103:454–8.

Surgical Management of Nasal Airway Obstruction

John F. Teichgraeber, MD[a], Ronald P. Gruber, MD[b], Neil Tanna, MD, MBA[c],*

KEYWORDS

- Nasal obstruction • Nasal breathing • Septal deviation • Nasal valve narrowing
- Turbinate hypertrophy

KEY POINTS

- The management and diagnosis of nasal airway obstruction requires an understanding of the form and function of the nose.
- Nasal airway obstruction can be structural, physiologic, or a combination of both.
- Anatomic causes of airway obstruction include septal deviation, internal nasal valve narrowing, external nasal valve collapse, and inferior turbinate hypertrophy.
- Thus, the management of nasal air obstruction must be selective and carefully considered.
- The goal of surgery is to address the deformity and not just enlarge the nasal cavity.

INTRODUCTION

The management and diagnosis of nasal airway obstruction requires an understanding of the form and function of the nose. Nasal airway obstruction can be structural, physiologic, or a combination of both. Thus, the management of nasal airway obstruction must be selective and often involves medical management. The goal of surgery is to address the deformity and not just enlarge the nasal cavity. This article reviews airway obstruction and its treatment.

ANATOMY

The nasal airway is both a dynamic and rigid structure. It begins at the external nasal valve, which is composed of the caudal edge of the lower lateral cartilages, caudal septum, nostril sill, and the soft tissue alae. The septum and the bone walls provide the rigid structure of the nose. The septum is made up of quadrilateral cartilage, nasal spine, frontal spine, perpendicular plate of the ethmoid, vomer, and maxillary crest. The narrowest portion of the nose is the internal nasal valve (10°–15°), which is formed by the septum, the inferior turbinate, and the upper lateral cartilage. Short nasal bones, a narrow midnasal fold, and malposition of the alar cartilages all predispose patients to internal valve incompetence.

The lateral wall of the nose contains 3 to 4 turbinates (inferior, middle, superior, supreme) and the corresponding meatuses that drain the paranasal sinuses. The nasolacrimal duct drains through the inferior meatus, whereas the maxillary, frontal, and anterior ethmoid sinuses articulate with the middle meatus. The posterior ethmoid sinus opens into the superior meatus. The nasal cavity ends at the choanae as the airflow passes into the nasopharynx.

FUNCTION

The nose is not only a conduit for inspired air but also an air conditioner that cleans, humidifies,

Disclosures: The authors have no financial disclosures.
[a] Division of Plastic & Reconstructive Surgery, University of Texas Health Science Center at Houston, 6410 Fannin Street #1400, Houston, TX 77030, USA; [b] Division of Plastic & Reconstructive Surgery, Stanford University, Stanford, California, USA; [c] Division of Plastic & Reconstructive Surgery, North Shore – LIJ Health System, 1991 Marcus Avenue, Suite 102, Lake Success, NY 11042, USA
* Corresponding author.
E-mail address: ntanna@gmail.com

Clin Plastic Surg 43 (2016) 41–46
http://dx.doi.org/10.1016/j.cps.2015.09.006
0094-1298/16/$ – see front matter © 2016 Elsevier Inc. All rights reserved.

and warms the inspired air. It is also involved in olfaction and speech. Inspired air passes through the nose at 200 kph (125 mph) in a parabolic curve moving vertically through the roof of the nasal vestibule and then through the internal nasal valve. The nose is the site of nearly half of the total respiratory resistance; a third of the resistance occurs at the external valve and two-thirds occur at the internal valve. The gatekeeper of nasal airflow is the internal valve, which aids in respiration by limiting the flow of air so that it does not exceed the nose's ability to process it. On deep inspiration the nostril enlarges and the internal valve narrows, whereas on expiration the nostril narrows and the internal valve enlarges. Complete closure of the internal valve is prevented by the action of the alae, which flare outward and upward exerting a checkrein action on the connective-tissue aponeurosis of the upper lateral cartilages.

CAUSES

Nasal obstruction can be physiologic and/or structural. The differential diagnosis of physiologic nasal obstruction includes infections, allergies, medications, vasomotor rhinitis, endocrine disorders, and chemical irritants.

The common cold is the most frequent cause of physiologic nasal obstruction. It is usually self-limiting and treated with antihistamines and decongestants. Allergic rhinitis can be seasonal or perennial. Seasonal symptoms can be managed with antihistamines, decongestants, and topical and/or systemic steroids. Perennial allergic rhinitis requires a work-up, which includes nasal cytology, blood tests for immunoglobulin E levels, and skin test.

Rhinitis medicamentosa is most frequently seen in patients who use long-term nasal sprays or drops. However, it can also result from oral medications such as reserpine, propanol, and chlorpromazine. Its treatment requires stopping the offending medication and providing airway support with decongestants and systemic and/or topical steroids.

Pregnancy is a common endocrine cause of nasal obstruction. However, rhinitis of pregnancy usually resolves with the end of pregnancy. Interim treatment depends on the stage of the patient's pregnancy and the approach that the patient's obstetrician has toward therapy during pregnancy.

Persistent irritants can cause chronic allergic rhinitis, and pollution is the most common environmental cause. Other causes are primarily occupational, which include dust, fumes, and chemicals. The treatment is preventative and avoidance of the irritants.

DIAGNOSIS

The diagnosis of nasal obstruction begins with a complete history, including several key elements, including (1) duration and frequency of the symptoms, (2) whether they are unilateral or bilateral, (3) whether they are perennial or seasonal, (4) history of trauma, (5) history of surgery, (6) presence of allergic symptoms, and (7) medication usage. Examination of the patient's nasal cavities requires good illumination and adequate decongestion. The patient is initially observed at rest without a speculum. The external nasal valve is first examined and noted for alar collapse. The internal valve is also evaluated without a speculum, checking for mucosal scarring and the relationship of the upper lateral cartilage to the septum. The Cottle test is used to evaluate nasal valve disorder. While the patient breaths quietly, the cheek is retracted laterally in order to open up the nasal valve. If the patient's breathing is improved, the Cottle test is positive, indicating that the nasal valve is a factor in the patient's respiratory symptoms. However, if the valve is scarred, the maneuver may not alter the symptoms, and the test results are designated as false-negative. In this case, a Q-tip may be used to retract the nasal valve laterally. Although the Cottle test is specific for nasal valve collapse, false-positive tests are seen in patients with flaccid valves. Gruber and colleagues also described the use of a Breathe Right strip test to evaluate the internal and external valves separately.

The nasal structures are then examined with a nasal speculum. The nasal septum is evaluated for deviation, whereas the turbinates are evaluated for hypertrophy (**Fig. 1**). The caudal end of the septum is examined and deviations of the quadrilateral cartilage and bony septum are noted (**Fig. 2**). The nasal mucosa is examined for scarring or thinning. In addition, both inferior and middle turbinates are evaluated.

TREATMENT

Correction of the nasal airway obstruction is directed toward the anatomic source of obstruction. For septal deviation, a septoplasty can be considered. The goal of the septoplasty is the correct septal deviation while at the same time preserving as much of the septum anatomy as possible.

The septum can be approached endonasally through a hemitransfixion or Killian incision. Alternatively, an open approach can be used. In complex nasal airway cases, the septum is best treated with an open rhinoplasty. The open

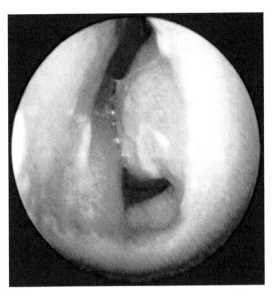

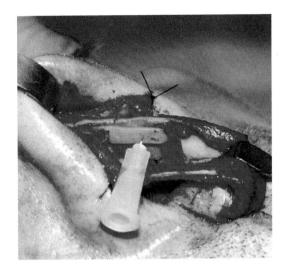

Fig. 3. A spreader graft being placed to correct internal nasal valve dysfunction.

Fig. 1. Septal deviation and left turbinate hypertrophy.

approach allows the surgeon to simultaneously approach the caudal and dorsal septum. The upper lateral is separated from the septum after a submucosal tunnel is developed on both sides of the nose. The quadrilateral cartilage is usually approached dorsally through a mucoperichondrial flap that is connected to a mucoperiosteal flap. The quadrilateral cartilage is separated from the perpendicular plate of the ethmoid, the vomer, and the maxillary crest. Bilateral mucoperiosteal flaps are developed, isolating the bony septum. The obstructing bone is fractured with double-action scissors and repositioned. Cuts in the bony septum are usually high on the perpendicular plate of the ethmoid and along the floor of the nose. The septal cut on the ethmoid is to prevent fracturing of the cribriform plate.

Once the bony septum is repositioned, the quadrilateral cartilage is approached. The quadrilateral cartilage is usually left attached to the anterolateral mucoperichondrium unless the caudal

septum needs repositioning. In this case, the caudal septum is freed from the ipsilateral and/or contralateral mucoperichondrium as far as needed. Vertical septal angulation is treated with vertical resection and horizontal angulation with horizontal resection. The thickened cartilage is shaved and, if the deformity persists, it may be necessary to weaken the deformed segment with cross-hatching or conservative morcellation. The area of deflection along the caudal and dorsal borders of quadrilateral cartilages is managed with incisions within 2 mm of the affected border. Although this helps straighten the quadrilateral cartilage it may also weaken it. In order to prevent loss of nasal support, grafts (3 mm × 10–20 mm) of septal cartilage or ethmoidal bone are sutured to the concave side of the caudal and/or dorsal septal borders, which helps reinforce and straighten the septum as well as fixing it in the midline. The authors have also used absorbable plates made of polylactic and polyglycolic acid (Synthes) (3 mm × 20 mm) to reinforce or

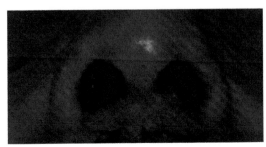

Fig. 2. Caudal septal deflection obstructing the left nasal cavity.

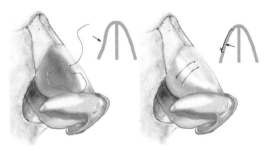

Fig. 4. A suspension suture can also be used to correct internal nasal valve narrowing.

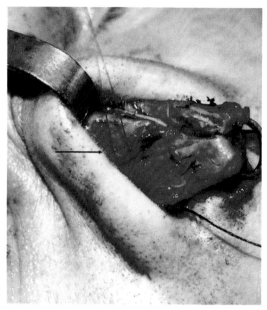

Fig. 5. A mattress suture is placed to improve the internal nasal valve.

straighten the deviated septum. The plates are sutured through preexisting holes to the quadrilateral cartilages with through-and-through polydioxanone sutures. Following the septoplasty, a septal suture of 4-0 plain on a Keith needle is used to coapt the mucosal flaps.

After the septum is corrected, the upper lateral cartilages and internal valve are approached. The lower lateral cartilages have already been separated submucosally from the septum. Abnormalities of the medial portion of the upper laterals may require conservation resection. If the internal valve has collapsed, a spreader flap and/or spreader grafts are used to laterally displace the cartilages, in order to open up the internal valve. The spreader grafts maybe be harvested from the septum, ear, and/or rib in order of preference. The grafts (2–4 mm × 20–30 mm) are sutured 2 mm below the septal border with polydioxanone sutures (**Fig. 3**). Subsequently, the upper laterals are sutured back to the septum with the same suture. A composite graft from the ear is used in patients with internal nasal collapse from mucosal scarring. An alternative method to correct internal nasal valve narrowing is to use a permanent mattress suspension suture (**Figs. 4** and **5**).

The external valve is usually obstructed because of a malposition of the lower lateral cartilage, inadequate underlying support, and/or mucosal scarring. Reconstruction of the external valve and nasal tip begins with a columellar strut, which is harvested from the septum, ear, or rib. It is sutured

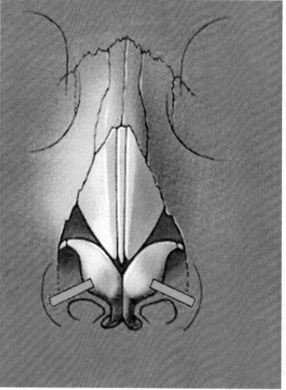
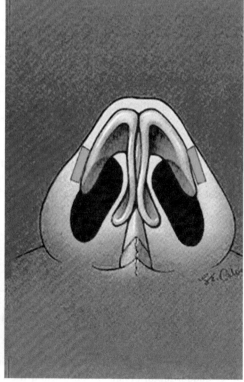

Fig. 6. Rim grafts can be used to treat external nasal valve collapse.

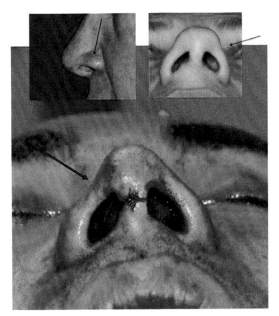

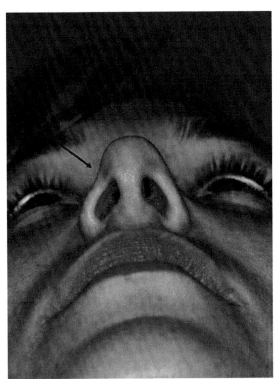

Fig. 7. Rim grafts can be considered when concavity of the rim exists.

between the medial crura with a polydioxanone suture. Once the central limb of the tripod is stabilized, attention is directed to its lateral limbs. In patients with adequate lower lateral cartilage,

repositioning of the lower lateral cartilage to the upper lateral cartilages and septum often stabilizes the lower lateral cartilages and opens up the valve. If the lateral crura are over-resected or weak, they are reinforced with lateral crura spanning grafts from the septum or ear. These grafts are placed lateral to the dome running one-half to one-third the length of the lateral crura (1.0–1.5 cm) and sandwiched between the lower lateral cartilages and the nasal lining. They are sutured with polydioxanone sutures. Rim grafts have also been advocated for supporting the external nasal valve (**Figs. 6–8**).

If its external valve needs further opening or support, a lateral crural spanning graft is used. The graft is usually harvested from the septum or the ear (2 mm × 16–18 mm) and helps expand the intercrural space. The position of the nasal valve and lateral crural spanning grafts are adjusted by stabilizing the structures with two 27-gauge needles and redraping the retracted skin. When both vestibular skin and cartilage are needed, a composite graft from the ear is used.

The inferior turbinate often plays a major role in nasal obstruction. The anterior third of the turbinate forms the internal valve, the narrowest portion of the nasal airway. A multitude of destructive and nondestructive turbinotomy techniques have been

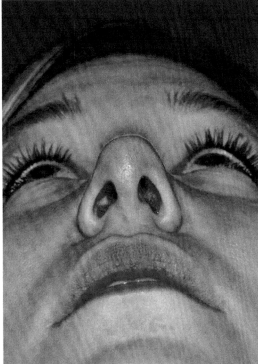

Fig. 8. Preoperative (*left*) and postoperative (*right*) results with rim graft placement. The arrow shows the area of preoperative external nasal valve narrowing.

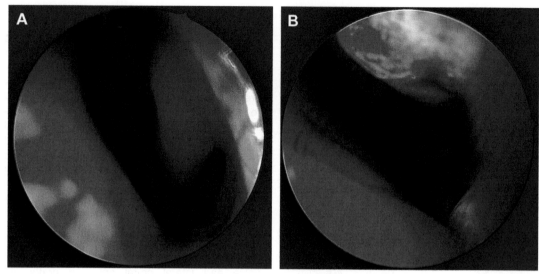

Fig. 9. Intranasal view before (*A*) and after (*B*) septoplasty and turbinate reduction.

described to treat the enlarged turbinates. Treatment approaches include turbinectomy, submucous resection (**Fig. 9**), turbinate outfracture (**Fig. 10**), radiofrequency ablation, submucous diathermy, laser cautery, cryosurgical reduction, and septoturbinotomy.

Septoturbinotomy is a noninvasive procedure used to correct turbinate hypertrophy and septal deviation. It can expand the nasal vault with insertion of a large and long speculum that outfractures the turbinates and also centralizes the bony septum when the handles are compressed. Alternatively, a large clamp can be passed into the nasal cavity and expanded (in reverse nutcracker fashion) to achieve a similar result. Mechanical dilation (expansion) of the nasal vault with the speculum or large clamp improves the airway diameter of the nasal vault and may preclude the need for further work on the turbinates. The nasal vault is not necessarily expanded to the maximal diameter that could be achieved with resection procedures, but it may be to achieve satisfactory air flow.

An enlarged middle turbinate can also cause nasal obstruction and necessitate endoscopic surgery. In some patients, nasal obstruction results from the loss of boney support. In these patients medial and lateral osteotomies with bilateral spreader grafts are used to lateralize the upper lateral cartilages and nasal bones. In some cases, a cantilever costochondral graft is required.

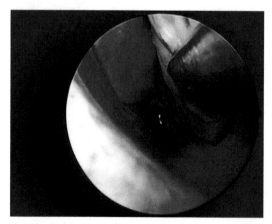

Fig. 10. Turbinate outfracture is performed by lateralizing the turbinate.

SUMMARY

The management of nasal obstruction requires a clear understanding of nasal anatomy and function. Nasal obstruction can be physiologic, anatomic, or a combination of both. The operative treatment is aided by the open approach, which allows clear visualization of the nasal structures, and enables surgeons to precisely address the underlying anatomic deformities. Even though the septum is the key to treating nasal obstruction, attention must also be given to the internal and external nasal valves and the turbinates.

Dorsal Hump Reduction and Osteotomies

Babak Azizzadeh, MD[a],*, Michael Reilly, MD[b]

KEYWORDS

- Osteotomy • Dorsal hump • Nasal profile • Surgical technique • Rhinoplasty

KEY POINTS

- Consider the relationship of the nose to the other elements of the facial profile when planning dorsal hump takedown.
- Be prepared to use temporalis fascia for disguising osteotomy sites and nasal dorsal contour irregularities in thin-skinned patients.
- Preventatively address issues with post-hump-takedown middle nasal vault collapse with the use of spreader grafts.
- An onlay graft can be used to disguise the hump accentuation caused by a deep radix.

INTRODUCTION

Western ideals of nasal beauty have evolved around the leptorrhine nose, which consists of a thinner dorsum and more slender nostrils than the other 2 general nasal types, platyrrhine (broad) and mesorrhine (intermediate). Among leptorrhine noses, the Greek subtype (straight profile) has persisted as the most esthetically desirable variant over the Roman (convex) or Armenoid (convex with ptotic tip) subtypes.

The reasons for the desirability of the Greek nasal type are most likely 3-fold: esthetic, cultural, and evolutionary.[1,2] The esthetic harmony of the face is based on the concept of vertical facial fifths and horizontal facial thirds, first described by the ancient Greeks.[3] This concept ascribes the face with the unique role of serving as a communication portal with the world and suggests that a balanced appearance will be best received by others. The cultural contribution to our beauty ideals stem from popular figures and messages in our given society, usually dictated by the dominant class.[4–6] The fact that the Greeks were the first to describe the concept of facial harmony may not be entirely unrelated to why the Greek nose remains the preferred leptorrhine subtype. The evolutionary reasons for the development of a specific nasal esthetic are most likely related to a desire for highlighting the femininity or masculinity of a given subject, which conveys sexual attractiveness.[7,8] Women generally have a lower nasal dorsum due to the absence of exposure to testosterone, which exerts anatomic influence over the development of masculine facial features such as a lower, more prominent brow, stronger jaw, and more prominent nasal dorsum. Given that the overwhelming majority of patients seeking rhinoplasty surgery have been women, it is no surprise that there has been an emphasis on feminizing the nose through dorsal hump reduction.[9] For male patients, the driver to reduce a dorsal hump is likely more cultural.

No relevant disclosures pertaining to this topic and article.
[a] Department of Head & Neck Surgery, The Center for Advanced Facial Plastic Surgery, David Geffen School of Medicine at UCLA, 9401 Wilshire Boulevard, Suite 650, Beverly Hills, CA 90212, USA; [b] Department of Otolaryngology–Head & Neck Surgery, Georgetown University Medical Center, 3800 Reservoir Road Northwest, 1st Floor Gorman Building, Washington, DC 20007, USA
* Corresponding author.
E-mail address: drazizzadeh@gmail.com

plasticsurgery.theclinics.com

Men are faced with the decision of potentially increasing their attractiveness based on cultural norms, but must be cautious about the potential to sacrifice masculinity in the process.

TREATMENT GOALS AND PLANNED OUTCOMES

The goal of dorsal nasal hump reduction is to effectively improve the esthetic, cultural, and evolutionary attractiveness of the nose, which involves rendering the nose closer to the modern esthetic of the balanced and harmonious face.[10]

PREOPERATIVE PLANNING AND PREPARATION

Despite the relatively common desire of patients to reduce their prominent nasal dorsum, there are great variations in the anatomic specifics for each patient. Skin type and thickness, height and width of the hump, relationship of the dorsal hump to the other defining profile points, and the esthetic desires of the patient, including gender appropriateness, are all important variables to consider in the planning and execution of dorsal hump reduction.[11,12]

Rhinoplasty surgeons must possess a mastery of the inherent nasal anatomy (**Fig. 1**) as well as an ability to perform a comprehensive assessment of surrounding nasal structures in 3 dimensions. Ideal nasal and facial angles must be considered in the context of the overall facial profile, including forehead shape, nasofrontal angle, radix height, nasofrontal angle, supratip break, tip-defining points and projection, infratip break, nasolabial angle, length of upper lip, dental occlusion, and chin projection. A change to any one of the above regions may result in a relative change to the other sites as well. On anterior view, changes in the nasal dorsum will frequently lead to an altered appearance of the dorsal esthetic lines, which are one of the most important aspects of nasal beauty (**Fig. 2**).

Taking all of these data points into consideration, the surgeon will identify a treatment plan that will most accurately execute the desired results.

PATIENT POSITIONING

Positioning for rhinoplasty surgery should optimize unimpeded access to the patient for both physician and assistant. The patient's airway should be established in such a way as to avoid distorting the lip anatomy and to avoid encroaching on the physician's maneuverability. The authors recommend using an oral RAE endotracheal tube taped to the midline of the lower lip in order to accomplish the above. In cases where an external approach will be used, it is advisable to prepare the patient's facial skin preoperatively with Betadine or another antiseptic solution. Draping should be performed in such a way as to include the patient's entire facial profile, from the hairline superiorly to below the cervicomental angle inferiorly.

PROCEDURAL APPROACH

Dorsal hump reduction is typically performed in combination with other nasal alterations. Although

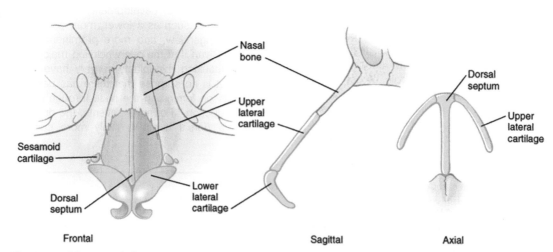

Fig. 1. Nasal framework from anterior, lateral, and base views. (*From* Numa W, Johnson CM. Surgical anatomy and physiology of the nose. In: Azizzadeh B, Murphy MR, Johnson CM, et al, editors. Master techniques in rhinoplasty. Philadelphia: Elsevier; 2011; with permission.)

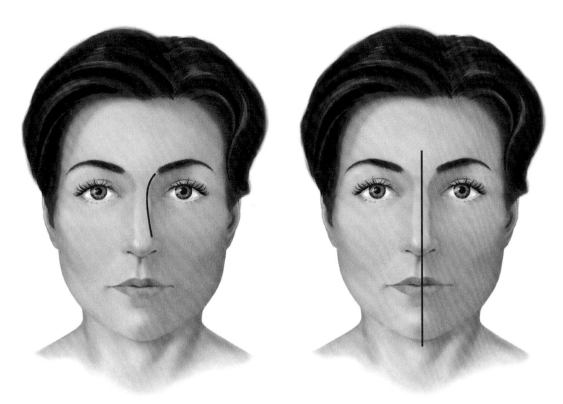

Fig. 2. The dorsal esthetic line should follow a gentle curve from the medial brow to the nasal tip. (*From* Swamy RS, Most SP. Nasal osteotomies. In: Azizzadeh B, Murphy MR, Johnson CM, et al, editors. Master techniques in rhinoplasty. Philadelphia: Elsevier; 2011; with permission.)

surgeon preference is variable for determining the order of the procedure, it is often appropriate to perform the tip refining steps of the procedure before executing the dorsal hump reduction.[13–15] Tip refining can aid in ensuring proper harmony between the ultimate dorsal reduction and the overall nasal form and can be particularly important when caring for patients with saddle nose deformity who are also undergoing bony hump reduction (**Fig. 3**).

Tip-refining aspects of the procedure should be completed based on preoperative planning for desired tip projection, rotation, and shape. Tip rotation can significantly alter the extent of dorsal hump modification and therefore must be considered carefully.[16–19] Once this has been executed, the cartilaginous and bony dorsal hump are taken down. Conservative primary excision is advisable at the outset of the procedure because additional excision is always possible.

There are several different techniques for addressing the dorsal hump.[20–23] Some authors recommend en-bloc reduction of the cartilaginous vault, whereas others advocate component reduction by first separating the upper lateral cartilages

from the nasal septum in order to maintain the transverse portions of the upper lateral cartilages.[24–27] Regardless, the cartilaginous portion of the hump is traditionally taken down sharply with a 15-blade or truncated 11-blade scalpel (**Fig. 4**). Limiting the resection at the rhinion can help prevent a concave nasal profile, while placement of a radix graft can help disguise a hump in select patients by easing the transition from the nasal dorsum to frontal bone (**Fig. 5**).

For mild to moderate bony reduction, a pull nasal rasp may be used to reduce the bony portion of the dorsal hump (**Fig. 6**). For large dorsal humps, a 10-mm Rubin osteotome is inserted underneath the transected cartilaginous hump and used to complete the hump reduction en-bloc and simultaneously create the medial osteotomies. If the hump reduction has not resulted in freely mobile medial nasal bones, completion medial osteotomies may be required (**Fig. 7**).

The authors recommend that these medial osteotomies be planned with surgical markings on the skin in order to guide the direction of the controlled fractures. After the hump resection and medial osteotomies are complete but before

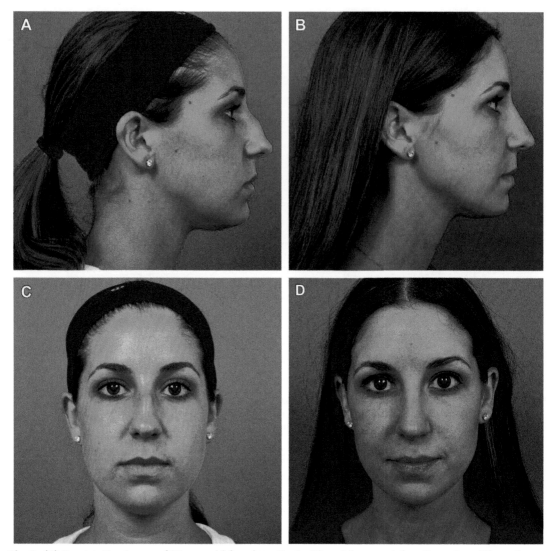

Fig. 3. (*A*) Preoperative image of 26-year-old female patient with saddle nose deformity and small bony hump. (*B*) Postoperative image following bony and cartilaginous hump resection, correction of septal deviation, crushed cartilage graft to the nasal tip, left-sided spreader graft, and dome-binding suture. (*C*) Anterior view of same patient before surgery, and (*D*) postoperative view showing significant improvement in dorsal aesthetic lines.

performing any destabilizing intermediate or lateral osteotomies, nasal rasps can be further used to soften any jagged, asymmetrical, or irregular edges that are evident. The use of temporalis fascia or thoroughly morselized cartilage to camouflage irregularities is always considered in individuals with thin, aging, or inelastic skin (**Fig. 8**). There are also automated oscillating instruments that can accomplish the same goal. Regardless of method, rasping technique should be used in an alternating fashion from side to side in order to prevent overreduction or asymmetry.

Following hump reduction, there is most often an open book deformity, which then needs to be addressed and corrected by performing lateral osteotomies with or without intermediate osteotomies.[28] The decision to proceed with intermediate osteotomies is made based on the curvature of the nasal bones and the width of the dorsal hump. For convex bones and a wide base to the bony nasal vault, intermediate

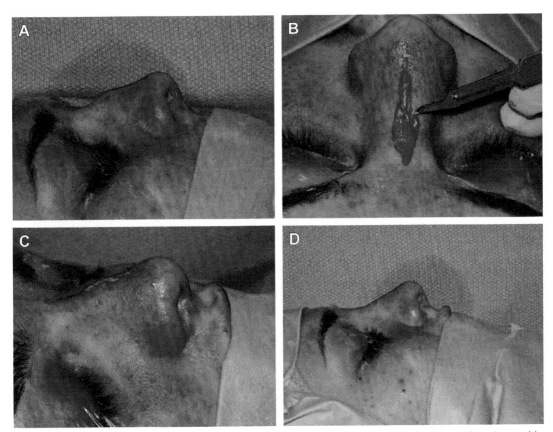

Fig. 4. 19-year-old female patient undergoing dorsal hump reduction: (*A*) Patient before undergoing en-bloc bony and cartilaginous dorsal hump reduction, (*B*) after dorsal takedown with 15-blade scalpel, (*C*) three-quarter view of reduced hump with overlying en-bloc resection, and (*D*) profile after hump reduction.

osteotomies are often useful to facilitate a more natural-looking and graduated closure of the open roof.

Like the medial osteotomies, the authors advise surgically marking the sites of the desired lateral ± intermediate osteotomies before proceeding with this portion of the procedure. Intermediate osteotomies are executed through a small stab incision in the pyriform aperture on each side made with a 15-blade scalpel. A straight guarded osteotome is then placed through this incision, taking care not to engage the nasal mucosa. The cutting edge of the osteotome is then typically engaged around the midpoint of the inferior border of the nasal bone. The osteotomy then proceeds superiorly along a straight path in order to meet with the superior aspect of the medial osteotomy.

The lateral osteotomies are then carried out with a similar technique. This time, the osteotome is engaged further laterally, taking care to remain superior to the anterior aspect of the inferior turbinate in order to prevent medialization of the turbinate bones and potential airway compromise. Curved guarded osteotomes are used to facilitate a high-low-high (or anterior-posterior-anterior) trajectory, with the low point being just low and lateral to the nasofacial junction in order to prevent possible visible or palpable step-off deformities and to facilitate optimal contour of the dorsal esthetic lines (**Fig. 9**).

Although executing both intermediate and lateral osteotomies, manual palpation of the guarded tip is used to guide the osteotome along the correct path. It is important to recognize that the guarded tip of an osteotome is typically 6 to 8 mm distal to actual point of bony engagement, which is particularly important when determining where to finish the osteotomy. A useful method for determining the superior extent of the osteotomy is to listen for a change in the sound of the audible fracture to a lower frequency. This audible sound typically indicates that the osteotome has engaged with the thicker bone of the radix. Caution should be exercised at this point in order to prevent potential rocker deformity from proceeding too far superiorly (**Fig. 10**).

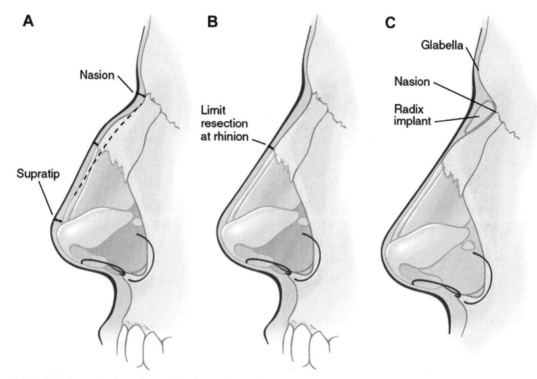

Fig. 5. (*A*) Schematic of a patient with a deep radix and a strong dorsal hump. (*B*) A slightly more conservative resection at the rhinion should be done in order to account for the thinner skin in this area. (*C*) An onlay graft can be used to disguise the hump accentuation caused by a deep radix. (*From* Swamy RS, Most SP. Nasal osteotomies. In: Azizzadeh B, Murphy MR, Johnson CM, et al, editors. Master techniques in rhinoplasty. Philadelphia: Elsevier; 2011; with permission.)

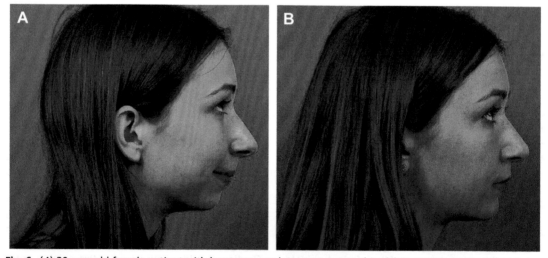

Fig. 6. (*A*) 20-year-old female patient with large nose and severe retrognathia. (*B*) Postoperative image at 1 year after undergoing surgery for overall reduction in nasal size with bony and cartilaginous hump reduction, cephalic trim, septoplasty, lateral crural straightening suture, dome-binding suture, and chin implant.

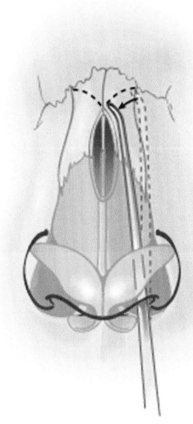

Fig. 7. Medial osteotomies can be done either in a straight path parallel to the septum or at an oblique angle of 15° laterally to help with the mobilization of the nasal bone once the lateral osteotomy is completed. (*Adapted from* Most SP, Murakami CS. A modern approach to nasal osteotomies. Facial Plast Surg Clin North Am 2005;13:85–92; with permission.)

Intermediate and lateral osteotomies may also be performed percutaneously using a straight, thin and narrow, sharp osteotome. A stab incision is made by an 11-blade scalpel at the junction of the lateral nasal wall and maxilla. The osteotome is then used to fracture in a stamplike fashion the desired areas on the nasal bone. Manual manipulation is used to complete the fracture line.

COMPLICATIONS

In addition to the rocker deformity mentioned above, there are several other complications that can occur from dorsal hump reduction. These complications include the development of an inverted-V deformity, Polly beak deformity, ski slope deformity, and open roof deformity.

An inverted-V deformity is due to disruption of the dorsal esthetic lines that can occur when the midvault is not properly supported following hump reduction. Essentially, there is a lack of continuity between the upper lateral cartilages and the nasal bones, which creates a visible triangular shadowing of the midvault on anterior view. This complication can be prevented by the routine use of spreader grafts prophylactically in the setting of hump removal. The nuances of the various different types of spreader grafts and the technique for each are beyond the scope of this chapter.

Polly beak deformity can result from either overresection of the bony dorsum, underresection of the cartilaginous dorsum, or relative deprojection of the lower nasal third. The tripod concept of the lower nasal third has been widely discussed. This concept should be used as a guiding force to set the nasal tip projection and rotation before proceeding with dorsal hump reduction. Once the tip has been set in its desired location, the necessary dorsal reduction can be completed to ensure that the tip stands proud to the middle vault and that there is a discernible supratip break. Oftentimes, the anterior septal angle needs to be further reduced in order to provide optimal supratip definition.[29]

Saddle nose deformity occurs because of either excessive hump reduction or concave hump reduction. The nasofrontal angle, starting point of the dorsum, supratip break, and tip projection should be used as guidance for appropriate dorsal resection. An important practice to aid in the prevention of this complication is to use frequent application of topical cold compresses with significant digital pressure in order to ensure accurate judgment of the final profile appearance. If the edema of the skin and soft tissue envelope is not routinely compressed throughout surgery, the surgeon may misjudge the degree of reduction and proceed with further hump reduction when it is not indicated. Furthermore, the surgeon must be aware that the intraoperative evaluation of dorsal hump resection is more challenging in external rhinoplasty due to the lack of tension on the nasal skin. The external incision should be closed temporarily to ensure an appropriate reduction.

Persistent open roof deformity is characterized by the palpable or visible separation of the nasal bones medially; this is most often the result of greenstick/incomplete lateral osteotomies, preventing complete closure of the open roof. It is more common with reduction of a larger dorsal hump because the required angle of closure is greater. When a hump reduction necessitates more than 3 to 5° of closure on each side to correct the open roof deformity, the surgeon should

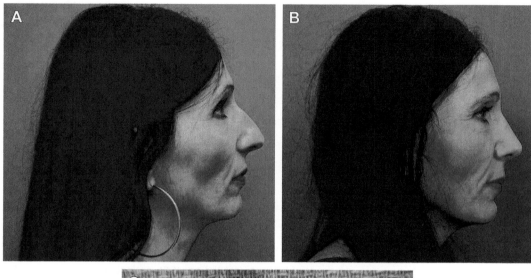

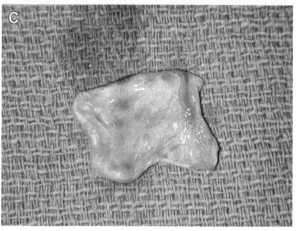

Fig. 8. (*A*) 53-year-old female patient with dorsal hump and thin dorsal skin. (*B*) 1 year postoperative image following dorsal hump reduction, cephalic trim, medial and lateral osteotomies, spreader grafts, septoplasty, and placement of temporalis fascia along the nasal dorsum. (*C*) Temporalis fascia placed along the nasal dorsum to help disguise any irregularities.

consider placing intermediate osteotomies in order to smooth this adjustment and refine the contour change.

POSTPROCEDURAL CARE

Following rhinoplasty, it is necessary to stabilize and protect the nasal bones and to provide compression to minimize postoperative edema. The nose is typically dressed with quarter-inch adhesive strips, which traverse the entire dorsum and cross the nasofacial junction bilaterally. The inferior extent of these compressive bandages should be at the supratip break, in order to prevent blunting of this transition point and to prevent tethering of the inferior third of the nasal vault. An external thermoplastic or Denver nasal splint (Summit Medical Inc, St. Paul, MN, USA) is then applied. The splint is typically cut to shape and size and then lightly rested on the desired nasal contour. If there is any concern about collapse or excessive medialization of the nasal bones, additional internal support for the nasal architecture can be achieved with the placement of a conservative amount of absorbable packing material internally at the apex of the bony pyramid. If this technique is required, care must be taken to consider the potential expansion of the absorbable material in order to prevent lateralization and potential open roof deformity.

A drip pad is often placed under the nares to collect blood and mucous drainage following the procedure. This drip pad is typically useful for 1 to 3 days, depending on individual patient

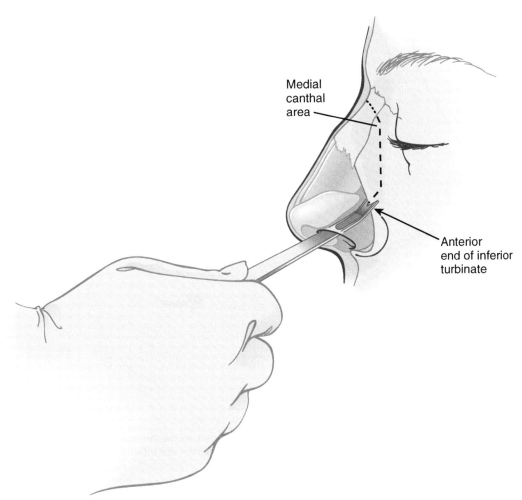

Medial canthal area

Anterior end of inferior turbinate

Fig. 9. The lateral osteotomy is begun at the anterior edge of the inferior turbinate and is performed in a high-low-high direction. (*From* Swamy RS, Most SP. Nasal osteotomies. In: Azizzadeh B, Murphy MR, Johnson CM, et al, editors. Master techniques in rhinoplasty. Philadelphia: Elsevier; 2011. p. 137; with permission.)

characteristics and the extent of surgery. Patients are instructed to avoid blowing their nose and to maintain a moist nasal environment in the postoperative period, which can be accomplished by a combination of ambient humidification or the topical application of nasal saline, antibiotic ointment, petroleum, or sterile mineral oil.

REHABILITATION AND RECOVERY

On postoperative day 7 (±1 day), the nasal splint and adhesive dressings are removed. If a septoplasty has been done concomitantly, the septal splints are also removed at this time. Patients are advised to exercise caution for a period of 6 weeks after surgery in order to allow ossification of the osteotomy sites. During this period, contact sports should be avoided and caution should be taken while engaging in any activity that may subject the nose to an accidental blow. Patients should be educated about expectations for the resolution of edema, 90% of which is typically resolved within 3 to 4 weeks after surgery. The remaining nasal refinement will occur over a period of approximately 1 to 2 years following surgery, depending on the extent of the surgery and nature of skin thickness.

OUTCOMES

Outcomes measures in rhinoplasty surgery are limited to patient satisfaction, surgeon satisfaction, and complication rates (**Table 1**). Tools for

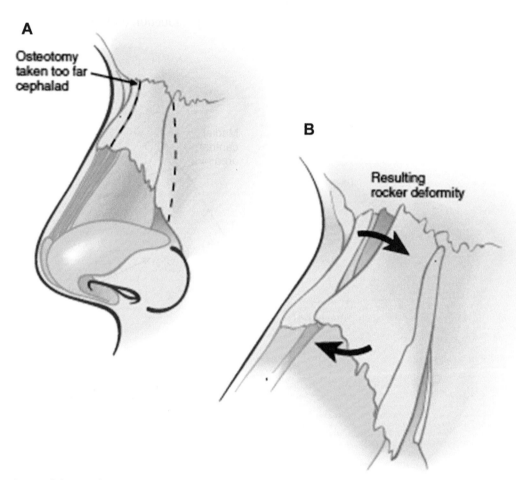

Fig. 10. (*A*) Lateral osteotomies that proceed too far superiorly into the frontal bone can result in (*B*) rocker deformity, where the superior nasal bone is pushed outward when the inferior nasal bones are medialized. (*Adapted from* Toriumi DM, Hecht DA. Skeletal modifications in rhinoplasty. Fac Plast Surg Clin North Am 2000;8:413–23; with permission.)

Table 1
Summary of the medical literature as it pertains to dorsal hump reduction

Authors	Topic	Findings
Palhazi et al,[27] 2015	Osseocartilaginous vault anatomy	Length of dorsal keystone = 8.9 mm (range 4–14 mm) Width of keystone area = 4.9 mm (range 3–9 mm)
Pearson & Adamson,[8] 2004	Ideal nasal profile	Compared with the average white female profile, the ideal profile appears to have a slight decrease in dorsal height, slight overrotation, and slight underprojection
Mowlavi et al,[5] 2003	Ideal nasion position	Nasion level preferred at supratarsal fold, ciliary margin, or mid-pupil; not preferred at the lower limbus Nasion height preferred at 10 mm (>13 mm > 7 mm)
Springer et al,[9] 2008	Gender and nasal shape	Optimal female noses showed a horizontally and vertically lower nasion and were concave to straight Optimal male noses showed a vertically and horizontally higher nasion and a straight profile
Ponsky et al,[28] 2010	Frequency of dorsal hump reduction	Dorsal hump reduction performed in approximately 84% of cosmetic rhinoplasty patients
Mojallal et al,[30] 2011	Dorsal line symmetry	Dorsal line symmetry improved from 68% preoperatively to 94% postoperatively
van Heerbeek et al,[31] 2009	3-Dimensional imaging to measure dorsal hump reduction	Decreased height of the nasal dorsum ranged from 0.8 to 4.4 mm following reduction rhinoplasty

postoperative patient satisfaction following cosmetic surgery have been developed and can be used to provide a standardized measure of the results from surgery. Practice standards encourage surgeons to perform assessments of the rates of postoperative bleeding, prolonged swelling and bruising, and other undesirable outcomes. There is a trend toward using the evaluations of third-party sources to validate results and to serve as a guide for technique adjustment when necessary.

SUMMARY

The goal of dorsal nasal hump reduction is to effectively improve the attractiveness of the nose based on esthetic, cultural, and evolutionary influences. Although surgical techniques for reducing the dorsal hump remain widely unchanged, this article outlines the nuances of this procedure that must be considered in order to produce optimal results for each patient.

REFERENCES

1. Powell N, Huphreys B. Proportions of the aesthetic face. New York: Theime-Stratton; 1984.
2. Azizzadeh B, Reilly MJ. Primary caucasian female rhinoplasty. In: Shiffman MA, Di Giuseppe A, editors. Advanced aesthetic rhinoplasty. New York: Springer; 2013. Chapter 13. p. 147–62.
3. Farkas LG, Hreczko TA, Kolar JC, et al. Vertical and horizontal proportions of the face in young adult North American Caucasians: revision of neoclassical canons. Plast Reconstr Surg 1985;7:328–38.
4. Enquist M, Arak A. Symmetry, beauty, and evolution. Nature 1994;372:169–72.
5. Mowlavi A, Meldrum DG, Wilhelmi BJ. Implications for nasal recontouring: nasion position preferences as determined by a survey of white North Americans. Aesthetic Plast Surg 2003;27(6):438–45.
6. Leong SC, White PS. A comparison of aesthetic proportions between the oriental and caucasian nose. Clin Otolaryngol Allied Sci 2004;29(6):672–6.
7. Leong SC, White PS. A comparison of aesthetic proportions between the healthy Caucasian nose and the aesthetic ideal. J Plast Reconstr Aesthet Surg 2006;59(3):248–52.
8. Pearson DC, Adamson PA. The ideal nasal profile: rhinoplasty patients vs the general public. Arch Facial Plast Surg 2004;6(4):257–62.
9. Springer IN, Zernial O, Nölke F, et al. Gender and nasal shape: measures for rhinoplasty. Plast Reconstr Surg 2008;121(2):629–37.
10. Yellin SA. Aesthetics for the next millenium. Facial Plast Surg 1997;13(4):231–9.
11. Rowe-Jones J, Carl van Wyk F. Special considerations in northern European primary aesthetic rhinoplasty. Facial Plast Surg 2010;26(2):75–85.
12. Fitzpatrick TB. Soleil et peau. J Med Esthet 1975;2: 33–4.
13. Larrabee WF. The tripod concept. Arch Otolaryngol Head Neck Surg 1989;115(10):1168–9.
14. Adamson PA, Litner JA, Dahiya R. The M-Arch model: a new concept of nasal tip dynamics. Arch Facial Plast Surg 2006;8(1):16–25.
15. Papel ID. Interlocked transdomal suture technique for the wide interdomal space in rhinoplasty. Arch Facial Plast Surg 2005;7:414–7.
16. Peck GC. The onlay graft for nasal tip projection. Plast Reconstr Surg 1983;71(1):27–39.
17. Sheen JH. Tip graft: a 20-year retrospective. Plast Reconstr Surg 1993;91(1):48–63.
18. Soliemanzadeh P, Kridel RWH. Nasal tip overprojection: algorithm of surgical deprojection techniques and introduction of medial crural overlay. Arch Facial Plast Surg 2005;7:374–80.
19. Kridel RWH, Konior RJ. Controlled nasal tip rotation via the lateral crural overlay technique. Arch Otolaryngol Head Neck Surg 1991;117:411–5.
20. Cobo R. Correction of dorsal abnormalities in revision rhinoplasty. Facial Plast Surg 2008;24: 327–38.
21. Skoog T. A method of hump reduction in rhinoplasty. A technique for preservation of the nasal roof. Arch Otolaryngol 1966;83:283–7.
22. Toriumi DM, Johnson CM. Open structure rhinoplasty featured technical points and long-term follow-up. Facial Plast Surg Clin North Am 1993;1: 1–22.
23. Sykes JM, Tapias V, Kim JE. Management of the nasal dorsum. Facial Plast Surg 2011;27(2): 192–202.
24. Roostaeian J, Unger JG, Lee MR, et al. Reconstitution of the nasal dorsum following component dorsal reduction in primary rhinoplasty. Plast Reconstr Surg 2014;133(3):509–18.
25. Halewyck S, Michel O, Daele J, et al. A review of nasal dorsal hump reduction techniques, with a particular emphasis on a comparison of component and composite removal. B-ENT 2010;6(Suppl 15): 41–8.
26. Rohrich RJ, Muzaffar AR, Janis JE. Component dorsal hump reduction: the importance of maintaining dorsal aesthetic lines in rhinoplasty. Plast Reconstr Surg 2004;114(5):1298–308 [discussion: 1309–12].
27. Palhazi P, Daniel RK, Kosins AM. The osseocartilaginous vault of the nose: anatomy and surgical observations. Aesthet Surg J 2015;35(3):242–51.
28. Ponsky D, Eshraghi Y, Guyuron B. The frequency of surgical maneuvers during open rhinoplasty. Plast Reconstr Surg 2010;126(1):240–4.

29. Park SS. Fundamental principles in aesthetic rhinoplasty. Clin Exp Otorhinolaryngol 2011;4(2): 55–66.

30. Mojallal A, Ouyang D, Saint-Cyr M, et al. Dorsal aesthetic lines in rhinoplasty: a quantitative outcome-based assessment of the component dorsal reduction technique. Plast Reconstr Surg 2011;128(1):280–8.

31. van Heerbeek N, Ingels KJ, van Loon B, et al. Three dimensional measurement of rhinoplasty results. Rhinology 2009;47(2):121–5.

Management of the Nasal Dorsum
Construction and Maintenance of a Barrel Vault

R. Laurence Berkowitz, MD[a],*, Ronald P. Gruber, MD[b,c]

KEYWORDS

• Middle vault • Spreader flaps • Spreader grafts • Barrel vault • DDAVP • Power instrumentation

KEY POINTS

- Preoperative patient preparation is paramount to ensure optimal outcomes.
- The operative technique for the management of the nasal dorsum requires several key steps:
  - Component separation to permit preservation of all structural layers and parts.
  - Modification of structural components.
  - Reassembly of components to mimic the natural state.
- Spreader flaps and grafts are used as needed to achieve a straight, symmetric, and functional nose.
- Power instrumentation may be used to refine tissue modification and facilitate the procedure.

INTRODUCTION

Properly executed rhinoplasty is probably the most valuable of all aesthetic procedures done by plastic surgeons. However, there is also no other esthetic procedure less forgiving than nasal surgery. The results of rhinoplasty must be judged over time. The inadequacies of the procedure may not be evident for months or even years. As edema subsides, the skin envelope shrinks, and tissues atrophy as a result of surgical manipulation and the aging process. Management of the cartilaginous or middle vault is critical to controlling the entire rhinoplasty process. It is addressed first before contouring the bony vault or refining the nasal tip. A poorly managed middle vault is a terrible liability that can leave a legacy of esthetic and functional disability. A successful approach to the middle vault and the nasal dorsum is demonstrated here. As is seen, the natural components of the nose are organized as a barrel vault and not a pyramid as a concept in order to engineer one of nature's most beautiful structures.

Ideally, one would like to demineralize all of the nasal hardscape, reshape and mold as a sculpture, and then harden the tissues again! This is not yet feasible. One is therefore left with reshaping bone and cartilage with cuts and tools, sutures, and adhesives. Power instrumentation provides one of the most efficient, controllable, and least traumatic modalities for remodeling the hard structures. Sutures allow the surgeon to control the more elastic cartilage. Adhesives are used (by the primary author) to seal tissue planes (fibrin sealants) or to fixate grafts (cyanoacrylates).

Disclosure: The authors have no disclosures.
[a] Aesthetic & Reconstructive Plastic Surgery, 3803 South Bascom Avenue, Suite 100, Campbell, CA 95008, USA;
[b] Division of Plastic & Reconstructive Surgery, University of California, San Francisco, Oakland, CA, USA;
[c] School of Medicine, Stanford University, Stanford, CA, USA
* Corresponding author.
E-mail address: rlberkowitz@gmail.com

ANATOMY

The cartilaginous or the middle vault is architecturally similar to a barrel vault (**Fig. 1**) confluent with the vertical upright of the septum. It consists of lateral alar cartilages, also known as the upper lateral cartilages, which are contiguous with the quadrangular septal cartilage. Aside from the cartilaginous components to define the middle vault, the nasalis muscle also plays an important role in compressing the cartilage and flaring the nostrils. The middle vault, while usually described as containing valves, is actually in its entirety an elastic and dynamic valve in itself that controls airflow.

Skin

The skin of the middle vault is usually thicker than that of the bony vault. It varies depending on size and structures of skin adnexae (eg, oil glands) and can vary in thickness regardless of ethnicity. The adnexae arise within the fatty layer, a thin carpet layer of fat that atrophies as a result of the aging process, surgical manipulation, or disruption of blood supply. The adherent muscle layer or nasalis muscle is also subject to trauma by injudicious blind elevation.

Cartilage

The middle vault consists of upper lateral cartilages, which are contiguous with the quadrangular septal cartilage. As a trapezoidal shape, the upper lateral cartilages arise from the face of the maxilla laterally by ligamentous attachment and extend medially toward the dorsum, where they become confluent with the dorsal edge of the quadrangular septal cartilage (**Fig. 2**). From a basal view, one can see that the upper lateral cartilages fuse with the septum and create an angle of approximately 15° according to traditional teachings (**Fig. 3A**). Actually, the upper lateral cartilage moves directly away from the septum at 80° to 90° for a very short distance before curving around to make that acute angle. In reality, there is more of a barrel vault arrangement to the upper lateral cartilage and septum (**Fig. 3B**).

This junction is anatomically recognized as the valve of Minx—the loss of which is responsible for alar collapse and airflow restriction. Cephalically, these cartilages underlap the nasal bones as a shingle relationship. Preservation of the upper lateral cartilage from beneath the nasal dorsum is an important step for spreader flap extension. Caudally, the upper lateral cartilage provides a lip or scroll from which the greater alar cartilages or lower lateral cartilages of the nasal tip will

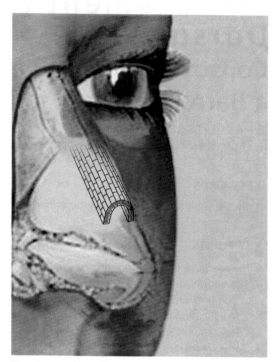

Fig. 1. Barrel vault, an architectural approach to rhinoplasty.

couple. This scroll of cartilage is architecturally an I-beam. It supports the valvular mechanism, and excision of this structure can also contribute to airflow restriction. The bony or upper vault consists of the nasal bones and is also structurally a

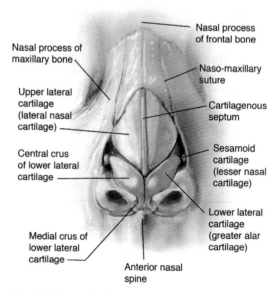

(bones/cartilages)

Nasal process of frontal bone

Nasal process of maxillary bone

Naso-maxillary suture

Upper lateral cartilage (lateral nasal cartilage)

Cartilagenous septum

Central crus of lower lateral cartilage

Sesamoid cartilage (lesser nasal cartilage)

Lower lateral cartilage (greater alar cartilage)

Medial crus of lower lateral cartilage

Anterior nasal spine

Fig. 2. Skeletonized nasal anatomy.

barrel vault. The 2 bones arise laterally from suture lines along the buttress of bone along the maxilla. The nasal bones, while thin, gradually thicken along this nasomaxillary process. The base width of the nose is defined not so much by the nasal bones, but by the elevation of these maxillary processes as they arise from the face of the maxilla. It is here that bone cuts may be required. Medially, these 2 bones fuse in a suture line confluent with the vertical plate of ethmoid, a thin bony structure that fuses or often overlaps on one side or the other with quadrangular septal cartilage. Cephalically, the nasal bones form suture lines with the frontal process. Behind this frontal process lies the frontal sinus. Caudally, the nasal bones bifurcate as they join the upper lateral cartilages in a forklike fashion overlapping that cartilage. Central to this bifurcation is the keystone region of the nasal hump, where the cartilaginous septum, vertical plate of the ethmoid, upper lateral cartilages, and the nasal bones fuse in an overlapping relationship like grooved shingles. When bone flaps are cut, it is the firm attachment of the upper lateral cartilages laterally that suspend them to the fixed upright of the dorsal septum and vertical plate of ethmoid.

Mucosa

The nasal mucosa provides blood supply to the bone and cartilage, and it functions to provide moisture that humidifies and warms the incoming air. Uninterrupted and carefully preserved nasal lining will serve to ensure nasal function, the loss of which by devascularization and resultant scarring can cause considerable disability.

Inferior Turbinates

Although these appendages of the nasal airway will be treated more thoroughly along with the septum elsewhere in this issue, it is important to recognize the reflective and cooperative relationship these structures bear to the septum, maxillary and pyriform processes, and the middle vault as a whole. The size of these structures is dynamic in relation to all of the bordering structures that must be addressed accordingly because they are baffles that humidify, warm, and regulate airflow in cooperation with the musculocartilaginous function of the middle vault within which they lie.

PREOPERATIVE PATIENT EVALUATION

A thorough examination of the nose including the nasal airway is imperative. Evaluation of the structures and potential problems must be elicited by history and illuminated inspection. Vasoconstricted examination aided by oxymetazoline will permit a more thorough inspection and provides a test for airway resistance as to whether it is structural or congestive. A computerized

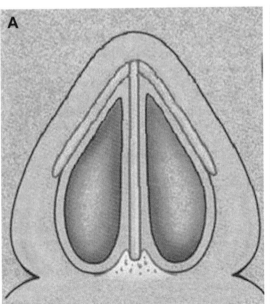
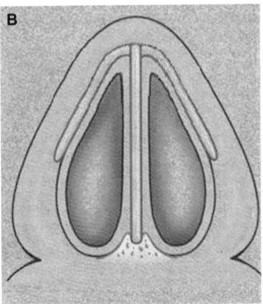

Fig. 3. (*A*) From a basal view, one can see that the upper lateral cartilages fuse with the septum and create an angle of approximately 15° according to traditional teachings. (*B*) Actually, the upper lateral cartilage moves directly away from the septum at 80° to 90° for a very short distance before curving around to make that acute angle. In reality, there is more of barrel vault shape to the upper lateral cartilage.

tomographic 3-dimensional scan is advisable in cases of deviated noses or posttraumatic deformities. This scan will provide information regarding bone thickness, displacement, and causes of airway obstruction. Although digital photographic documentation has been shown to be a valuable tool in presentation[1,2] to the patient of potential results, the primary author still prefers a 1:1 (life-size) black-and-white photograph taken in the Frankfort horizontal for surgical planning. These photographs by onlay or drawing on the reverse side with a light box permit an accurate life-size blueprint for nasal addition and subtraction. This blueprint will permit precise rhinoplasty.

PREOPERATIVE PATIENT PREPARATION

Two weeks before surgery, a meeting is scheduled with the patient to review the photographs and surgical plan. A comprehensive history and physical examination are done to elicit risk factors and to educate the patient. For the ensuing 2 weeks before surgery, the patient is instructed to refrain from all nonsteroidal anti-inflammatory drugs, supplements, vitamins, and herbal and hormonal therapy, including, most importantly, oral contraceptives. Women of childbearing age are instructed to use barrier protection during intercourse for this 2-week period and for 1 month following surgery after oral contraceptives are reinstated because many medications and the interruption of the hormonal therapy can place female patients at greater risk of conception. Five days preoperatively, the patient is instructed to apply mupirocin ointment 2% twice daily to the nostrils in complicated cases where extensive grafting is anticipated or if there has been a prior history of staphylococcal, or specifically, methicillin-resistant *Staphylococcus aureus* (MRSA) infection. It is also used for all health care workers that are exposed to MRSA. In other routine rhinoplasties in low-risk populations, the use of povidone-iodine ointment can be used in place of the more costly mupirocin. Cautious facial cleansing twice daily during these 5 days with chlorhexidine in an off-label use with appropriate caution to the eyes and mucous membranes is instituted. The patient is asked to refrain from trimming, waxing, or plucking of any nasal hairs in the perioperative period. The patient is also instructed to not have any food or liquids by mouth after midnight. If the surgery is scheduled for the afternoon, the patient is permitted to have clear liquids until 2 to 4 hours before surgery to avoid dehydration. The patient may benefit from self-administration of an antiemetic

before leaving home on day of surgery to prevent postoperative emesis. The primary author prefers 40 mg aprepitant given 3 hours before surgical start time.

In the preoperative area, an intravenous line is begun early to hydrate the patient. Through that same venipuncture, 30 cc of blood is withdrawn, and following strict Harvest System protocol (Harvest Technologies, Lakewood, CO, USA), 10 cc of platelet-poor and 6 cc of platelet-rich plasma are prepared for intraoperative use to reduce ecchymosis and to accelerate wound healing—in the primary author's cases. Clonidine 0.1 mg in older patients and 0.2 mg orally in adolescents and young adults reduce response to vasoconstrictive agents and circulating catecholamines associated with youth. It also helps to reduce perception of postoperative pain. Dexamethasone 4 mg is administered intravenously as a second drug treatment for antiemetic effect, to reduce postoperative edema, and to improve overall well-being following surgery. Infrequent cases of steroid dysphoria have been observed in the older population.

Faber and colleagues[2] pioneered and demonstrated the effectiveness of desmopressin (DDAVP) for orthognathic surgery and epistaxis. The primary author has been using DDAVP routinely for the past 10 years unless a hypercoagulable state has been identified before surgery by history or laboratory tests.[3] An amount of 0.3 μg/kg (14–24 μg range given as 4 μg/mL) administered 30 minutes before surgery will diminish or eliminate postoperative ecchymosis and provide a remarkably dry field for the operator. In the secondary author's practice, DDAVP is given at the first sight of a less than ideally dry operative field or for a case in which bleeding is anticipated, such as very thick nasal bones. A low dose (0.1 μg/kg) is given initially. If, after 20 minutes, the field is not satisfactorily dry, a second dose is given. A third dose is given if the field is still not ideally dry after yet another 20 minutes. The total dose should not exceed 0.3 μg/kg. Finally, a broad-spectrum antibiotic, such as cefazolin (1 or 2 g) or clindamycin (600 mg if penicillin-sensitive), is given. Vancomycin (500 mg to 1 g) is used if there is a history of previous staphylococcal infection, if the patient is a known MRSA carrier, or if extensive grafting is to be done. The anesthesiologist examines the patient, and a determination of proper airway management is determined. Thigh-high T.E.D. stockings (Covidien, Minneapolis, MN, USA) are applied in all patients, and the patient is taken to the operating room from the preoperative area fully alert and unsedated.

Operating Room

In the operating room, the unsedated alert patient is included in the briefing of the surgical plan with all members of the team included. All members must be in agreement. The operative consent is read aloud to confirm, and any corrections, emissions, or additions are then done.

The anesthesiologist may use general anesthesia or monitored anesthesia care. The authors prefer TIVA (total intravenous anesthetic) using propofol exclusively to minimize malignant hyperthermia and vasodilation that can be experienced with inhalational agents. A flexible laryngeal mask airway is usually used. For longer cases, high-risk cases for aspiration, or anticipated bleeding, a soft flexible armored silicone Rusch endotracheal tube (Teleflex, Morrisville, NC, USA) is used and secured to the central incisors with dental tape. The eyes are immediately covered with Tegaderm polyurethane patches (3M, Maplewood, MN, USA). Sequential compression devices are applied to the calves, and a pillow is placed under the knees. A Foley catheter (Bard Medical, Covington, GA, USA) is rarely placed unless the procedure is expected to extend more than 4.5 to 5 hours; DDAVP also serves to reduce urinary output. The arms are wrapped with circumferential silicone gel pads and placed on the patient's lap, comfortably supported by articulating arm supports. A shoulder to toe forced-air heating blanket is applied to maintain euthermia. Temperature is monitored with either axillary or esophageal probes. The table is placed into reflex "chaise" position, and the patient is grounded. The skin is first prepared with 20% isopropyl alcohol to remove any oils, and then markings are done with an indelible single-use gentian violet Write-Site surgical marker (Aspen Surgical, Caledonia, MI, USA). The surgical plan is transferred to the nose by careful measurement taken from the 1:1 photographs placed near the head of the bed for constant reference.

Outlines of the bone and cartilages and proposed addition and subtraction of the substructure are marked, and a W-plasty or an inverted V is designed at the junction of the columella and the upper lip over the anterior nasal spine or where skin thickness changes abruptly from thin to thick. Any alar base reduction incisions are marked as well. The markings in gentian violet are preparation-resistant, and there is no need for tattooing.

The nose is then anesthetized with 4% cocaine-soaked pledgets (1/2 × 2-inch neuro patties). Six pledgets are placed, one in each concha on each side. The tails of the pledgets are tied together so that all 6 will be accounted for during the procedure. No throat packing is done to avoid irritation and increased risk of aspiration, and with open procedures, it should not be required.

Then, 1% lidocaine with epinephrine blocks the infraorbital and infratrochlear nerves and elevates the planes of the nasal dorsum, tip, and columella, usually requiring 12 mL of solution. An additional 3 mL is used on each side internally to elevate the mucoperichondrium off the undersurface of the upper lateral and lower lateral cartilages. The mucoperiosteum is also elevated under the bony hump. If septal or vomer work is done, another 3 mL on each side is expected to be used to lift the mucoperichondrium off the quadrangular septal cartilage and the mucoperiosteum off the vomer. A total of 24 mL may be used in these cases. All injections are done with a 3-mL syringe with a 1-inch 30-gauge needle. Then, 6 mL of the local anesthetic will be reserved on the back table from the 30-mL bottle to be used for turbinates when treated. The secondary author uses a local anesthetic consisting of 2/3 lidocaine HCl (Xylocaine) and 1/3 bupivacaine (Marcaine) with 1:70,000 fresh epinephrine.

The nasal vibrissae are shaved with a disposable handle Bard Parker number 15 blade (ACE Surgical Supply Co., Inc, Brockton, MA, USA), which is a thinner, more flexible blade than the detachable blades. As described by Sheen, the internal nose is prepared with applicators soaked with 10% povidone-iodine. The entire face is then prepared with chlorhexidine cautiously and as an off-label use. Alternatively, 5% povidone-iodine or baby shampoo can be used. The patient is then draped.

SURGICAL PROCEDURE

Powder-free latex-free gloves are used by all members of the operating team to reduce inflammation and for the possibility of a latent latex allergy regardless of history. The field is exposed. The nose is opened by connecting rim incisions to the W or inverted V incision along the edge of the columella within its portion of the limen vestibulare. A meticulous identification of the medial edge of the medial crura is done just on the perichondrium. In secondary cases, a subperichondrial plane is sought because it is usually previously undissected and will facilitate a cleaner identifiable structure. All soft tissue is preserved within the nasal flap, including the depressor muscle from the columella to maintain thickness and blood supply to this long flap. Bipolar cautery is used judiciously at all times to both flap and structural surfaces to maintain an unstained and dry field. Dissection extends onto the tip and lateral crura of the lower lateral cartilages, then onto the upper lateral cartilages, and then to the bony dorsum, where the periosteum is included within the flap. Extensive undermining is performed laterally to the face of the maxilla to allow redraping of the skin envelope, improve visibility of all planned bone cuts and surgical maneuvers, as well as permit the introduction of power tools,[4–6] which are more space-occupying than traditional hand tools. Being able to visualize the bony dorsum in its entirety will permit less opportunity for asymmetry. The only place that dissection is limited is over the bony radix, where, if a graft is planned, the tunnel will be kept intentionally narrow to hold the graft in position. When the tissue is elevated, hemostasis is checked again. The wound is then irrigated with saline solution, to which gentamicin has been added 80 mg per liter of normal saline.

COMPONENT SEPARATION

Middle vault surgery is conducted in many ways by many surgeons.[7–18] In the authors' case, the middle vault and bony vault are then divided into their respective components. Mucosa is undermined from underneath the valve of Minx, where the upper lateral cartilage fuses to the dorsal septum. Openings are made on either side of the caudal edge of the septum, while the tip cartilages are retracted in the caudal direction for exposure. When the subperichondrial plane is clearly identified, a Cottle elevator easily strips a tunnel of mucosa and perichondrium from this cartilaginous junction and continues contiguously as a subperiosteal dissection from under the nasal bones of the hump (**Fig. 4**). Right-angle turbinectomy scissors facilitate the separation of the upper lateral cartilage from the dorsal septum. At the nasal bones, a number 15 blade cuts through the ligamentous attachment of the nasal bones over the upper lateral cartilages. A Woodson elevator is then used to pry the extension of the upper lateral cartilage from underneath the nasal hump no more than 4 to 5 mm wide. The greater portion of the upper lateral cartilage is left attached to the nasal bones laterally as this will act as a handle to control final nasal bone position. The upper lateral cartilages are then scored longitudinally once or twice on each side to mimic barrel staves that will easily

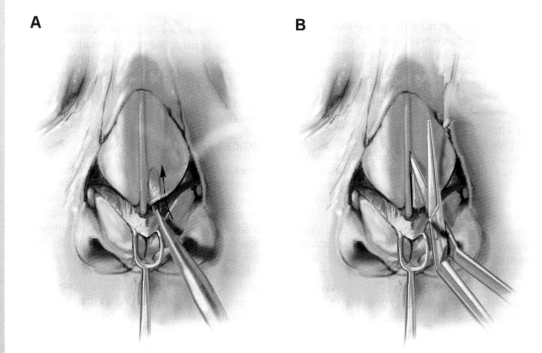

A

B

Fig. 4. (*A*) When the subperichondrial plane is clearly identified, a Cottle elevator easily strips a tunnel of mucosa and perichondrium from this cartilaginous junction and continues contiguously as a subperiosteal dissection from under the nasal bones of the hump (*Arrow* indicates rotation of cartilage flaps inward). (*B*) Cottle scissors separating upper lateral cartilages from septum.

curve into the desired shape. Sutures may be required to maintain the appropriate shape of the newly formed spreader flap (**Fig. 5**). The cartilage underneath the nasal hump will be an extension of the spreader flap. At this point, if septoplasty or vomer remodeling is required, further dissection is done from above to expose these structures. In cases of vomer spurs, a 4-mm egg-shaped burr on a Saber Drill (Stryker, Kalamazoo, MI, USA) is used to smooth this bony spur and thin the vomer into the midline. The vomer is not resected; this greatly eliminates the pain, bleeding, and central incisor numbness that can often result from wholesale resection of the vomer. The tissue planes are again irrigated, and then platelet-poor plasma fibrin sealant (a preference of the primary author) from Harvest Technologies is sprayed into the wound; the tissues are gently compressed.

The dorsal edge of the septum is then marked for the proposed reduction, taking the measurements from 1:1 black-and-white photographs of the plan. A caliper, whose tips have been dipped in methylene blue, will allow an accurate straight-line marking from the supratip to the bony junction. This dorsal cartilage is resected with right-angled dorsal scissors. The resected piece is peeled

from the dorsal ligament that has tied it to the nasal bones, and then this strip of cartilage is preserved in a covered cup of antibiotic irrigation for graft potential.

BONY VAULT

Humpectomy has been approached in several ways.[19–21] In the authors' case, it is incorporated into the reconstruction of the internal valves. The upper lateral cartilages having been scored will fold inward and out of the way by laying a Cottle elevator on each side of the septum to protect them while the bony hump is reduced with the power tool (**Fig. 6**). The amount of bone to be reduced in the anterior-posterior dimension is again marked with the calipers dipped in methylene blue, taking direction from the operative plan. Again, the 4-mm oval- or egg-shaped burr is used on the Stryker drill to reduce the dorsal bone precisely to the level of the septum, bringing the vertical plate of ethmoid with it.

Depending on the ultimate dorsal width required, triangles of the now thinned dorsal nasal bone can be snipped from either side of the vertical plate of ethmoid to allow medial movement of the bone. Osteectomy bone snippers are used for this process. L-shaped bone cuts are then marked on each nasal bone extending from the roof of the nose vertically or slightly obliquely toward the medial canthus and then running horizontally along the face of the maxilla. This technique is usually referred to as a "medial oblique osteotomy" (**Fig. 7**). The cuts are almost complete to allow easy movement of the bone, because this is a flap and not a greenstick fracture. Fracture lines are avoided to reduce bleeding and to avoid possible unwanted extension. Stabilization of these bones is maintained by the underlying mucoperiosteum that is undisturbed by these ultrahigh-frequency saws. Specifically, a right-angle 4-mm saw blade is used on the Stryker sagittal saw. Alternatively, a saber-shaped blade attached to the reciprocating Stryker saw may be introduced from a pyriform or intraoral puncture. The end result of this particular osteotomy is commonly referred to as a low-to-low osteotomy, which connects to the vertical/oblique ("medial oblique") osteotomy. In cases where it is undesirable to change the width of the base of the nasal bones, but still necessary to close the open dorsum, a transverse cut closer to the dorsum will accomplish this, which is referred to as a "keystone fracture" to signify that only the keystone region is being altered. The extended cartilaginous spreader flaps are then reintroduced into the medial bone dorsal complex to maintain

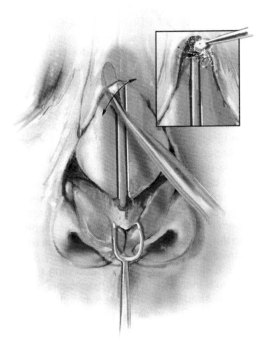

Fig. 5. The upper lateral cartilage separated underneath the nasal hump (*inset*) Power burr reducing dorsal hump (*Arrow* indicates rotation of cartilage flaps inward).

A

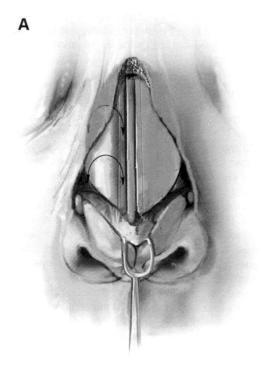

B

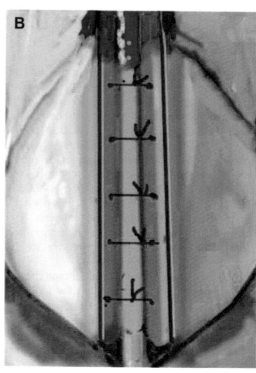

Fig. 6. (*A*) Folding of upper lateral cartilages (*Arrows* indicate rotation of cartilage flaps inward). (*B*) Spreader flaps sutured to septum.

the desired width of the bridge by trimming and folding as needed and then suturing them in place to the cartilaginous dorsal septum with 5-0 PDS Plus suture (Ethicon, Somerville, NJ, USA) using an atraumatic round needle.

REASSEMBLY

The middle vault is then reassembled by reattaching the medial edges of the upper lateral cartilages

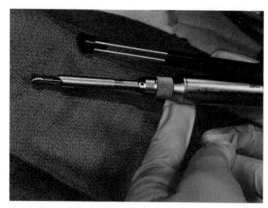

Fig. 7. The Stryker saber drill with 4-mm oval-shaped burr is used to remove the bony hump. (*Courtesy of* Stryker, Inc, Kalamazoo, MI; with permission.)

(now spreader flaps) to the dorsal septum (**Fig. 8**). The authors use 5-0 PDS Plus suture (Ethicon) on a round atraumatic needle. This suture is dyed violet for easy visibility and impregnated with triclosan to resist infection; the suture will absorb in a few months. The authors discourage the use of permanent nylon or polypropylene sutures due to the potential for intranasal exposure that can occur. Horizontal mattress sutures secure the cartilage edge directly to the septum, trimming the excess as needed to achieve the desired width, which can be up to 10 to 12 mm total. This suturing should be done in harmony with the bony dorsum to maintain the same width. Sometimes, the excess can be infolded as a lapel flap as described by Lerma[12] to help maintain the required space to keep the internal nasal valve open, but this will be a narrower spreader usually.

It is during this process of rebuilding the middle vault that many other maneuvers can be accomplished. In cases of asymmetry, cartilage can be trimmed on either side to help bring the septum into the midline or spreader grafts inserted to straighten, widen, or lengthen the middle vault. Mattress sutures can be used for compression to straighten a concavity within the dorsal septal line as well. As the upper lateral cartilages are reattached to the septum, this will

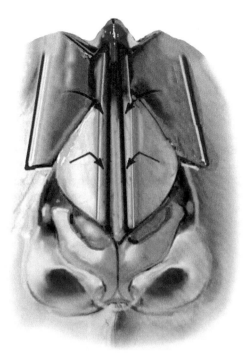

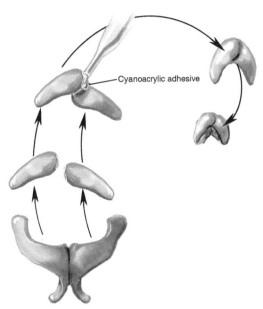

Cyanoacrylic adhesive

Fig. 9. Butterfly radix graft (*Arrows* indicate rotation of cartilage flaps inward).

Fig. 8. Depending on the ultimate dorsal width required, triangles of the now thinned dorsal nasal bone can be snipped from either side of the vertical plate of ethmoid to allow medial movement of the bone. Osteectomy bone snips are used for this process. Bone cuts are then marked on each nasal bone extending from the roof of the nose slightly obliquely toward the medial canthus and then running horizontally along the face of the maxilla. This is usually referred to as a medial oblique osteotomy (*Arrows* indicate rotation of cartilage flaps inward).

by extension stabilize the mobilized nasal bone flaps as well.

After the assembly is complete, the power burr can then be used on high speed to polish the junction of the bone and cartilage as needed without fear of disruption (a common potential problem with a hand rasp). The wound is again irrigated to cleanse the field of any bone dust to reduce postoperative inflammation. It is then sprayed with a platelet-poor fibrin sealant while tip work is completed, and a radix graft, if required, is prepared.

RADIX GRAFT WHEN NEEDED

After the tip is completed, a radix graft is secured in cases where elevation of the radix is preferred to complete resection of the hump. The primary author's preference is to fuse 2 pieces of the cephalic cartilage (that is often a remnant of tip reduction when available) by applying a drop of Indermil cyanoacrylate adhesive (**Fig. 9**). The graft is

made into a butterfly shape that lays over the radix as a soft flexible saddle. It can safely be secured there with an additional drop of the adhesive. When thinned, these grafts are compliant and rarely palpable or problematic. If greater thickness is required, an appropriate piece of septal cartilage can be added as a third layer beneath the softer tip cartilage again secured with glue. When larger grafts are required for the radix, diced cartilage in fascia would be preferred.

The entire pocket is then sprayed with a thin layer of platelet-rich fibrin sealant as a wound-healing accelerant and final sealant. The trunk of the columella is secured with a buried mattress suture of 5-0 PDS Plus to attach at the upper lip junction and intranasal sutures of 5-0 chromic catgut to close the rim incisions. The W plasty of the columella is sealed with a few drops of the adhesive.

A few other maneuvers should be mentioned. Alar base incisions if used when required are treated also with buried 5-0 PDS and then the Indermil. The cuts for alar base reduction are made at the beginning of the procedure when the W plasty is incised to avoid these marks becoming smeared or lost. The primary author prefers that inferior turbinates are treated at the time of septoplasty with the Somnus radiofrequency device (Olympus Medical, Center Valley, PA, USA) with or without outfracturing as the anatomy dictates.

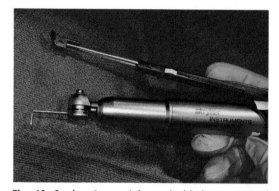

Fig. 10. Stryker 4-mm right-angle blade on sagittal saw. (*Courtesy of* Stryker, Inc, Kalamazoo, MI; with permission.)

The nose is not packed, but nostril retainers from Stryker Medical or Sientra (Santa Barbara, CA, USA) are selected by size of the nose and placed to maintain the internal shape of the nose and to separate the inferior turbinates from potential adherence to the septum during the edema phase that can result in synechiae. The nose is then taped with 1/4-inch Steri-Strips for the nasal tip and $^1/_2$-inch for the nasal dorsum. No Mastisol or Benzoin is used by the primary author due to rare, but debilitating, cases of reactions to these substances. A thermoplastic fiberglass cast is then applied. The authors avoid squeezing the tissues to avoid pressing blood through the tissue planes that can result in periorbital ecchymosis.

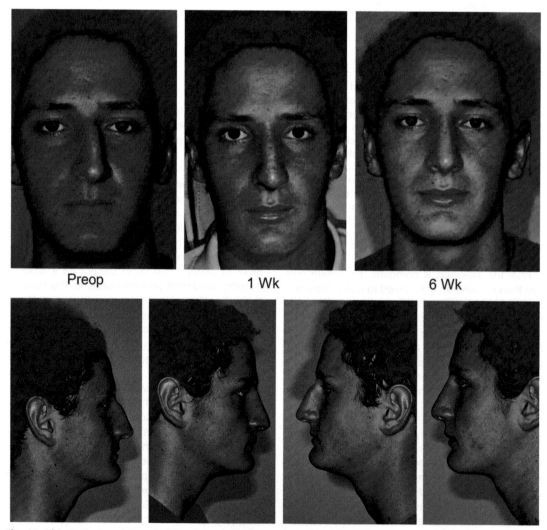

Preop   1 Wk   6 Wk

Fig. 11. This patient underwent rhinoplasty, including osteotomies. DDAVP was used to minimize bruising and ecchymosis. Note how little there is early postoperatively as well as at 6 weeks.

POSTOPERATIVE CARE

The patients are instructed in the postoperative area to keep their backs elevated approximately 15° and to avoid bending or lifting for the next 7 to 10 days. A snuffer is placed under the nose, and the patients are instructed to change it as needed in the event that there could be some postoperative bleeding because reactive vasodilatation occurs following the metabolization of the vasoconstricting agents. More often than not, there is little to no bleeding in uncomplicated cases. The patients are also advised to use cold compresses to the eyes for the next 72 hours to reduce swelling. The maximum edema is generally reached between 48 and 72 hours, and during that time, the eyes will commonly swell as will the cheeks. There may be the appearance of chemosis in the lower eyelids, which the patient might interpret as bruising, but will subside quickly and in fact in most cases there is little or no ecchymoses (**Figs. 9** and **10**). The 2 patients in **Figs. 9** and **10** underwent rhinoplasty, including osteotomies. DDAVP was used to minimize bruising and ecchymoses. Note how little bruising and ecchymoses there are early postoperatively as well as at 6 weeks. Long-term results have been satisfactory in the authors' hands also (**Figs. 11–13**). This patients in **Fig. 11** underwent primary rhinoplasty including humpectomy. Note the improved profile, but also the appropriate width of the nasal bones at 14 months postoperatively.

The nostril retainers that were placed will often become quite loose on the fourth or fifth day and

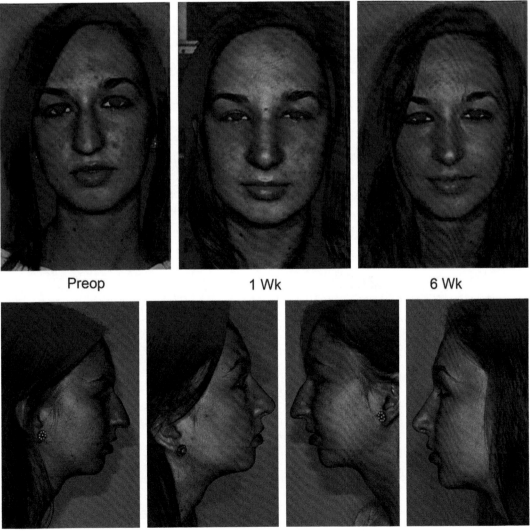

Preop   1 Wk   6 Wk

Fig. 12. This patient had a standard rhinoplasty, including osteotomies and DDAVP. Here, too, there is minimal ecchymosis and swelling during the early phase postoperatively.

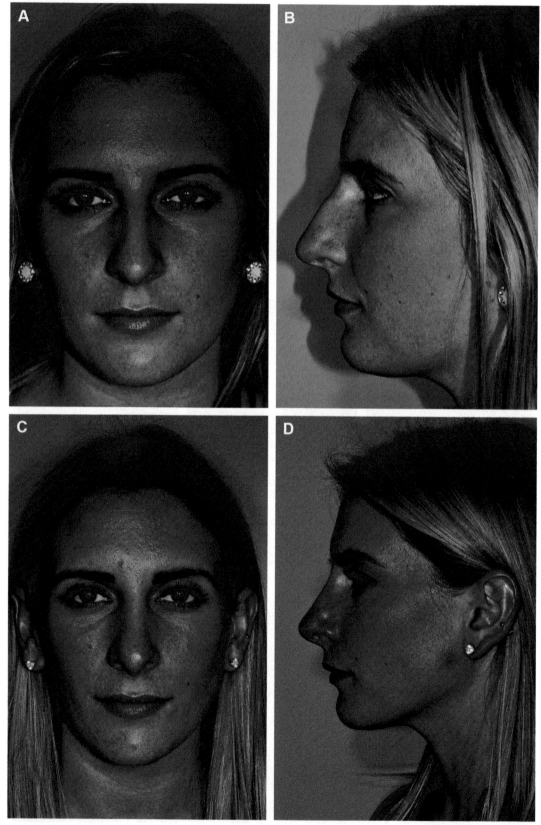

Fig. 13. This patient (preoperatively *A*, *B*) underwent primary rhinoplasty, including humpectomy. Note the improved profile but also the appropriate width of the nasal bones at 14 months postoperatively (*C*, *D*).

may slide out while the patient is at home before their first postoperative visit at 7 days. At 7 days, if the nostril retainers have not come out on their own, they are removed, and the dressing is removed from the nose. The nose is cleansed with Detachol (Eloquest Healthcare, Ferndale, MI, USA) and then wiped gently with 20% isopropyl alcohol to dry the nose. The nose is inspected internally and externally and then an application of 1/2-inch beige-colored Micropore Surgical Tape (3M) is applied to the nose and left in place for a second week undisturbed. At the end of the second week, the patient returns; the tape is removed; the nose is cleansed; and the patient is instructed on taping the nose at night to help eliminate edema. The same Micropore Surgical Tape can be used for night taping, or Blenderm Surgical Tape (3M) can be used if the patient prefers a clear, more elastic tape. Nostril retainers can be trimmed to a shorter length, and the patient can use them for orthorhinotics as needed to shape the nostrils; otherwise, they can be dispensed with if necessary. Internal nasal edema is expected to subside within 2 weeks with maximum improvement noted at approximately 6 weeks. Residual edema in the nose is expected for up to 1 year and in thicker noses up to 2 years.

COMPLICATIONS
Functional

If, at the end of 6 weeks, the patient is experiencing airway resistance, it is important to evaluate to see if there is untreated turbinate hypertrophy or if synechiae have caused the inferior turbinate to attach to the septum and will then need to be treated accordingly. There should be no airway problems if a correct barrel vault had been reconstructed, but it is understandable that in some cases additional spreader grafts may be required to open the airway with the understanding that this will widen the middle vault accordingly on either or both sides as the grafts are inserted between the septum and upper lateral cartilages.

Aesthetic

The most common aesthetic problem that is noted is asymmetry of the upper lateral cartilages. One cartilage may be more concave than the other and can often be treated with the principle of orthorhinotics. Elastic tape (3M) applied to one side of the middle vault and then stretched to reach the cheek on the other side of the nose is a way of applying mild pressure to reshape the nose. The patient is asked to wear that tape from dinner to bed time for several weeks if he or she is not going out that night or not having

visitors. On occasion, hyaluronic acid fillers for the concave side can be used until enough postoperative time has elapsed to allow permanent correction with a cartilaginous graft. Overcorrection of the dorsum (ie, depressed) can be corrected with an onlay graft of cartilage or fascia at the appropriate postoperative time. If the depression is a functional problem, a spreader graft would be a better choice.

Final results in any type of dorsal and middle vault surgery cannot be adequately assessed, however, for up to 1 year or even longer in most cases, and it is imperative the patients understand that there is an acceptable rate of reoperation in rhinoplasty procedures of up to 20%. The authors hope that following the measures that have been described will help to reduce that percentage in the practice of their colleagues.

REFERENCES

1. Daniel RK, Farkas LG. Rhinoplasty: image and reality. Clin Plast Surg 1988;15:1–10.
2. Faber C, Larson K, Amirlak B, et al. Use of desmopressin for unremitting epistaxis following septorhinoplasty and turbinectomy. Plast Reconstr Surg 2011;128(6):728e–32e.
3. Gruber RP, Zeidler KR, Berkowitz RL. Desmopressin as a hemostatic agent to provide a dry intraoperative field in rhinoplasty. Plast Reconstr Surg 2015; 135:1337.
4. Avsar Y. Nasal hump reduction with powered micro saw osteotomy. Aesthet Surg J 2009;29:6.
5. Berkowitz RL. "Power instrumentation in rhinoplasty." The Rhinoplasty Society Annual Meeting. Lecture. New York. May 2012.
6. Gerbault O. "Power assisted osteotomies—are we ready?" The Rhinoplasty Society Annual Meeting. San Francisco. April 2014. Panel Discussion.
7. Constantian MB, Clardy RB. The relative importance of septal and nasal valvular surgery in correcting airway obstruction in primary and secondary rhinoplasty. Plast Reconstr Surg 1996;98:38–54.
8. Gunter JP, Rohrich RJ. Correction of the pinched nasal tip with alar spreader grafts. Plast Reconstr Surg 1992;90:821–9.
9. Rohrich RJ, Hollier LH. Use of spreader grafts in the external approach to rhinoplasty. Clin Plast Surg 1996;23:255–62.
10. Oneal RM, Berkowitz RL. Upper lateral cartilage spreader flaps in rhinoplasty. Aesthet Surg J 1998; 18(5):370–1.
11. Seyhan A. Method for middle vault reconstruction in primary rhinoplasty: upper lateral cartilage bending. Plast Reconstr Surg 1997;100:1941.
12. Lerma J. Reconstruction of the middle vault: the "lapel" technique. Cir Plast Ibero Latinoam 1995;21:207.

13. Fayman MS, Potgieter E. Nasal middle vault support—a new technique. Aesthetic Plast Surg 2004;28:375–80.

14. Sciuto S, Bernardeschi D. Upper lateral cartilage suspension over dorsal grafts: a treatment for internal nasal valve dynamic incompetence. Facial Plast Surg 1999;15:309–16.

15. Byrd HS, Meade RA, Gonyon DL Jr. Using the autospreader flap in primary rhinoplasty. Plast Reconstr Surg 2007;119:1897–902.

16. Neu BR. Use of the upper lateral cartilage sagittal rotation flap in nasal dorsum reduction and augmentation. Plast Reconstr Surg 2009;123:1079.

17. Gruber RP, Perkins S. Humpectomy and spreader flaps. Clin Plast Surg 2010;37:285.

18. Gruber RP, Park E, Newman J, et al. The spreader flap in primary rhinoplasty. Plast Reconstr Surg 2007;119:1903–10.

19. Rohrich RJ, Muzaffar AR, Janis JE. Component dorsal hump reduction: the importance of maintaining dorsal aesthetic lines in rhinoplasty. Plast Reconstr Surg 2004;114:1298.

20. Ishida J, Ishida LC, Ishida LH, et al. Treatment of the nasal hump with preservation of the cartilaginous framework. Plast Reconstr Surg 1999;103:1729.

21. Becker DG, Toriumi DM, Gross CW, et al. Powered instrumentation for dorsal reduction. Facial Plast Surg 1997;13:291–7.

Nasal Bone Osteotomies with Nonpowered Tools

Ronald P. Gruber, MD[a],*, Rebecca M. Garza, MD[b], Gerald J. Cho, MD[c]

KEYWORDS

- Osteotomy • Osteotome • Low-to-low osteotomy • Medial oblique osteotomy • DDAVP
- Nasal bones

KEY POINTS

- Nasal bone issues can be classified into broad dorsum, broad base, and both broad dorsum and base.
- There is a zone of dense bone that should be avoided when doing osteotomies to minimize bleeding and spicule formation. Proper vasoconstriction minimizes bleeding after osteotomy.
- A low-to-low osteotomy results in mobilization of the base. The bone tends to migrate medially, but can be manipulated into a more lateral position.
- There is a learning curve to the use of the low-to-low osteotomy. One has to know where the guard of the osteotome is located at all times.
- Osteotomy results are independent. Dorsal changes can be made independently and separately from base changes.

INTRODUCTION

Nasal bone osteotomies have a complicated history.[1–9] The problems plastic surgeons have been struggling with include (a) an inability to achieve the proper shape (eg, sufficient reduction in width), (b) an inability to maintain that shape over time (recurrence of deformity), (c) avoiding excessive bleeding during and after surgery, (d) improper location of osteotomy sites with resultant step-off deformities, (e) spicule formation, and (f) collapse of the nasal bones.

There has been a great deal of controversy regarding choice of osteotomy sites, for example, medial oblique, low-to-high lateral osteotomy, high-to-low lateral osteotomy, and medial osteotomy that is perpendicular to the long axis of the bone. It has been recognized that an osteotomy that is too wide, for example, wider than 3 mm, can damage the periosteum, causing excessive bleeding. It is also known that there is a region of dense bone that one should avoid to minimize bleeding and spicule formation—a zone 30° off the midline[10,11] where the bone is excessively thick. The actual nasal bones are relatively thin plates.

Various access sites for osteotomies have been used including percutaneous, intranasal, and the buccal sulcus. Bleeding has been a formidable problem but mitigated in large part by smaller osteotomies. This requires a certain manual skill that comes from some practice—a significant but not insurmountable learning curve. Without acquiring that skill, the surgeon can have great difficulty executing the cut in the proper location (eg, low-to-low) and can have great difficulty even making the cut completely in the patient with very dense bones. Although possible, the potential for damage to the medial canthal region or structures cephalad to the nasion (intracranial) is remote. The issue is

[a] Division of Plastic & Reconstructive Surgery, University of California, San Francisco, 3318 Elm Street, Oakland, CA 94609, USA; [b] Division of Plastic & Reconstructive Surgery, Stanford University, Stanford, CA, USA; [c] Division of Plastic & Reconstructive Surgery, University of California, San Francisco, San Francisco, CA, USA
* Corresponding author.
E-mail address: rgrubermd@hotmail.com

Clin Plastic Surg 43 (2016) 73–83
http://dx.doi.org/10.1016/j.cps.2015.09.019

more one of getting the actual bone cut in the lowest (most posterior) location as possible to avoid a step-off and to truly narrow the entire nasal bone width. The medial oblique osteotomy does not require as much of a learning curve.

Today, there is a movement underway to use power tools[12] because these tools can make the actual bone separation an easier process. Physical restraint of the hand is not required, as is the case when using osteotomes. The principal disadvantage of the osteotome is that the surgeon must maintain a high degree of tension on the tool with his or her hand to prevent it from suddenly slipping forward out of control when struck by the mallet. There is also the assertion that there is less bleeding associated with power tools. The main disadvantage of power tools, of course, is cost, and in some situations, the need to do a wider dissection to get exposure for introduction of the larger power tool.

For those who do not have power tools, we offer a technique that in our hands has resulted in minimal bleeding and, most important, full control of the bones in a highly reproducible fashion.

CLASSIFICATION OF NASAL BONE DEFORMITIES AND PERTINENT ANATOMY

Nasal bone issues can be classified into (a) type I, broad base, (b) type 2, broad base and dorsum,

and (c) type 3, broad dorsum only. In **Fig. 1A**, the patient has a broad base. Clearly, any method to reduce the base is going to solve the problem. Unlike the low-to-high approach, the low-to-low approach goes more cephalically and has the potential to reduce the more cephalic (upper) part of the nasal bone. In **Fig. 1B**, the patient has a broad dorsum and broad base. In **Fig. 1C**, the dorsum is broad (as is the middle one-third of the nose), but the base is not. This is not uncommonly seen after a lateral osteotomy that reduces the base but typically fails to reduce the dorsum. The result is that the nasal bone plates are parallel to one another, which gives the nasal bone region a "hot dog" shape. The purpose of classifying bones in this fashion is to appreciate what is and what is not required surgically to correct each deformity. Thus, the broad dorsum patient does not need a base reduction, for example, and therefore does not need a lateral osteotomy.

The triangular area in the medial aspect near the nasion is the zone of dense bone that should be avoided when doing osteotomies to minimize bleeding and spicule formation (**Fig. 2**). The bone in this region can be 3 to 6 mm in thickness, and it is rich with blood vessels. The typical "medial osteotomy" runs parallel to the septum and runs into this dense bone and its blood vessels. When outfractured, an unwanted spicule of bone typically results. This spicule is extremely difficult to set

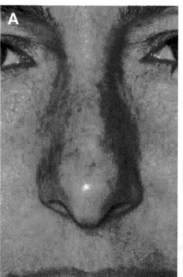 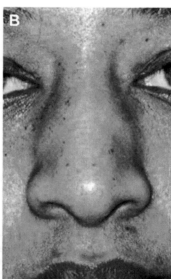 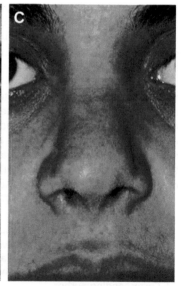

Fig. 1. (*A*) Broad nasal base (type 1). (*B*) Broad nasal base and dorsum (type 2). (*C*) Broad nasal dorsum only (type 3). This occurs occasionally after lateral osteotomy only procedures in which the base was narrowed without regard to the dorsum.

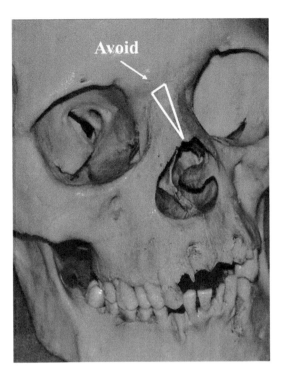

Fig. 2. There is a zone of dense bone in the cephalic central part of the nasal bones near the nasion filled with blood vessels. It lies within a region 30° off the vertical. To avoid spicule formation, bleeding, and simply difficult bone manipulation, it is wise to avoid the territory within that 30° zone. A medial osteotomy traditionally goes straight through it and can result in those problems. A medial oblique osteotomy skirts this zone.

back into position to give a smooth surface. It is best to simply avoid this region of the bony anatomy. Exclusive of this dense zone, the nasal bones are simply thin plates attached medially to the dorsum, laterally to the maxilla, and cephalically to the area adjacent to the nasion.

The surgical concept that is key to success is to conceptualize the nasal bones as plates that need to be released from their medial and lateral attachments to be manipulated into any desired position. By leaving a small cephalic bony attachment or an intact periosteum deep to the nasal bone plate, the plates will have a greenstick quality and will not collapse.

VASOCONSTRICTION

Proper vasoconstriction minimizes bleeding after osteotomy. This includes direct injection of epinephrine deep to the nasal bones. For general anesthesia cases, a mixture of xylocaine

(Lidocaine) and bupivacaine (Marcaine) with fresh epinephrine is used. Twenty milliliters of xylocaine and 15 mL of bupivacaine are mixed with 0.5 mL of 1:1000 epinephrine to make a solution that has a 1:70,000 concentration of epinephrine. This is a concentrated solution and therefore must be injected incrementally for the entire nose at the beginning of the case. Later during the surgery, the inside of the nasal bones are infiltrated with the solution at least 7 minutes before the osteotomy. The injection is performed along the inside of the nose where the turbinates are located. In essence, the local anesthetic solution fills some of the turbinates and migrates up along the medial wall of the bone.

One of the most important recent additions to our protocol is the use of desmopressin as a routine part of rhinoplasty (**Fig. 3**). Guyuron and colleagues[13] have pioneered use of this drug for maxillofacial surgery and for epistaxis treatment. Gruber and associates[14] have used it routinely for rhinoplasty to minimize postoperative ecchymosis and edema. The recommended dose is 0.3 µg/kg, and it is given at least 20 minutes before the desired effect. There are very few reported complications and no reported cases of thrombosis we are aware of at this time. We use it routinely for all rhinoplasty cases if the field is not hemostatic to our satisfaction for whatever the reason. We use a smaller dose, however (0.1 µg/kg and increase it 20 minutes later if needed, and again 20 minutes after that if needed). We use the full dose for most patients who require osteotomy because they are likely to experience a good deal of ecchymosis.

TECHNIQUE
Osteotomes

Straight osteotomes work well, but should be less than 3 mm[15] wide to minimize injury to the periosteum and allow support in the event both the medial oblique and lateral low-to-low osteotomy does not leave a small cephalic bridge of bone (**Fig. 4**). It is also wise to sharpen the osteotome at the operating table just before use.

Medial Oblique Osteotomy

The medial oblique osteotomy begins in the lateral aspect of the open roof (**Fig. 5**A). So doing allows the nasal plate to migrate medially. Placing the bone cut flush up against the septum (the medial aspect of the open roof) precludes the bone from moving and frustrates the surgeon that the osteotomy is not working. The medial oblique osteotomy skirts this dangerous zone medial to the 30° line.

A

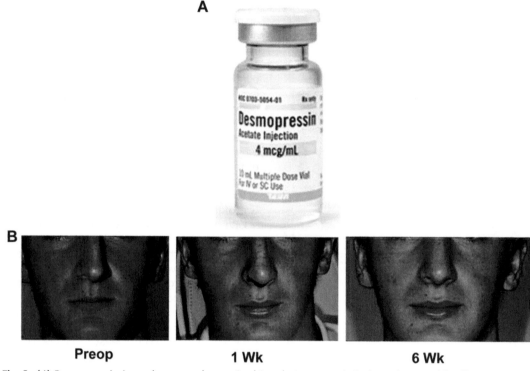

B

| Preop | 1 Wk | 6 Wk |

Fig. 3. (*A*) Desmopressin is used more and more in rhinoplasty as prophylaxis to decrease bleeding, minimizing postoperative ecchymosis, and maintain a dry operative field. It can be given in the maximum dose (0.3 μg/kg) or incrementally as needed to attain a dry operative field. In the latter situation, it is given at a dose of 0.1 μg/kg q20 minutes for a maximum of 3 doses. Image *B* shows the effectiveness of the drug.

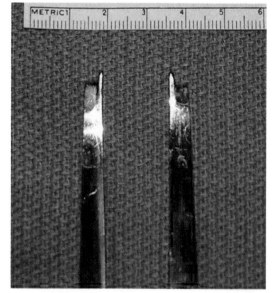

Fig. 4. Osteotomes should be less than 3 mm wide to minimize damage to the periosteum. They should be sharpened at the operating table just before use.

Angling it at 45° work well (such as toward the medial canthus) or even at 60°. The important point is that the directed angle of the osteotomy be more than 30°. The length of the bony cut need only be several millimeters (**Fig. 5**B). When dense bone is heard or felt, one need not proceed deeper. It only takes a few millimeters of bone cut to achieve some mobilization. The osteotome or a Freer inserted into the osteotomy site is used to gently twist the bone, greenstick it, and manipulate it into proper position (**Fig. 5**C). If it is not malleable at this point, the osteotome should be reinserted and a deeper cut made. The medial aspect of the bone typically slips deep to the dorsal bone that remains. This can be visualized in the open approach. The palpable dorsal edge that results is then rasped smooth.

Lateral Osteotomy

A low-to-low osteotomy results in mobilization of the bony base (**Fig. 6**). The bone tends to migrate medially. But if needed, it can be manipulated into

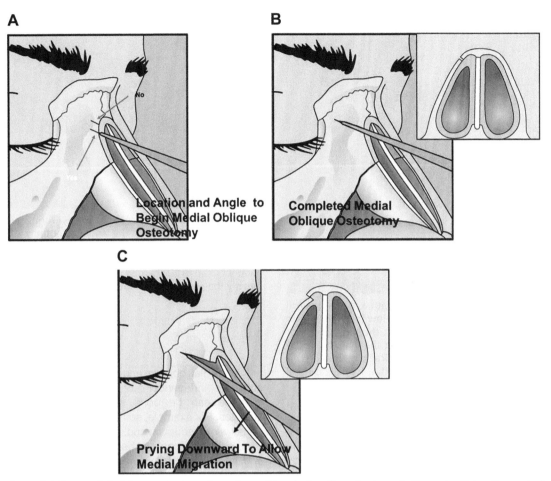

Fig. 5. (*A*) The medial oblique osteotomy is performed by placing the osteotomy in the outer (lateral) aspect of the open roof. This allows the bony plate to migrate medially. (*B*) After penetrating several millimeters, the osteotome (or a Freer) is used to loosen the bone. (*C*) That allows it to migrate medially and deep to the dorsal bone. A small bony ridge (edge) results that is then smoothed with a rasp.

a more lateral position—for example, in those cases where there is complete collapse of the nasal bone after a prior rhinoplasty. Both the buccal sulcus (**Fig. 7**) and the intranasal (intravestibular) approaches for the low-to-low osteotomy work well. The advantage of the buccal sulcus approach is that in some cases, the surgeon may want to visualize the entire osteotomy site by widening the entry incision, inserting an elevator, and being certain that the cut is in the correct location (eg, not too far laterally near the infraorbital foramen or too anterior causing a step-off deformity). The buccal sulcus approach was originally developed to allow the blood from the osteotomy site to drain through the mouth, not the nostril. At most, 1 absorbable stitch may be needed to close the buccal opening.

The most difficult and challenging part of the nasal bone paradigm provided here is the actual bone cut. It begins by marking the site externally (see **Fig. 6**) for the osteotome guard to follow subsequently. After local anesthesia is administered to the underside of the nasal bone and turbinate region at least 7 minutes before, an incision is made in the buccal sulcus near the ala. The osteotome is placed in the most posterior and lateral part of the pyriform aperture. A decisive move is made to drive the osteotome toward the region just a few millimeters anterior to the medial canthal ligament (**Fig. 8**A). The tool can be removed at any time and reinserted if it is done gently. This is sometimes done to convince the surgeon that the tool is in the correct location. A change in sound quality is heard as the very dense nasion

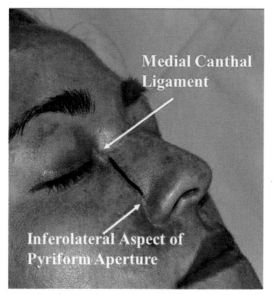

Fig. 6. A line should be drawn with a marking pencil to indicate where the low-to-low osteotomy site should be. The line is placed at the most posterior aspect of the bony plate. It is at the junction of the maxilla and nasal bone. Cephalically, it should be a few millimeters anterior to the medial canthal ligament.

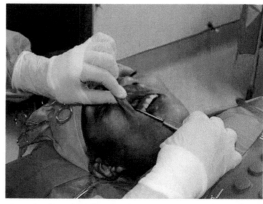

Fig. 7. A buccal sulcus approach to the pyriform aperture and the starting site of the lateral osteotomy is as good a way to perform the osteotomy. In some cases, it has been useful to expand the entry site so it is large enough to insert a narrow speculum and visualize directly the completed osteotomy.

bone is reached, at which point the osteotomy is stopped. A slight prying action (**Fig. 8**B) with the osteotome in the anterior direction will not only allow the tool to be removed easily, but causes the nasal plate to move medially; the more the prying, the more the medial migration. Practice on cadavers is ideal if that opportunity affords itself.

The medial oblique and lateral osteotomy results are independent of one another. Dorsal changes can be done separately from base changes. For example, some patients only require dorsal width reduction and, therefore, a medial oblique osteotomy only. When both medial oblique and lateral osteotomy are performed, the bony plates are not only freed up for a position change (eg, moving medially), but their slope can be adjusted by simple manipulation with forceps (**Fig. 9**).

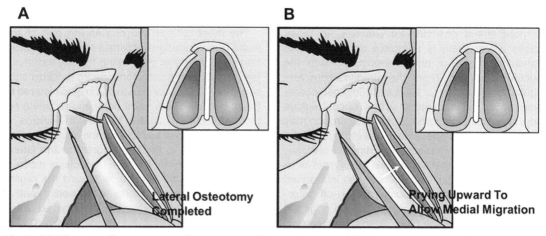

Fig. 8. (A) Schematically, one can see the osteotomy drive up the course of the posterior aspect of the nasal bone plate. (B) When a change in sound is heard, the tool is pried slightly anterior to not only remove it, but to displace the bone plate medially. The more the osteotome is pried, the more the bone migrates medially.

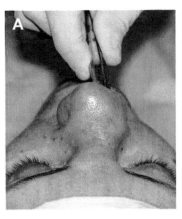
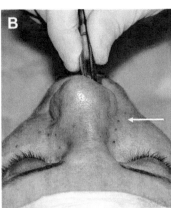

Fig. 9. After an oblique and lateral osteotomy is performed the bony plate tends to be cephalically detached or is at least held in place by the intact mucos (by not using an osteotome more than 3 mm in width). Therefore it is possible, if desired, to manipulate the slope of the nasal bone. It is grasped with Brown-Adson forceps (A) and twisted into the desired slope (B).

On occasion, the crooked nose is so severe that the bony septum (perpendicular plate) needs to be reduced. In most cases, if the bony septum is not midline, it will not matter because the lateral bones camouflage the bony septum, and the cartilaginous septum can be straightened separately. However, some bony septa will need centralization. This is done by a partial osteotomy at the cephalic end of the bony plate (**Fig. 10**). The bony septum is then greensticked into a more central position. So doing allows the entire bony–cartilaginous septum to become more centralized.

PATIENT EXAMPLES

The patient in **Fig. 11** exhibited a broad nasal bone base and dorsum (type 2). She underwent a medial oblique osteotomy and a low-to-low lateral osteotomy through the buccal sulcus approach. A humpectomy and other maneuvers not germane to this discussion were also performed. The result at well over a year postoperative demonstrates the improvement in width of the nasal bone plates.

The patient in **Fig. 12** exhibited a right nasal bone that was medially displaced at its caudal end. The left nasal bone was displaced laterally at the dorsal end causing the bony plate to be somewhat perpendicular (with an improper slope). In this case, bilateral medial oblique and lateral osteotomies were performed to allow complete freedom to reposition the nasal bone plates in a greenstick fashion. The bony septum was off to the left somewhat, too. An osteotomy and greensticking maneuver was performed to manipulate the bony septum into a more central position, one that would not impinge on the adjacent

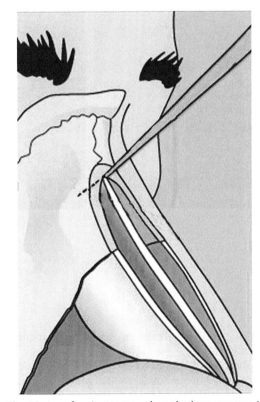

Fig. 10. In a few instances, when the bony septum is extremely displaced and pushes one of the nasal bones laterally, it is necessary to centralize it. This is done by making an osteotomy at the bony septum region for several millimeters and greensticking it. With gentle digital manipulation, the bony septum (with the trailing cartilaginous septum) can be manipulated easily into a more central position.

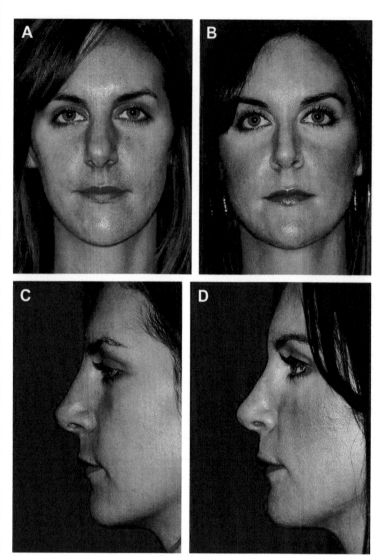

Fig. 11. (*A*, *C*) This patient exhibited a broad nasal bone base and dorsum. She underwent a medial oblique osteotomy and a low-to-low lateral osteotomy through the buccal sulcus approach. A humpectomy and other maneuvers not germane to this discussion were also performed. (*B*, *D*) The result at well over a year postoperative demonstrates the improvement in width of the nasal bone plates.

nasal bone. The result is seen at 11 months postoperative.

The patient in **Fig. 13** exhibited a broad nasal dorsum only (type 3) as a result of a prior lateral osteotomy that ignored the wide dorsum. She underwent a medial oblique osteotomy only. The middle third of the nose (the upper lateral cartilages) was shaved medially to reduce the width as well. The postoperative result demonstrates that osteotomies can manipulate different regions of the bone. A lateral osteotomy here would have only made matters worse.

DISCUSSION

Nasal bone osteotomies require (1) a classification to determine what the appropriate osteotomy should be, (2) an awareness of the anatomy pitfalls, (3) an aggressive means to vasoconstrict, and (4) a surgical concept that permits complete manipulation of the bones into the desired anatomic structure. Then, surgeons must climb the learning curve and achieve a reproducible means of executing the lateral osteotomy in a consistent manner.

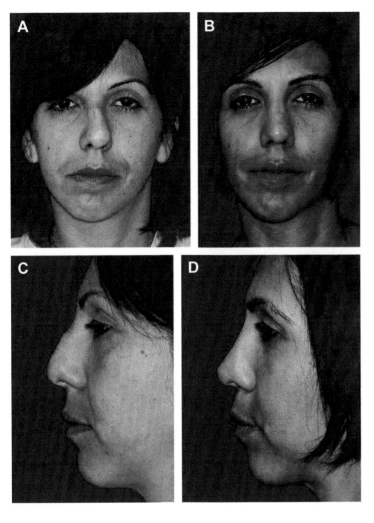

Fig. 12. (*A, C*) This patient exhibited a right nasal bone that was medially displaced at its caudal end. The left nasal bone was displaced laterally at the dorsal end causing the bony plate to be somewhat perpendicular (with an improper slope). In this case, bilateral medial oblique and lateral osteotomies were performed to allow complete freedom to reposition the nasal bone plates in a greenstick fashion. The bony septum was off to the left somewhat, too. An osteotomy and greensticking maneuver was performed to manipulate the bony septum into a more central position, one that would not impinge upon the adjacent nasal bone. (*B, D*) The result is seen at 11 months postoperative.

In years past, problems with osteotomies included lack of hemostasis, bony collapse, step-off deformity, and simple inability to narrow the nasal bones. However, the method and maneuvers described herein should serve the novice rhinoplasty surgeon well. The methods we recommend here are, of course, not the only way to achieve successful results. They are, however, the results of many years of trial and error and collaboration with other colleagues. We are grateful to them for their input without which our technique would not serve us well.

SUMMARY

Performing nasal bone osteotomies can be less intimidating and a more pleasant experience for the rhinoplasty surgeon today with several improvements in technique. The nonpower osteotomy technique has stood the test of time. Before initiating it, however, it is important to appreciate the pertinent anatomy. This means recognizing that increased dorsal width is independent of the bony base width, and that each can be treated separately. The nasal bones can be thought of as 2 thin plates, and the purpose of the osteotomies is to release them in such a way that they can be moved into any position required. Vasoconstriction is exceedingly important and improved dramatically with prophylactic desmopressin. There is a learning curve when it comes to the actual use of the osteotomy tool. However, once that skill is acquired, the rhinoplasty surgeon will find that control of nasal bones structure is truly within his or her grasp.

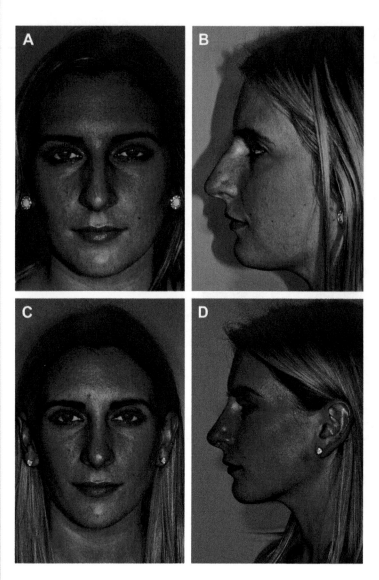

Fig. 13. (*A, B*) This patient exhibited a broad nasal dorsum only as a result of a prior lateral osteotomy that ignored the wide dorsum. She underwent a medial oblique osteotomy only. (*C, D*) The middle third of the nose (the upper lateral cartilages) were shaved medially to reduce their width as well.

REFERENCES

1. Rohrich RJ, Krueger JK, Adams WP Jr, et al. Achieving consistency in the lateral nasal osteotomy during rhinoplasty: an external perforated technique. Plast Reconstr Surg 2001;108:2122.
2. Tebbetts JB. Primary rhinoplasty. St Louis (MO): Mosby; 1998. p. 249.
3. Murakami CS, Larrabee WF Jr. Comparison of osteotomy techniques in the treatment of nasal fractures. Facial Plast Surg 1992;8:209.
4. Tardy ME, Toriumi DM, Hecht DA. Philosophy and principles of rhinoplasty. In: Papel ID, editor. Facial and plastic reconstructive surgery. New York: Thieme; 2002. p. 384–9.
5. Gunter JP, Rohrich RJ, Adams WP Jr, editors. Dallas rhinoplasty: nasal surgery by the masters. 3rd edition. CRC Press; 2014.
6. Guyuron B. Nasal osteotomy and airway changes. Plast Reconstr Surg 1998;102:856.
7. Rohrich RJ, Janis JE, Adams WP, et al. An update on the lateral nasal osteotomy in rhinoplasty: an anatomic endoscopic comparison of the external versus the internal approach. Plast Reconstr Surg 2003;111:2461.

8. Becker DG, Mclaughlin RB Jr, Loevner LA, et al. The lateral osteotomy in rhinoplasty. Plast Reconstr Surg 2000;105:1806.

9. Daniel RK. Mastering Rhinoplasty: a comprehensive atlas of surgical techniques with integrated video clips. Berlin: Springer-Verlag; 2010.

10. Harshbrger RJ, Sullivan PK. The optimal medial osteotomy: a study of nasal bone thickness and fracture patterns. Plast Reconstr Surg 2001;108: 2114.

11. Harshbarger RJ, Sullivan PK. Lateral osteotomies: implications of bony thickness on fracture patterns. Ann Plast Surg 1999;42:365.

12. Avsar YI. The oscillating micro-saw: a safe and pliable instrument for transverse osteotomy in rhinoplasty. Aesth Surg J 2012;32:700–8.

13. Guyuron B, Vaughan C, Schlecter B. The role of DDAVP (Desmopressin) in orthognathic surgery. Ann Plast Surg 1996;37(5):516–9.

14. Gruber RP, Zeidler KR, Berkowitz RL. Desmopression as a hemostatic agent to provide a dry intraoperative field in rhinoplasty. Plast Reconstr Surg 2015;135:1337–40.

15. Gryskiewicz JM, Gryskiewicz KM. Nasal osteotomies: a clinical comparison of the perforating methods versus the continuous technique. Plast Reconstr Surg 2004;113:1445.

Surgical Treatment of the Middle Nasal Vault

Amir Allak, MD, MBA, Stephen S. Park, MD*

KEYWORDS

- Middle nasal vault • Internal nasal valve • Nasal obstruction • Valve collapse
- Upper lateral cartilage • Spreader graft

KEY POINTS

- The middle nasal vault is a critical region of the esthetics and function of the nose.
- Internal valve collapse is associated with abnormalities that arises in the middle vault.
- The thinnest nasal skin is over the middle third, and irregularities are often not well masked.
- Proper resuspension of the upper lateral cartilages during rhinoplasty will prevent postoperative cosmetic deformities and nasal obstruction.
- Dorsal hump reduction may unmask underlying middle vault abnormality and should be accompanied by appropriate grafting when indicated.

INTRODUCTION

Successful rhinoplasty is contingent on the appropriate evaluation of matching anatomic deformities to surgical strategies. The surgeon must understand the structurally sensitive regions of the nose and the implications of surgical alteration to both cosmesis and nasal function. The middle nasal vault is a critical anatomic region for the esthetics of the middle third of the nose as well as for maintaining nasal airflow. In patients evaluated for secondary rhinoplasty, middle third visual deformity and obstruction account for 2 of the 3 most common findings.[1] In both primary and revision rhinoplasty, special consideration must be dedicated to addressing deformities and preserving supporting structures of the middle vault because this is an important point in the prevention of postoperative complications.

ANATOMY

The middle nasal vault is difficult to understand because of its complex 3-dimensional anatomy and dynamic alteration with nasal airflow. The middle vault is also referred to as the cartilaginous vault and comprises cutaneous tissue, a musculoaponeurotic layer, upper lateral cartilages (ULC), dorsal septum, and intranasal mucosa.

The cutaneous tissue is often the thinnest over the middle third of the nasal envelope. The superficial musculoaponeurotic system (SMAS) over the nose contains the transverse nasal and levator alaeque nasi and has fascial insertions inferiorly along the anterior septum, the lower lateral cartilages (LLCs), and the columella.[2] The paired ULC are deep to the SMAS and anchored superiorly to the undersurface of the nasal bones in the so-called K-area. Inferiorly, they are attached to the

The authors have nothing to disclose.
Department of Otolaryngology–Head and Neck Surgery, University of Virginia, PO Box 800713, Charlottesville, VA 22908, USA
* Corresponding author.
E-mail address: ssp8a@virginia.edu

plasticsurgery.theclinics.com

LLCs in the scroll region, and laterally, the soft tissue of the sidewall connects them to the piriform aperture. The ULC medially articulates with the dorsal edge of the cartilaginous septum, where the dorsal septum is often wider, forming a T- or Y-shaped orientation. When progressing toward the caudal aspect of the ULC, the angle between the septum and sidewall becomes more and more acute, narrowing the nasal airway.[3] At this level, the reported normal angle in Caucasians is 10 to 20°.[4] Intranasal mucosa is fixed to the undersurface of the ULC and is continuous with the septal mucosa.

The internal nasal valve is bound by the caudal aspect of the ULC anterolaterally, septum medially, and inferior turbinate posterolaterally (**Fig. 1**). Because of its low cross-sectional area, nasal airflow is physiologically subject to the highest resistance in this area, as dictated by Poiseuille's law. When accounting for Bernoulli effect, the high air velocity causes collapse at the internal valve, which can be pathologic if there is a lack of adequate structural support. In fact, approximately 1 in 6 patients with chronic nasal obstruction will have collapse of the internal nasal valve.[5] When considering that the cross-sectional area of the internal nasal valve decreases by 25% after reduction rhinoplasty, it is not surprising that many patients have postoperative obstruction.[6] Therefore, it is essential to address the middle vault effectively to avoid causing iatrogenic weakening of the nasal valve or exacerbating stenosis in patients with unfavorable anatomy.

PREOPERATIVE PLANNING AND PREPARATION

Evaluation of the rhinoplasty patient is paramount before any surgical intervention is planned. The surgeon should be thorough in inquiry of desires and expectations of the patient and differentiate functional and cosmetic concerns. The patient should relay which specific esthetic features are bothersome and the anticipated change. Surgery should be avoided if the patient's expectations are unrealistic or there is any indication of significant psychological abnormality suggesting body dysmorphic disorder. Preoperative photographs should be taken and reviewed with the patient to facilitate discussion and education of the areas of concern. Morphing imaging software can be additionally helpful in demonstrating a reasonable result and if that is an acceptable outcome for the patient.

A detailed history should be taken regarding nasal obstruction with laterality, alleviating or exacerbating factors, prior interventions, and any concomitant sinonasal disease. Prior nasal surgery, facial trauma, history of severe diabetes, granulomatous or bleeding/clotting diseases, smoking, and intranasal drug use are also important to document. The surgeon should always inquire regarding anticoagulation use, including supplements that alter the clotting cascade and heavy nonsteroidal anti-inflammatory drug use. In the case of revision surgery, review of prior operative reports is beneficial if records are available.

Physical examination should include facial and nasal esthetics as well as a functional analysis. The middle vault correlates externally with the middle third of the nose and is best viewed from the frontal and lateral views. General observation should include patient height, facial proportions, overall skin quality and thickness, scars, and obvious deformities. Special consideration is given to the skin overlying the middle vault because it is often the thinnest of any region of the nose. The frontal view will reveal a narrow or wide middle vault, or asymmetry/deviation of the middle third that could indicate dorsal septal deviation or twisting (**Fig. 2**). A lack of appropriate shadowing along the dorsum would suggest

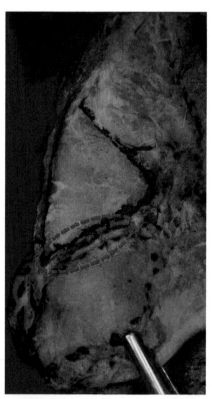

Fig. 1. Cadaveric dissection with blue demarcation of the ULC and LLC. The red oval indicates the area that corresponds with the internal valve in the middle vault.

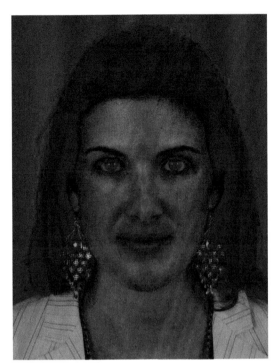

Fig. 2. Frontal view displaying a narrow or pinched middle third indicating middle vault abnormality.

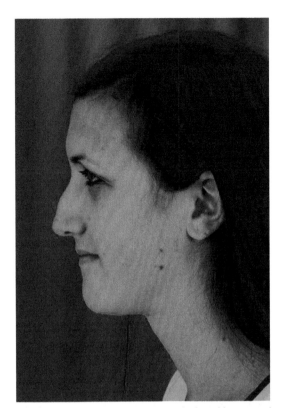

Fig. 3. Lateral view in a patient with dorsal hump and middle third overprojection.

underprojection. In patients with prior surgery, the hourglass or inverted V deformity is visible from the frontal view and would create an interruption of the smooth brow-tip line, indicating poor middle vault support.

The lateral view shows projection and shape of the middle third. Ideally, the nasal dorsum should be a straight line from the radix to the tip in male patients and in females, a very slight concavity present for the supratip break.[7] Overprojection is often a result of a dorsal hump, essentially overdevelopment of the cartilaginous dorsal septum, especially the anterior septal angle (**Fig. 3**). Tip rotation/projection and radix height should be noted because tip ptosis and a low radix produce a pseudohump (**Fig. 4**).[8] Inadequate chin projection can have a similar effect in creating the illusion of a larger nose. Pollybeak deformity is also apparent on lateral view and refers to the situation when the supratip projects farther than the tip. This can be a result of addressing the bony but underresection of the cartilaginous portion of a dorsal hump and can also be due to fibrous tissue formation at the supratip after cartilaginous dorsal hump and anterior septal angle overresection. Underprojection of the middle third can be a result of prior overaggressive dorsal hump reduction, dorsal cartilage resection during septoplasty, or a septal perforation causing a saddle nose deformity (**Fig. 5**).

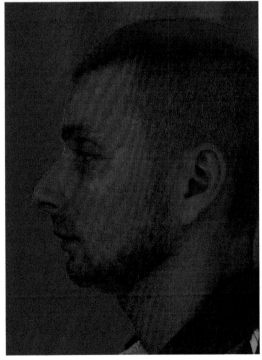

Fig. 4. Lateral view displaying a low radix creating the illusion of a pseudohump. This patient has both a low radix and a true dorsal hump.

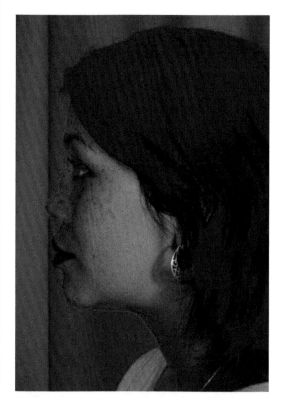

Fig. 5. Lateral view in a patient with saddle nose and middle third underprojection.

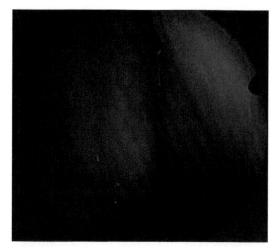

Fig. 6. Intranasal view of middle vault collapse.

Palpation of the nose provides adjunctive information to the visual examination, including skin quality, dorsal hump composition, nasal bone length, and lateral nasal wall support. Also, placement of a gloved thumb and second finger on either side of the intranasal dorsal septum can give additive information about intrinsic septal deviation.

The functional examination focuses on the intranasal static and dynamic aspects of inspiratory airflow. A static examination should include identification of septal deviation or perforation, ULC collapse, inferior turbinate hypertrophy, as well as any nasal bone or external valve/intervalve abnormality (**Fig. 6**). While occluding the contralateral naris, the surgeon asks the patient to inhale through the nose with mild force to evaluate for dynamic collapse. Inadequate force may not unmask collapse, whereas an overly forceful inhalation will cause there to be collapse that may not be pathologic. Careful assessment of the true location of obstruction is critical to addressing the correct level of collapse with the appropriate surgical strategy. In lieu of the Cottle maneuver, the surgeon places a small-tipped instrument (eg, cerumen loop) to support specifically the area of objective collapse while the patient repeats the inhalation to assess for subjective improvement.

PROCEDURAL APPROACH

Although endonasal approaches exist for certain aspects of middle vault surgery, the surgical exposure is best optimized with the external rhinoplasty approach. For the purposes of this article, the open technique is highlighted, as are the areas where an endonasal approach is feasible.

Preparation

- Patients undergo induction of general anesthesia and endotracheal intubation. The head is placed in a neuro headrest in a neutral position. The endotracheal tube is sewn to the precise midline mentum to facilitate intraoperative visual assessments of symmetry and to avoid pulling the nose to one side. The surgical lights are also placed in the midline so as not to cast asymmetric shadows.
- Lidocaine 1% with 1:100,000 epinephrine is injected into the nasal soft tissue envelope and septal mucosa with a portion submucosally for hydrodissection. Pledgets soaked in 1% tetracaine/0.05% oxymetazoline are placed in the nasal cavity. Mineral oil/petrolatum ophthalmologic lubricant is placed in the eyes.
- The face and neck are prepared with Poloxamer 188–containing wash and povidone-iodine 10% solution, and a head wrap is placed with a sterile towel. Appropriate sterile draping is performed.

External Approach

- An inverted V columellar incision is carried out with a number-15-c blade midway between the alar base and anterior aspect of the naris, taking care not to injure the medial crura of the LLC. Vertical columellar incisions are performed. While retracting the ala with a skin hook and everting the lateral crus, marginal incisions are performed at the caudal aspect of the lateral crura. The marginal and columellar incisions are joined while maintaining 3-point countertraction, and the nasal envelope is dissected from the LLCs in a submuscular plane.

- The anterior septal angle is identified, and the submuscular dissection is carried out over the dorsal septum where the ULC and the middle vault are exposed. The dissection plane should be just superficial to the cartilage to ensure adequate thickness of the overlying soft tissue.
- Standard open septoplasty can be performed at this point for resection of deviated septal elements and cartilage harvest for grafting.
- If a bony hump is to be reduced, a Joseph periosteal elevator is used to create a subperiosteal pocket. In the case that osteotomies are expected, this dissection should not be carried out laterally to preserve soft tissue support of the nasal bones.
- At the termination of the case, closure is performed with a single 5-0 polydioxanone (PDS) deep stitch in the midline columella, 6-0 fast absorbing gut interrupted stitches for the skin of the inverted V incision, and 5-0 chromic for marginal incisions when grafts are placed.

Widening of the Narrow Middle Vault

- Spreader grafts are the mainstay of widening the middle vault. Using septal cartilage either from open septoplasty or via a hemitransfixion incison, unilateral or bilateral grafts are created in a long rectangular shape with beveled ends. These grafts should be 1 to 2 cm in length, 1 to 4 mm in width, and no more than 5 mm in height so as not to impinge on the nasal airway.[9]
- Mucosa is elevated from the dorsal septum and the undersurface of the ULC, wherein the ULC are carefully disarticulated from the dorsal septum with a Freer or Cottle periosteal elevator. The graft or grafts are placed between the anterior aspect of the ULC and the dorsal septum (**Fig. 7**). These grafts can be held in place with either Brown-Adson forceps or a 27-gauge needle placed through all 3 structures. Several 5-0 nylon sutures are then used to secure the graft in place (**Fig. 8**).
- Auto-spreaders, also known as spreader flaps, have become more popular in recent

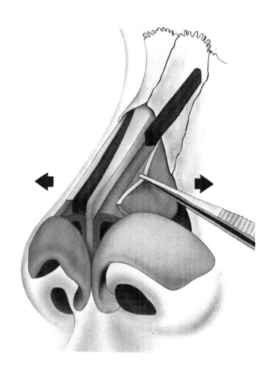

Fig. 7. Schematic illustration of spreader placement. Note the location between ULC, dorsal septum, and middle vault nasal mucosa.

years. Auto-spreaders entail mucosal elevation as with normal spreader grafts, then use of the medial aspect of the ULC themselves as a spreader; this is accomplished with either complete separation, a partial thickness incision and hinged placement, or folding of the medial aspect of the cartilage without any incisions. Auto-spreaders are secured in the same fashion as standard spreaders.[10]

- Additional cartilage grafts can be also be placed to assist in stiffening the structure of the ULC adjacent to the internal valve to prevent collapse. Conchal cartilage is used with the concave face down, superficial to the caudal aspect of the ULC as a butterfly graft or deep to it as an ULC splay graft. These grafts are suture fixed with a 5-0 PDS or clear nylon and act almost as an implantable breathe-strip.[11,12]
- Flaring sutures are also used to improve the internal valve by increasing the angle of the ULC in relation to the dorsal septum. A 5-0 clear nylon suture is placed in a vertical mattress fashion across the caudal aspect of the ULC and tied across the nasal dorsum, effectively using it as a fulcrum for flaring of

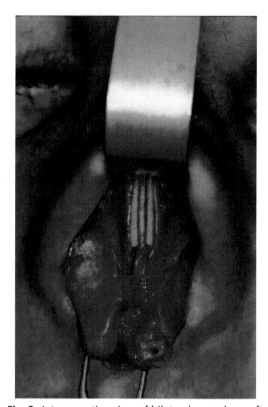

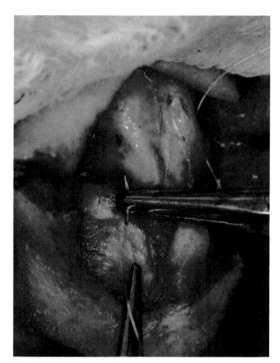

Fig. 9. ULC flaring suture.

Fig. 8. Intraoperative view of bilateral spreader graft inset.

the narrow portion of the valve (**Fig. 9**). This portion of the cartilage is often difficult to visualize and can be delivered with an intranasal cotton tipped applicator.[13]

- When placed in isolation, it is technically feasible to place spreader grafts with a closed approach after careful elevation of submucosal pockets through an intercartilaginous incision. However, when spreader grafts are often placed along with other interventions, the open approach provides better visualization and ability to suture the grafts to the dorsal septum and to place extended spreader grafts.

Narrowing of the Wide Middle Vault

- In patients with wide middle vaults, coexisting nasal obstruction is not common, and conservative dorsal width reduction is a feasible option.
- The so-called reverse spreader technique has been described and can be performed via open or closed approaches (intercartilaginous and partial transfixion incisions). After disarticulation of the ULC from the dorsal septum, a narrow strip of the medial aspect of the ULC is resected. The cross-sectional shape is a

wedge bevel so as to take more of the external redundant ULC and less of the intranasal aspect to prevent valve collapse. The cartilage is then reapproximated with 5-0 Vicryl.[14]

- Often a wide middle vault is accompanied by wide nasal bones, and osteotomies should be performed when indicated.

Dorsal Hump Reduction for Overprojection

- Submucoperichondrial elevation is carried out between the dorsal septum and intranasal mucosa with a Cottle periosteal elevator. The mucosa is then dissected from the undersurface of the ULC and carried out under the nasal bones, taking care not to disrupt the k-area and lose the anchoring point of the ULC. The ULC are disarticulated from the dorsal septum to allow for separate reduction and prevent overresection.
- In the case of an isolated dorsal hump, the closed approach can be used with an intercartilaginous incision.
- The cartilaginous hump is then sharply excised with a number 11 or number 15 blade (**Fig. 10**). This portion is either removed or kept attached to the caudal aspect of the nasal bones for engagement of a Rubin osteotome for bony resection (**Figs. 11–13**). Care is taken not to disrupt the ULC attachments to the undersurface of the nasal bones.

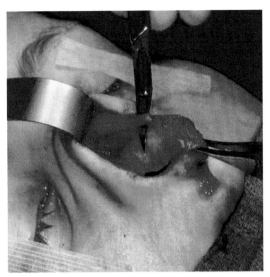

Fig. 10. The cartilaginous portion of the dorsal hump is excised sharply with a number 11 blade.

- Alternatively, the cartilaginous portion is removed, and rasps are used to reduce the nasal bones. Coarse rasping should be followed by a fine diamond rasp for contouring of fine irregularities as the nasal skin is thinnest at the rhinion and does not tolerate even subtle deformity. Rasping should be performed at an oblique angle to again avoid loss of ULC attachment and direct trauma to the ULC themselves.
- In cases of isolated bony hump deformities, powered burrs or rasps can be used with good success and minimal collateral tissue damage when used properly.

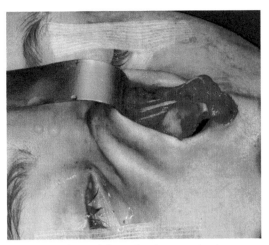

Fig. 12. Resulting defect after hump reduction.

- The wound is irrigated to remove bony debris, and the nasal soft tissues are redraped. Firm pressure is applied to the nose with saline-soaked gauze. A moistened fingertip is used to palpate the dorsum for any persistent irregularities. Further resection or rasping should be performed if necessary. Autologous temporalis fascia or crushed cartilage can be placed for further masking of subtle deformity.
- Spreader grafts can be placed at this point if deemed necessary. ULC are then resuspended to the new dorsal edge of the septum with a 5-0 clear nylon suture. It should be noted that resection of the dorsal aspect of the septum may unmask a septal deviation, which may cause asymmetry if not addressed before ULC resuspension.
- If an open roof deformity is created from bony hump resection, lateral osteotomies should

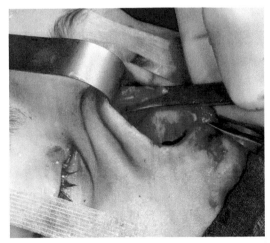

Fig. 11. The Rubin osteotome is used to engage and resect the bony portion of the dorsal hump through the cartilaginous incision.

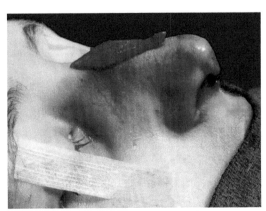

Fig. 13. Excised dorsal hump placed on the nasal envelope.

be performed to reapproximate the medial aspect of the nasal bones.

Dorsal Augmentation for Underprojection

- External or endonasal (via intercartilagenous incision) approaches can be used for placement of a dorsal onlay graft for augmentation. Dissection along the dorsum should be limited to the area where the graft is to be placed and should be submuscular. Excessive lateral dissection may lead to graft displacement.
- A coarse rasp can be used to abrade and prepare the dorsum for optimal biointegration of grafted material.
- Septal, auricular, or rib cartilage can be used. Costochondral rib graft can be an option in case there is significant dorsal deficit that includes the nasal bones (**Fig. 14**). In the absence of ideally contoured autograft material, cartilage can be morselized and wrapped in temporalis fascia. If desired, additional fascia or acellular dermis can be overlaid to smooth any irregularities.
- If autografted material is chosen, appropriate contouring should include a concavity on the deep aspect, smooth convexity on the superficial surface, and slightly tapered cephalic and caudal tips (**Fig. 15**). This contouring can be performed with cold or powered instrumentation.
- Once appropriate shape and contour are achieved, the graft is placed into the pocket (**Fig. 16**) and occasionally secured to the underlying structure with sutures or even percutaneous titanium screws or K-wires. A moldable rigid nasal splint and tape should secure the reconstruction externally to minimize graft movement. Excellent dorsal projection can be achieved with this technique (**Fig. 17**).

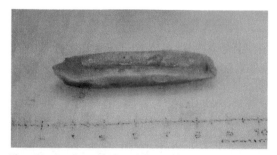

Fig. 15. Carving of the deep surface of the dorsal augmentation graft in a concave fashion for articulation with the nasal dorsum.

Correcting the Deviated/Twisted Middle Vault

- After disarticulation of the ULC and complete septal mucosal elevation, the septum should be examined for deviation and intrinsic curvature (**Fig. 18**). If excessive length is observed, a conservative strip of the inferior aspect of the cartilaginous septum can be resected to release it from the floor. Mild higher dorsal deviations can also be addressed with scoring of the concave surface or conservative full-thickness cartilaginous incisions to weaken the structure.
- If spreader grafts are deemed necessary, a unilateral spreader can be used to straighten the dorsal deviation. Alternatively, variable thickness bilateral spreader grafts can be constructed and placed.
- For persistent deviations or dorsal septal deflections, an extracorporeal septoplasty can be performed and reimplanted in an orientation providing a midline anchor for the ULC. In addition, the twisted cartilage can be fixed

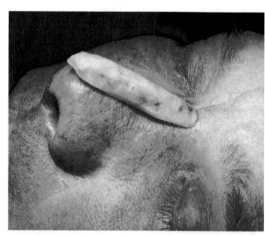

Fig. 16. Proposed placement of dorsal augmentation graft.

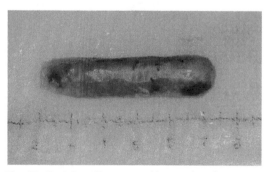

Fig. 14. Costal cartilage carved into a dorsal augmentation graft.

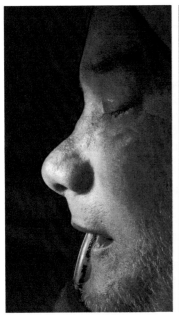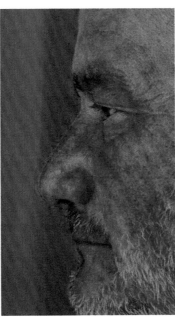

Fig. 17. Before and after dorsal augmentation.

to explanted ethmoid bone or a perforated polydioxanone plate (0.15 mm thickness) with 4-0 PDS suture. If ethmoid bone is used, holes can be hand drilled with an 18-gauge needle to prevent cracking.

- In cases when the middle vault is underprojected and there is a recalcitrant dorsal septal deviation, an overlay graft can be placed with the lateral aspects suture fixed to the ULC

with a 5-0 nylon suture so it will also function as an onlay spreader graft. A camouflage graft can be fixed on the overlay to enhance projection and set the dorsum midline.[15]

POSTPROCEDURAL CARE

Cutaneous taping is performed on all patients with 0.5-in paper tape; external splints are applied for osteotomies, and intranasal Doyle splints and intranasal packs are used sparingly. Patients are given prophylactic antibiotics to cover general skin flora and strict activity restrictions until the first postoperative appointment at 1 week. At that time, dressings and splints are removed (as are K-wires or screws for dorsal augmentation). Full activity is resumed at 2 to 4 weeks postoperatively.

POTENTIAL COMPLICATIONS AND MANAGEMENT

- Low dorsal height and saddle nose
  - Cause: Overresection of dorsal hump
  - Consequence: Cosmetic deformity, may lead to nasal obstruction and static/dynamic valve collapse
  - Treatment: dorsal augmentation
- Pollybeak and supratip deformity
  - Cause: Blood filling the potential space of the supratip after dorsal hump overresection, which incites an inflammatory reaction and fibrosis obscuring the supratip break.

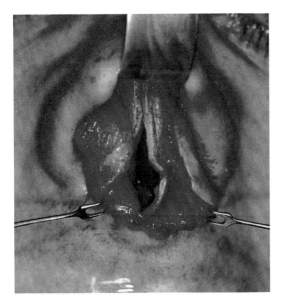

Fig. 18. Deviation and curvature of the dorsal septum causing a twisted nose and middle vault collapse.

Also caused by cartilaginous under-resection and residual anterior septal angle
- ○ Consequence: Cosmetic deformity
- ○ Treatment: Initially taping, deep steroid injections as early as 6 to 8 weeks, and revision surgery only after 6 to 12 months. Re-resection if anterior septal angle remains
- Inverted V deformity
  - ○ Cause: Collapse of ULC at internal valve after inadequate resuspension or loss of suspensory support at K-area
  - ○ Consequence: Cosmetic deformity, nasal obstruction
  - ○ Treatment: Resuspension, possible spreader grafts
- Open roof deformity
  - ○ Cause: Inadequate reapproximation of nasal bones after bony dorsal hump reduction
  - ○ Consequence: Cosmetic deformity
  - ○ Treatment: Lateral osteotomies, possible small dorsal onlay if inadequate bone remains to cover the defect
- Graft infection
  - ○ Cause: Bacterial colonization and infection of implanted materials
  - ○ Consequence: Delayed healing, graft loss, or need for explant
  - ○ Treatment: Initially antibiotics and local wound care; operative explant for persistent infections and future revision
- Graft migration (dorsal augmentation)
  - ○ Cause: Inadequate securing of graft to underlying dorsum
  - ○ Consequence: Cosmetic deformity
  - ○ Treatment: Repeat suspension with taping, wires, or screws. May require revision if graft fixes in improper location
- Nasal valve collapse
  - ○ Cause: Improper ULC suspension, underestimation of graft size, persistent septal deviation
  - ○ Consequence: Nasal obstruction
  - ○ Treatment: May eventually require surgical revision

SUMMARY

Understanding the middle nasal vault is important for rhinoplasty surgeons. Given its complex 3-dimensional anatomy and vulnerability to esthetic deformity and internal valve collapse, consideration should always be given to the effect that common rhinoplasty maneuvers will have on the middle third of the nose. Identifying and addressing potential pitfalls of the middle vault during primary rhinoplasty will lead to better outcomes and more satisfied patients.

REFERENCES

1. Yu K, Kim A, Pearlman SJ. Functional and aesthetic concerns of patients seeking revision rhinoplasty. Arch Facial Plast Surg 2010;12:291–7.
2. Saban Y, Amodeo CA, Hammou JC, et al. An anatomical study of the nasal superficial musculoaponeurotic system. Arch Facial Plast Surg 2008; 10(2):109–15.
3. Toriumi DM. Management of the middle nasal vault in rhinoplasty. Op Tech Plast Reconstr Surg 1995; 2(1):16–20.
4. Kasperbauer JL, Kern EB. Nasal valve physiology: implications in nasal surgery. Otolaryngol Clin North Am 1987;20:699–719.
5. Constantian MB. Differing characteristics in 100 consecutive secondary rhinoplasty patients following closed versus open surgical approaches. Plast Reconstr Surg 2002;109(6):2097–111.
6. Grymer LF. Reduction rhinoplasty and nasal patency: change in the cross-sectional area of the nose evaluated by acoustic rhinometry. Laryngoscope 1995;105(4 Pt 1):429–31.
7. Taub PJ, Baker SB. Operative atlas of rhinoplasty. New York: McGraw-Hill, Inc; 2011.
8. Mowlavi A, Meldrum DG, Wilhelmi BJ. Implications for nasal recontouring: nasion position preferences as determined by a survey of white North Americans. Aesthetic Plast Surg 2003;27(6):438–45.
9. Toriumi DM, Johnson CMJ. Open structure rhinoplasty: featured technical points and long-term follow-up. Facial Plast Surg Clin North Am 1993;1: 1–22.
10. Byrd HS, Meade RA, Gonyon DL Jr. Using the autospreader flap in primary rhinoplasty. Plast Reconstr Surg 2007;119(6):1897–902.
11. Clark JM, Cook TA. The 'butterfly' graft in functional secondary rhinoplasty. Laryngoscope 2002;112: 1917–25.
12. Guyuron B, Michelow BJ, Englebardt C. Upper lateral splay graft. Plast Reconstr Surg 1998; 102(6):2169–77.
13. Park SS. The flaring suture to augment the repair of the dysfunctional nasal valve. Plast Reconstr Surg 1998;101:1120–2.
14. Prendiville S, Zimbler MS, Kokoska MS, et al. Middle-vault narrowing in the wide nasal dorsum: the "Reverse Spreader" technique. Arch Facial Plast Surg 2002;4(1):52–5.
15. Murakami C. Nasal valve collapse. Ear Nose Throat J 2004;83:163–4.

Surgical Treatment of the Twisted Nose

Dirk Jan Menger, MD, PhD

KEYWORDS

- Rhinoplasty • Twisted nose • Crooked nose • Osteotomies • Septoplasty • Realignment

KEY POINTS

- Key in the surgical procedure is that all structures of the nasal skeleton need to be dissected free, mobilized, repositioned, and stabilized.
- Important surgical steps are intermediate osteotomies on the contralateral side of the deviation for the upper nasal third.
- Important surgical steps include, for the mid nasal third, a unilateral spreader graft or splint on the nondeviated side, and for the lower nasal third, fixation of the caudal septum to the anterior nasal spine.

 Videos of the steps in the correction of the twisted nose accompany this article at http://www.plasticsurgery.theclinics.com/

INTRODUCTION

The nasal septum plays an essential role in the twisted nose. Cottle's dictum, "as the nasal septum goes, so goes the nose," is true and implies that a successful correction of a crooked nose starts with accurate septoplasty. Isolated cartilaginous deviations, including the nasal septum and upper lateral cartilages (ULCs), are rare, and in most cases, the nasal bones are involved in the deformity with a need for additional osteotomies. Usually, the deformity is caused by nasal trauma; sometimes, however, the cause is unknown.

Typically on the ipsilateral side of the deviation, the twisted nose has a shorter and steeper bony and cartilaginous nasal sidewall. On the contralateral side of the deviation, the nasal bone usually is longer and has a more gradual angle with the cheek area; this has important implications for the osteotomies, which should be performed in an asymmetric manner. Because the ULC and nasal septum form a T-bar, if the middle nasal vault appears to be deviated, then by definition the dorsal septum is also deviated. In contrast,

the basal part of the nasal septum is usually deviated to the contralateral side with or without a deviation of the premaxilla and anterior nasal spine. Therefore, both sides of the nasal airway can be blocked partially or completely in patients with a twisted nose. These patients have a functional and esthetic problem of the nose.

The nasal septum, ULCs, and nasal bones should be brought into midline in order to straighten a twisted nose. Therefore, all structures of the nasal skeleton need to be dissected free, mobilized, repositioned, and stabilized.[1] Because the upper and middle third of the twisted nose are asymmetric, the right and left side of the nose require a different surgical technique. In most cases, the open, or external approach, provides the best exposure to the anatomic regions in the nose for optimal reconstruction.

TREATMENT GOALS AND PLANNED OUTCOMES

The goal of surgery is to realign the bony and cartilaginous nasal skeleton in order to create

---

Disclosures: None.
Department of ENT/FPRS, University Medical Center Utrecht, Heidelberglaan 100, 3584 CX, Utrecht, The Netherlands
E-mail address: D.J.Menger@Gmail.com

Clin Plastic Surg 43 (2016) 95–98
http://dx.doi.org/10.1016/j.cps.2015.08.004

symmetry in the face and to restore nasal patency. Despite the highest personal effort of the surgeon, the patient should understand that a perfectly straight nose is not always possible due to nonsurgical factors. These factors include other asymmetries of the face, wound healing, scar tissue or stresses, trauma in the postoperative phase, and so on.

PREOPERATIVE PLANNING AND PREPARATION

A standardized rhinoplasty protocol is essential for a successful outcome. This protocol includes standardized preoperative documentation using an assessment and surgical rhinoplasty sheet. The medical history should be reported including the use of medication. Medication that can influence blood coagulation should be stopped before surgery. Inhalation allergies should be tested and treated as needed with antihistamines and nasal corticosteroids. Inspection of the nasal airway using an endoscope might be required in selected cases. Standardized preoperative rhinoplasty photographs (frontal, oblique, lateral, basal, and bird's eye view) should always be performed and documented. Sometimes 3dimensional imaging or computer-simulated imaging is helpful in the communication with the patient. In all cases, a written informed consent with all possible side effects of the surgery and postoperative period should be given and signed by the patient.

PATIENT POSITIONING

The patient is preferably placed supine into slight reverse Trendelenburg position because this position reduces bleeding. Surgery is usually performed under general anesthesia in combination with a local infiltration anesthetic and topical application of 200 mg of cocaine in order to promote vasoconstriction and prevent bleeding. The local anesthetic should be given at least 10 minutes before starting surgery.

PROCEDURAL APPROACH

Surgical correction of the twisted nose can be divided into 4 steps:

1. External approach rhinoplasty
   a. Full dissection of the nasal skeleton (Videos 1 and 2)
   b. Releasing the mucoperichondrium on both sides of the nasal septum (Video 3)
   c. Separation of the ULCs from the nasal septum
2. Osteotomies

a. Endonasal or percutaneous microosteotomies: on both sides (medial, lateral, and oblique; Video 4)
   b. Intermediate osteotomies: on the contralateral side of the deviation because the nasal bone usually is longer on this side. Intermediate osteotomies can also be applied in patients with a complex posttraumatic fracture pattern of the nasal bones. The intermediate osteotomies should be performed before the lateral and oblique osteotomies.
   c. Percutaneous root (frontal beak) osteotomies in severe cases
3. Septoplasty and realignment of the middle nasal vault
   a. An L-strut is created of the nasal septum with a dorsal and caudal part of approximately 1.5 cm (Video 5)
   b. The premaxilla and anterior nasal spine are mobilized and realigned in cases where there is deviation from the midline
   c. Partial thickness scoring is performed of the dorsal and caudal part of the L-strut. The scoring is performed on the concave side to relieve intrinsic binding forces.
   d. The dorsal or caudal part of the septum is splinted with a strong cartilaginous or bony (with predrilled holes) batten or spreader graft. In order to create symmetry, this is performed on the contralateral side of the deviation. Depending on the amount of deviation and asymmetry, bilateral or asymmetric spreader grafts are applied (Videos 6 and 7).
   e. Dissolvable polydioxanone (PDS) plate can be used to restore the L-strut in the case of multiple fractures of the cartilaginous and bony nasal septum. A PDS plate (0.15 mm) can act as a temporary template for suturing and stabilizing cartilage pieces[2] (Video 8).
   f. The caudal part of the septum is secured to the anterior nasal spine through a predrilled hole with a (semi) permanent suture (Video 9).
   g. The ULCs are stabilized and fixed to the straightened L-strut using mattress sutures.
   h. Septal mattress sutures are applied to prevent dead space and septal hematoma.
   i. Extracorporeal septoplasty can be performed in severe deviations. The nasal septum can be scored and splinted with cartilaginous or bony battens on the table and reinserted in between the mucoperichondrium layers. Securing the septum to the dorsum is critical to prevent subsequent

collapse and postoperative saddle nose deformity[3] (Video 8).

j. Onlay grafts of lightly crushed or diced cartilage can be applied to camouflage residual asymmetries of the upper and middle third.

4. Packing and dressing
   a. Two-centimeter gauze with antibiotic ointment in the nasal cavity for 24 to 48 hours.
   b. Taping of the nose and a nasal splint for 1 week (Video 10).

POTENTIAL COMPLICATIONS AND MANAGEMENT OF THEM

Potential complications of this procedure include a staircase phenomenon when the lateral osteotomies are carried out too far medially. The contralateral side of the deviation is especially at risk because the nasal bone is longer. The L-strut can accidentally be disrupted in the keystone area leading to collapse and saddle nose deformity. As with the extracorporeal technique, this can be prevented by firm fixation of the dorsal part of the septum with (semi) permanent sutures to the bony compartment by drilling one or more holes and fixation to the ULCs. Scoring of the nasal septum without the use of splinting grafts will lead to unpredictable results and subsequent redeviation of the middle and lower part of the nose.

POSTPROCEDURAL CARE

Oral and written instructions are of great importance to reduce postoperative complications. The instructions are similar to regular rhinoplasty protocol. The nasal packing is usually removed after 24 to 48 hours. Antibiotic-containing ointment can be administered to prevent crusts, local inflammation, and infection. The external dressing and sutures can be removed after 1 week. Additional taping or dressing of the nose is not necessary, and the patient should prevent trauma of the nose.

REHABILITATION AND RECOVERY

After diminishing of the ecchymosis and edema, most patients can continue their daily activities within 10 to 14 days. Care should be taken to avoid direct sun exposure and intensive sports and other activities that can traumatize the nose. The complete healing phase will take approximately 1 year; the nose, however, is stable enough after 6 weeks to permit wearing spectacles and more intensive physical activities.

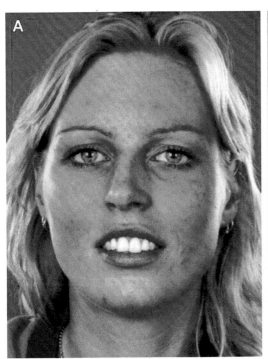
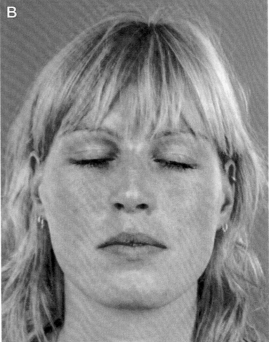

Fig. 1. (A) Preoperative frontal view of a 25-year-old female patient. There was a severe deviation of the nose to the right side. (B) Postoperative view. Realignment of the nasal skeleton was performed through an external approach rhinoplasty.

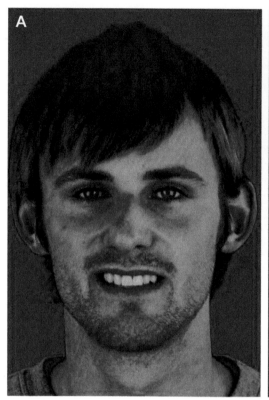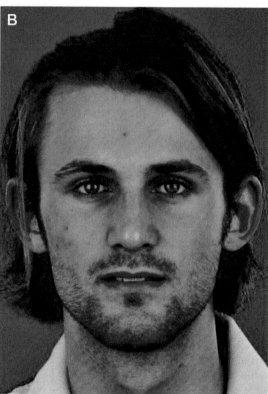

Fig. 2. (*A*) Preoperative frontal view of a 27-year-old male patient. The nasal skeleton was deviated to the right side. (*B*) Postoperative view after an external rhinoplasty. During the procedure, lateral and oblique osteotomies were performed bilaterally, while intermediate osteotomy was done on the left side only. The dorsal part of the nasal septal L-strut was scored and splinted with an internal cartilage on the left side. The caudal septum was fixated on the nasal spine with a permanent 4-0 suture.

OUTCOMES

With the described surgical technique of destabilization, realignment, fixation, and stabilization, the reconstructed nasal skeleton of the twisted nose deformity is predictable and stable for a satisfying long-term postoperative result (**Figs. 1** and **2**).

SUMMARY

The twisted nose is one of the most challenging procedures in rhinoplasty. The goal of surgery is to realign the nasal skeleton in order to create symmetry in the face and to restore nasal patency. Key in the surgical procedure is that all structures of the nasal skeleton need to be dissected free, mobilized, realigned, and stabilized. Important surgical steps are intermediate osteotomies on the contralateral side of the deviation for the upper nasal third. For the middle nasal vault, a unilateral spreader graft or splint on the nondeviated side may be necessary. For the lower nasal third, fixation of the caudal septum to the anterior nasal spine is often required.

SUPPLEMENTARY DATA

Supplementary data related to this article can be found online at http://dx.doi.org/10.1016/j.cps. 2015.08.004.

REFERENCES

1. Park SS. Fundamental principles in aesthetic rhinoplasty. Clin Exp Otorhinolaryngol 2011;4(2): 55–66.

2. Menger DJ, Tabink IC, Trenité GJ. Nasal septal abscess in children: reconstruction with autologous cartilage grafts on polydioxanone plate. Arch Otolaryngol Head Neck Surg 2008;134(8):842–7.

3. Gubisch W. Extracorporeal septoplasty for the markedly deviated septum. Arch Facial Plast Surg 2005; 7(4):218–26.

The Crooked Nose

Jamil Ahmad, MD, FRCSC[a],*, Rod J. Rohrich, MD, FACS[b]

KEYWORDS

- Crooked nose • Deviated nose • Twisted nose • Septal deviation

KEY POINTS

- Both esthetic and functional issues are typically present in patients with this deformity.
- A major septal deformity is almost always a component of severely deviated noses.
- The crooked nose results from extrinsic and intrinsic forces that produce distortion of the nasal structures and nasal deviation.
- The exposure afforded by the open approach allows maximal accuracy in diagnosis and control in achieving optimal repair of the crooked nose.
- The osteocartilaginous framework can be modified and reconstituted under direct visualization through the open approach, resulting in more predictable correction of the crooked nose.

INTRODUCTION

Correction of a crooked nose is one of the most common requests from patients presenting for rhinoplasty. The crooked nose is also referred to as the deviated or the twisted nose. The nose can appear crooked for several reasons (**Fig. 1**):

1. The nose or parts thereof deviate from the vertical midline of the face
2. The nose has asymmetries and irregularities that create an unbalanced and crooked appearance.

The crooked nose may be congenital or acquired secondary to trauma or previous surgery. Both esthetic and functional issues are typically present in patients with this deformity. Severely crooked noses are particularly challenging because multiple nasal structures, both external and internal, are commonly involved.[1–9] A major septal deformity is almost always a component of severely deviated noses.[1–4,9]

The crooked nose results from extrinsic and intrinsic forces that produce distortion of the nasal structures and nasal deviation.[1–3] Extrinsic forces include congenitally asymmetrical attachments of the osteocartilaginous skeleton, including attachments between the bony pyramid, the upper lateral cartilages, the lower lateral cartilages, and the septum, and can also be secondary to scar contracture following trauma or surgery. Intrinsic forces are those inherent to the septal cartilage as well as the upper and lower lateral cartilages.

Given the underlying structural deformities that are commonly observed in the crooked nose, the open approach is particularly useful and is the focus of this article.[1–11] Outlined are principles for treating the crooked nose to improve predictability and reliability of rhinoplasty for this challenging problem.

TREATMENT GOALS AND PLANNED OUTCOMES

Attaining consistently good esthetic and functional results when correcting the crooked nose requires a thorough understanding of nasal anatomy and physiology, accurate preoperative clinical analysis

[a] The Plastic Surgery Clinic, 1421 Hurontario Street, Mississauga, Ontario L5G 3H5, Canada; [b] Department of Plastic Surgery, University of Texas Southwestern Medical Center at Dallas, 1801 Inwood Road, Dallas, TX 75390-9132, USA
* Corresponding author.
E-mail address: drahmad@theplasticsurgeryclinic.com

Clin Plastic Surg 43 (2016) 99–113
http://dx.doi.org/10.1016/j.cps.2015.08.005
0094-1298/16/$ – see front matter © 2016 Elsevier Inc. All rights reserved.

plasticsurgery.theclinics.com

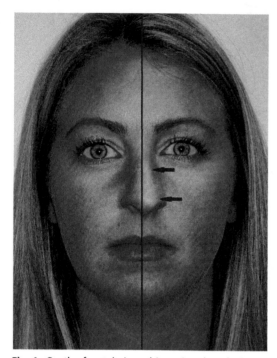

Fig. 1. On the frontal view, this patient has deviation of the bony vault, midvault, and nasal tip from the vertical midline of the face (*black vertical line*). In addition, she has irregular dorsal esthetic lines (*black arrow*) and an asymmetric nasal tip (*black arrow*) that contribute to the crooked appearance of her nose.

and intraoperative diagnosis, and the knowledge and skill to precisely execute a variety of surgical techniques required to predictably create an attractive and straight nose with a patent and functional nasal airway.[1–12] When performing rhinoplasty for the crooked nose, the goal should be to achieve both esthetic and functional goals in one surgery because the external deformity is often intimately related to the functional problems with nasal airflow.

PREOPERATIVE PLANNING AND PREPARATION

The preoperative consultation serves as an opportunity to understand the patient's concerns and expectations for surgery and to identify the nasal deformities and disproportions and formulate the goals of surgery.[10–12] Critical components of the history include age, history of trauma, nasal airway complaints, previous nasal surgery, smoking history, and any other medical comorbidities.

Clinical analysis is a key factor to successful outcomes in rhinoplasty. Evaluating nasofacial proportions and using a systematic nasal analysis

will allow for thorough and accurate identification of all structural abnormalities and deformities contributing to the crooked nose.[10–13] The external examination should include a systematic nasal analysis from frontal, lateral, and basal views. Particular emphasis is placed on identifying the abnormalities that contribute to the crooked nose. Asymmetries and irregularities of the bony vault, dorsal esthetic lines, nasal tip, and nostrils, as well as deviation of these structures from the facial midline, should be noted.

Standardized photography with frontal, oblique, lateral, and basal views should be obtained for all patients. Careful evaluation of these photographs will often reveal subtle deformities that were not appreciated during physical examination. Reviewing these photographs with the patient can facilitate communication and help the patient to fully understand the deformities that are present and the goals of surgery. In addition, photographs are a key component of the medical record and can be used as a reference postoperatively.

The frontal view allows evaluation of the nasal asymmetries and its relationship to facial asymmetries. In some instances, nasal asymmetries are secondary to asymmetries of the facial skeleton, and rhinoplasty will have a limited effect on full correction of these. The basal view is especially important for assessing caudal septal deviation, tip deviation, and asymmetries of the nostrils related to the columella and alar rims.

There are 3 basic types of nasal deviation, 2 of which have subtypes[1–3]:

1. Caudal septal deviation
   Straight septal tilt
   S-shaped septal tilt
2. Concave deformity
   C-shaped dorsal deformity
   Reverse C-shaped deformity
3. Concave/convex dorsal deformity.

The internal examination is performed to evaluate for anterior septal deviations and the status of inferior turbinates.[4,9–12,14–16]

After evaluating the patient, the goals of surgery should be reviewed with the patient. The patient should understand the esthetic goals of surgery and if there will be any improvement in nasal airflow. There should be a frank discussion about what can be realistically achieved when performing rhinoplasty for the crooked nose: it is impossible to create a perfectly straight and symmetric nose. Setting the patient's expectations preoperatively is critical to avoid dissatisfaction postoperatively.[10–12]

PRINCIPLES FOR TREATING THE CROOKED NOSE

Correction of the crooked nose is based on the 8 key operative principles (**Box 1**).[1–3]

Wide Exposure of Deviated Structures

The open approach is preferred for the management of the crooked nose.[1–3,10,11] The exposure afforded by the open approach allows maximal accuracy in diagnosis and control in achieving optimal repair of the crooked nose. The crooked nose results from extrinsic and intrinsic forces that produce distortion of the nasal structures and nasal deviation. The open approach is particularly advantageous for releasing attachments between the soft tissue and osteocartilaginous framework that are creating extrinsic deforming forces. Following release of these extrinsic forces, intrinsic forces contributing to distortion of each anatomic part can be fully appreciated without distortion from the overlying soft tissue envelope. The osteocartilaginous framework can be modified and reconstituted under direct visualization through the open approach, resulting in more predictable correction of the crooked nose (**Fig. 2**).

Wide Release of Mucoperichondrial Attachments

The mucoperichondrial attachments are preserved when possible to maintain the blood supply to the cartilage to minimize resorption.[1–4,10,11,14] However, septal deviation frequently occurs as part of the crooked nose, and the mucoperichondrial attachments to the deviated portion of the septum must be widely released before the septum can be returned to the midline. Beginning at the anterior septal angle, bilateral

---

Box 1

Key operative principles for treating the crooked nose

1. Wide exposure of deviated structures
2. Wide release of mucoperichondrial attachments
3. Straightening the deviated septum and septal reconstruction
4. Correcting caudal septal deviation
5. Correction of dorsal septal deviation
6. Restoration of septal support
7. Inferior turbinate surgery
8. Nasal osteotomies

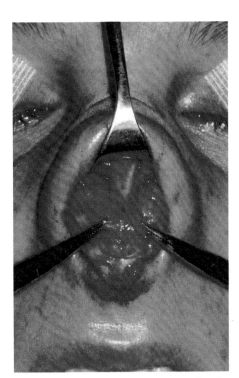

Fig. 2. Intraoperative view shows visualization of dorsum with open approach.

submucoperichondrial flaps are elevated and a submucoperichondrial dissection is performed using a Cottle elevator to free the septum from the overlying mucosa. In the case of caudal septal deviation, the mucoperichondrium must be released all the way to the anterior nasal spine. Bilateral mucoperichondrial tunnels are dissected deep to the upper lateral cartilages, and a scalpel is used to separate the upper lateral cartilages from the dorsal septum (**Fig. 3**). If the deformity exists because asymmetrical upper lateral cartilages are causing twisting of the septum, this will result in straightening of the septum. Once this has been done, the septum can be visualized to accurately assess for any intrinsic forces causing septal deviation.

If extrinsic forces are causing distortion of the lower lateral cartilages and upper lateral cartilages at the scroll, these can be released through a direct incision through the scroll area, or if the lateral crura require modification using techniques such as cephalic trim and lower lateral crural turnover flaps.

Straightening the Deviated Septum and Septal Reconstruction

Once the deviated septum has been widely exposed and separated from the upper lateral cartilages, it must be straightened by addressing and

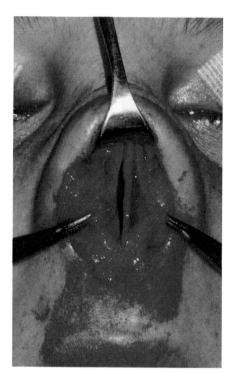

Fig. 3. Intraoperative view shows component approach to dorsum with separation of upper lateral cartilages from dorsal septum.

Fig. 4. Intraoperative view shows reduction of dorsal septum.

correcting the intrinsic deforming forces.[1–4,10,11,14] The goal is to straighten the septum and return the septum to the midline while ensuring that the remaining anterior septum has adequate strength for dorsal nasal support.

Before septal reconstruction, the component dorsal hump reduction should be performed (**Fig. 4**). After setting the dorsal profile, the deviated portion should be resected, taking care to preserve at least 10 mm of an L-strut. However, this will depend on the strength of the septal cartilage, and in many instances, a width of 15 mm or more may be required to ensure long-term support (**Fig. 5**). The resection may include septal cartilage, maxillary crest, vomer, and perpendicular plate of the ethmoid. The L-strut should remain attached to the perpendicular plate at the keystone area and the anterior nasal spine and maxillary crest area. In addition, curving the transition points between the perpendicular plate of the ethmoid and the dorsal L-strut and, also, between the dorsal and caudal L-strut can help to strengthen the construct.

Septal reconstruction involves returning the deviated septum to the midline. The principle of cartilage preservation is paramount. Cartilaginous septum that is deviated or required for grafting should be removed. When addressing the bony

septum, the septum can be microfractured and returned to the midline. In cases of C- or S-shaped craniocaudal deviation, there is vertical excess of the septum, and removing the inferior aspect of the septum allows for microfracture of the remaining septum and return to the midline. Microfracture should be performed in a careful and controlled manner to avoid uncontrolled fractures into the superior nasal septum and cribriform plate. This is particularly important in posttraumatic cases where there may have been a prior septal fracture. Bony spurs of the septum can be removed using Takahashi forceps. Septal cartilage or bone should be removed with ease; if there is any resistance, residual soft tissue attachments should be completely released.

Correcting Caudal Septal Deviation

Following reconstruction of the posterior septum, if there is persistent deviation of the anterior septum, this is commonly due to vertical excess of the anterior septum (**Fig. 6**).[1–4,10,11,14] Vertical excess of the septum is associated with caudal septal deviation, and the caudal septum can be found seated on one side or the other of the anterior nasal spine and maxillary crest as opposed to directly articulated with these structures.

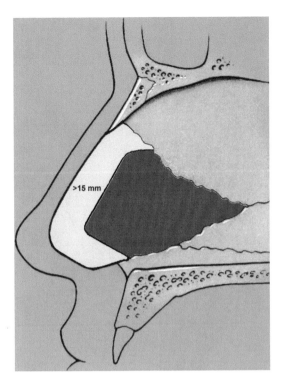

Fig. 5. In many instances, the width of the dorsal and caudal L-strut should be 15 mm or more to ensure long-term support. Curving the transition points between the perpendicular plate of the ethmoid and the dorsal L-strut and between the dorsal and caudal L-strut can help add strength. (*From* Constantine FC, Ahmad J, Geissler P, et al. Simplifying the management of caudal septal deviation in rhinoplasty. Plast Reconstr Surg 2014;134:380e; with permission.)

Correction of vertical excess of the septum and caudal septal deviation is performed by disarticulating the caudal portion of the L-strut from the osteocartilaginous junction with the anterior nasal spine and maxillary crest. The degree of vertical excess is assessed, and this is excised to allow the previously deviated septum to be returned to midline. A 5-0 polydioxanone (PDS; Ethicon US, LLC, Somerville, NJ, USA) suture is used to suture the caudal septum down to the periosteum of the anterior nasal spine (**Fig. 7**). When the anterior nasal spine is located away from the midline, it may be necessary to perform an osteotomy to the anterior nasal spine to return it to the midline or excise the anterior nasal spine and suture the septum down to the periosteum of the maxilla. Excessive resection of the anterior nasal spine can damage the anterior maxillary nerve and subsequently cause some upper lip numbness. When extensive work has been done to the caudal septum, it is usually necessary to place several through-and-through horizontal mattress 5-0 chromic gut sutures in the caudal septum to reapproximate the caudal mucoperichondrial flaps to the midline, allowing the flaps to scar down in the midline position and providing extra long-term support.

In some instances, it is necessary to be more aggressive in correcting severe deformities of the anterior septum. Scoring or partial-thickness wedge excisions coupled with the application of splinting grafts may be required to establish a straight and stable L-strut.[1–4,10,11,14] Similarly, deformities of the anterior septum stemming from

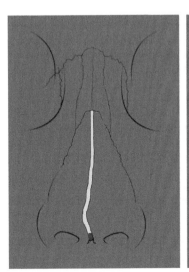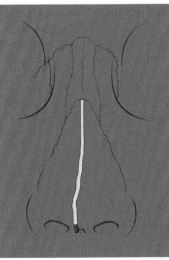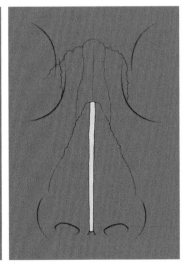

Fig. 6. (*left*) Cranial caudal septal deviation due to vertical excess shown in red. (*center*) Release of the caudal L-strut from the maxillary crest shows amount of vertical excess in red. (*right*) Repositioning of the caudal L-strut to the midline after excision of the excess caudal L-strut. (*From* Constantine FC, Ahmad J, Geissler P, et al. Simplifying the management of caudal septal deviation in rhinoplasty. Plast Reconstr Surg 2014;134:381e; with permission)

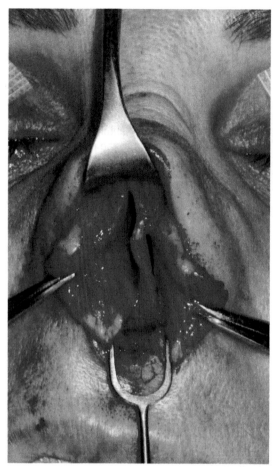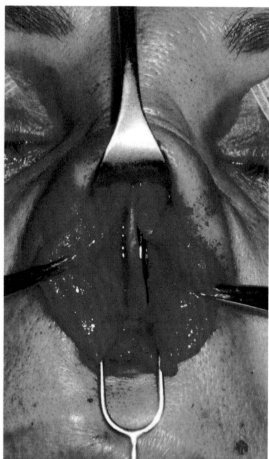

Fig. 7. Intraoperative views show correction of vertical excess of the septum (*left*) before release of the caudal L-strut and shortening followed by (*right*) repositioning to the midline by suturing to the anterior nasal spine.

previous fracture lines, such as sharp angulations or overlapping segments, also require more complex maneuvers to first weaken or divide the L-strut and then reinforce or reconstruct the L-strut into a straight construct. Other techniques, such as splinting grafts, tongue-in-groove grafts, drill-hole fixation, or medial crural footplate excision, may be necessary for adequate correction of severe caudal septal deviations. These techniques may require more cartilage than present in the septum and necessitate ear or rib cartilage harvest.

Correction of Dorsal Septal Deviation

Correction dorsal septal deviations will vary. In the case of a high dorsal septal deviation, placement of a pushing spreader graft on the same side as that the dorsal septum is deviated to, between the bony vault and upper lateral cartilage laterally, and dorsal septum, medially, can help move the septum to the midline (**Fig. 8**).[1–4,10,11,14] Deviation of the dorsal septum at the midvault may require placement of a spreader graft on the concave side to camouflage any residual deformity. Cartilage scoring techniques may be necessary to help straighten more severe dorsal septal deviation.

If a significant deformity persists despite these techniques, sequential inferior full-thickness cuts in the deviated portion of the dorsal septal cartilage are made up through 50% of the remaining dorsal L-strut (**Fig. 9**),[1–4] permitting straightening of the deviated septum, but also weakening its support. Bilateral spreader grafts may be necessary to maintain support and restore the dorsal esthetic lines.[15,16]

After the septum has been straightened, the upper and lower lateral cartilages are reassessed for symmetry. Any remaining asymmetries should be addressed by trimming and securing the upper lateral cartilages by suturing them to the dorsal septum before performing a lower lateral cartilage manipulation. Autospreader flaps can also be used

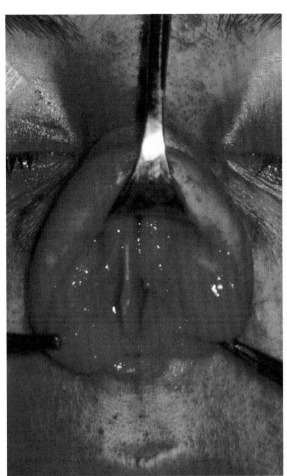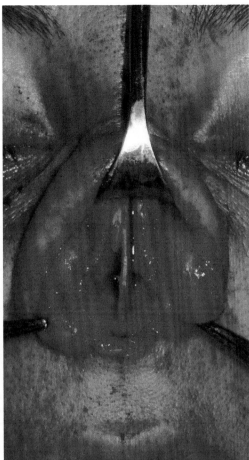

Fig. 8. Intraoperative view of high septal deviation to right before (*left*) and after (*right*) placement of a pushing spreader graft.

to smooth and straighten the dorsum as well as camouflage any residual midvault deformity.[17–19] It may be necessary to perform clocking sutures from the upper lateral cartilage to the dorsal septum to help reposition the L-strut in the midline.[20]

Restoration of Septal Support

The midvault should be reconstituted with upper lateral cartilage tension-spanning sutures.[20] In some instances, autospreader flaps can also be used to smooth and straighten the dorsum as well as camouflage any residual midvault deformity.[15,16] If the dorsal septum is weak, long-term support is restored by buttressing the dorsal septum with spreader grafts.[17–19] The spreader grafts serve to maintain or restore the integrity of the internal nasal valves, to restore the dorsal esthetic lines, and to strengthen and maintain long-term septal support. The spreader grafts are

secured with two or three 5-0 PDS mattress sutures either unilaterally or bilaterally parallel to the dorsal septum according to the deformity being addressed. Asymmetrical (unilateral) placement will camouflage of any residual deviation.[21] Following spreader graft placement, the midvault should be reconstituted with upper lateral cartilage tension-spanning sutures (**Fig. 10**).[20]

Inferior Turbinate Surgery

Septal deviation can be a developmental abnormality or may occur after trauma and is commonly associated with nasal airway problems.[1–4,10,11,14] Septal deviation can lead to compensatory inferior turbinate hypertrophy and typically occurs on the contralateral side of the septal deviation.[1–4,10,11,14,22,23] Even if the patient does not complain of nasal airway obstruction preoperatively, straightening of the septal deviation may lead to narrowing of the anterior nasal airway if

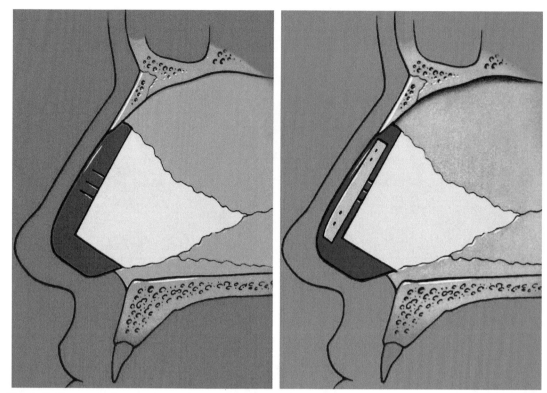

Fig. 9. (*left*) For significant deformities, sequential inferior full-thickness cuts up through 50% of the deviated portion of the septum are made. This will weaken the cartilage sufficiently to allow it to be straightened. (*right*) Support is restored by securing spreader grafts with 5-0 PDS mattress sutures. (*From* Rohrich RJ, Gunter JP, Deuber MA, et al. The deviated nose: optimizing results using a simplified classification and algorithmic approach. Plast Reconstr Surg 2002;110:1513; [discussion: 1524–5]; with permission.)

inferior turbinate hypertrophy is present. In most cases of mucosal hypertrophy, the inferior turbinate can be outfractured. In some cases of inferior turbinate hypertrophy, bony hypertrophy is present and submucous microfracture and resection of the hypertrophied anterior inferior turbinate are performed to allow for an adequate postoperative airway.

Nasal Osteotomies

Nasal osteotomies are commonly required to straighten and improve symmetry of both the superior dorsal esthetic lines and the bony nose-cheek junction (**Fig. 11**).[1–4,10,11,21,24–27] Accurately planned lateral and medial nasal osteotomies will restore symmetry to the bony vault. Before performing osteotomies, the dorsal profile must be reassessed to determine whether dorsal reduction of the bony vault is necessary. The orientation of the nasal bones must be considered when reducing the bony hump when there is asymmetrical bony deviation. Less bone will need to be excised or rasped from the nasal bone on the

deviated side that is more vertically oriented; this will prevent excessive reduction in nasal bone dorsal height of that side after the nasal bone is infractured and medialized.

Lateral osteotomies alone will be sufficient only in the settings of bony vault deviation with symmetric nasal bones or a significant open roof. In some cases where significant bony asymmetries are present, medial osteotomies may also be required to allow adequate repositioning of the bony vault.[21,24–27] These medial osteotomies are required to allow independent movement of the nasal bones. If required, medial osteotomies should be performed before the lateral osteotomies are done. If bony vault convexity is present, double-level osteotomies will be necessary. The surgeon should be careful not to excessively free up the periosteum of the nasal bones, because comminution can result from multiple osteotomies and the periosteum can prevent the displacement of these comminuted fragments.

The dorsal profile should be reassessed after osteotomies to ensure that repositioning on the

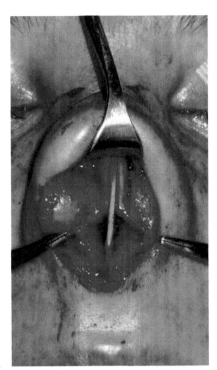

Fig. 10. Intraoperative view shows reconstitution of the nasal dorsum with bilateral autospreader flaps and upper lateral cartilage tension-spanning sutures.

nasal bones has not created any dorsal irregularity. Only minimal bony rasping and incremental cartilage reduction can be performed after the osteotomies.

PROCEDURAL APPROACH

The open approach is used with a stairstep transcolumellar incision connected to bilateral infracartilaginous incisions.[1–4,10,11,28] The soft tissue is elevated off of the osteocartilaginous framework. At the bony vault, only enough exposure should be performed to allow manipulation of the dorsum so that the lateral soft tissue attachments are preserved for bony stability if osteotomies are required.

A component dorsal approach to the dorsum is performed as follows[10,11,28–33]:

1. Release of the upper lateral cartilages from the dorsal septum
2. Resection of the dorsal septum incrementally
3. Rasping of the bony dorsum
4. Restoration of the dorsal esthetic lines.

The anterior septal angle is exposed and scored. Bilateral mucoperichondrial flaps are elevated using the Cottle elevator beginning.[1–4,10,11,14,28–31] Bilateral mucoperichondrial

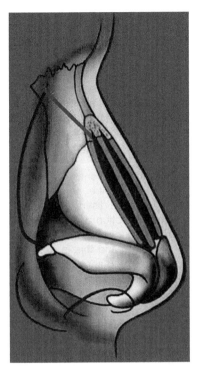

Fig. 11. Preferred location of low-to-low lateral nasal osteotomy (*black*) and superior oblique osteotomy (*red*). These are percutaneous discontinuous osteotomies. If no open roof is present, then a medial osteotomy will be required to address an asymmetric bony vault. (*From* Rohrich RJ, Gunter JP, Deuber MA, et al. The deviated nose: optimizing results using a simplified classification and algorithmic approach. Plast Reconstr Surg 2002;110:1514; [discussion: 1524–5]; with permission.)

tunnels are dissected deep to the upper lateral cartilages, and then both are separated from the dorsal septum using a scalpel. If dorsal reduction is required, component dorsal hump reduction is performed. The dorsal septum is incrementally reduced. The bony hump is reduced using a rasp. If the nasal bones are asymmetric, rasping must be performed obliquely, taking care to reduce the side of the more vertically oriented bone to a lesser degree so that the nasal bones are symmetric after lateral osteotomies. Three-point digital palpation of the dorsum, right and left dorsal esthetic lines and midline, is performed until the dorsum and keystone are smooth.

Septal reconstruction and cartilage graft harvesting are performed through a dorsal approach after the bilateral mucoperichondrial flaps are elevated posteriorly to expose the cartilaginous and, if necessary, the bony septum.[1–4,10,11,14,28–31] Posterior septal deviation is repositioned to the midline or resected, taking care to maintain at least a 10- to 15-mm L-strut dorsally and caudally. If possible, a wider L-strut should be preserved. The septal resection may include septal cartilage, maxillary crest, vomer, and perpendicular plate of the ethmoid.

If the remaining anterior caudal septum is deviated off the anterior nasal spine and maxillary crest but does not have a dorsal deviation or vertical excess of the septum, it is anatomically reduced and secured in position with a figure-of-8 suture of 5-0 PDS to the periosteum of the contralateral anterior nasal spine.[1–4,10,11,14] If a significant intrinsic deviation is present, this is typically due to vertical excess of the septum. The caudal portion of the L-strut is disarticulated from the osteocartilagenous junction with the anterior nasal spine and maxillary crest. The degree of vertical excess is assessed, and this is excised to allow the previously deviated septum to be returned to midline. A 5-0 PDS suture is used to suture the septum down to the periosteum of the anterior nasal spine.

If the septum still remains deviated, posterior full-thickness parallel cuts through 50% of the dorsal L-strut are made to remove these intrinsic forces.[1–3] If present, any remaining cartilaginous asymmetries are now addressed by trimming the upper lateral cartilages and performing autospreader flaps or spreader grafts.[1–4,14–19] If required, spreader grafts are fashioned from the harvested septum and contoured to 4 to 6 mm in height and 30 to 32 mm in length. They are secured to the L-strut with at least two 5-0 PDS horizontal mattress sutures to restore support and internal nasal valve integrity. Asymmetric spreader grafts may be used if necessary to camouflage any residual deformity to accurately restore the dorsal esthetic lines.

In some cases, correction of the deviated nose does not require spreader grafts. Instead, autospreader flaps may be used to both camouflage residual concavity of the dorsal septum and restore the internal valve.[14–20] In addition, clocking sutures can be placed to the autospreader flap to control residual septal deviations.

If the dorsal septum remains straight without the use of spreader grafts or autospreader flaps, then the midvault and dorsal esthetic lines should be restored using upper lateral cartilage tension-spanning sutures.[20,29–31]

The inferior turbinates are now assessed. If mucosal hypertrophy of the anteroinferior turbinate is present, outfracture is performed.[4,10,11,14,22,23] If bony hypertrophy is present, limited submucous microfracture and resection of the hypertrophied bone anteriorly are performed with preservation of the overlying mucosa.

If a bony vault deviation or asymmetry is present or there is an open roof, then percutaneous perforated lateral nasal osteotomies are performed using the 2-mm osteotome.[1–3,10,11,21,24–27] Generally, lateral osteotomies are performed, but medial osteotomies will be necessary in the absence of an open roof or in the presence of asymmetric nasal bones that must be moved independently. For convex deformities of individual nasal bones, double-level osteotomies are performed. The periosteum is preserved as much as possible so that displacement of any fragments does not occur in the event of comminution. Three-point digital palpation of the dorsum should be performed after osteotomies to ensure no dorsal irregularities are remaining.

Tip refinement is performed using a variety of techniques.[10,11,28,34–36] A columellar strut graft may be required and helps to unify the tip complex and also control and contour the basal esthetic lines.[10,11,28,37–42] The length and strength of the alar rims and lateral crura are assessed.[10,11,28,43,44] Most commonly, alar contour grafts are used to strengthen the alar rims and soft triangles. The nostrils and alar bases are assessed, and if there is asymmetry of nostril size or alar flaring, alar base excisions are performed to correct these.[1,3,10,11]

The incisions are closed, and antibiotic ointment–coated Doyle internal nasal splints are placed in each nostril.[10,11,45] Steri-Strips are applied to the dorsum from the supratip to the radix, and a firmly contoured Denver dorsal nasal splint is applied.

POSTPROCEDURE CARE

Postoperative management of rhinoplasty patients is an important component of rhinoplasty and an extension of what was performed in the operating room. The external and internal splints as well as the sutures are removed 1 week following surgery.[10,11,45] The nasal skin can be taped with Steri-Strips following removal of the external splint to help control edema. It is essential to provide support during this interval and reassure patients that what they are seeing is a normal part of the recovery process. Ultimately, the final results after open rhinoplasty can take more than 1 year to appreciate. In patients with thick skin, edema may take even longer to fully resolve.

OUTCOMES

A 29-year-old primary rhinoplasty patient had a history of a deviated nose and nasal airway obstruction (**Fig. 12**). She had a high dorsal septal

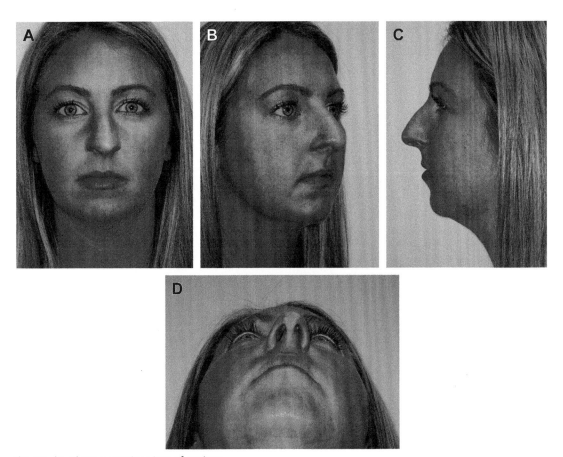

Fig. 12. (*A–D*) Preoperative view of patient.

deviation and a bulbous tip deviated to the left. The frontal view demonstrates the high dorsal septal deviation, irregular dorsal esthetic lines, and a bulbous tip that is deviated to the left. On the lateral view, the patient exhibits a prominent dorsal hump, supratip fullness, and an overprojected tension tip with blunting of the columellarlobular angle. The basal view demonstrates caudal septal deviation, nostril asymmetry, and a bulbous tip deviated to the left.

The surgical plan consisted of the following (**Fig. 13**):

1. Open rhinoplasty
2. Component dorsal hump reduction
3. Septal reconstruction and septal graft harvest with preservation of 30-mm-wide L-strut
4. Correction of vertical excess with resection of caudal septal excess and fixation of caudal L-strut to anterior nasal spine with 5-0 PDS suture
5. Bilateral inferior turbinate outfracture
6. Right spreader graft
7. Bilateral autospreader flaps
8. Clocking upper lateral cartilage tension-spanning sutures to draw the dorsal septum-right spreader graft complex to the right
9. Unification of tip complex with a columellar strut graft secured with intercrural sutures
10. Cephalic incision of lateral crura preserving a 6-mm alar rim strip and allowing cephalic edge of lateral crura to fall deep to alar rim strip
11. Interdomal and transdomal sutures to shape tip
12. Right lateral crus transection and overlap to draw the tip complex to the right
13. Bilateral percutaneous discontinuous lateral nasal osteotomies
14. Bilateral alar contour grafts to correct alar weakness.

The patient is shown 9 months postoperatively (**Fig. 14**). Note the straight nasal dorsum with balanced dorsal esthetic lines. The asymmetric, bulbous tip has been corrected. The lateral view reveals a straight dorsum with slight supratip

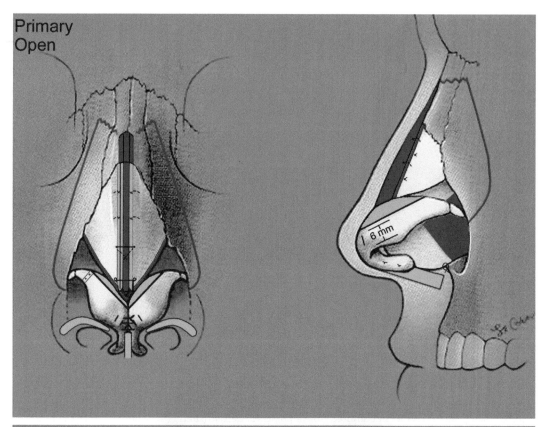

Primary
Open

6 mm

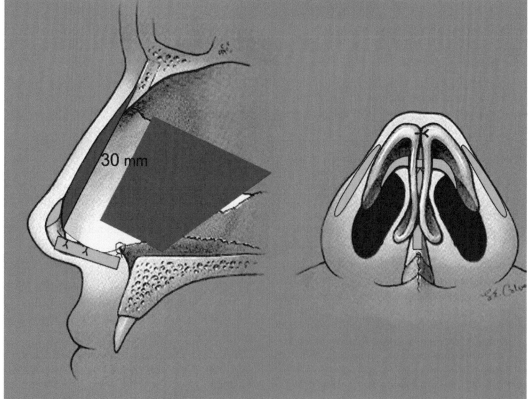

30 mm

Fig. 13. Gunter diagram illustrating surgical plan.

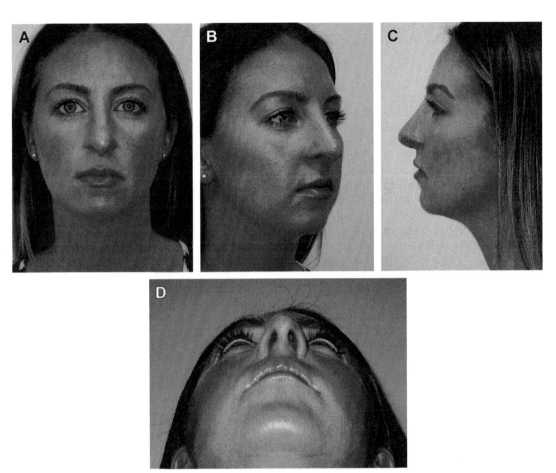

Fig. 14. (*A–D*) Nine-month postoperative view of patient.

break and correction of the tension tip with an improved nasal tip-upper lip transition as well as restoration of the columellar-labial angle. The basal view shows the significant correction of the leftward tip deviation and bulbosity and improved symmetry of the nostrils.

SUMMARY

The crooked nose is a common and challenging problem. Both esthetic and functional issues are typically present. There are several key operative principles for treating the crooked nose that lead to consistent outcomes. The exposure afforded by the open approach allows maximal accuracy in diagnosis and control in achieving optimal repair of the crooked nose. The open approach is particularly advantageous for releasing attachments between the soft tissue and osteocartilaginous framework that are creating extrinsic deforming forces. The osteocartilaginous framework can be modified and reconstituted under direct visualization through the open approach, resulting in more predictable correction of the crooked nose.

REFERENCES

1. Rohrich RJ, Gunter JP, Deuber MA, et al. The deviated nose: optimizing results using a simplified classification and algorithmic approach. Plast Reconstr Surg 2002;110:1509–23 [discussion: 1524–5].
2. Constantine FC, Ahmad J, Geissler P, et al. Simplifying the management of caudal septal deviation in rhinoplasty. Plast Reconstr Surg 2014;134: 379e–88e.
3. Rohrich RJ, Gunter JP, Adams WP Jr, et al. Comprehensive management of the deviated nose. In: Rohrich RJ, Adams WP Jr, Ahmad J, et al, editors. Dallas rhinoplasty: nasal surgery by the masters. 3rd edition. St Louis (MO): Quality Medical Publishing, Inc; 2014. p. 1029–63.
4. Ahmad J, Rohrich RJ, Lee MR. Safe management of the nasal airway. In: Rohrich RJ, Adams WP Jr, Ahmad J, et al, editors. Dallas rhinoplasty: nasal surgery by the masters. 3rd edition. St Louis (MO): Quality Medical Publishing, Inc; 2014. p. 975–98.
5. Ahmad J, Rohrich RJ, Lee MR. The aesthetics and management of the nasal base. In: Rohrich RJ, Adams WP Jr, Ahmad J, et al, editors. Dallas

rhinoplasty: nasal surgery by the masters. 3rd edition. St Louis (MO): Quality Medical Publishing, Inc; 2014. p. 641–63.

6. Gunter JP, Rohrich RJ. Management of the deviated nose. The importance of septal reconstruction. Clin Plast Surg 1988;15:43–55.

7. Byrd HS, Salomon J, Flood J. Correction of the crooked nose. Plast Reconstr Surg 1998;102:2148–57.

8. Guyuron B, Behmand RA. Caudal nasal deviation. Plast Reconstr Surg 2003;111:2449–60.

9. Guyuron B, Uzzo CD, Scull H. A practical classification of septonasal deviation and an effective guide to septal surgery. Plast Reconstr Surg 1999;104: 2202–9 [discussion: 2210–2].

10. Rohrich RJ, Ahmad J. Rhinoplasty. Plast Reconstr Surg 2011;128:49e–73e.

11. Rohrich RJ, Ahmad J. A practical approach to rhinoplasty: leading edge CME. Plast Reconstr Surg, in press.

12. Rohrich RJ, Ahmad J. Preoperative concepts for rhinoplasty. In: Rohrich RJ, Adams WP Jr, Ahmad J, et al, editors. Dallas rhinoplasty: nasal surgery by the masters. 3rd edition. St Louis (MO): Quality Medical Publishing, Inc; 2014. p. 63–83.

13. Rohrich RJ, Ahmad J, Gunter JP. Nasofacial proportions and systematic nasal analysis. In: Rohrich RJ, Adams WP Jr, Ahmad J, et al, editors. Dallas rhinoplasty: nasal surgery by the masters. 3rd edition. St Louis (MO): Quality Medical Publishing, Inc; 2014. p. 85–110.

14. Howard BK, Rohrich RJ. Understanding the nasal airway: principles and practice. Plast Reconstr Surg 2002;109:1128–46.

15. Sheen JH. Spreader grafts: a method of reconstructing the roof of the middle nasal vault following rhinoplasty. Plast Reconstr Surg 1984;73:230–9.

16. Rohrich RJ, Hollier LH. Use of spreader grafts in the external approach to rhinoplasty. Clin Plast Surg 1996;23:255–62.

17. Byrd HS, Meade RA, Gonyon DL. Using the autospreader flaps in primary rhinoplasty. Plast Reconstr Surg 2007;119:1897–902.

18. Gruber RP, Park E, Newman J, et al. The spreader flap in primary rhinoplasty. Plast Reconstr Surg 2007;119:1903–10.

19. Gruber RP, Perkins SW. Humpectomy and spreader flaps. Clin Plast Surg 2010;37:285–91.

20. Geissler PJ, Roostaeian J, Lee MR, et al. Role of upper lateral cartilage tension spanning suture in restoring dorsal aesthetic lines in rhinoplasty. Plast Reconstr Surg 2014;133:7e–11e.

21. Rohrich RJ, Janis JE. Osteotomies in rhinoplasty: an updated technique. Aesthet Surg J 2003;23:56–8.

22. Rohrich RJ, Krueger JK, Adams WP Jr, et al. Rationale for submucous resection of hypertrophied inferior turbinates in rhinoplasty: an evolution. Plast Reconstr Surg 2001;108:536–44.

23. Pollock RA, Rohrich RJ. Inferior turbinate surgery: an adjunct to successful treatment of nasal obstruction in 408 patients. Plast Reconstr Surg 1984;74:227–36.

24. Rohrich RJ, Adams WP Jr, Ahmad J. Nasal osteotomies. In: Rohrich RJ, Adams WP Jr, Ahmad J, et al, editors. Dallas rhinoplasty: nasal surgery by the masters. 3rd edition. St Louis (MO): Quality Medical Publishing, Inc; 2014. p. 249–73.

25. Rohrich RJ, Minoli JJ, Adams WP, et al. The lateral nasal osteotomy in rhinoplasty: an anatomic endoscopic comparison of the external versus the internal approach. Plast Reconstr Surg 1997;99:1309–12.

26. Rohrich RJ, Krueger JK, Adams WP Jr, et al. Achieving consistency in the lateral nasal osteotomy during rhinoplasty: an external perforated technique. Plast Reconstr Surg 2001;108:2122–30.

27. Rohrich RJ, Janis JE, Adams WP, et al. An update on the lateral nasal osteotomy in rhinoplasty: an anatomic endoscopic comparison of the external versus internal approach. Plast Reconstr Surg 2003;111:2461–2.

28. Rohrich RJ, Ahmad J. Getting rhinoplasty right the first time. In: Rohrich RJ, Adams WP Jr, Ahmad J, et al, editors. Dallas rhinoplasty: nasal surgery by the masters. 3rd edition. St Louis (MO): Quality Medical Publishing, Inc; 2014. p. 159–76.

29. Rohrich RJ, Ahmad J, Roostaienen J. Evaluation and surgical approach to the nasal dorsum: component dorsal hump reduction and dorsal reconstitution. In: Rohrich RJ, Adams WP Jr, Ahmad J, et al, editors. Dallas rhinoplasty: nasal surgery by the masters. 3rd edition. St. Louis (MO): Quality Medical Publishing, Inc; 2014. p. 219–48.

30. Rohrich RJ, Muzaffar AR, Janis JE. Component dorsal hump reduction: the importance of maintaining dorsal aesthetic lines in rhinoplasty. Plast Reconstr Surg 2004;114:1298–308.

31. Roostaeian J, Unger JG, Lee MR, et al. Reconstitution of the nasal dorsum following component dorsal reduction in primary rhinoplasty. Plast Reconstr Surg 2014;133:509–18.

32. Lee MR, Unger JG, Rohrich RJ. Management of the nasal dorsum in rhinoplasty: a systematic review of the literature regarding technique, outcomes, and complications. Plast Reconstr Surg 2011;128:538e–50e.

33. Mojallal A, Ouyang D, Saint-Cyr M, et al. Dorsal aesthetic lines in rhinoplasty: a quantitative outcome-based assessment of the component dorsal reduction technique. Plast Reconstr Surg 2011; 128:280–8.

34. Gunter JP, Lee MR, Ahmad J, et al. Basic nasal tip surgery: anatomy and technique. In: Rohrich RJ, Adams WP Jr, Ahmad J, et al, editors. Dallas rhinoplasty: nasal surgery by the masters. 3rd edition. St Louis (MO): Quality Medical Publishing, Inc; 2014. p. 321–50.

35. Rohrich RJ, Janis JE, Ghavami A, et al. A predictable and algorithmic approach to tip refinement and projection. In: Rohrich RJ, Adams WP Jr, Ahmad J, et al, editors. Dallas rhinoplasty: nasal surgery by the masters. 3rd edition. St Louis (MO): Quality Medical Publishing, Inc; 2014. p. 441–71.

36. Ghavami A, Janis JE, Acikel C, et al. Tip shaping in primary rhinoplasty: an algorithmic approach. Plast Reconstr Surg 2008;122:1229–41.

37. Rohrich RJ, Kurkjian TJ, Hoxworth RE, et al. The effect of the columellar strut graft on nasal tip position in primary rhinoplasty. Plast Reconstr Surg 2012; 130:926–32.

38. Unger JG, Lee MR, Kwon RK, et al. A multivariate analysis of nasal tip deprojection. Plast Reconstr Surg 2012;129:1163–7.

39. Rohrich RJ, Hoxworth RE, Kurkjian TJ. The role of the columellar strut in rhinoplasty: indications and rationale. Plast Reconstr Surg 2012;129:118e–25e.

40. Lee MR, Malafa M, Roostaeian J, et al. Soft-tissue composition of the columella and potential relevance to rhinoplasty. Plast Reconstr Surg 2014; 134:621–5.

41. Lee MR, Tabbal G, Kurkjian TJ, et al. Classifying deformities of the columella base in rhinoplasty. Plast Reconstr Surg 2014;133:464e–70e.

42. Geissler PJ, Lee MR, Roostaeian J, et al. Reshaping the medial nostril and columellar base: five-step medial crural footplate approximation. Plast Reconstr Surg 2013;132:553–7.

43. Rohrich RJ, Raniere J Jr, Ha RY. The alar contour graft: correction and prevention of alar rim deformities in rhinoplasty. Plast Reconstr Surg 2002;109: 2495–505.

44. Janis JE, Trussler A, Ghavami A, et al. Lower lateral crural turnover flap in open rhinoplasty. Plast Reconstr Surg 2009;123:1830–41.

45. Rohrich RJ, Ahmad J. Postoperative management of the rhinoplasty patient. In: Rohrich RJ, Adams WP Jr, Ahmad J, et al, editors. Dallas rhinoplasty: nasal surgery by the masters. 3rd edition. St Louis (MO): Quality Medical Publishing, Inc; 2014. p. 133–46.

Reshaping of the Broad and Bulbous Nasal Tip

Karan Dhir, MD[a], Ashkan Ghavami, MD[b],*

KEYWORDS

- Bulbous nasal tip • Broad nasal tip • Boxy nasal tip • Nasal tip surgery • Nasal tip reshaping
- Tip sutures • Nasal tip grafting • Ethnic rhinoplasty

KEY POINTS

- The ideal nasal tip is achieved when there is a balanced interaction between the soft tissue covering and underlying nasal framework.
- Contouring maneuvers that establish, and maintain, aesthetically pleasing highlights and shadowing around the nasal tip region are mandatory for the overall balance of a truly refined nasal appearance.
- Comprehensive management of the broad nasal tip requires maneuvers that allow for a favorable contour extending from the lateral dome region to the alar margins.
- Surgical changes to the nasal framework dynamically alter the relationship between the tip structures, dorsum, and overlying soft tissues and must be evaluated preoperatively and intraoperatively to direct surgical maneuvers.

INTRODUCTION

Obtaining an aesthetically harmonized nasal tip complex remains one of the most challenging aspects of both primary and revision rhinoplasty. The ideal nasal tip is achieved when there is a balanced interaction between the soft tissue covering and underlying nasal skeleton.[1–7] It has been well described that contouring maneuvers that establish, and maintain, aesthetically pleasing highlights and shadowing around the nasal tip region are mandatory for an overall balance of a truly refined nasal appearance.[8,9] These expectations are exponentially challenged by nasal tips that are broad or bulbous/boxy. The skin envelope in the nasal tip region can further frustrate even the most experienced surgeon in its unpredictable long-term behavior.

During the perioperative planning period, it is important not only to design a surgical plan to obtain the desired result but also to recognize and document potential difficulties that may arise, because surgical changes to the nasal skeleton dynamically alter the relationship between the tip structures, dorsum, and overlying soft tissue.[2,4–6] In dealing with a broad nasal tip, it is imperative to use maneuvers that allow for a favorable contour extending from the lateral dome region to the alar margins bilaterally to prevent undertreatment as well as an overly narrowed/artificial tip appearance.[8,9]

Factors that inhibit this balance include skin thickness (thick or thin), lower lateral cartilage inherent strength and position, retracted soft tissue triangle facet, tip support, sufficient caudal septal support, domal architecture, and contractile forces that occur during the healing process.[10,11]

For example, a retracted soft tissue triangle facet may necessitate additional rim grafting or direct soft triangle support at the marginal incision

Conflict of Interest Disclosures: Dr K. Dhir and Dr A. Ghavami have no financial disclosures.
[a] Department of Head and Neck Surgery, Harbor-UCLA Medical Center, 433 North Camden Boulevard, Suite 780, Beverly Hills, CA 90210, USA; [b] Department of Plastic and Reconstructive Surgery, David Geffen School of Medicine, University of California, Los Angeles, 433 North Camden Boulevard, Suite 780, Beverly Hills, CA 90210, USA
* Corresponding author.
E-mail address: rose@ghavamiplasticsurgery.com

plasticsurgery.theclinics.com

once the necessary tip projection and refinement are attained.[12]

The contribution of the lower lateral crura to the projection, position, and contour flow from the paradomal region to the more lateral alar rim region is often underestimated.[8,9] The orientation, strength, and position of the lower lateral crura have a direct impact on the limitations and successes in overall tip shaping.[13–16] For example, cephalic orientation of the lateral crura is defined as lateral crura that are positioned 30° or less from the midline. This creates a vertical fullness of the nasal tip that interrupts the brow-tip aesthetic line.[17–20] Once the domal architecture is surgically manipulated with proper suturing techniques, lateral crural repositioning/reshaping with or without lateral crural strut grafts can improve cephalically malpositioned lower lateral cartilages, retracted alae, and a pinched nasal tip.[18,20,21]

The broad, bulbous, or wide nasal tip continues to challenge the most proficient rhinoplasty surgeon. Central to this inherent dilemma is that there may be a tendency to sacrifice tip-to-alar rim balance and support at the expense of excessive or poorly supported nasal tip narrowing.[22] Conceptually, this is an operation of contour and reshaping to exploit proper nasal tip visible aesthetics—not simply narrowing of a wide tip. If surgical approaches take into account the appropriate magnitude of nasal tip narrowing balanced with alar rim support and soft tissue contributions, then outcomes are improved and revision rates reduced.[1–6,8–12,20] With proper planning during preoperative assessment and a comprehensive understanding of structural rhinoplasty maneuvers, surgeons can effectively treat the wide array of broad nasal tips in a reproducible and predictable fashion.

PREOPERATIVE ANALYSIS

To harmonize nasal form with facial balance, the nose must be both analyzed and treated via multiple views. Although debatable, treating the primary and secondary nasal tip, with all its complexities, effectively may be best achieved via the open approach. Tip shape is best viewed from frontal and base views, whereas projection and tip position are viewed from the lateral and basal views. Dynamic (animated and inspiratory) views are also helpful in analyzing collapse of the nasal valve regions as well as noting active depressor septi nasi hyperactivity resulting in nasal tip ptosis.[12]

Proper photography guidelines have been well described in the literature. On lateral view, the Frankfort horizontal plane that extends from the inferior margin of the bony orbit to the superior margin of the external auditory canal is used as the proper plane the parallels the Earth.[2,4,6] This view is also important in establishing a nose-lip-chin plane (NLCP) for analysis and notation of chin and tip projection. A plumb line is drawn vertically (perpendicularly) from the Frankfort horizontal plane inferiorly extending adjacent to the most projecting portion of the upper lip. In women, the chin lies approximately 3 mm posterior to this vertical line. Tip projection can also be assessed with this method. Proper nasal tip projection is defined when 50% to 60% of the tip extends anterior to this vertical line. If the tip lacks proper projection, less than 50% of the tip extends to this line. Additionally, tip projection can successfully be measured as two-thirds (0.67 times) the ideal nasal length[2,4,23,24] (Fig. 1).

On basilar view, nostril aperture size and shape should also be considered. The ideal nostril/tip ratio has been described as 55:45 on lateral view.[24] Studies using the basilar view to define a proportional aesthetic balance historically have described the infratip lobule to measure 33% of the columellar length.[24–26] Recent observations regarding basilar view proportions mimic the lateral view findings and are consistent with a 60:40 to 55:45 ratio.[23,24]

Also, some investigators stress importance of photographing patients twice, one with a single flash and the second with double light sources. This allows for proper analysis of highlights and shadows formed from the complex areas of convexities and concavities that surround the external nasal tip complex.[8]

The nasolabial angle and alar-columellar balance should also be evaluated and noted. Maneuvers that increase tip projection intimately affect these angles, and other factors may be needed to take into consideration. By recognizing a premaxillary deficiency, proper tip projection may be achieved by simple premaxillary or caudal septal extension grafting and should be discussed in the surgical plan.[27]

Tip balance relative to overall alar base width should be scrutinized relative to the alar base width. Although numeric values have been contemplated, the authors think it is best to evaluate on a case-by-case basis. Alar flaring and interalar width should be taken into account because these dimensions may require simultaneous modifications. Alar soft tissue modifications are performed at the end of the operation, mandating a keen understanding of the dynamic implications of alar width and nasal tip width. It is not uncommon for alar narrowing to be lessened

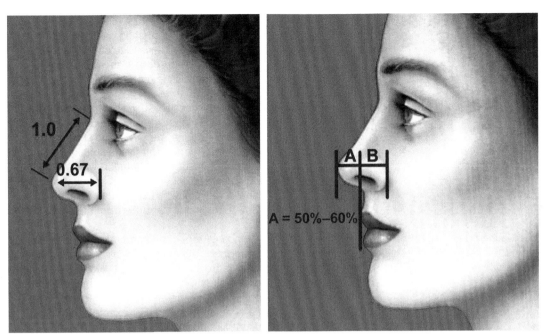

Fig. 1. (*Left*) Proper projection can be successfully measured as two-thirds (0.67 times) the nasal dorsal length. (*Right*) Ideal tip projection can also be defined when 50% to 60% of the tip extends anterior to the NLCP. (*From* Janis JE, Ghavami A, Rohrich RJ. A predictable and algorithmic approach to tip refinememt and projection. In: Gunter JP, Rohrich RJ, Adams WP, editors. Dallas rhinoplasty: nasal surgery by the masters. vol. 1. 2nd edition. St Louis (MO): QMP; 2007. p. 339.)

or completely unnecessary as the medializing forces from tip complex narrowing and refinement may achieve this goal.[28]

SKIN AND SOFT TISSUE

Evaluation of the overlying skin envelope assists in preoperative planning of the tip structure needed to appropriately drape the skin for an elegant tip. Fibrofatty tissue is found in the alar lobules and less in the nasal tip.[8,9] The nasal tip and skin envelope should be examined, massaged, and palpated for proper evaluation. Medium skin thickness bodes well in the nasal tip region to successfully mask the underlying tip cartilaginous structure without hiding the provided definition form tip grafting.

In contrast, thick skin overtly conceals definition and can lead to an amorphous tip lacking refinement. A thick blanket of skin can hide the numerous tip-shaping maneuvers as well as creating a trapdoor-like effect with long-term dynamic edema and an amorphous tip appearance, regardless of all the structural alterations. Understanding this concept may lead a surgeon to plan for debulking techniques that effectively, and safely, allow for more definition of the tip complex. Additional tip definition may require more

aggressive grafting when indicated. The nasal tip blood supply should be understood in detail to protect from complications arising from devascularization of the skin via violation superficial to the subdermal plexus.[13,29–31] There should remain a thick uniform cobblestone appearance to the soft tissue left behind after debulking the tip skin. Maintaining trepidation during the debulking process is imperative to protect from excessive thinning, scarring, and skin loss. Moreover, active smokers yield a significantly higher risk for postoperative fibrosis of skin flap, scarring, and columellar skin incision complications. The authors recommend extreme caution during the decision-making process of whether to operate on patients with active tobacco use. Debulking techniques are indicated for noses with ethnic features, including, but not limited to, those of patients of Middle Eastern, African American, Indian, or Hispanic (Mestizo) descent[32–34] (**Fig. 2**).

Conservation of the subdermal plexus and a thick uniform cobblestoned appearance of the subcutaneous tissue left behind are imperative for safety. By adhering to this principle, soft tissue necrosis or skin loss should be avoided. Additional grafts, such as various tip onlay and infratrip shied grafts, may be placed to help further reduce the

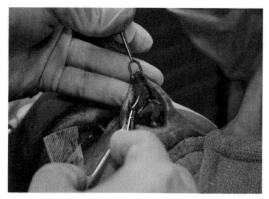

Fig. 2. A curved scissors is used to debulk the soft tissue of a thick skin envelope. It is imperative to not dissect superficially past the subdermal plexus. Debulking techniques are indicated in noses with ethnic features, including, but not limited to, those of patients of Middle Eastern, African American, Indian, or Hispanic (Mestizo) descent.

interference of a thick skin envelope by providing visible grafts.[19,35] By creating a heavier footprint on the overlying skin sleeve, subtle aesthetic highlights are not blunted. Selective soft tissue thinning at the apices of these onlay grafts assists with proper soft tissue draping and can be performed

with curved scissors to excise the loose areolar fatty tissue. Lastly, crushed cartilage and cephalic rim remnants can be used to camouflage any graft or native cartilage edges as well as prevent unwanted soft tissue contracture in thin-skinned noses (**Fig. 3**).

Finally, excessively thin skin results in the opposite effect during the healing process. The underlying imperfections, step-offs, and sharp angles may be visualized once soft tissue shrink wrapping occurs. Soft tissue augmentation with temporal fascia (preferred) or AlloDerm (LifeCell, Branchburg, New Jersey) may be used in these regions to allow for a harmonious transition from the dorsum to the tip.[12]

Once a proper and comprehensive evaluation is performed, the surgical goals are noted and the plan is reviewed with the patient to manage expectations. It is important to review details, in particular, in the selfie-obsessed era, of exact tip-shaping nuances. For example, some patients might like and have an attachment to their deep soft triangle facets or bifid tip and may want it preserved. When a surgical plan necessitates significant cartilage grafting, the patient should be notified of the likelihood of stiffness of the nasal tip, effects on smiling, and the ability to palpate the grafts during manipulation.

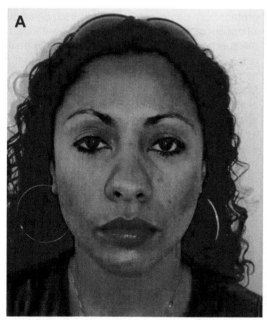
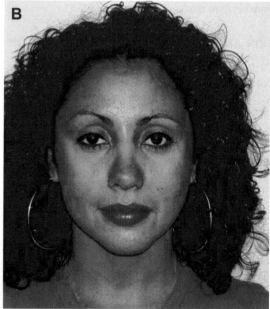

Fig. 3. (*A*) Preoperative frontal view demonstrates thick skin envelope with a very wide bulbous nasal tip. (*B*) Postoperative frontal view demonstrates importance of alar rim shaping and positioning with concomitant correction of a broad nasal tip with multiple modalities, including tip suturing, tip grafts, alar contour graft, and soft tissue debulking maneuvers.

TIP SUTURING

Previous tip suturing techniques historically sacrificed the integrity of the lateral crural cartilages, and maneuvers were aimed toward augmenting the medial crural cartilages for projection and height for tip definition.[22,36] Postoperative fibrosis and retraction of specific nasal subunits after disrupting the lateral tip support mechanisms ensued, resulting in less than desirable results, including supratip fullness, tip drop, alar retraction, and tip asymmetry. Although cephalic trim is often necessary as a precursor to effective broad tip correction via suturing and grafting techniques, it may not always be necessary. Assessment of native lower lateral crural size, strength, and position is required before using a typical knee-jerk approach to routine cephalic trimming.[3,8,9,12,18,19,35]

Modern-day tip suturing maneuvers describe methods that reshape and reposition the tip support components as opposed to the classically described reduction techniques of the past.[22] Currently, the arsenal of tip sutures includes the medial crural suture, the middle crura suture, the interdomal suture, the transdomal suture, the lateral crura suture, the medial crural anchor suture, the tip rotation suture, the medial crura footplate suture, and the lateral crura convexity control suture.[10,11,14,17,22,37,38]

By precise placement and control of tension, the suture techniques specifically address both the medial and lateral tip components for a well-supported and defined tip complex. Intraoperative analysis is paramount in formulating a surgical plan. The lateral crura are assessed for symmetry, position, degree of convexity/concavity, length, width, dimension, and strength. The medial crura are assessed for length and strength, both of which determine tip projection and support. Finally, the domal region is assessed for domal arch width, degree of divergence, and degree of symmetry.

One of the first articles to publish an algorithmic methodology regarding the nuances of tip suturing describes a 4-stage approach that serves useful today.[14,15] To obtain success in tip surgery, it is important to understand the various tip suturing techniques, and this 4-stage algorithm serves as a guide of when to use each suture maneuver once proper intraoperative evaluation is completed.

In stage 1, the soft tissue envelope is dissected from the underlying lower lateral cartilages in an open or closed technique. The lateral crural rim strips are manipulated for symmetry either by scoring or conservative trimming of the cephalic border. In stage 2, the medial crura are positioned and the medial arch is unified with medial crura

sutures placed cephalically. Transdomal, interdomal, and medial crura sutures can be used during this stage to properly position the domal cartilages, control caudal flaring, and secure an interdomal strut when necessary (**Fig. 4**). Medial crura footplate sutures may also be used to address asymmetries from long-standing caudal septal deflections.

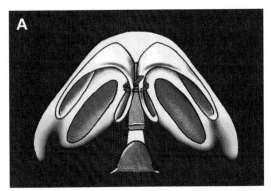

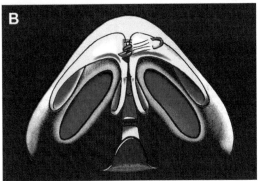

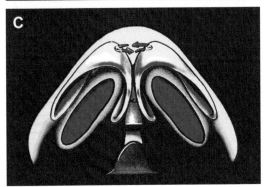

Fig. 4. (*A*) Medial crural suture securing columellar strut to medial crura providing support and also increased projection when necessary. (*B*) Transdomal sutures reposition the domal cartilage subunits into proper shape and position. (*C*) Interdomal sutures properly position the domal cartilages in a more unified position, address asymmetries, and control caudal flaring.

In stage 3, a columellar strut is placed, secured and shaped. The increased projection and repositioning of the medial crural components support the tripod of the nose. At this point, the lateral crura are examined for convexities, or concavities. Lateral crural spanning sutures are deployed to reposition lateral crural convexities as noted in the boxy, or trapezoid, tip. Finally, stage 4 addresses the final positioning of the unified, symmetric tip complex. A medial crural anchoring suture may control projection by securing the tip complex to the septum as well as advancing the tip anteriorly or posteriorly. Other described suture techniques that may be used during this stage include septocolumellar sutures, tongue-in-groove sutures, and tip rotation sutures. Tip rotation sutures are passed through the cephalad edge of the medial crura and secured to the dorsal septum near the septal angle to maintain tip rotation.

In broad nasal tips, cephalic lower lateral crural reduction via excision or with overlapping techniques can be useful in eliminating fullness as well as correcting residual convexities of the alar margin. It is common for lower lateral convexity to become exaggerated after release of the scroll ligaments and cephalic trim. If unrecognized, 2 problems can be created. One is that the necessity to narrow and augment the tip may be overestimated to compensate for the full-appearing alar rims and paradomal regions. Second, proper broad or boxy tip reshaping may be thwarted as a result of lower lateral crura convexity persistence.

Tip suturing techniques that reposition and support the nasal tip complex are the mainstay of providing an elegant tip. The decision for tip cartilage grafting, soft tissue augmentation, and lateral crural strengthening/repositioning is dependent on the preoperative evaluation of the soft tissue and intraoperative lateral crural dynamic changes that occur. **Fig. 5** shows an easy-to-follow general guide in approaching tip refinement with suturing and grafting techniques.

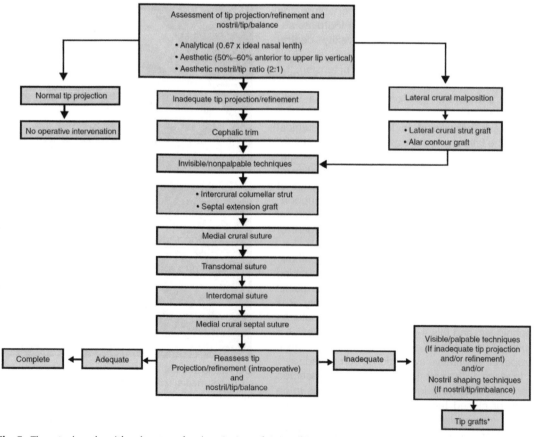

Fig. 5. Tip suturing algorithm (see text for description of tip grafting options). (*From* Janis JE, Ghavami A, Rohrich RJ. A predictable and algorithmic approach to tip refinememt and projection. In: Gunter JP, Rohrich RJ, Adams WP, editors. Dallas rhinoplasty: nasal surgery by the masters, vol. 1, 2nd edition. St Louis (MO): QMP; 2007. p. 339.)

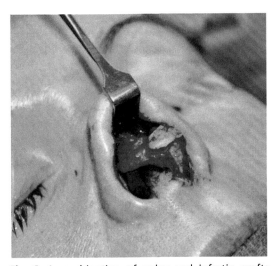

Fig. 6. A combination of onlay and infratip grafts further refines the nasal tip complex by harmoniously transitioning from the nasal tip to the columella as well as appropriately enhancing the lateral genu and paradomal region.

TIP GRAFTS

If the final tip components provide smooth and aesthetic breakpoints from the domal structure extending laterally to the ala, then grafting may not be necessary. Tip sutures alone, however, are not always sufficient in providing the necessary desired tip projection and shape.

Columellar Strut

The columellar strut is often placed as the surgeon proceeds through stage 3 of the tip suturing algorithm. This graft remains a powerful tool in maintaining or strengthening tip support and in increasing tip projection. Generally, the strut graft is invisible as it is placed between the medial crura and secured with a medial crural suture. The graft can be positioned, however, to be visible for the purpose of augmenting the infratip lobule or increasing columellar show when necessary. A colmellar strut is a key foundation in supporting any further tip-shaping techniques, particularly in situations where the medial curua are weak and insufficient.[35]

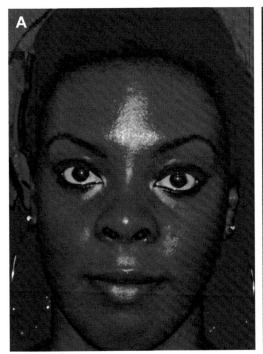

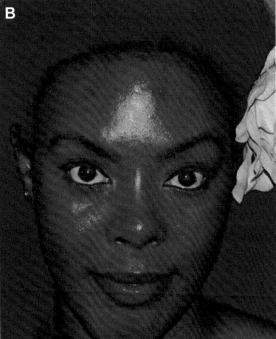

Fig. 7. (A) Preoperative frontal view—alar rim position is underappreciated in the comprehensive management of the broad nasal tip. (B) Postoperative frontal view—comprehensive techniques, including tip suturing, trip grafting, soft tissue debulking, crushed soft tissue triangle grafting, lateral crural strut grafting, and alar rim grafting, provide refinement of the broad nasal tip as well as improving alar margin position.

Onlay Tip Grafts and Infratip Grafts

Although there are many types of tip grafts of various shapes and sizes described in the literature, the most common types of grafts can be generally designated as onlay grafts and infratip grafts. It is imperative that the grafting material is of appropriate thickness and beveled/crushed at the edges.[19,35]

The authors secure onlay tip grafts with 5.0 polydioxanone sutures at multiple fixation points to prevent migration, rotation, or buckling during fibrosis and soft tissue shrink wrapping. Ultimately, this allows for a smooth transition from the supratip breakpoint to the tip region with the added benefit of improving tip projection. Double-layer grafting and grafts of various thicknesses should be used when indicated. Experience improves the intraoperative instincts on which the degree of shape and thickness these grafts should be fashioned when contending with the entire spectrum of wide and bulbous nasal tips.

A combination of an onlay graft with an infratip graft further refines the nasal tip complex by harmoniously transitioning from the nasal tip to the columella.[39] Infratip grafts are indicated when infratip volume and projection are lacking or when the breakpoints are dull and weak.[19] The shield graft must have an appropriate width to abscond from a displeasing heavy tip. Furthermore, scoring the cartilage at its superior edge to effectively bend itself at a predictable breakpoint has been described.[12] Placement of the shield graft can be variable. It can either be fixated at the level of the domal cartilage apex or can extend

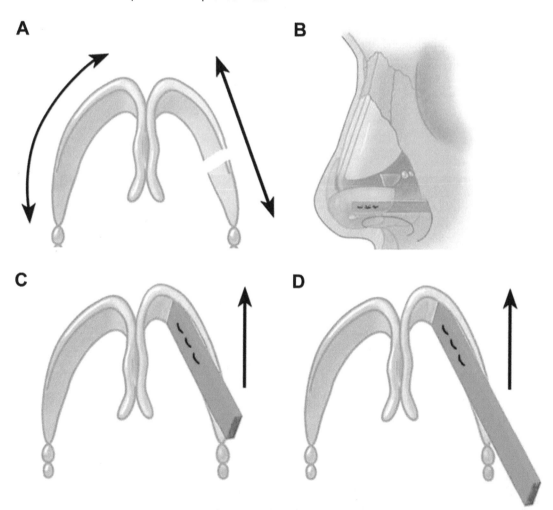

Fig. 8. (*A*) Lateral crural transection for the correction of severe convexities of the lateral crura. (*B*) Lateral crural strut with repositioning in a more caudal position accompanied with comprehensive tip refining modalities enhances tip support and definition. (*C, D*) Lateral crural strut length may vary depending desired tip projection and for manipulation of alar position. (*D*) Demonstrates increased projection by increasing length of graft. This provides further support for tip-shaping maneuvers and can avoid unwanted steal phenomenon.

beyond this point. Thick-skinned individuals lend themselves to more aggressive grafting techniques for increased projection and shape (**Fig. 6**). The visible edges are more likely to be camouflaged due to the inherent virtues of a thick skin envelope, as discussed previously.

Alar Contour Grafts

Before discussing the more complex technique of lower lateral crural strut grafting and repositioning, the alar contour graft is discussed as an option to prevent undesirable notching at the nasal ala and soft tissue triangle subunit.[40,41] Although creation of a soft tissue pocket and securing of the graft with sutures are not technically difficult, these grafts often mobilize postoperatively. Their importance, however, is stressed with maneuvers that significantly increase tip projection, cause a depression, or result in a retraction point from the nasal tip to the alar rims. Therefore, it is critical

to secure the graft at 2 points to prevent migration. After fixation, crushed cartilage, cephalic trim remnants, or cartilage graft harvest remnants may be placed at the soft tissue triangle to camouflage and provide a continuous smooth transition.

Modified alar contour grafts that are secured to the lateral aspects of the domes can be powerful in both aesthetics and support of tip-to-alar transition contour and highlights. Soft triangle facets may also require direct grafting when they are deep or in vertical excess despite alar contour grafts (**Fig. 7**). In some cases, alar contour grafts can be avoided if soft triangle grafting of various forms are used.[12]

Lower Lateral Crurual Strut and Repositioning

A contemporary review of rhinoplasty maneuvers that aim to achieve a favorable nasal tip contour is not complete without a discussion regarding the lateral crural cartilage contribution to proper

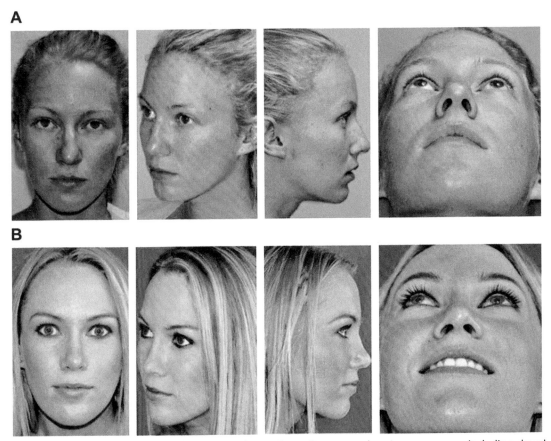

A

B

Fig. 9. (A) Preoperative patient. (B) Postoperative patient after comprehensive maneuvers, including dorsal reduction, tip elevation and projection, and finesse tip shaping using transdomal, interdomal, and medial crural sutures without a columellar strut; an onlay sunglass graft for the domes; and a soft, crushed infratip lobular shield graft to define the breakpoints.

tip shadowing, structure, and protection from a pinched nasal tip.[8,9] The original description of the lateral crural steal effect of tip string forces medializing and drawing the lower lateral crura centrally still hold true today.[42] With all the tip suturing methods and grafts at a surgeon's disposal, it is a critical concept to understand when approaching the wider nasal tips. Previous techniques that focused on tip projection and narrowing of the domal tip, while sacrificing the lateral crura structure, yielded results with retracted and

deeper soft tissue triangle facets, pinched nasal ala, increased columellar show, and unfavorable shadowing due to uneven transition points between the newly narrowed tip complex and the lateral alar regions.[8,9,22]

Lateral crural strut grafts are lateral crural repositioning are important to discuss separately as well as in combination. If exaggerated convexities or concavities are present and the desired tip projection and contour are achieved, then lateral crural strut grafts and/or alar rim grafts are

A

B

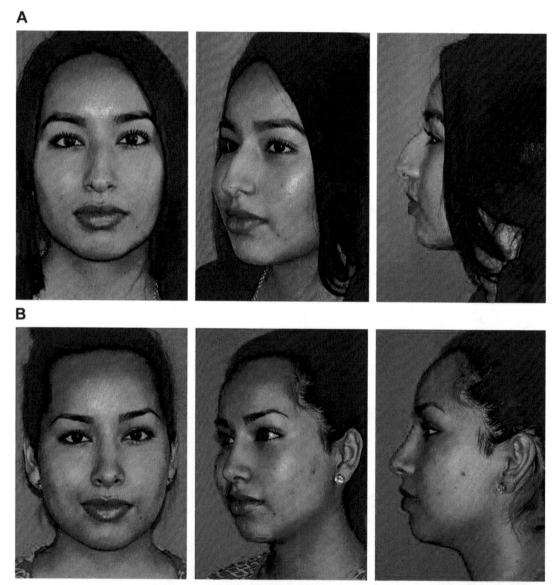

Fig. 10. (*A*) Preoperative patient with a very nasal tip complicated by exaggerated soft triangle facets, strong dorsal hump, and tip ptosis. (*B*) Postoperative patient after comprehensive maneuvers, including soft triangle grafts used to offset the facets that otherwise would have been exaggerated with the narrowing and refinement of the wide tip; tip suturing methods, dorsal hump reduction, caudal septal resection, spreader grafting, correction of alar malposition by placement of alar contour grafts, and resection of depressor nasi septi muscle.

deployed to support the ala and protect from retraction.[7–9,18,20] The caudal and cranial border must lie in the same plane. These grafts are fashioned from septum, concha, or rib with preference in that order. Strut grafts are fashioned to be rigid, but attempts should be made to fashion and secure an unpalpable graft and to critically evaluate for unwanted thickening of the alar rim tissue. A thickened alar rim can have deleterious functional consequences. Regarding placement, the medial end of the graft can extend to the lateral genu or the domal apex if increased tip projection is warranted. The grafts do not always have to extend to the pyriform region. They can be inserted in a proper alar rim soft tissue pocket or sutured free to the soft tissues laterally and/or the native lower lateral crura. Discussion of the decision to transect and reposition the lower lateral crura is beyond the scope of this article but it is a powerful tool that, when indicated, can enhance overall tip-to-rim balance.

When the caudal margin is below the cephalic margin (lower lateral cartilage malposition), the resulting appearance is a parenthesis tip deformity that may require repositioning of the lateral crura by transecting laterally adjacent to the accessory chain.[19] Constantian[43] simplified this definition and describes orientation by the axis of the crus lateral to the lateral genu. Orthotopic lateral crura were described as running toward the lateral canthus of the ipsilateral eye, whereas cephalically malpositioned lateral crura ran toward the medial canthus. A lateral crural strut graft is used for the purpose of strengthening the crura and may vary in length depending on the goal of positioning and for manipulation of alar position in cases of asymmetry.[20] The lateral crural grafts may extend past the lateral transected border and be placed into a pocket that may extend to the maxilla when necessary. It is advised to secure with sutures to maintain position during healing if a proper pocket is not achievable (**Fig. 8**).

SUMMARY

This article presents a contemporary overview of tip suturing and tip structural grafting techniques used to refine the wide nasal tip. Previous reductive techniques have proved to produce unnatural results over time. Preoperatively, it is imperative to correctly evaluate the nose and assess all possible pitfalls before outlining a surgical plan. Intraoperatively, an algorithmic approach helps obtain a reproducible and refined yet properly narrowed domal tip region with graceful contours that extend laterally to the alar lobule with proper shadowing (**Figs. 9** and **10**).

REFERENCES

1. Rohrich RJ, Deuber MA, Adams WP Jr. Pragmatic planning and postoperative management. In: Gunter JP, Rohrich RJ, Adams WP, editors. Dallas rhinoplasty: nasal surgery by the masters, vol. 1, 1st edition. St Louis (MO): QMP; 2002. p. 72–104.
2. Gunter JP, Hackney FL. Clinical assessment and facial analysis. In: Gunter JP, Rohrich RJ, Adams WP, editors. Dallas rhinoplasty: nasal surgery by the masters, vol. 1, 1st edition. St Louis (MO): QMP; 2002. p. 53–71.
3. Janis JE, Ghavami A, Rohrich RJ. A predictable and algorithmic approach to tip refinememt and projection. In: Gunter JP, Rohrich RJ, Adams WP, editors. Dallas rhinoplasty: nasal surgery by the masters, vol. 1, 2nd edition. St Louis (MO): QMP; 2007. p. 339.
4. Byrd HS, Hobar PC. Rhinoplasty: a practical guide for surgical planning. Plast Reconstr Surg 1993;91:642.
5. Tebbetts JB. The next dimension: rethinking the logic, sequence, and techniques of rhinoplasty. In: Gunter JP, Rohrich RJ, Adams WP, editors. Dallas rhinoplasty: nasal surgery by the masters, vol. 1, 1st edition. St Louis (MO): QMP; 2002. p. 219–53.
6. Byrd HS, Burt JD. Dimensional approach to rhinoplasty: perfecting the aesthetic balance between the nose and chin. In: Gunter JP, Rohrich RJ, Adams WP, editors. Dallas rhinoplasty: nasal surgery by the masters, vol. 1, 1st edition. St Louis (MO): QMP; 2002. p. 117–31.
7. Gunter JP, Hackney FL. Basic nasal tip surgery: anatomy and Technique. In: Gunter JP, Rohrich RJ, Adams WP, editors. Dallas rhinoplasty: nasal surgery by the masters, vol. 1, 1st edition. St Louis (MO): QMP; 2002. p. 193–218.
8. Toriumi DM, Checcone M. New concepts in nasal tip contouring. Facial Plast Surg Clin North Am 2009;17:55–90.
9. Angelos PC, Been MJ, Toriumi DM. Contemporary review of rhinoplasty. Arch Facial Plast Surg 2012;14:238–47.
10. Daniel RK. Middle eastern rhinoplasty in the United States: part I. Primary rhinoplasty. Plast Reconstr Surg 2009;124(5):1630–9.
11. Daniel RK. Middle Eastern rhinoplasty in the United States: part II. Secondary rhinoplasty. Plast Reconstr Surg 2009;124(5):1640–8.
12. Ghavami A. Tip shaping in primary rhinoplasty. In: Shiffman MA, Di Giuseppe A, editors. Advanced aesthetic rhinoplasty: art, science, and new clinical techniques. Berlin: Springer-Verlag GmbH; 2012. p. 853–68.
13. Adams WP Jr, Rohrich RJ, Hollier LH, et al. Anatomic basis and clinical implications for nasal tip support in open versus closed rhinoplasty. Plast Reconstr Surg 1999;103:255.

14. Tebbetts JB. Shaping and positioning the nasal tip without structural disruption: a new systematic approach. Plast Reconstr Surg 1994;94:61–77.

15. Tebbetts JB. Secondary tip modification: shaping and positioning the nasal tip using nondestructive techniques. Chapter 10. In: Tebbets JB, editor. Primary rhinoplasty: a new approach to the logic and the techniques. St Louis (MO): C. V. Mosby; 1998. p. 261–441.

16. Janeke JB, Wright WK. Studies on the support of the nasal tip. Arch Otolaryngol 1971;93:458.

17. Tardy ME. Rhinoplasty: the art and the science. Philadelphia: WB Saunders CO; 1996.

18. Gunter JP, Friedman RM. Lateral crural strut graft: technique and clinical applications in rhinoplasty. Plast Reconstr Surg 1997;99(4):943–52.

19. Sheen J. Aeshtetic rhinoplsty. 2nd edition. St Louis (MO): CV Mosby; 1987.

20. Toriumi DM, Asher SA. Lateral crural respositiong for treatment of cephalic malposition. Facial Plast Surg Clin North Am 2015;23:55–71.

21. Gruber RP. Suture techniques. In: Gunter JP, Rohrich RJ, Adams WP, editors. Dallas rhinoplasty: nasal surgery by the masters, vol. 1, 1st edition. St Louis (MO): QMP; 2002. p. 254–70.

22. Behmand RA, Ghavami A, Guyuron B. Nasal tip sutures part I: the evolution. Plast Reconstr Surg 2003; 112:1125.

23. Guyuron B, Ghavami A, Wishnek S. Components of the short nostril. Plast Reconstr Surg 2005;116:1517.

24. Daniel RK. Rhinoplasty: large nostril/small tip disproportion. Plast Reconstr Surg 1874;107:2001.

25. Goldman IB. Rhinoplasty manual. New York: Restricted Publication; 1968.

26. Powell N, Humphreys B. Proportions of the aesthetic face. New York: Thieme; 1984. p. 28–31.

27. Toriumi DM. Caudal septal extension graft for correction of the retracted columella. Operat Tech Otolaryngol Head Neck Surg 1995;6:311–8.

28. Planas J, Planas J. Nosril and alar reshaping. Aesthetic Plast Surg 1992;17:139.

29. Toriumi DM, Mueller RA, Grosch T, et al. Vascular anatomy of the nose and the external rhinoplasty approach. Arch Otolaryngol Head Neck Surg 1996;122:24.

30. Rohrich RJ, Muzaffar AR, Gunter JP. Nasal tip blood supply: confirming the safety of the transcolumellar incision in rhinoplasty. Plast Reconstr Surg 2000; 106:1640.

31. Rohrich RJ, Muzaffar AR. Rhinoplasty in the African-American patient. Plast Reconstr Surg 2003;111(3): 1322.

32. Rohrich RJ, Ghavami A. Rhinoplasty for middle eastern noses. Plast Reconstr Surg 2009;123:1343.

33. Ghavami A, Rohrich RJ. The ethnic rhinoplasty. In: Aston SJ, Steinbrech DS, Walden JL, editors. Aesthetic plastic surgery. London: Saunders; 2009. p. 531–54.

34. Daniel RK. Hispanic rhinoplasty in the United States with emphasis on the Mexican American nose. Plast Reconstr Surg 2003;112(1):244.

35. Ghavami A, Janis JE, Acikel C, et al. Tip shaping in primary rhinoplasty: an algorithmic approach. Plast Reconstr Surg 2008;122:1229.

36. Goldman IB. Surgical tips on the nasal tip. Eye Ear Nose Throat Mon 1954;33:583.

37. Gruber RP, Peled A, Talley J. Mattress sutures to remove unwanted convexity and concavity of the nasal tip: 12 year follow-up. Aesthet Surg J 2015; 35(1):20–7.

38. McCollough EG, English JL. A new twist in nasal tip surgery: an alternative to the Goldman tip for the wide or bulbous lobule. Arch Otolaryngol 1985; 111:524.

39. Brenner MJ, Hilger PA. Grafting in rhinoplasty. Facial Plast Surg Clin North Am 2009;17(1):91–113.

40. Rohrich RJ, Raniere J Jr, Ha RY. The alar contour graft: correction and prevention of alar rim deformities in rhinoplasty. Plast Reconstr Surg 2002;109: 2495.

41. Boahene KD, Hilger PA. Alar rim grafting in rhinoplasty: indications, technique, and outcomes. Arch Facial Plast Surg 2009;11(5):285–9.

42. Kridel RW, Konior RJ, Shumrick KA, et al. Advances in nasal tip surgery. the lateral crural steal. Arch Otolaryngol Head Neck Surg 1989;115(10):1206–12.

43. Constantian MB. The boxy nasal tip, the ball tip, and alar cartilage malposition: variation on a theme- a study in 200 consecutive primary and secondary rhinoplasty patients. Plast Reconstr Surg 2005;116(1): 268–81.

Alar Rim Deformities

Ali Totonchi, MD[a], Bahman Guyuron, MD[b],*

KEYWORDS

- Alar rim • Nose • Deformity • Rhinoplasty

KEY POINTS

- The alar rim plays an important role in nasal harmony.
- Alar rim flaws are common following the initial rhinoplasty.
- Classification of the deformities helps with diagnosis and successful surgical correction.
- Diagnosis of the deformity requires careful observation of the computerized or life-sized photographs.
- Techniques for treatment of these deformities can easily be learned with attention to detail.

BACKGROUND

Alar rim harmony plays an important role in the nasal base balance. Inherited or iatrogenic deformities disturb the balance of this zone and engender a displeasing appearance. Retraction is the most common alar abnormality, and was the hallmark of rhinoplasties done in the 1960s and 1970s. Gunter and colleagues[1] classified alar rim abnormalities into 6 distinct subgroups based on two-dimensional observation. In 2001, Guyuron[2] modified the classification with a three-dimensional concept. This article describes deformities of the alar rim and the surgical techniques to correct them.

CLASSIFICATION
Profile View

By connecting a line from the apex of the nostril to the nadir of the nostril, if the alar rim is within 1.5 to 2 mm cephalic to this line, then the ala is in an optimal position. If this distance is more than 2 mm, the ala is retracted, and if the distance is shorter than 1.5 mm then patient has a hanging ala (Fig. 1).

Basilar View

In a basilar view of the optimal nose, the 2 alar rims and nasal base create an equilateral triangle. In this triangle, each ala is positioned in a straight line that constitutes a limb of the triangle. The 2 types of disharmony that might be observed in this view are concave and convex alar rims.

If the alar outline is medial to the leg of the triangle, then the ala has a concave shape. This condition is often a consequence of inappropriate interruption of the lower lateral cartilage, improper application of the tip graft that extends lateral to existing dome, a transdomal suture that is too tight, or excessive resection of the lower lateral cartilage.

If the ala is lateral to this triangle, then it is referred to as a convex ala. Two conditions may cause this abnormality: too much convexity to the lower lateral cartilage, or excessively thick ala (Fig. 2).

SURGICAL CORRECTION OF THE DEFORMITIES

The hanging ala can be easily corrected by removing an elliptical alar lining along with a proportionate amount of subcutaneous tissue and leaving the skin intact (Fig. 3). This procedure is extremely simple. However, the hanging ala is a rare condition.

The most common abnormality of the ala in the lateral view is a notched or retracted ala. A variety

[a] Plastic Surgery Division, MetroHealth Medical Center, 2500 MetroHealth Drive, Cleveland, OH 44109, USA;
[b] Zeeba Clinic, 29017 Cedar Road, Lyndhurst, OH 44124, USA
* Corresponding author.
E-mail address: Bahman.Guyuron@gmail.com

Clin Plastic Surg 43 (2016) 127–134
http://dx.doi.org/10.1016/j.cps.2015.09.014
0094-1298/16/$ – see front matter © 2016 Elsevier Inc. All rights reserved.

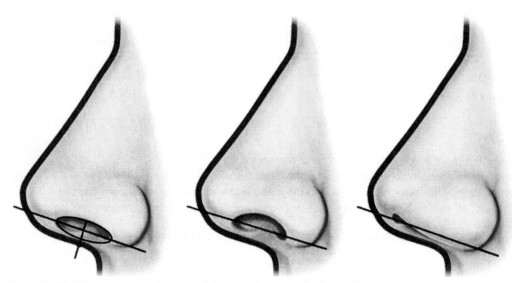

Fig. 1. (*Left*) A line connecting the apex of the nostril to its nadir divides the nostril into 2 equal halves. (*Center*) A retracted or notched ala exists when the distance from this line to the alar rim is greater than 1.5 to 2 mm. (*Right*) A hanging columella occurs when the distance is less than 1.5 to 2 mm. (*Adapted from* Gunter JP, Rohrich RJ, Friedman RM. Classification and correction of the alar-columellar discrepancies in rhinoplasty. Plast Reconstr Surg 1996;97:643; and Guyuron B. Alar rim deformities. Plast Reconstr Surg 2001;107(3):856–63, with permission.)

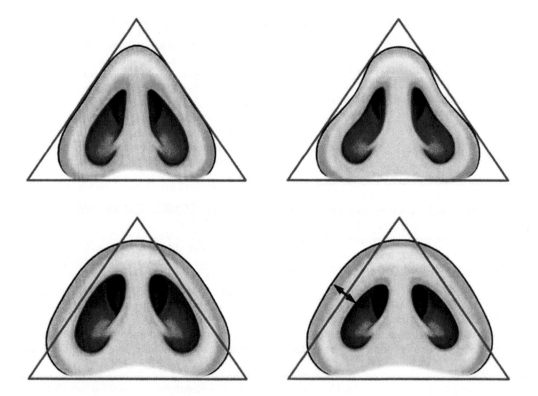

Fig. 2. In a pleasing basilar view, the alar rims are located within an equilateral triangle (*above, left*). Artistic renderings of a concave ala (*above, right*), a convex ala caused by excessively convex lower lateral cartilage (*below, left*), and a convex ala caused by excessively thick ala (*below, right*). (*Adapted from* Guyuron B. Alar rim deformities. Plast Reconstr Surg 2001;107(3):856–63; with permission.)

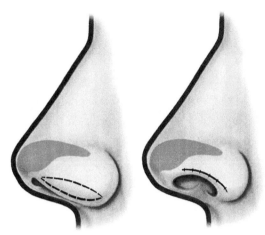

Fig. 3. Removal of an elliptical piece of tissue from the lining along with a proportionate amount of subcutaneous tissue to correct hanging ala. (*Adapted from* Guyuron B. Alar rim deformities. Plast Reconstr Surg 2001;107(3):856–63; with permission.)

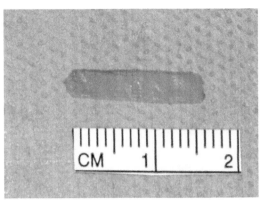

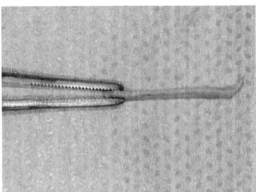

Fig. 4. A piece of cartilage 15 to 16 mm by 2 to 3 mm is used as the alar rim graft. The posterior end is rounded to facilitate its insertion and the anterior end is beveled to reduce its visibility. (*Adapted from* Guyuron B, Bigdeli Y, Sajjadian A. Dynamics of the alar rim graft. Plast Reconstr Surg 2015;135(4):981–86; with permission.)

of techniques have been used to correct this deformity. Each is effective with some nuances, with the magnitude of the alar retraction dictating the surgical course.

If the retraction is minimal (≤1.5–2 mm), results in a weakness of the external valve, and is noted as a concavity in the basilar view, our corrective approach of choice is the placement of an alar rim graft. This graft can be readily accomplished either in conjunction with other nasal procedures or independently. A septal, conchal, or costal cartilage graft approximately 2 to 3 mm wide, 1 to 1.5 mm thick, and 15 to 16 mm long is prepared in an almost rectangular shape (**Fig. 4**). The ends are beveled and rounded to avoid visible irregularities and to facilitate its insertion. Next, a rim incision is made close to the apex of the nostril internally. The incision is extended to the subcutaneous tissue as close to the rim as possible, avoiding penetration of the skin. Using a pair of iris scissors, a pocket is created along the alar rim and then a graft is introduced into the pocket (**Fig. 5**). The length or the width of the graft may require alteration for optimal results. The wound is then repaired using 6-0 or 5-0 plain catgut suture. If this procedure is performed during an open rhinoplasty, then, through the anterior portion of the incision, a pocket is created in the posterior direction. Again, the cartilage is prepared, placed in position, and sewn to the nostril lining to avoid dislodgment in the process of healing. In a recent article by Guyuron and colleagues,[3] a few dynamic changes were observed after the insertion of each graft, including (1) correction of the concavity of the ala, (2) caudal advancement

of the alar rim, (3) elongation of nostril, and (4) widening of the nostril.

If the alar rim is retracted more than 1.5 to 2 mm, there are several options. The choice of a composite graft was introduced and discussed by Ellenbogen.[4] Another technique that has been successful in the senior author's (BG) practice is an internal V to Y advancement. The clinician should ascertain the necessity of this technique before making the open rhinoplasty incision. In this case, the flap design can be incorporated in the vestibular incision design. The V is designed starting from the apex of the nostril and extending cephalically to the intercartilaginous line, which is then angled toward the most posterior portion of the nostril (**Fig. 6**). A flap is developed in the subperichondrial level and is extended caudally. Many patients requiring this type of surgery have had either transection or resection of the lateral crus. The dissection is extended toward the alar rim and the flap is unfolded like a book page. It is crucial to continue the dissection as far caudally as possible to facilitate unfolding the flap along

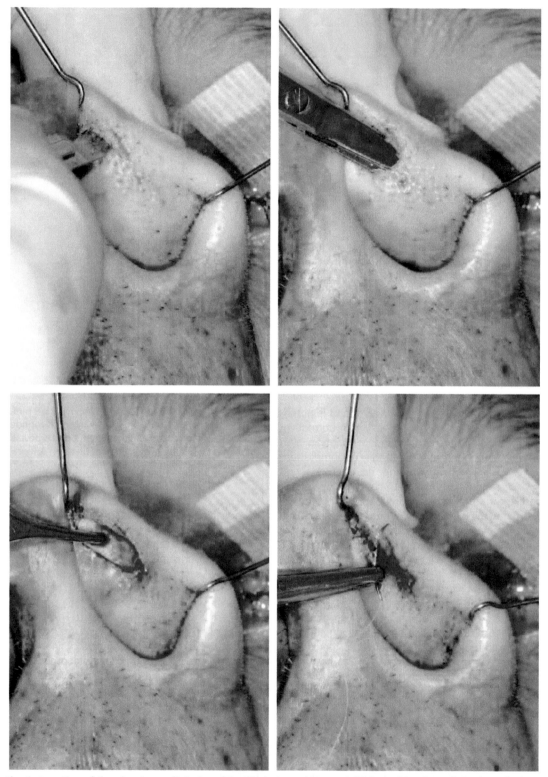

Fig. 5. Insertion of the alar rim graft during closed technique. (*Above, left*) An incision is made in the soft tissue triangle lining close to the most anterior portion of the nostril rim. (*Above, right*) Using iris scissors, the pocket is created to accept the graft while the skin hooks stretch the alar rim. (*Below, left*) insertion of the alar rim graft. (*Below, right*) Repair of the rim incision using 6-0 fast-absorbing catgut suture. (*Adapted from* Guyuron B, Bigdeli Y, Sajjadian A. Dynamics of the alar rim graft. Plast Reconstr Surg 2015;135(4):981–86; with permission.)

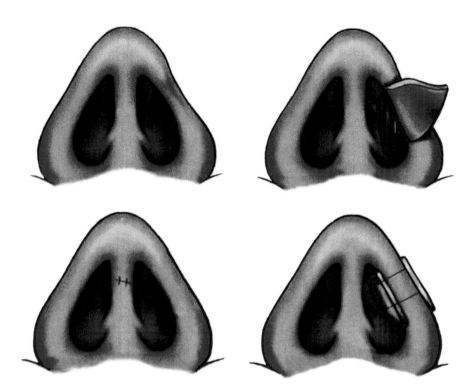

Fig. 6. The V design of the flap starts from the apex of the nostril and extends cephalically to the intercartilaginous line, which is then angled toward the most posterior portion of the nostril (*above, left*). The flap is unfolded like a book page after careful dissection (*above, right*). Cartilage graft is used if alar cartilage is missing or is transected. The Y advancement is sewn in position with 5-0 chromic interrupted sutures (*below, left*). The alar complex is sandwiched in between 2 pieces of simple stents (Xomed) (*below, right*). (*Adapted from* Guyuron B. Alar rim deformities. Plast Reconstr Surg 2001;107(3):856–63; with permission.)

to the alar rim without penetrating the skin surface. If the lateral crural cartilage is missing, using a septal or conchal cartilage graft can emulate a normal anatomy. Placing a cartilage graft adjacent to the existing dome and extending it laterally to the stump of the lower lateral cartilage can accomplish this goal. If the cartilage is present but transected, a simple approximation of the transected lateral crus to the dome is often insufficient. A Gunter lateral crus strut is inserted and the graft is fixed in position using an absorbable suture such as 6-0 Vicryl.

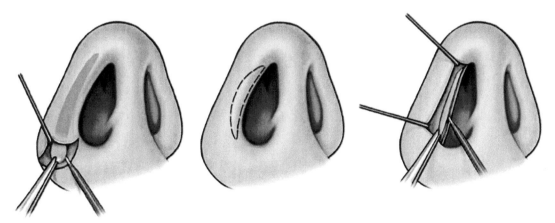

Fig. 7. Reduction of alar thickness using the alar base incision (*left*), the design for removing excessive subcutaneous tissue (*middle*), and removal using a blade for the skin and subcutaneous tissue and microneedle cautery (*right*). (*Adapted from* Guyuron B. Alar rim deformities. Plast Reconstr Surg 2001;107(3):856–63; with permission.)

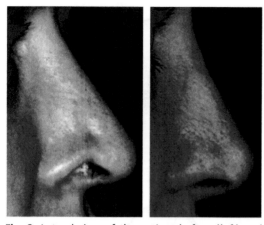

Fig. 8. Lateral view of the patient before (*left*) and after (*right*) correction of alar retraction using a V to Y advancement. The patient's nasal tip was also augmented using an onlay graft. (*Adapted from* Guyuron B. Alar rim deformities. Plast Reconstr Surg 2001;107(3):856–63; with permission.)

After completion of the rhinoplasty, the flap that was incised as a V and dissected is now folded further caudally and Y advancement is accomplished. The lining is then sewn in position using 5-0 chromic interrupted sutures. As the internal incision (where the V is converted to Y) is repaired, the lateral nasal wall cephalic to the alar rim becomes tighter and the previous depression is eliminated. Next, the alar complex is sandwiched between the 2 pieces of Simple Splints (Xomed, Jacksonville, FL), which eliminates the dead space and avoids excessive thickness in the alar rim from scar formation. The internal stent is pentagonal and is smaller than the external stent, which is often trapezoid. The stents are then supported in position using a through-and-through 5-0 Prolene U-shaped suture, which is removed 5 to 7 days after surgery. It is important not to tie these sutures tightly, otherwise necrosis of the alar rim can occur. Retractions of as much as 5 mm can be corrected with this technique.

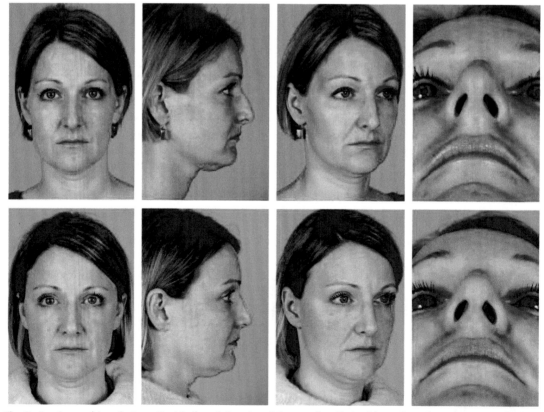

Fig. 9. A primary rhinoplasty patient before (*above*) and 1 year after (*below*) insertion of an alar rim graft along with use of transdomal suture and the removal of the cephalic margin of the lower lateral cartilage. Preoperatively, this patient showed some alar retraction and concavity. Placement of alar rim graft widened and elongated the nostril, prevented further alar concavity, and then reversed the minor alar retraction. (*Adapted from* Guyuron B, Bigdeli Y, Sajjadian A. Dynamics of the alar rim graft. Plast Reconstr Surg 2015;135(4):981–6; with permission.)

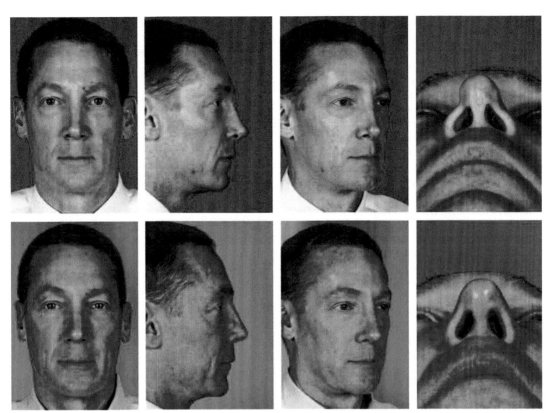

Fig. 10. Secondary rhinoplasty patient before (*above*) and 5 years after (*below*) insertion of an alar rim graft, showing correction of alar retraction and concavity, widening of the nostril (dust external valve), and elongation of the nostril. (*Adapted from* Guyuron B, Bigdeli Y, Sajjadian A. Dynamics of the alar rim graft. Plast Reconstr Surg 2015;135(4):981–6; with permission.)

The senior author has not observed retractions of more than 5 mm.

When the convexity of the ala is a result of excessive thickness of the ala there are 2 options. If an alar base reduction is planned concomitantly, the alar thickness is reduced through the alar base incision by removing excessive tissue between the lateral skin and internal lining, as described by Matarasso.[5] If alar reduction is not part of this aesthetic goal, an alar rim incision is used to reduce alar rim thickness and an elliptical incision is made along the thick ala as close to the medial nostril rim as possible. A combination of skin and subcutaneous tissue is removed (**Fig. 7**). The incision is repaired using fast-absorbing 6-0 plain catgut. Again, a stent similar to those discussed for V-Y advancement serves here to avoid the collection of blood and recurrence of the thickness.

If the convexity is the consequence of bulging cartilage, then transection and overlap of the lateral crura posteriorly often corrects this disharmony. Unless the lateral crus is thick, a Gunter strut should be placed for a better functional

and aesthetic outcome. However, if the defect is associated with an excessively curved cartilage or a boxy tip, the transdomal sutures or a Gruber lateral crura spanning suture may correct the excessive convexity of the ala more successfully.

DISCUSSION

Identifying and correcting alar imbalances adds significantly to nasal harmony, and, perhaps more importantly, improves the function of the external valve (see **Fig. 7**; **Figs. 8–10**). Thus, the surgeon's ability to identify and correct these imperfections is extremely important.

Rhinoplasty demands a more detailed analysis and greater surgical finesse than most other procedures in plastic surgery. The key to successful surgical correction is detection, which is only possible through careful clinical analysis combined with either computer or life-sized photography assessment.

Adherence to the criteria discussed earlier leads to identification of nasal base and alar abnormalities and should provide a successful outcome in most situations. However, in rhinoplasty, 100% elimination of disharmony remains an elusive goal for many surgeons, despite their efforts to achieve this rate of improvement. It is hoped that, in the future, surgeons can overcome all of these unpredictable elements.

The techniques discussed here are simple, but any operation has potential risks. For example, a small area of necrosis along the alar rim can occur if the U suture is too tight. Other possible complications include overcorrection, undesirable scarring, and temporary paresthesia in the area, although there have been no reports of complete numbness in our practice.

The potential complications of alar rim graft placement include cartilage visibility, warping, and excessive fullness of the alar rim. Some patients also complain about stiffness and palpable thickness after surgery.

The simplicity of these procedures and attention to detail will help junior surgeons reduce or eliminate these minor complications.

Although most retracted and/or concave alae are the product of alar interruption, suture techniques commonly used to reshape the lateral crus harbor a high risk of creating a convex, and possibly retracted, ala. This risk makes familiarity with these techniques, and particularly the alar rim graft, paramount.

REFERENCES

1. Gunter JP, Rohrich RJ, Friedman RM. Classification and correction of the alar-columellar discrepancies in rhinoplasty. Plast Reconstr Surg 1996;97:643.

2. Guyuron B. Alar rim deformities. Plast Reconstr Surg 2001;107(3):856–63.

3. Guyuron B, Bigdeli Y, Sajjadian A. Dynamics of the alar rim graft. Plast Reconstr Surg 2015;135(4): 981–6.

4. Ellenbogen R. Alar rim lowering. Plast Reconstr Surg 1987;79:50.

5. Matarasso A. Alar rim excision: a method of thinning bulky nostrils. Plast Reconstr Surg 1996;97:828.

Nasal Tip Deficiency

Nazim Cerkes, MD

KEYWORDS

- Nasal tip deficiency • Tip projection • Tip grafting • Lateral crural lengthening
- Lateral crural grafting • Lateral crural graft • Bended lateral crural graft • Lateral crural steal

KEY POINTS

- Structural grafting of alar cartilages strengthens the tip framework, reinforces the disrupted support mechanisms, and controls the position of the nasal tip.
- Columellar strut is a very useful tool in stabilizing the nasal base and correcting medial crural deformities. When a significant increase in tip projection is desired, a longer and stronger columellar strut can be used, and medial crura are advanced on the strut with sutures.
- Lateral crural grafts are indicated in the correction of cephalic malposition of lateral crura, alar rim retraction, strengthening of the weak lateral crura, and elongation of short lateral crura.
- In secondary cases with overresected nasal tip framework, tip projection is usually lost and can be reestablished using a columellar strut, a caudal septal extension graft, and/or a tip graft. Lateral crural grafts are used to strengthen and replace missing segments of lateral crura.

Videos of strengthening of a deficient nasal tip; correction of cephalic malposition; elongation of short alar cartilages; and bending technique for lateral crura and dome reconstruction using rib cartilage accompany this article at http://www.plasticsurgery. theclinics.com/

INTRODUCTION

The lower third of the nose has a tripodlike support structure that is made up of the conjoined medial crura and lateral crural complex based bilaterally on the piriform aperture.[1–16] The medial crura together form 1 leg of the tripod, and each lateral crus makes up the other 2 legs. In rhinoplasty, the tripod should be maintained and/or restored to provide tip support and a normal-appearing nasal tip shape (**Fig. 1**).

One of the vital steps of a rhinoplasty operation is to control the nasal tip projection and position. The length and strength of the medial crura is critical for tip projection and definition. Short and weak medial crura can lead to loss of supratip definition due to decreased differential between dorsal height and domal peak. This becomes an important issue, particularly in cases with thick nasal tip skin.

The shape and the stability of the lateral crura are important factors for aesthetic and functional reasons. Poorly supported lateral nasal walls may collapse with negative airway pressure during inspiration, thereby causing nasal airway obstruction.

TREATMENT GOALS AND PLANNED OUTCOMES

Nasal tip deficiency can be congenital or secondary to previous nasal surgeries. Preservation or reconstitution of a stable, well-defined nasal tip framework is essential for a successful rhinoplasty outcome. Structural grafting of alar cartilages strengthens the tip framework, reinforces the disrupted support mechanisms, and controls the position of the nasal tip to resist the scar forces of the healing phase in the long term.

Disclosure Statement: Adviser, Marina Medical Company, Florida, USA. Cerkes Video Series, Quality Medical Publishing, St Louis, Missouri, USA.
Private Practice, Hakki Yeten Cad No: 17/6, Fulya, Besiktas, Istanbul 34365, Turkey
E-mail address: ncerkes@hotmail.com

Clin Plastic Surg 43 (2016) 135–150
http://dx.doi.org/10.1016/j.cps.2015.09.011

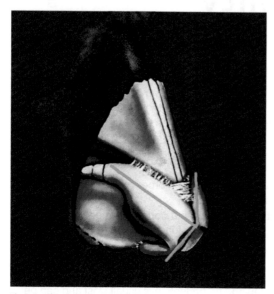

Fig. 1. The lower third of the nose has a tripodlike support structure that is made up of the conjoined medial crura and lateral crural complex based bilaterally on the piriform aperture.

Autologous cartilage is the best material for structural grafting of the nasal tip. If available, septal cartilage is the graft of choice for autologous cartilage grafting because it is rigid, relatively straight, and in the same operative field. It can be used as a columellar strut to support the nasal tip or replace parts of the lower lateral cartilage complex. However, septal cartilage is often insufficient in secondary operations. Auricular cartilage can be used to replace lateral crural defects. Onlay tip grafts and shield-type tip grafts can be prepared from concha, but flaccidity and convolutions inherent in its structure limit its use in structural grafting. If significant support is required, autologous rib cartilage is the graft of choice. Rib offers unlimited amount of cartilage for structural grafting. Long and straight struts can be prepared from the rib cartilage for reinforcement or reconstruction of the alar complex. Rib cartilage is less calcified and more elastic in young individuals and this allows the preparation of thin grafts for alar cartilage reconstruction.

The open rhinoplasty approach provides better visualization without distortion of cartilages, leading to accurate diagnosis and treatment.

PROCEDURAL APPROACH
Increasing Tip Projection and Stabilizing the Columellar Base

Underdeveloped alar cartilages usually present with loss of tip projection and ill-defined nasal tip contours. In these patients, cartilage grafting is usually required to increase tip projection and improve tip contours.

Columellar strut graft
Columellar strut is a versatile and powerful tool to stabilize the columellar base, strengthening the weak medial and intermediate crura, increasing tip projection, and changing rotation. It is placed in a pocket between medial and intermediate crura, keeping a bed of soft tissue above the nasal spine. When a considerable increase in tip projection is desired, a longer and stronger columellar strut should be used and medial crura are advanced on the strut with sutures. The columellar strut is also useful in changing columella-lobule angle, controlling the length of the medial or middle crural segments and correcting intercrural deformities or asymmetries of the lateral crura.

If a significant increase of the tip projection is needed, advancing the lateral crura medially with a spanning suture (lateral crural steal) and the simultaneous use of a long and strong columellar strut give consistent results (**Fig. 2**). Strong columellar strut grafts can be prepared from the thicker portions of the septal cartilage or lamination of 2 struts from septal cartilage side-to-side suture (**Fig. 3**). In primary patients who do not have thick septal cartilage and in secondary rhinoplasty patients without sufficient septum cartilage, columellar strut can be fabricated from rib cartilage. The columellar strut is placed between the medial crura, and medial crura are advanced on the strut with sutures to achieve the desired tip projection. In cases with short medial crura and long lateral crura, lateral crural steal procedure is a very useful technique that elongates the medial crura, shortens the lateral crura, and increase the tip projection. This technique also rotates the nasal tip upward, augments the infratip lobule, and changes infratip lobule angle.

Tip graft
After placement of the columellar strut, if additional increase in tip projection and further refinement is needed, a tip graft can be used to increase tip projection and improve the tip contour. Shield-type tip grafts are particularly useful in patients with short infratip lobule and in secondary cases.

Caudal septal extension graft
Caudal septal extension graft is a rectangular cartilage that is extended off of the caudal septum and sutured between the medial crura. It is a useful

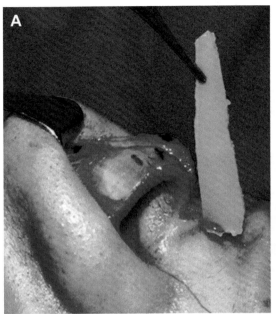
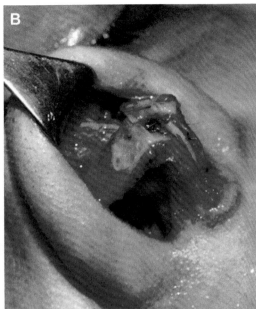

Fig. 2. (A) The original and new domal points are marked to create new domes using spanning sutures, and a long and strong columellar strut is prepared from the septum cartilage. (B) Tip projection is increased with lateral crural steal and advancement of medial crura on a strong columellar strut.

method to increase projection and rotation of nasal tip. To maximize stability and avoid asymmetries, it should be stabilized to existing dorsal septum with bilateral spreader grafts. Then the medial crura are stabilized to the caudal margin of the graft to achieve the desired tip projection and rotation. In this method, first needles are passed through the medial crura and septal extension graft to judge the position of the tip, then medial crura are fixated to the septal extension graft with tongue-in-groove fashion horizontal mattress sutures.

Strengthening the Lateral Crura

If lateral crura are congenitally weak, a structural grafting should be considered. In the presence of a weak lateral crural strip, any surgical intervention may accentuate an external nasal valve collapse. In mild cases of lateral crural weakness, a lateral crura turn-in flap can be used for support. Alar contour graft is another method to reinforce the alar rim in mild to moderate weakness of the lateral crura. Lateral crural strut graft is the most effective method to support weak lateral crura, adding stability to the nostril rim and external nasal valve.

Case analysis
A 20-year-old patient presented with dorsal hump, underprojected tip, acute nasolabial angle, and retracted alae. Her lateral crura were weak, alar rims were not well supported, and domes were weak and pointed. Intranasal examination revealed a deviated septum obstructing the airway (**Fig. 4**A–D).

Using the open rhinoplasty technique, septoplasty and septal cartilage harvest were performed. Bony and cartilaginous humps were reduced and medial oblique and lateral osteotomies were performed. Spreader flaps were used

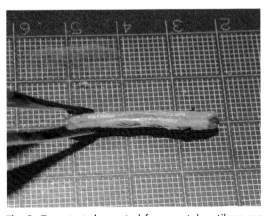

Fig. 3. Two struts harvested from septal cartilage are laminated with side-to-side sutures to create a stronger columellar strut.

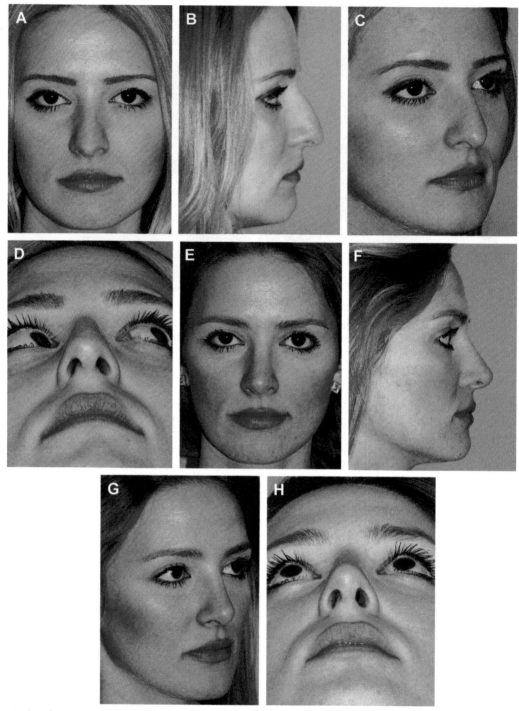

Fig. 4. (*A–D*) A 20-year-old patient presented with dorsal hump, underprojected tip, acute nasolabial angle, and retracted alae. Her lateral crura were weak, alar rims were not well supported, and domes were weak and pointed. (*E–H*) The patient is shown 2 years postoperatively. The dorsal hump is removed, resulting in a smooth and straight dorsum. Tip projection is increased, the nasal tip is well supported, and alar rim retraction is corrected.

to establish the cartilaginous dorsum. To increase tip projection, the lateral crura were advanced medially with spanning sutures. A long columellar strut was prepared from the harvested septum and the medial crura were advanced on the columellar strut with 3 sutures. A subdomal graft was placed to reinforce and widen the weak domes. A thin onlay tip graft was placed for further increase in tip projection. Alar contour grafts were placed bilaterally to support alar rims (Video 1).

The patient is shown 2 years postoperatively. The dorsal hump is removed, and a smooth, straight dorsum is achieved. Tip projection is increased, nasal tip is well supported, and alar rim retraction is corrected (**Fig. 4**E–H).

Cephalic Malposition of Lateral Crura

In patients who have cephalic malposition of the lateral crura, the alar rim is not supported, causing a parenthesis deformity of the nasal tip. The malpositioned lateral crus does not parallel the alar rim, resulting in weakness. The degree of cephalic malposition may differ from mild to severe. In mild and moderate malposition, a lateral crural strut graft or an alar rim graft can be placed parallel to the alar rim without caudal transposition of the lateral crura, so as to support the alar rim and correct the supra alar notching. However, in severe cephalic malposition, lateral crural transposition should be the method of choice. In this technique, the malpositioned lateral crus is separated from accessory cartilages and transposed caudally. If the lateral crura are not long and strong enough, it is wiser to strengthen and elongate the lateral crura with a lateral crural strut graft for the predictability of the reconstruction. The lateral end of the graft is placed in a pocket undermined caudal to the accessory cartilages.

Case analysis
A 32-year-old patient presented with dorsal hump, hanging columella, and severe cephalic malposition of the lateral crura (**Fig. 5**A–D).

Minimal bony and cartilaginous hump reduction was performed and spreader flaps were used to reconstruct cartilaginous dorsum. Lateral crura were separated from the accessory cartilages. Medial crura were fixated to the caudal septum with a tongue-in-groove suture. Crural struts from septal cartilage were placed underneath the lateral crura. New pockets were undermined caudal to the accessory cartilages, then lateral crura were transposed into the new pockets (Video 2).

Fifteen months postoperatively, the pictures reveal corrected lateral crura positions and well-supported alar rims (**Fig. 5**E–H).

Elongation of Short Alar Cartilages

Short alar cartilages usually present with decreased tip projection and ill-defined nasal tip contours. If overall length of alar cartilages are short, they must be elongated with cartilage grafts. In patients with short alar cartilages, the lateral crural steal technique and advancement of medial crura on a columellar strut can be used to elongate the medial crura and increase tip projection. However, this maneuver further shortens and weakens the lateral crura. In this case, the lateral crura can be divided from the accessory cartilages and advanced medially, then a lateral crural graft is placed between the lateral crura and the accessory cartilage to bridge the gap and reconstitute a stable nasal tip tripod. With this method, both medial and lateral crura are elongated and tip framework is strengthened.

Case analysis
A 19-year-old patient presented with dorsal hump, decreased tip projection, and ill-defined nasal tip. Her medial crura were short and footplates were not extending down to the nasal base. The lateral crura were weak, alar rims were not well supported, and she had weak dome support (**Fig. 6**A–D).

Using the open rhinoplasty technique, the nasal dorsum and nasal tip were exposed. After harvesting the septal cartilage, the bony and cartilaginous hump was removed. Spreader flaps were used to establish the cartilaginous dorsal width. Medial crura were separated and caudal septum was exposed down to the nasal spine. The anterior nasal spine was reduced. A transfixing suture was placed to set back the medial crura on the caudal septum. Lateral crura were divided from the accessory cartilage junction. Lateral crura were advanced 5 mm medially with spanning sutures (lateral crural steal). A long columellar strut was placed between the medial crura to increase the tip projection. Lateral crural grafts were placed on both sides between the lateral crura and the accessory cartilage to reconstitute a stable nasal tip tripod (**Fig. 6**E–H, Video 3).

The patient is shown 1 year postoperatively. The dorsal hump is removed, tip projection is increased, medial crura are set back to the nasal base, the short medial crura are lengthened, the nasal tip is well supported, and alar rim retraction is corrected (**Fig. 6**I–L).

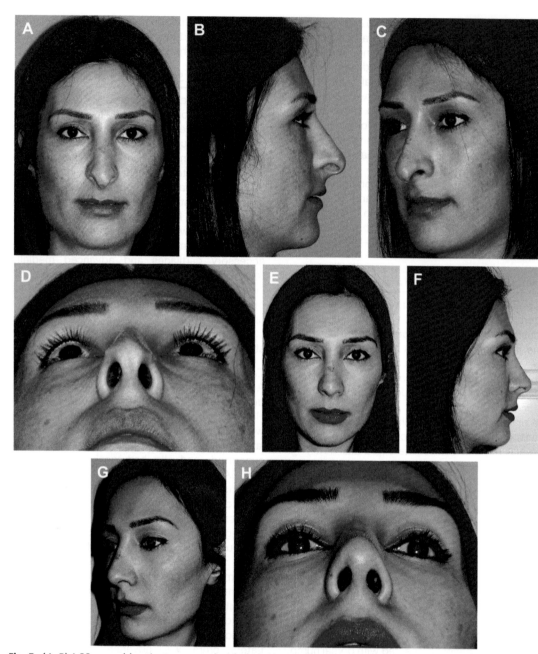

Fig. 5. (*A–D*) A 32-year-old patient presented with dorsal hump, hanging columella, and severe cephalic malposition of the lateral crura. (*E–H*) Fifteen months postoperatively, the pictures reveal corrected lateral crura positions and well-supported alar rims.

Congenital Absence or Asymmetries of the Alar Cartilages

Congenital asymmetries or absence of alar cartilages can be reconstructed with structural grafting principles. Tip projection can be reestablished by using a columellar strut, a caudal septal extension graft, and/or a tip graft.

Lateral crural grafts can be used to replace lateral crural defects and correct lateral crural asymmetries.

Case analysis

A 23-year-old patient presented with maxillo-nasal dysplasia (Binder syndrome). She had low tip

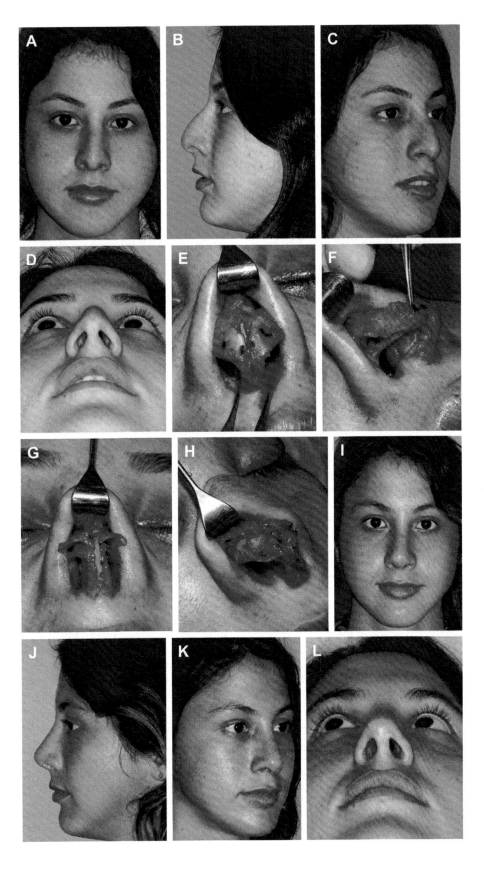

projection and underdeveloped, infantile alar cartilages and septum cartilage (**Fig. 7**A–D).

The sixth rib cartilage was harvested. Five cartilage strip grafts were prepared for septal L-strut reconstruction and alar cartilage reconstruction. First, septal L-strut reconstruction was performed with placement of 2 struts dorsally and 1 strut caudally. The caudal strut was placed more caudally as a septal extension graft. Two long cartilage grafts were prepared for alar cartilage reconstruction. These grafts were thinned to less than a millimeter in thickness to make them pliable. Medially, the cartilage grafts were sutured to the caudal septal extension graft reconstructing the medial crura. The grafts were bent with spanning sutures and new domes were created. The lateral segments of the grafts were extended to the piriform aperture. The vestibular skin is then secured to the lateral crural grafts. A dome equalization suture was placed to approximate the lateral crural grafts and to create dome-defining points (**Fig. 7**E–H).

Nine months after surgery, a structured approach allowed anatomic reconstruction of the nasal tip and the septum. Tip projection is increased significantly and alar rims are well supported (**Fig. 7**I–L).

Secondary Deformities of the Alar Cartilages

If the principles of the structural rhinoplasty are not taken into consideration at the time of the primary rhinoplasty, there usually is a loss of the tip-supporting mechanisms. Excessive removal of the tip cartilages and inadvertent use of sutures further accentuates the problem. The septal integrity might be lost and this increases the tip-support problems. A stable and straight septum cartilage is essential for tip support and septum reconstruction should precede any tip reconstruction.

Anatomic reconstruction of the weakened or interrupted alar cartilages and reconstitution of a stable nasal tip tripod must be performed for a predictable outcome. The newly reconstructed cartilaginous framework should be strong enough to withstand the even greater forces of wound contraction during the healing period.

Establishing tip projection and position

In secondary cases with overresected nasal skeleton, tip projection is usually lost, which has to be reestablished. The typical polly beak deformity due to overresected nasal skeleton can be corrected with adjusting the tip projection.

Structural grafts for tip projection include the columellar strut, the caudal septal extension graft, and tip grafts.

Columellar strut grafts strengthen the existing tip support, provide stability, and increase tip projection when medial crura are advanced on it.

If septum cartilage was overresected or weakened in the primary operation, a caudal septal extension graft stabilized with spreader grafts provide septal stability, and medial crura can be fixated to the septal extension graft to establish tip projection and position (**Fig. 8**).

Tip grafts can be used to increase the tip projection and improve the tip contour. In revision cases, shield-type tip grafts are preferred to achieve tip definition and hide tip asymmetries. If the shield graft is prepared from rib cartilage, visibility of the sharp edges of the cartilage can be a problem in the long term; hence, is camouflaged using fascia or perichondrial grafts (**Fig. 9**).

Lateral crural reconstruction

Overzealous resection of the lateral crura may result in alar rim collapse because of severe attenuation or interruption of lateral crural rim strip. Patients usually present with narrow nostrils and pinching deformity. In many cases, airway obstruction due to external nasal valve collapse accompanies this deformity.

Weak, misshapen, malpositioned, or segmentally deficient lateral crura must be reconstructed to achieve a stable nasal tip tripod for an aesthetically pleasing outcome and the efficiency of the external and internal nasal valves. The lateral crural graft is a versatile tool for reshaping, repositioning, or replacing the missing segments of the

Fig. 6. (*A–D*) A 19-year-old patient presented with dorsal hump, decreased tip projection, and ill-defined nasal tip. Her medial crura were short and footplates were not extending down to the nasal base. The lateral crura were weak, alar rims were not well supported, and she had weak dome support. (*E*) A transfixing suture was placed to set back the medial crura on the caudal septum. (*F*) Lateral crura were divided from the accessory cartilage junction. (*G*) Lateral crura were advanced 5 mm medially with spanning sutures. A long columellar strut was placed between the medial crura to increase the tip projection. (*H*) Lateral crural grafts were placed on both sides between the lateral crura and the accessory cartilage to reconstitute a stable nasal tip tripod. (*I–L*) The patient is shown 1 year postoperatively. The dorsal hump is removed, tip projection is increased, medial crura are set back to the nasal base, the short medial crura are lengthened, the nasal tip is well supported, and alar rim retraction is corrected.

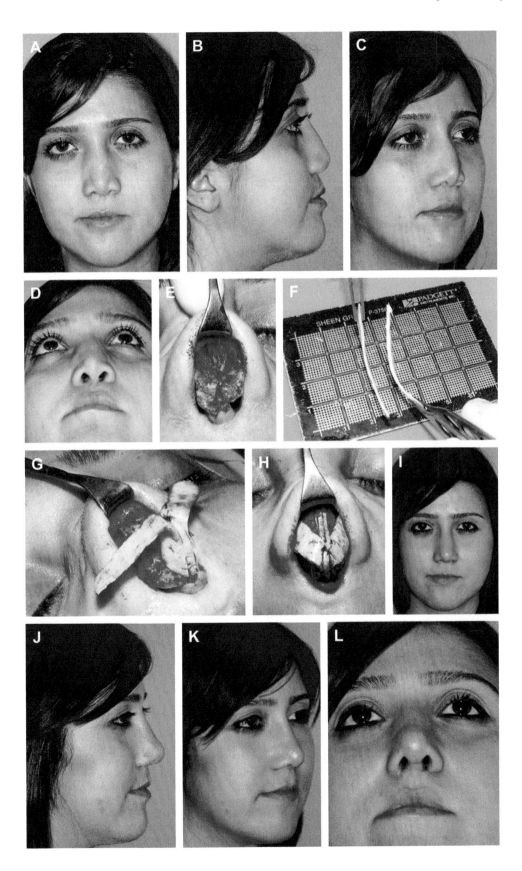

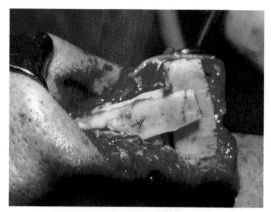

Fig. 8. The caudal septal extension graft is stabilized to the septum with bilateral spreader grafts.

lateral crura. The grafts can be prepared from septum, auricle, or rib cartilages.

If the deformity is not severe, such as attenuated lateral crura or a missing small segment, replacing or strengthening the deformed segment with a lateral crural graft is the preferred method of reconstruction to establish the shape and stability of the lateral crura (**Fig. 10**).

If the lateral crura are missing but the medial crura and domes are intact, the vestibular skin is dissected off of the undersurface of each dome to fixate lateral crural grafts. Lateral crural grafts, prepared from septum cartilage or rib cartilage, are then sutured to the undersurface of each dome to replace the missing lateral crura (**Fig. 11**).

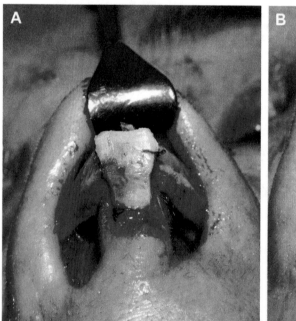
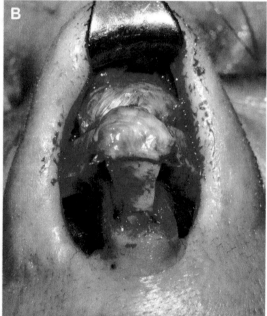

Fig. 9. (*A*) A shield-type tip graft is prepared from rib cartilage. (*B*) A double-layer rectus abdominis fascia graft is placed on top of the shield-type tip graft to camouflage sharp edges.

Fig. 7. (*A–D*) A 23-year-old patient presented with maxillo-nasal dysplasia. She has low tip projection, and underdeveloped, infantile alar cartilages and septum cartilage. (*E*) Skin flap was elevated. The alar cartilages were soft and underdeveloped like infantile cartilages. The septum cartilage was absent. (*F*) Sixth rib cartilage was harvested. Two long cartilage grafts were prepared for alar cartilage reconstruction. These grafts were thinned to less than a millimeter in thickness to make them pliable. (*G*) Septal L-strut reconstruction was performed with placement of 2 struts dorsally and 1 strut caudally. The lateral crural grafts were first sutured to the septal extension graft and then bent to recreate the genu with spanning sutures. (*H*) The lateral segments of the grafts were extended to the piriform aperture. A dome-equalization suture was placed to approximate the grafts and to create dome-defining points. (*I–L*) Nine months after surgery. A structured approach allowed anatomic reconstruction of the nasal tip and the septum. Tip projection is increased significantly and alar rims are well supported.

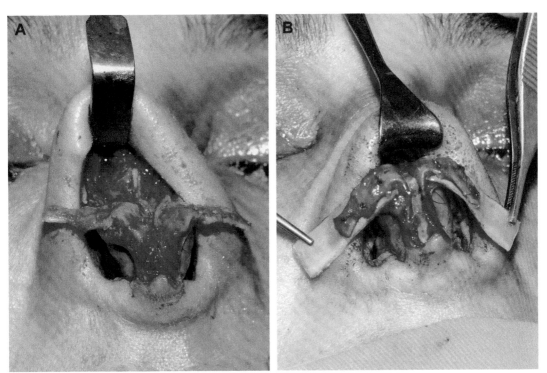

Fig. 10. (*A*) In a secondary case, lateral crura of alar cartilages are attenuated and deformed. (*B*) Reconstruction of the lateral crura is performed with placement of lateral crural grafts.

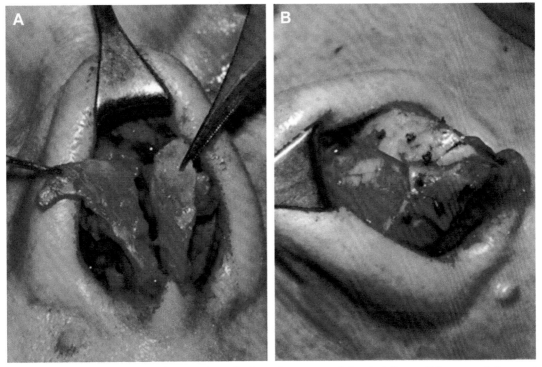

Fig. 11. (*A*) In a secondary rhinoplasty patient, the lateral crura are missing but the medial crura and domes are intact. The vestibular skin is dissected off the undersurface of each dome to fixate lateral crural grafts. (*B*) Lateral crural grafts, prepared from septum cartilage, are sutured to the undersurface of each dome to replace the missing lateral crura.

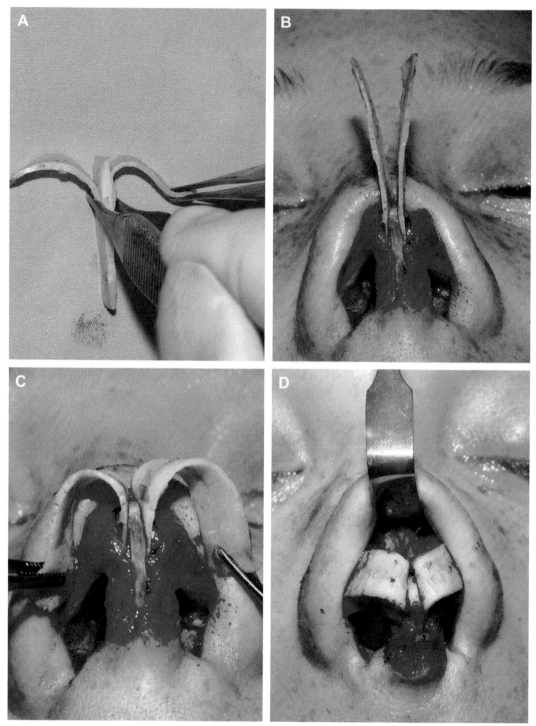

Fig. 12. (*A*) A columellar strut and 2 lateral crural grafts are prepared from rib cartilage to reconstruct nasal tip tripod. The lateral crural grafts can be bent to create the domes. (*B*) Columellar strut is placed between medial crura, and lateral crural grafts are fixated to the upper end of the columellar strut with 2 sutures. (*C*) Lateral crural grafts are bent to create domes and achieve an anatomic reconstruction. (*D*) The domes are created with spanning sutures. The newly created domes are approximated with a dome equalization suture. These sutures help to create 2 tip-defining points and a supratip break point.

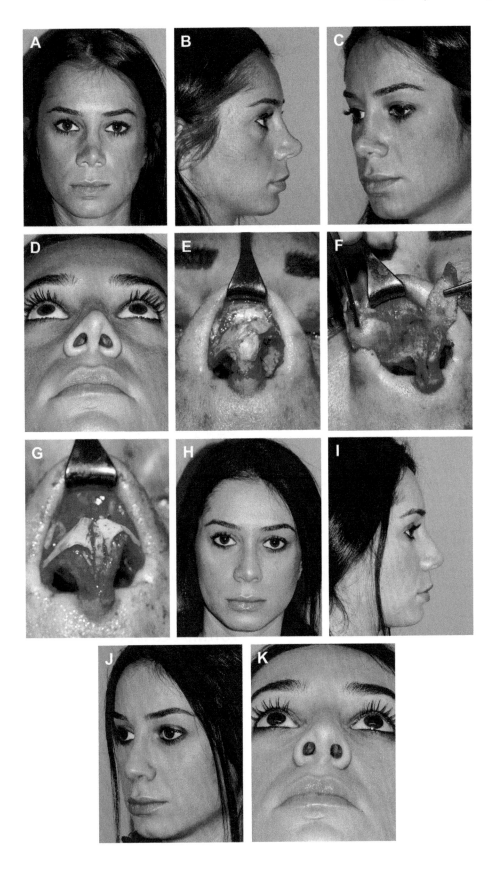

If the domes and lateral crura are missing or severely deformed, a columellar strut is placed to reconstruct the caudal leg of the tripod and fixated to the medial crural remnants. Long lateral crural grafts are prepared from the rib cartilage (usually the length of the septum cartilage is not sufficient) and thinned, to allow the graft to bend. The lateral crural grafts are fixated to the columellar strut with 2 sutures approximately 4 to 5 mm below the upper end of the columellar strut. Then, lateral crural grafts are bent and domes are created with dome-spanning sutures. The newly created domes are approximated with a dome-equalization suture. These sutures help to create 2 tip-defining points and supratip break point (**Fig. 12**, Video 4).

Case analysis

After one prior rhinoplasty, this 23-year-old patient presented with overprojected pinched tip, low nasal dorsum, narrow midvault, and functional nasal problems (**Fig. 13**A–D).

The deformed lateral crura were resected. The sixth rib cartilage and 4×4-cm rectus abdominis fascia graft were harvested. Bilateral spreader grafts were placed to reconstruct the internal nasal valves. A columellar strut was placed between the medial crural remnants. Two long lateral crural grafts were prepared in 0.5-mm in thickness from the rib cartilage. The lateral crural grafts were first sutured to the columellar strut. Then they were bent and extended laterally. Dome-spanning sutures and an interdomal suture were placed to create new domes and tip-defining points. A thin diced cartilage-rectus abdominis fascia graft was placed to camouflage dorsal irregularities (**Fig. 13**E–G).

The patient is shown 2 years after the surgery. Tip projection is decreased, and a structured nasal tip is achieved with functional improvement. The nasal dorsum is smoothed and augmented (**Fig. 13**H–K).

In some patients and the elderly, the rib cartilage is more calcified and rigid, and it is not usually possible to carve thin lateral crural grafts, which are pliable enough to create new domes with spanning sutures. In these cases, the lateral

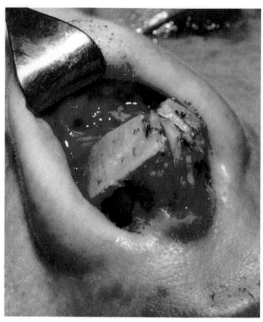

Fig. 14. In a patient with calcified rib cartilage, the lateral crural grafts are sutured to the tip of the columellar strut to reconstitute the nasal tip tripod.

crural grafts are sutured to the tip of the columellar strut to reconstitute the nasal tip tripod. The grafts are extended laterally to the pyriform aperture. The angle between the columellar strut and lateral crural graft is kept at approximately 45° (**Fig. 14**). To create the tip-defining points and camouflage the sharp edges of the columellar strut and lateral crural grafts, a tip graft can be placed on top of the junction (**Fig. 15**). To avoid the visibility of the sharp edges of the tip graft, an onlay rectus fascia graft or a perichondrial graft is placed on the newly reconstructed dome (**Fig. 16**).

POTENTIAL COMPLICATIONS AND MANAGEMENT

Tip asymmetries can be seen due to uneven placement of structural grafts. Maximum care should be

Fig. 13. (A–D) After one prior rhinoplasty, this 23-year-old patient presented with overprojected and pinched tip, low nasal dorsum, narrow midvault, and functional nasal problems. (E, F) The deformed lateral crura were resected. (G) A columellar strut was placed between the medial crural remnants. Two lateral crural grafts were prepared, 0.5 mm in thickness, from the rib cartilage and sutured to the columellar strut. The lateral crural grafts were bent, and dome-spanning sutures and an interdomal suture were placed to create new domes and tip-defining points. (H–K) The patient is shown 2 years after surgery. The nasal tip projection is decreased, and a structured nasal tip is achieved with functional improvement. The nasal dorsum is smoothened and augmented.

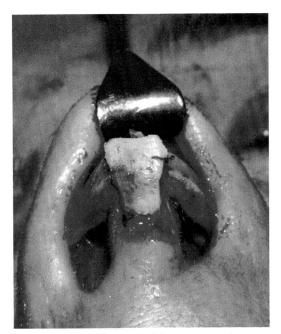

Fig. 15. To create the tip-defining points and camouflage the sharp edges of the columellar strut and lateral crural grafts, a tip graft is placed on top of the junction.

taken in placement of the grafts symmetrically at the time of surgery.

If the columellar strut is placed directly against the premaxilla, a displacement from the midline can be seen postoperatively. If the columellar strut

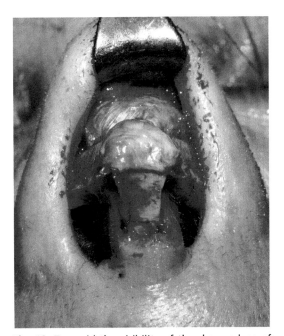

Fig. 16. To avoid the visibility of the sharp edges of the tip graft, a double-layer onlay rectus fascia graft is placed over the newly reconstructed dome.

overlaps the caudal septum, shifting from the midline can be seen. If a soft tissue pad is not protected in-between the columellar strut and the anterior nasal spine, the patient can experience a clicking sensation while smiling.

Lateral crural strut grafts may displace the vestibular skin medially and compromise the airway if they are not placed in proper position.

Caudal septal extension grafts may cause deviation of the nasal tip if stabilized in an overlapping fashion to the caudal septum. To avoid this, the caudal septal graft should be aligned end to end with existing caudal septum by using caudally extended spreader grafts.

If structural grafts for lower lateral reconstruction are thick, the thickness of the grafts may create a bulk around the tip and obstruct the airway. This is particularly true for the grafts prepared from the rib cartilage. The crural strut grafts prepared from the rib cartilage must be thinned enough to avoid this problem.

SUPPLEMENTARY DATA

Supplementary data related to this article can be found online at http://dx.doi.org/10.1016/j.cps. 2015.09.011.

REFERENCES

1. Anderson JR. A reasoned approach to nasal base surgery. Arch Otolaryngol 1984;110:349–58.
2. McCollough EG, Mangat D. Systematic approach to correction of nasal tip in rhinoplasty. Arch Otolaryngol 1981;107:12.
3. Sheen JH. Spreader graft: a method of reconstructing the roof of the middle nasal vault following rhinoplasty. Plast Reconstr Surg 1984;73:230.
4. Gunter JP, Freidman RM. Lateral crural strut graft: technique and clinical applications in rhinoplasty. Plast Reconstr Surg 1997;99:943.
5. Toriumi DM. Structure approach in rhinoplasty. Facial Plast Surg Clin North Am 2002;10:1.
6. DeRosa J, Watson D, Toriumi DM. Structural grafting in secondary rhinoplasty. In: Gunter JP, Rohrich RJ, Adams WP Jr, editors. Dallas rhinoplasty nasal surgery by the masters. St Louis (MO): Quality Medical Publishing, Inc; 2007. p. 719–40.
7. Gunter JP, Cochran CS. The tripod concept for correcting severely deformed nasal tip cartilages. In: Gunter JP, Rohrich RJ, Adams WP Jr, editors. Dallas rhinoplasty nasal surgery by the masters. St Louis (MO): Quality Medical Publishing, Inc; 2007. p. 841–50.
8. Rohrich RJ, Raniere J Jr, Ha RY. Alar contour graft: correction and prevention of alar rim

deformities in rhinoplasty. Plast Reconstr Surg 2002;109:2495.

9. Gunter JP, Freidman RM, Hackney FL. Correction of alar rim deformities: lateral crural strut grafts. In: Gunter JP, Rohrich RJ, Adams WP Jr, editors. Dallas rhinoplasty nasal surgery by the masters. St Louis (MO): Quality Medical Publishing, Inc; 2007. p. 757–72.

10. Petroff MA, McCollough EG, Hom D, et al. Nasal tip projection. Arch Otolaryngol Head Neck Surg 1991; 117:783.

11. Kridel RWH, Konior RJ, Shumrick KA, et al. Advances in nasal tip surgery: the lateral crural steal. Arch Otolaryngol Head Neck Surg 1989;115:1206.

12. Foda H, Kridel RWH. Lateral crural steal and lateral crural overlay. Arch Otolaryngol Head Neck Surg 1999;125:1365.

13. Gibson T, Dawis WB. The distortion of autogenous cartilage grafts: its causes and prevention. Br J Plast Surg 1958;10:257.

14. Sheen JH. Achieving more nasal tip projection by the use of a small autogenous vomer or septal cartilage graft. A preliminary report. Plast Reconstr Surg 1975;56:35.

15. Byrd S, Andodochick S, Copit S, et al. Septal extension grafts: a method of controlling tip projection, rotation and shape. Plast Reconstr Surg 1997; 100:999.

16. Cerkes N. Structural grafting of the nasal tip. In: Rohrich RJ, Adams WP Jr, Ahmad J, editors. Dallas rhinoplasty nasal surgery by the masters. 3rd edition. St Louis (MO); Boca Raton (FL): Quality Medical Publishing & CRC Press Inc; 2014. p. 393–440.

Projection and Deprojection Techniques in Rhinoplasty

Fazil Apaydin, MD

KEYWORDS

- Projection • Deprojection • Increasing projection • Decreasing projection • Shield graft
- Lateral crural steal • Septocolumellar suture • Tip graft

KEY POINTS

- Analyze the nose thoroughly to decide on the ideal projection of the nose.
- Discuss the alternatives of tip projection with the patient.
- If the patient's tip projection is satisfactory, the surgeon must prevent postoperative loss of tip support by using columellar struts, or septocolumellar or tongue-in-groove sutures.
- For overprojected tips, the surgeon must determine whether the issue is resulting from to the nasal septum or the lower lateral cartilages.
- The surgeon should try to put all the surgical techniques in his or her armamentarium and choose the ones that will work in each selected case.

 Videos of the major surgical steps to deproject the nose accompany this article at http://www.plasticsurgery.theclinics.com/

INTRODUCTION

There are 3 important parameters of the nose that the rhinoplasty surgeon and patients must take into account: nasal length, projection, and rotation of the tip (**Box 1**). All of these parameters are closely linked to each other. During the preoperative consultation, the surgeon should examine and analyze the nose thoroughly and discuss the available solutions with the patient.

In facial analysis, there are many methods to calculate the ideal projection of the nose. The simplest method, described by Simons,[1] states that the length of the upper lip equals the length of the subnasale to the tip. In Goode's formula, a line to the nasal tip drawn perpendicular to a line from the nasion through the alar–facial junction should be 55% to 60% of the dorsal nasal length

from the nasion to the tip.[2] Crumley and Lanser described the ideal nasal projection as a ratio equal to 0.2833 by comparing the length of the line from the nasion to the vermilion of the upper lip and the length of a perpendicular line to the tip defining point.[3] Similarly, Powell described that a line drawn from nasion to subnasale is correlated with a perpendicular line reaching to the tip defining point and found it to be approximately 2.8.[4] Byrd published in his research that tip projection should be approximately two-thirds (0.67) of the surgically planned or ideal nasal length[5] (**Fig. 1**).

Current concepts in tip support are based on Anderson's tripod concept.[6] He described the conjoined medial crura as 1 leg and each of the lateral crura as the other legs in the tripod that

---

No disclosures.
Department of Otolaryngology, Ege University Medical Faculty, Bornova, İzmir 35100, Turkey
E-mail addresses: fazil.apaydin@ege.edu.tr; fazil.apaydin@gmail.com

---

Box 1
Algorithm regarding projection of the nasal tip

1. Decreasing projection
   a. Shortening the long medial crura
      i. Septocolumellar or tongue-in-groove sutures
      ii. Medial crural steal
      iii. Footplate resection
      iv. Lipsett
      v. Medial crural overlay
      vi. Vertical dome division
      vii. Dome truncation
   b. Shortening the long lateral crura
      i. Lateral crural steal
      ii. Lateral crural overlay
      iii. Vertical dome division
      iv. Dome truncation
2. Keeping the projection
   a. Septocolumellar or tongue-in-groove sutures
   b. Columellar strut
3. Increasing projection
   a. Sutures
      i. Lateral crural steal
      ii. Vertical dome division
      iii. Septocolumellar or tongue-in-groove sutures
   b. Grafts
      i. The grafts used to increase the dimensions, change the shape and strength of the caudal septum
         1. Columellar strut
         2. Caudal septal extension graft
         3. L-strut graft
         4. Subtotal septal reconstruction
      ii. The grafts used to support or replace the existing lower lateral cartilages
      iii. The grafts used over the tip
         1. Shield graft
         2. Tip onlay graft

---

determines tip projection and rotation (**Fig. 2**). The projection of the nasal tip can be changed by changing the length of these legs or the pedestal on which the tripod rests.

TREATMENT GOALS

When dealing with the projection of the tip, there are 3 options that must be considered while performing rhinoplasty: whether to maintain,

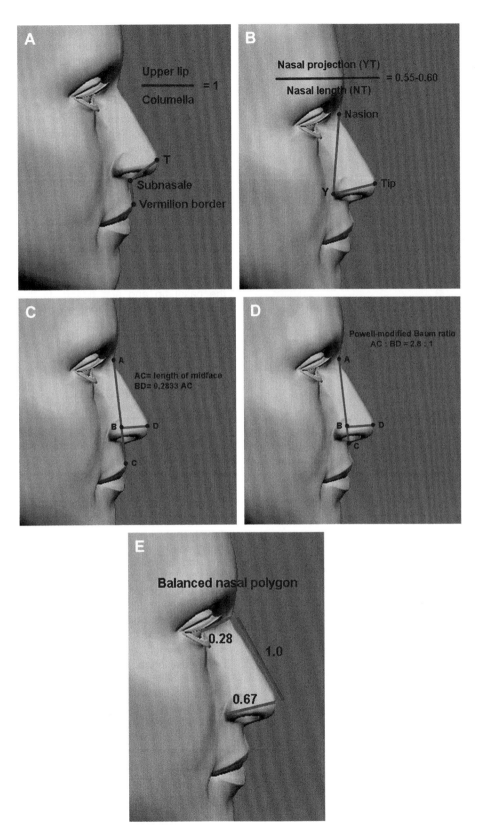

Fig. 1. The most popular methods to calculate the ideal projection of the nose. (*A*) Simons. (*B*) Goode. (*C*) Crumley and Lanser. (*D*) Powell. (*E*) Byrd. T, tip.

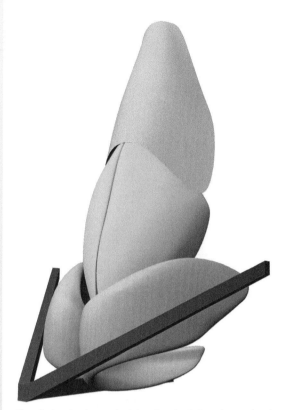

Fig. 2. In Anderson's tripod principle, the paired medial crura and 2 lateral crura serve as the 3 legs of the tripod. The projection, rotation, and shape of the tip can be changed by changing the length of these legs.

decrease, or increase the projection. In cases where the tip is overprojected or poorly projected, the surgeon should explore the underlying etiology. The 2 main factors in an overprojected nose are the lower lateral cartilages and/or the nasal septum, which acts as an important pedestal for the tip. In accordance with the results of facial analysis and examination, the surgeon should discuss his or her findings with the patient and try to find the best way to fulfill the patient's desires.

PREOPERATIVE PLANNING AND PREPARATION

The patient should be supplied with the general information on rhinoplasty and goals pertaining to their case. In revision cases, there may be a need for harvesting cartilage from the ear or rib. Preoperative photos must always be obtained. The author uses a studio with 2 flashes and a full-frame SLR camera with 105 mm macro lens to take life size 1:1 pictures. This is ideal for accurate aesthetic and photometric analysis as well as for postoperative comparison. These pictures are transferred typically into Rhinobase, a special program used to store patient data and enabling the surgeon to use an automated facial analysis tool.[7] The program is used to make 5 calculations relating to the patient's tip projection in accordance to Simons, Goode, Crumley and Lancer, and Powell and Byrd (**Fig. 3**). Morphing of the images is undertaken, taking into account the measurements but relying mostly on the aesthetic eye of the surgeon and desires of the patient. During the imaging session, the surgeon can modify the lateral and basal view to show the likely changes to the patient regarding their tip projection and rotation. Altering the basal view helps the patient to better understand how changes in the projection of the tip can alter the nasal tip and alar flaring. In this author's opinion, it is important to show different options to the patient to understand what the patient really wants.

PROCEDURAL APPROACH
Decreasing Tip Projection

The classic technique to address an overprojected tip is to perform a full transfixion leading to loss of a major tip support mechanism.[8] The author has not found this method to be predictable. More reliable and precise results can be achieved with external rhinoplasty techniques that directly address the relationship of the medial crura to the caudal septum. Septocolumellar suture techniques are excellent for addressing an overprojected tip in the author's practice.[9] The technique must take into consideration the length of the caudal septum as well as the degree of its connection and overlapping with the medial crura. A tongue-in-groove technique can be performed when the caudal septum is long enough, allowing easy overlapping with the medial crura.[10] The versatility of this technique lies in the freedom it gives the surgeon to attach the medial crura anywhere on the caudal septum depending on the need (**Fig. 4**). Of course, there is always a trade-off like any other surgical maneuver in rhinoplasty; the tip may become very stiff.

When the medial crura are longer than usual, 4 techniques can be used to deproject the nose:

1. Septocolumellar sutures may be used to lower the medial crura.[9]
2. A new deprojected dome can be created by stealing from the medial crus.[11]

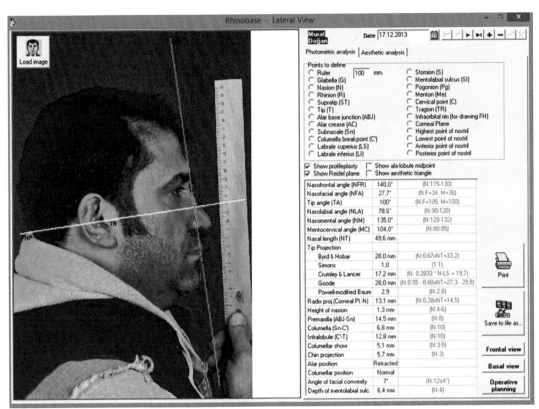

Fig. 3. This figure is captured from Rhinobase showing the screen in which all the measurements in terms of lengths and angles on the lateral view are calculated automatically after putting the landmarks on the patient's picture. The surgeon can see the results of 5 measurements regarding projection in this screen and compare the results by using his or her aesthetic eye.

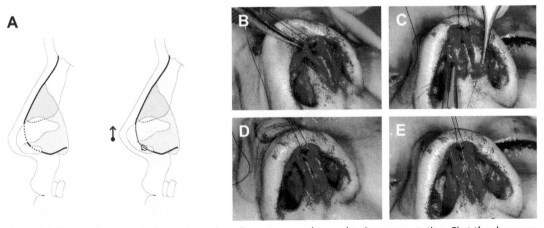

Fig. 4. (A) Shows schematically how septocolumellar suture can be used to increase rotation. First the domes are equalized by a transdomal suture (B). The first suture is passed from the caudal septum (C), then from the interior margin of the medial crura in a mattress fashion (D). A second septocolumellar suture further guarantees a better fixation of the medial crura to the caudal septum (E).

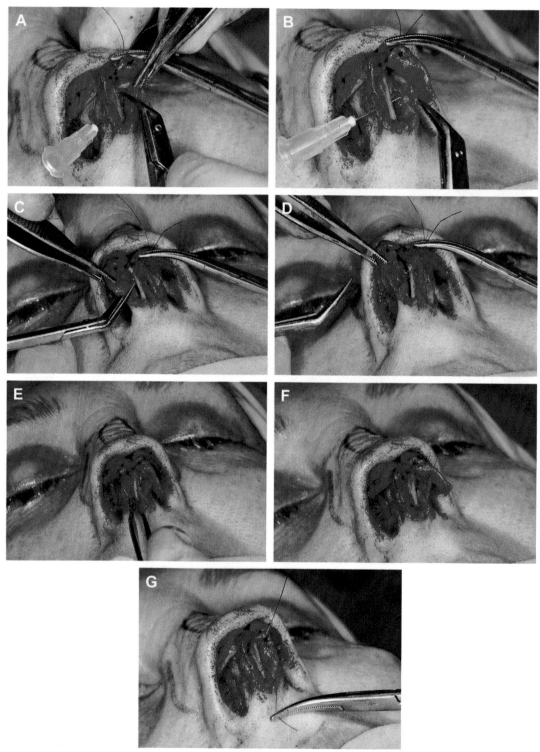

Fig. 5. When the medial crura are longer than usual, one of the best ways to reduce tip projection is to resect the medial crura (*A–D*), overlap and suture the cut edges (*E, F*), and suture the overlapped medial crura to the caudal septum (*G*).

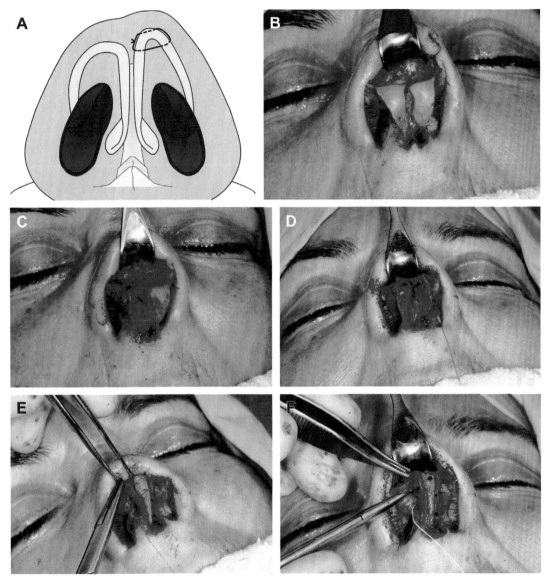

Fig. 6. Lateral crural steal is a suture technique that can be used to increase projection and rotation while obtaining a more favorable shape of the lateral crus (*A*). In this case, the patient has a droopy tip (*B*). Initially, a lateral crural turn-in flap is performed to get an improvement in shape and strength of the lateral crura. A lateral crural steal suture is then applied to increase the projection of the tip (*C*). The medial crura are attached to the caudal septum by septocolumellar suture (*D*) and then supported by a columellar strut (*E, F*). The preoperative and 14 months postoperative frontal, lateral, and basal views (*G–L*). When one looks at the picture with a nicely projected tip (*M*), it is clear that a loss of projection can sometimes happen (*J*) in the follow-up period.

3. The medial crus can be divided either segmentally with the cut edges sutured end to end[12] or with the edges overlapped and sutured without any resection[13] (**Fig. 5**).
4. Dome division or truncation can be performed to shorten the medial crura.[14,15]

Having tried all of these techniques, this author's preferred technique is to divide the medial crura and suture the cut edges as described by Kridel. This author usually cut 4 to 5 mm below the dome and overlap the cut fragments 2 to 5 mm depending on the amount of deprojection needed. The edges of the upper portion of the medial crura are maintained on the mucosal side and sutured with a 5-0 polydioxanone (PDS). Usually, this technique is combined with

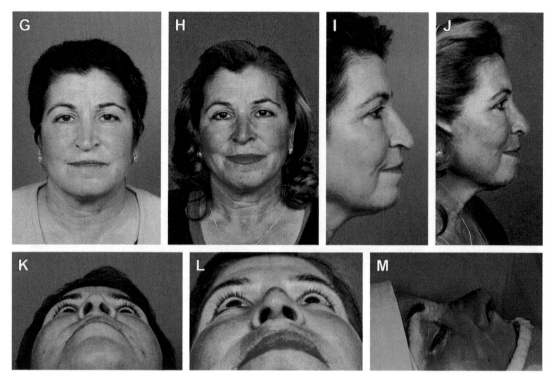

Fig. 6. (*continued*)

a septocolumellar suture and columellar strut to provide additional support and precision. In recent years, this author has also started using the new dome technique described by Pedroza[11] in selected cases, especially when the lateral crura are malpositioned or deformed. In fact, it can be called as "medial crural steal." This technique preserves the integrity of the lower lateral cartilages; however, it is technically challenging to recreate an uneventful relationship of the dome and lower lateral cartilage owing to complete separation of their mucosal attachments.

In cases where the lateral crura are longer than usual, the following techniques noteworthy.

1. Lateral crural steal[16] is a very versatile technique that can help the surgeon to address multiple issues at the same time. It can be used to shorten the lateral crus, give a more favorable shape to the lateral crus, decrease projection, increase rotation, and give a better definition to the dome (**Fig. 6**). Because the domes are not divided, it also gives more precision and symmetry than other options.

2. Lateral crural overlay[17] is a powerful technique to shorten the lateral crura. The difficulty is to get symmetry on both sides. Hydrodissection can facilitate the dissection of the cartilage from the vestibular mucosa. The width of the dissection depends on the amount of cartilage that would need to be overlapped. The lateral crura is typically divided 10 mm lateral to the dome and the medial segment is placed on top of the lateral segment. Usually a 2- to 5-mm overlap is performed (**Fig. 7**). In cases when the lateral crural overlay does not have enough strength to maintain a favorable shape, a lateral crural strut graft can be placed.[18] Lateral crural turn-in flap[19] and hinge flap[20] can also be combined with lateral crural overlay technique.

3. Lateral crural repositioning[21] is an excellent option to support external nasal valve and improve tip aesthetics in cases when the lateral crura are cephalically malpositioned, deformed, or asymmetric. A long lateral crural strut graft[18] or cephalic turn-in flap[19] is often needed with this maneuver (Video 2).

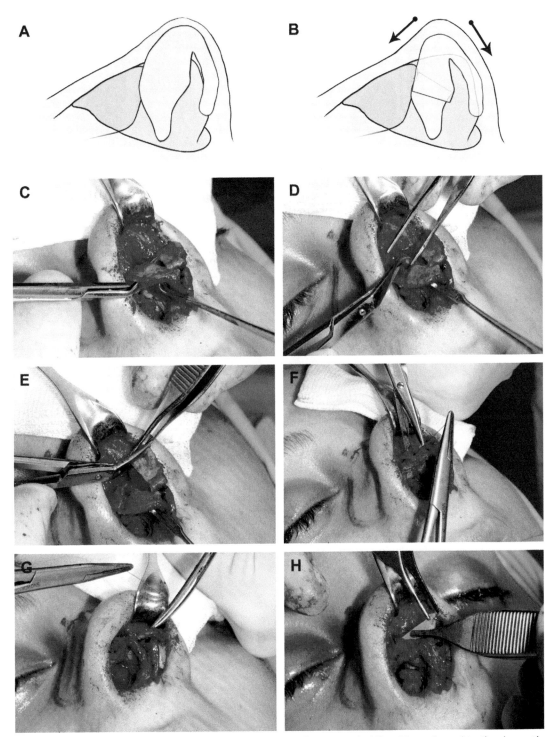

Fig. 7. Lateral crural overlay (*A, B*). After measuring and marking a vertical line 10 mm lateral to the dome, the skin under this line is dissected to free the cartilage (*C*). Then, full-thickness cuts are made bilaterally (*D, E*). The overlapped cartilages are sutured with a 5-0 PDS, keeping the medial fragment on top of the lateral fragment (*F, G*). To increase stability of the lateral crus, a lateral crural strut graft can also be inserted (*H*).

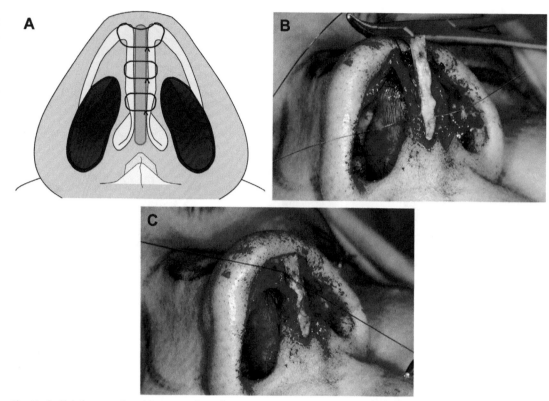

Fig. 8. A slightly curved and longer columellar strut is used that spans to the level of the domes while keeping them apart from each other as a spacer (A). It is sutured with multiple 5-0 PDS sutures for exact fixation (B, C).

Lateral crural repositioning is usually performed after the midline structures have been deprojected.

4. Dome division has historically been a very popular technique to reduce tip projection.[15] It is used less often by rhinoplasty surgeons currently owing to concerns about alar collapse, alar notching, and pinching of the tip.[22,23] These problems can be minimized by cartilage overlap techniques.[24]

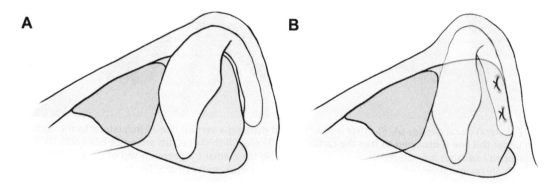

Fig. 9. The tongue-in-groove technique is used to obtain increased tip projection (A, B). The major trade-off is the rigidity it may cause.

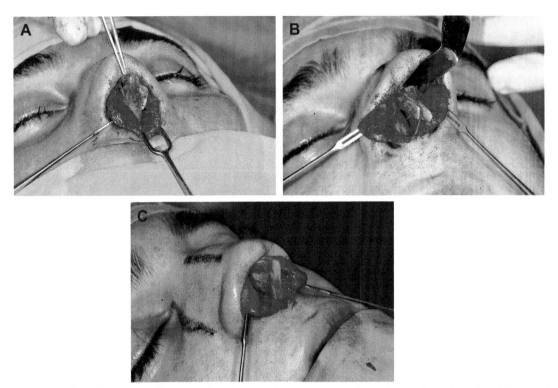

Fig. 10. A columellar strut can be secured to the caudal septum by a variety of ways. It can be sutured to caudal septum by multiple running sutures (*A*), or it can first sutured to a long splinting spreader graft (*B*, *C*).

Preserving Tip Projection

If a patient has adequate tip projection, its preservation can be challenging, especially in tip delivery or external rhinoplasty approaches that can damage the major tip support mechanisms. In these situations, this author refers to use a septocolumellar suture, columellar strut, or tongue-in-groove technique. A columellar strut is a very powerful implant to resist the contractual forces (**Fig. 8**).

Increasing Tip Projection

In cases with a poor projection, the following techniques can be considered. The selection depends on the severity of the projection, the expertise of the surgeon, and the individual characteristics of the patient.

Suture techniques

Lateral crural steal[17] or the new domes technique[11] is a very elegant way of increasing projection and rotation simultaneously. Because the lower lateral cartilage is not divided or separated from the vestibular mucosa, the suturing technique provides versatility and can be revised intraoperatively until the desired effect is achieved. It is possible to increase the tip projection by 2 to 4 mm, depending on the anatomy of the lower lateral cartilages. In the original technique described by Kridel, the mucosa under the dome is separated before the suturing of the lower lateral cartilage. As a modification, this author does not dissect the mucosa, which helps to preserve the strength of the lower lateral cartilage allowing for better positioning of the sutures. The mucosa also acts as a spacer under the dome to prevent an overly aggressive pinching of the dome.

Dome division[15] is also an option used to steal cartilage from the lateral crus by cutting and suturing them in the midline. This author prefers not to use this technique as originally described by Goldman because of the undesirable aesthetics. When the cartilage is overlapped and sutured as described by Adamson,[24] the risk of complications seems to be minimized.

Septocolumellar sutures[9] are very effective in increasing tip projection by about 2 to 4 mm, depending on the situation. This authors recommends putting at least two 4-0 PDS mattress sutures. However, if it is exaggerated, the subnasale can develop a web and the upper lip can rise excessively.

Similarly, the tongue-in-groove[10] technique (**Fig. 9**) is a very powerful option because the tip will be firmly secured wherever it is positioned intraoperatively. In this author's experience, this technique gives us the most predictable long-term tip projection results. The major drawback of this technique is the resultant rigidity of the tip.[25] This is a trade off that should be discussed with the patient before surgery.

Structural grafts

Midline grafts stabilize the nasal tip centrally and are used to improve the dimensions, shape and strength of the caudal septum and medial crural.

Columellar struts have been used for tip support in this author's practice for the past 16 years in the majority of cases.[26] In cases of malformed, buckled, or weak medial crura, columellar struts can help to reshape and strengthen the medial crura as well as increase tip projection.[27] Its shape can be modified from rectangular to slightly curved to adapt to the curvature of the columella. This author uses longer struts up to the level of the domes, which can act as a spacer to obtain a diamond shaped tip. Septocolumellar suture technique can be used with columellar

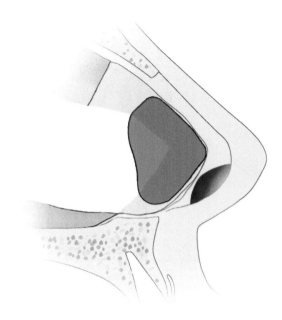

Fig. 12. An L-strut graft is used to splint the dorsal and caudal segment of the cartilaginous septum simultaneously.

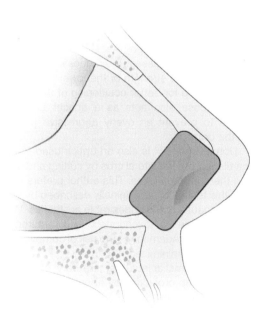

Fig. 11. Caudal septal extension graft creates a very strong platform on which the surgeon can tuck the medial crura in a tongue-in-groove fashion.

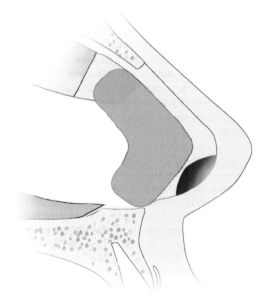

Fig. 13. There are cases with severe traumatic septal deviations that can be a cause of a deprojected tip. In these cases, complex subtotal septal reconstruction can be very helpful not only for function, but also to restore the projection.

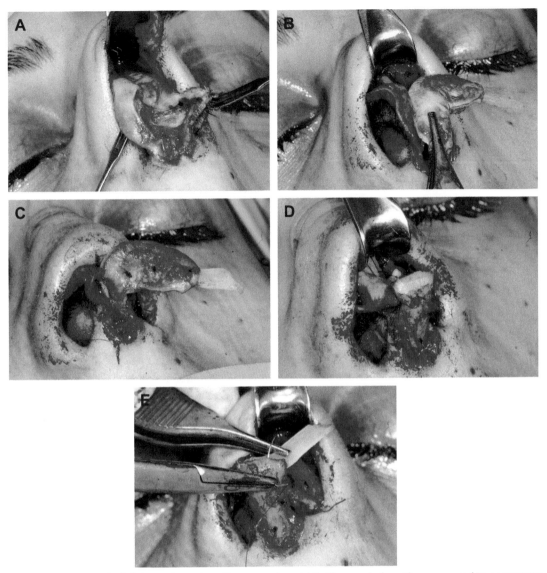

Fig. 14. In this case, the left lower lateral cartilage was absent (*A*). The conchal cartilage was used to reconstruct the lacking cartilage (*B*). It is supported by a longer lateral crural strut graft for better repositioning (*C*). Despite the best efforts, sufficient symmetry could not be achieved, so a shield graft (*D*) was used together with a left lateral crural graft (*E*). It is possible to see a better functioning nose with better tip projection (*F–K*).

struts sutured in place between the medial crura.[28] Not infrequently, this author will suture the columellar strut to the caudal end of the septal cartilage by passing multiple continuous simple sutures and sutures-of-eight or "shoe-lace" suturing[29] (**Fig. 10**A). This technique is a very efficient way of fixing the columellar strut to the caudal septum to elongate the caudal septum on which a tongue-in-groove technique can be applied. The third option is to anchor the columellar strut to unilateral or bilateral

splinting spreader grafts in addition to the caudal septum[29] (**Fig. 10**B, C).

A caudal septal extension graft[30] can be used in cases where the caudal end of the septum is weak, crooked, deviated, or fractured (**Fig. 11**). This is a very versatile graft not only to correct deformity, but also to support the caudal septum and act as a pedestal to suture the medial crura onto. In fact, its use is very popular in the Far East to increase projection and counterrotate the tip. Because it may cause thickening of the caudal

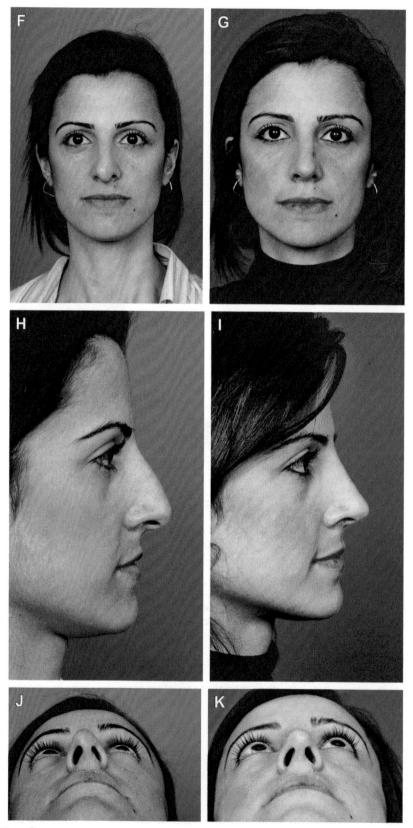

Fig. 14. (*continued*)

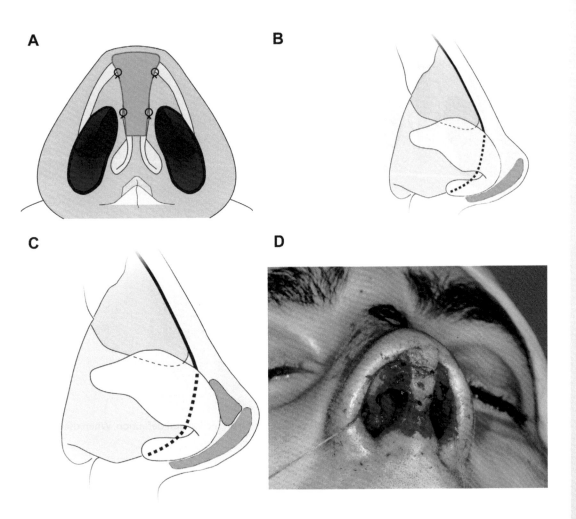

Fig. 15. The shield graft is sculptured according to the needs of the patient to reshape and/or increase the projection of the tip (*A, B*). It should be sutured from 4 points for better fixation (*A*). A buttress graft can be sutured cephalically to prevent its migration cephalically (*C*). Its edges should be beveled and softened to prevent its visibility (*D*).

septum, the surgeon must be cognizant to avoid overnarrowing the internal nasal valve area.

An L-strut graft[31] can be used in cases where the dorsal and caudal segment of the cartilaginous septum is severely deviated, underdeveloped, or overresected from a previous surgery (**Fig. 12**). This graft is usually obtained from the bony and/or cartilaginous septum. It serves as a multipurpose graft combining splinting spreader graft, caudal septal extension graft, and columellar strut.

Subtotal septal reconstruction[29,31] (**Fig. 13**) can be an excellent option in traumatic or revision cases. In these cases, a subtotal septal reconstruction is possible by using a single L-strut

cartilage or by using 2 pieces of cartilages as dorsal and caudal segments obtained from the septum or costal regions.

Structural grafts may be required to support and/or replace the existing or absent lower lateral cartilages, especially in revision or cleft rhinoplasty. These grafts can be septal, conchal, or costal cartilage.[32,33] The flexibility and resiliency of the lower lateral cartilages are unique and they should be preserved and supported. In this author's opinion, the conchal cartilage is the best option if total or subtotal reconstruction is required[32,34] (**Fig. 14**). Cartilage grafts placed over the existing lower lateral cartilages may be required to increase tip projection.

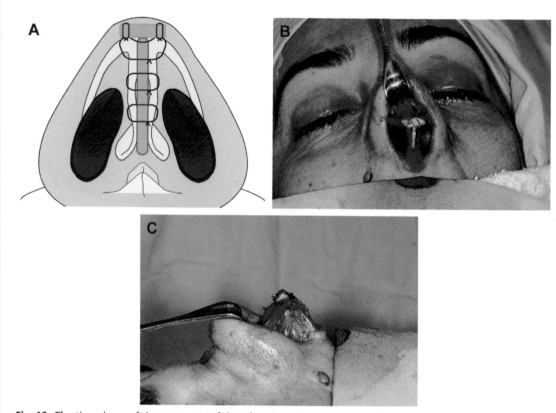

Fig. 16. The tip onlay graft is a very powerful graft to increase tip projection and definition. When used together with a long columellar strut, it is called as umbrella graft (*A–C*).

Shield grafts[35] were routinely used in all cases in this author's practice from 1999 to 2001 with great enthusiasm (**Fig. 15**). After following these patients long term, however, complications such as cartilage graft visibility owing to shrink wrapping of skin were noted. As a result, this author started using it only in selected cases, replacing its use with suture techniques. In daily practice, shield grafts can be used to reshape the tip and to increase tip projection. If it is used to increase the projection by 3 mm or more, then it should be supported by lateral crural grafts for a better transition from tip to alae.[36] Additionally, a buttress graft may also be needed to prevent cephalic migration of the shield graft and improve its transition to the supratip area.[36] Shield grafts should be used with extreme caution in individuals with thin skin or compromised skin soft tissue envelope. Its edges should be beveled and softened to prevent its visibility. Furthermore, shield grafts can also be camouflaged by temporalis fascia or costal perichondrium.

Tip grafts[37] are very versatile in increasing tip projection. Tip grafts can be single or multiple layers of cartilage with varying thickness. Its placement over the tip may change the nasal length. They can also be sutured on top of a long columellar strut creating an "umbrella graft" as described by Peck[38] (**Fig. 16**). Tip grafts, like shield grafts, should be camouflaged by soft tissue or thin slices of cartilage to prevent visibility.

SUMMARY

The projection of the nasal tip is one of the most important parameters in rhinoplasty. Obtaining an ideal tip projection can be a very challenging endeavor in rhinoplasty (**Fig. 17**). Suture techniques, lower lateral cartilage overlay techniques as well as cartilage grafting may be needed to change the projection and rotation of the tip. The surgeon must be adept at all of these approaches to be able to achieve excellent long-term results.

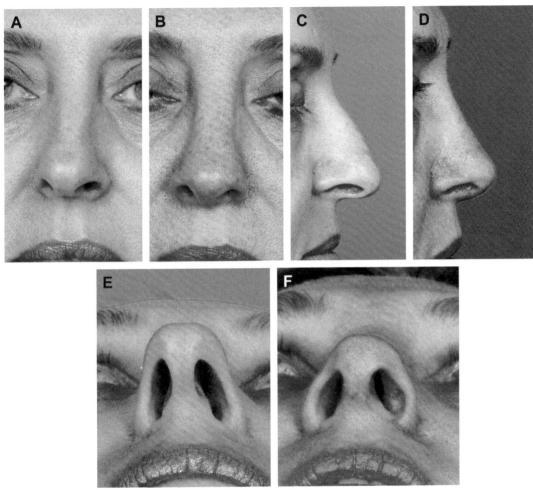

Fig. 17. The preoperative (*A, C, E*) and postoperative (*B, D, F*) frontal, lateral, and basal views of the patient with an overprojected tip is shown here. The major surgical steps to deproject the nose are shown in Video 1 and Video 2.

SUPPLEMENTARY DATA

Supplementary data related to this article can be found online at http://dx.doi.org/10.1016/j.cps. 2015.08.001.

REFERENCES

1. Simons RL. Nasal tip projection, ptosis and supratip thickening. Ear Nose Throat J 1982;61:452–5.
2. Goode RL. A method of tip projection measurement. In: Powell N, Humphreys B, editors. Proportions of the aesthetic face. New York: Thieme-Stratton; 1984. p. 15–39.
3. Crumley RL, Lanser M. Quantitative analysis of nasal tip projection. Laryngoscope 1988;98(2):202–8.
4. Powell N, Humphreys B. Proportions of the aesthetic face. New York: Thieme-Stratton; 1984.
5. Byrd HS, Hobar PC. Rhinoplasty: a practical guide for surgical planning. Plast Reconstr Surg 1993; 91(4):642–54.
6. Anderson JR. The dynamics of rhinoplasty. In: Bustamant GA, editor. Proceedings of the Ninth International Congress of Otorhinolaryngology, Mexico City, August 10-14, 1969. Amsterdam: Excerpta Medica; 1970.
7. Apaydin F, Akyildiz S, Hecht DA, et al. Rhinobase: a comprehensive database, facial analysis, and picture-archiving software for rhinoplasty. Arch Facial Plast Surg 2009;11(3):209–11.
8. Tardy ME Jr, Walter MA, Patt BS. The overprojecting nose: anatomic component analysis and repair. Facial Plast Surg 1993;9(4):306–16.
9. Porter JP, Toriumi DM. Surgical techniques for management of the crooked nose. Aesthetic Plast Surg 2002;26(Suppl 1):S1.

10. Kridel RW, Scott BA, Foda HM. The tongue-in-groove technique in septorhinoplasty. A 10-year experience. Arch Facial Plast Surg 1999;1(4):246–56.

11. Pedroza F. A 20-year review of the "new domes" technique for refining the drooping nasal tip. Arch Facial Plast Surg 2002;4(3):157–63.

12. Lipsett EM. A new approach to surgery of the lower cartilaginous vault. Arch Otolaryngol 1959; 70:42–7.

13. Soliemanzadeh P, Kridel RW. Nasal tip overprojection: algorithm of surgical deprojection techniques and introduction of medial crural overlay. Arch Facial Plast Surg 2005;7(6):374–80.

14. Goldman IB. The importance of medial crura in nasal tip reconstruction. Arch Otolaryngol 1957;65: 143.

15. Kridel RW, Konior RJ. Dome truncation for management of the overprojected nasal tip. Ann Plast Surg 1990;24(5):385–96.

16. Kridel RWH, Konior RJ, Shumrick KA, et al. Advances in nasal tip surgery: the lateral crural steal. Arch Otolaryngol Head Neck Surg 1989;115: 1206–12.

17. Kridel RW, Konior RJ. Controlled nasal tip rotation via the lateral crural overlay technique. Arch Otolaryngol Head Neck Surg 1991;117(4):411–5.

18. Gunter JP, Friedman RM. Lateral crural strut graft: technique and clinical applications in rhinoplasty. Plast Reconstr Surg 1997;99(4):943–52.

19. Apaydin F. Lateral crural turn-in flap in functional rhinoplasty. Arch Facial Plast Surg 2012;14(2):93–6.

20. Sazgar AA, Woodard C, Most SP. Preservation of the nasal valve area with a lateral crural hinged flap: a cadaveric study. Aesthetic Plast Surg 2012;36(2): 244–7.

21. Toriumi DM, Checcone MA. New concepts in nasal tip contouring. Facial Plast Surg Clin North Am 2009;17(1):55–90.

22. McCurdy JA. Surgery of the nasal tip: current concepts. Ear Nose Throat J 1977;56:238–48.

23. McCollough EG. Surgery of the nasal tip. Otolaryngol Clin North Am 1987;20:769–84.

24. Adamson PA, McGraw-Wall BL, Morrow TA, et al. Vertical dome division in open rhinoplasty. An update on indications, techniques, and results. Arch Otolaryngol Head Neck Surg 1994;120(4):373–80.

25. Guyuron B, Varghai A. Lengthening the nose with a tongue-and-groove technique. Plast Reconstr Surg 2003;111(4):1533–9.

26. Beaty MM, Dyer WK 2nd, Shawl MW. The quantification of surgical changes in nasal tip support. Arch Facial Plast Surg 2002;4(2):82–91.

27. Rohrich RJ, Hoxworth RE, Kurkjian TJ. The role of the columellar strut in rhinoplasty: indications and rationale. Plast Reconstr Surg 2012;129(1):118e–25e.

28. Toriumi DM, Tardy ME. Cartilage suturing techniques for correction of nasal tip deformities. Op Tech Otolaryngol Head Neck Surg 1995;6(4):245–330.

29. Apaydin F. Segmental reconstruction for nasal septal deviation. Facial Plast Surg 2013;29(6):455–63.

30. Toriumi DM. Caudal septal extension graft for correction of the retracted columella. Op Tech Otolaryngol Head Neck Surg 1995;6:311–8.

31. Toriumi DM. Subtotal reconstruction of the nasal septum: a preliminary report. Laryngoscope 1994; 104(7):906–13.

32. Burget GC. Aesthetic reconstruction of the tip of the nose. Dermatol Surg 1995;21(5):419–29.

33. Adelson RT, Karimi K, Herrero N. Isolated congenital absence of the left lower lateral cartilage. Otolaryngol Head Neck Surg 2008;138(6):7.

34. Pedroza F, Anjos GC, Patrocinio LG, et al. Seagull wing graft: a technique for the replacement of lower lateral cartilages. Arch Facial Plast Surg 2006;8(6): 396–403.

35. Johnson CMJ, Toriumi DM. Open structure rhinoplasty. Philadelphia: WB Saunders Co; 1989.

36. Toriumi DM. New concepts in nasal tip contouring. Arch Facial Plast Surg 2006;8(3):156–85.

37. Peck GC. The onlay graft for nasal tip projection. Plast Reconstr Surg 1983;71(1):27–39.

38. Peck GC Jr, Michelson L, Segal J, et al. An 18-year experience with the umbrella graft in rhinoplasty. Plast Reconstr Surg 1998;102(6):2158–65.

The Short Nose

Jeffrey D. Cone Jr, MD[a], P. Craig Hobar, MD[b],*

KEYWORDS

- Short nose • Lengthening the nose • Nasal elongation • Revision rhinoplasty
- Secondary rhinoplasty • Rib graft rhinoplasty

KEY POINTS

- Short nasal length and overrotation of the nasal tip (ie, increased nasolabial angle) define the short nose deformity.
- The first step in planning elongation of the short nose is to pinpoint the involved anatomy.
- Manual palpation can yield valuable insight into the quality and laxity of the nasal skin, the nasal lining, and the cartilaginous and skeletal framework.
- In patients with good skin quality and without lining deficiency, septal extension grafts can be considered to control tip projection and rotation. For stronger structural support, a rib graft is preferred.
- In cases of lining deficiency, complex nasal osteotomy lengthening should be considered.

INTRODUCTION

When a patient presents with a short nose, the diagnosis is fairly obvious. The challenge becomes correctly identifying the cause(s) of the deformity, ascertaining the anatomic components involved in the deformity, and then tailoring the surgery so that these each of these components is addressed. To this point, it cannot be overstressed that the short nasal deformity can involve asymmetries and/or deficiencies of all of the components of the nose, including skin, cartilage support, skeletal support, and mucosal lining. Moreover, the etiology can include a full spectrum from congenital malformations to acquired deformities.

Despite this great variability in etiology and in applied anatomy, the short nose is characterized by certain key findings: decreased nasal length, overrotation of the nasal tip, and associated increased nostril show.[1] This article is designed to elucidate involved anatomic asymmetries and deficiencies and then to tailor reliable techniques that address these asymmetries and deficiencies. Although the short nose presents elevated challenges, its correction offers elevated satisfaction to the patient and surgeon.

PREOPERATIVE PLANNING AND PREPARATION

The first step in evaluation is determining the etiology of a patient's short nose and the involved anatomy. Congenital short noses can be associated with craniofacial malformations or syndromes, such as cleft lip or Binder syndrome, and they can be familial.

Acquired short noses have an even more diverse background, and can include acute trauma or posttraumatic scarring and secondary rhinoplasty deformity (from overrotation of the nasal tip or overresection of the septum or dorsum). Rare causes include substance abuse (cocaine), syphilis, leprosy, or Wegener granulomatosis.

With such a diverse spectrum of etiologies, preoperative planning is focused on the following:

1. A thorough history, especially past trauma, surgeries, syndromes, and insults; and

The authors have nothing to disclosures.
a Wellspring Plastic Surgery, 911 West 38th Street, Suite 101, Austin, TX 78705, USA; b Medical City Children's Hospital, 7777 Forest Lane, B107, Dallas, TX 75230, USA
* Corresponding author.
E-mail address: phobar@gmail.com

Clin Plastic Surg 43 (2016) 169–176
http://dx.doi.org/10.1016/j.cps.2015.09.005

2. A physical examination, including intranasal examination, manual manipulation of the nose, and facial analysis.

Although the diagnosis is usually obvious, facial analysis is greatly beneficial for surgical planning and for framing a patient's expectations. The method we use is a simple soft tissue cephalometric analysis that can be performed in less than a minute.[2] Six measurements are taken:

1. Midfacial height (MFH); the distance from the glabella to the bottom of the ala.
2. Lower facial height: the distance from the subnasale to the menton.
3. Nasal length: The distance from the root of the nose at the level of the supratarsal fold to the tip projecting point.
4. Chin vertical: The distance from the stomion to the menton.
5. Tip projection: The distance from the junction of the cheek and the ala to the tip projecting point.
6. Chin projection: The distance from the anterior projecting point of the chin to a line drawn from the halfway point of the ideal nasal length and extending through and beyond the anterior projecting point of the upper lip.

Facial analysis is especially helpful in case of short nose because surgical correction of the short nose generates a significant change to the entire balance of the face. Thus, the optimal lengthening procedures take into account the proportions of the face. These measurements are meant to be a guide rather than a blueprint, and often "uncover" facial imbalances related to the short nose. When compared with ideal proportions, a short nose demonstrates a nasal length that is less than the chin vertical length (and <0.67 MFH). The nasolabial angle is increased from the normal values of 90° to 95° in men and women 95° to 105° in women, which generates an increased nostril show. Additional findings can include a deep radix, retracted alae, lack of cartilaginous or osseous support, and contraction of the soft tissue envelope.

Manual manipulation of the nose gives insight into skin quality, the strength of the cartilaginous and bony framework, and the anatomy (skin, cartilage, bone, and/or lining) that resists lengthening the nose. Another key aspect of the physical examination is an assessment of whether sufficient septal cartilage exists to elongate the nose or whether an additional cartilage donor site is required. If additional cartilage is required, our preference is to harvest rib, and specifically, the straight segment of the 10th rib. Although the 11th rib is often straight as well, it does not provide the length of the 10th rib. As known from cleft

rhinoplasty, the 10th rib provides roughly 33 mm for use as a columellar strut and 40 mm for a dorsal graft.[3] The information gained from a thorough physical examination and history allows a well-formulated plan that accounts for each patient's unique anatomy and challenges.

PATIENT POSITIONING

We perform an open approach for all cases involving a short nose. The patient is placed in a supine position with shoulder roll to create neck extension. If rib grafting is anticipated, this surgical site is prepped as an additional sterile field.

PROCEDURAL APPROACH

Various techniques have been described to elongate the short nose. This article outlines the 3 techniques that we prefer, because of their reproducibility and stability over the long term. These include (1) septal extension graft, (2) rib graft, and (3) complex osteotomy nasal lengthening. These techniques are assigned according to what anatomy is resisting elongation and to what degree it is resisting elongation.

For all 3 techniques, the procedure starts in a similar fashion. A transcolumellar incision allows elevation of the skin envelope off of the lower and upper lateral cartilages and the nasal bones. The septum is exposed by mobilization of the lower lateral cartilages from each other and the septum. This maneuver facilitates repositioning the domes of the lower lateral cartilages later in the procedure. Release of the lower lateral cartilages from the upper lateral cartilages can further enable downward rotation, as discussed elsewhere in this article.

The 2 reasons to resect the septum are to remove a functionally obstructive septum and/or to harvest graft material. The septal resection maintains at least 10 mm dorsal and caudal L-strut. If the septum does not cause obstruction and is not going to be used as graft material, it is kept intact. It is worth noting that a stable L-strut is a prerequisite for septal extension grafts, because these grafts are structural extensions from the L-strut. If the nasal lining is deficient but mild, the dissection over the lateral cartilages can be carried down in a preperichondrial plane to the piriform aperture. The nasal lining then can be released from the piriform aperture down to the anterior border of the turbinates.

TECHNIQUE

At this point, 1 of the 3 techniques is used to increase nasal length and decrease the nasolabial angle: septal extension grafts, rib graft, or complex osteotomy nasal lengthening.

Technique 1: Septal Extension Graft

In a patient with good nasal skin quality, no lining restriction, and adequate donor septal cartilage, a septal extension graft is a powerful and straightforward way both to lengthen the nose and to control tip projection.[4,5] The caudal end of the graft is placed beneath the domes of the lower lateral cartilages. If concern exists of broadening the mid vault, then the grafts can be placed posterior to the septal angle to prevent lateral displacement of the upper lateral cartilages.

Although the original extension graft descriptions refer to paired septal extension grafts, we now more commonly use a unilateral extension graft (both in cleft cases and in aesthetic ones). If internal nasal valve narrowing exists (especially in posttumor or posttrauma patients), then a spreader graft is placed on the opposite side. The 2 instances that use a paired septal extension grafts are (1) when the single septal extension graft is too weak and (2) if loading the domes of lower lateral onto the septal extension grafts generate deviation. In such situations, paired grafts can counterbalance each other and provide additional stability.

Case 1: primary rhinoplasty

A 27-year-old man sought surgical correction of a shortened, overrotated nose and improvement of what he perceived as a "weak chin." The MFH was used as the reference unit for both desired nasal length and chin vertical. An open approach was used. Adequate septal cartilage was harvested for graft material. The lower lateral cartilages were freed from the upper lateral cartilages. A septal extension graft was placed along the dorsal septum to allow 5 mm of nasal lengthening and control of tip projection. A sliding genioplasty was performed to gain 5 mm of increase in chin vertical and 8 mm of increase in anteroposterior projection. **Fig. 1** shows preoperative and postoperative photos.

Case 2: secondary rhinoplasty

A 28-year-old woman underwent a rhinoplasty as a teenager and had been living with a shortened, severely overrotated nose since that time. She had good skin quality and a large amount of good quality septum. Facial analysis showed her nose to be approximately 6 mm short in relation to both her MFH and chin vertical. An open approach was used, the lower lateral cartilages were mobilized and with the aid of a septal extension graft, 6 mm of lengthening was achieved. See **Fig. 2** for preoperative and postoperative photos.

Technique 2: Rib Graft

The use of a rib graft is an excellent technique when more strength is needed to overcome the soft tissue forces than can be provided with a septal extension graft. It is also our preferred technique when septum has been harvested previously or is inadequate. In fact, we rarely use costal cartilage in rhinoplasty. When a deficiency of the dorsum exists, a rib graft can be used as a cantilever graft, with the distal extension serving in a similar manner as the spreader graft but stronger. The authors prefer a straight segment of the 10th rib. The 11th rib is naturally straight, but often of inadequate length. Many prefer a rib located higher and supported with a K-wire, as has been popularized by Gunter.[6]

When the dorsum is adequate, a dorsal extension graft would interfere with an already adequate dorsum. In these cases, the 10th rib graft can be used as a columellar graft. The rib is placed just distal to the caudal septum and fixed to the anterior nasal spine of the maxilla with a threaded K-wire. If this produces excessive columellar show, an adequate adjacent portion of the caudal septum is resected. This form of rib graft controls nasal length and the angle off the maxilla and serves as another powerful tool for elongating the nose. Because the lower lateral cartilages are already mobilized from earlier dissection, their anterior aspect can be fixed either to the tip or over the tip of the precisely positioned rib.

Case 3: secondary rhinoplasty

A 44-year-old woman who had undergone a previous attempt at correction of a posttraumatic nasal deformity with a rib graft presented for secondary rhinoplasty. She presented with a visible step off at the superior edge of her rib graft and a shortened, overrotated nose. Facial analysis showed her nasal length to be short in relation to her midface by 5 mm and short in relation to her chin vertical by 6 mm. Through an open technique, the rib was removed and replaced with another rib graft contoured at the superior aspect to blend in with the normal bone at the radix. This new graft was also of adequate length to allow derotation of her lower lateral cartilages after separation from the upper lateral cartilages. The nose was lengthened by 5 mm (**Fig. 3**).

Technique 3: Complex Osteotomy Nasal Lengthening

This technique is reserved for the most complex type of nasal lengthening, usually related to posttraumatic or congenital etiologies. There is usually a lining deficiency that cannot be overcome with

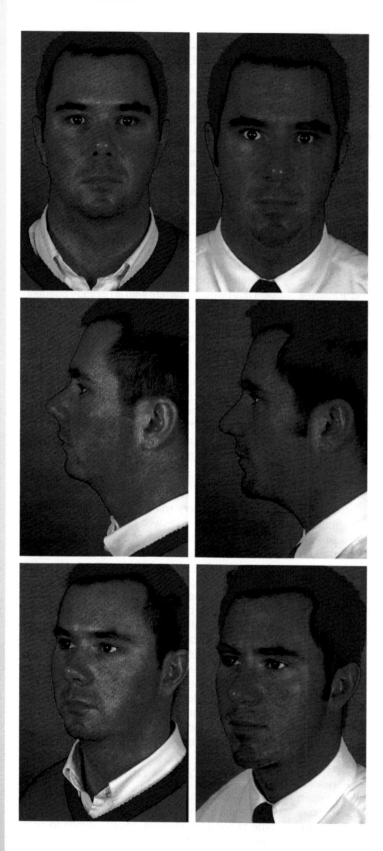

Fig. 1. Case 1. Preoperative (*left*) and postoperative photos (*right*) of septal extension graft technique used in a primary rhinoplasty to lengthen the short nose. A genioplasty was also performed.

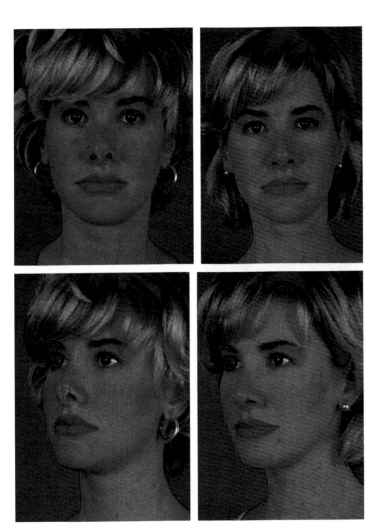

Fig. 2. Case 2. Preoperative (*left*) and postoperative photos (*right*) of septal extension graft technique used in a secondary rhinoplasty to lengthen the short, overrotated nose.

the 2 previously described methods. Grafts or lining flaps are of limited usefulness and usually not very rewarding for these difficult situations. If the lining is released high in the nasal cavity where the healing is quick and contracture is prevented by the bony surroundings, a powerful advancement of the lining can be achieved. We know this from the experience in Le Fort 3 osteotomies and advancements.

Wolfe[7] described a technique to achieve powerful nasal lengthening using cranial nasal separation based on techniques routinely used in craniofacial surgery, particularly the Le Fort 3 osteotomy. The senior author prefers a similar technique, but has modified it to allow the osteotomies to pass anterior to the nasolacrimal apparatus and medial orbit (**Fig. 4**).

As long as the osteotomy passes anterior to the turbinates, separation from the skull base and remainder of the face can be achieved safely. As the nose is lengthened, the caudal septum is impacted and distorted. This is a similar phenomenon, but from a reverse direction, that occurs in maxillary impaction for vertical maxillary excess. This is easily overcome by resecting an adequate amount of caudal septum. Rigid fixation with a small titanium plate and interposition bone grafts at the nasal root keeps the nose where it is positioned.

Case 4: secondary posttraumatic rhinoplasty

A 48-year-old woman presented with a posttraumatic nasal deformity. She has undergone multiple surgeries and previous attempts at nasal correction, but has a persistent severely shortened nose with excess rotation. Examination suggests she has a significant lining restriction and her overlying soft tissue envelope is scarred and suboptimal. A complex nasal osteotomy is performed with an 11-mm interposition bone graft and

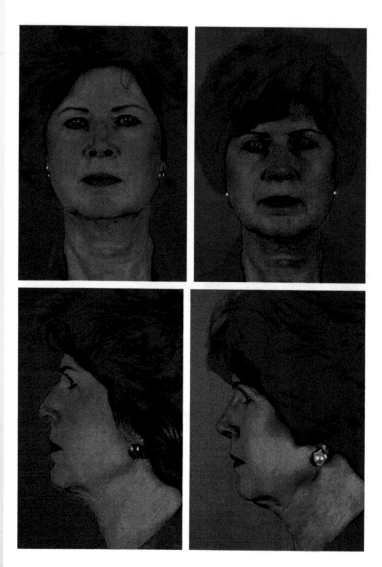

Fig. 3. Case 3. Preoperative (*left*) and postoperative photos (*right*) of rib graft technique used in a secondary rhinoplasty to lengthen the short, overrotated nose, and repair the step-off deformity.

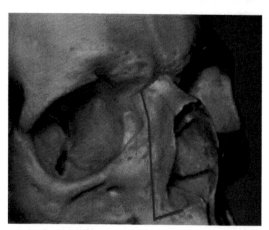

Fig. 4. Senior author's technique of complex nasal osteotomies for nasal elongation. This is indicated in particularly difficult posttraumatic or congenital deformities with a severe lining deficiency.

titanium plate fixation. Ultimately, 7 mm of external nasal lengthening is achieved (**Fig. 5**).

Case 5: posttraumatic rhinoplasty

A 26-year-old woman was involved in a devastating motor vehicle accident. She presented with severe secondary posttraumatic facial deformities, including a significantly shortened nose and contracted nasal lining. She underwent a complex osteotomy nasal reconstruction as described (**Fig. 6**).

POTENTIAL COMPLICATIONS AND MANAGEMENT OF THEM
Postprocedural Care

Afrin is used as needed for bleeding during the first 48 hours after surgery. Twice daily saline nasal

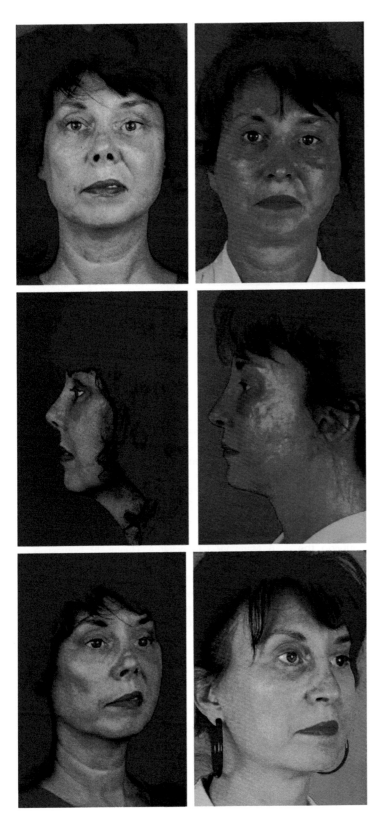

Fig. 5. Case 4. Preoperative (*left*) and postoperative photos (*right*) of the complex nasal osteotomy technique used in a secondary posttraumatic rhinoplasty.

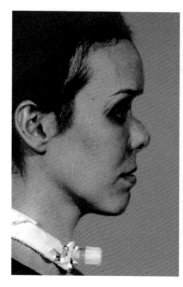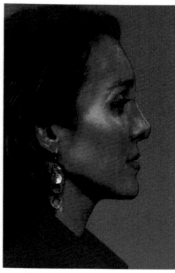

Fig. 6. Case 5. Preoperative (*left*) and postoperative photos (*right*) of the complex nasal osteotomy technique used in a secondary posttraumatic rhinoplasty.

spray is started on postoperative day 2 as needed. The customized Aquaplast cast (and underlying Steri-Strips and sutures) is removed at 5 to 7 days. Intranasal Doyle splints are kept intact for 1 to 2 weeks.

Rehabilitation and Recovery

Patients are kept on "nasal precautions" for 2 weeks, including no nose blowing, no heavy Valsalva, and no vigorous exercise, and then encouraged to gradually resume previous activities.

SUMMARY

The short nose presents unique challenges. An emphasis should be placed on identifying the involved anatomy that is causing the deformity, and then tailoring a surgical plan that addresses each of these causes. The selection between septal extension grafts, rib grafts, and complex osteotomies provide the rhinoplasty surgeon powerful tools in elongating the short nose.

REFERENCES

1. Gunter JP, Rohrich RJ. Lengthening the aesthetically short nose. Plast Reconstr Surg 1989;83:793–800.
2. Byrd HS, Hobar PC. Rhinoplasty: a practical guide for surgical planning. Plast Reconstr Surg 1993;91:642–54.
3. Ha RY, Cone JD, Byrd HS. Cleft rhinoplasty. In: Dallas rhinoplasty: nasal surgery by the masters. 3rd edition. Boca Raton (FL): CRC Press; 2014. p. 1305–31.
4. Byrd HS, Andochick S, Copit S, et al. Septal extension grafts: a method of controlling tip projection shape. Plast Reconstr Surg 1997;100(4):999–1010.
5. Ha RY, Byrd HS. Septal extension grafts revisited: 6-year experience in controlling nasal tip projection and shape. Plast Reconstr Surg 2003;112(7):1929–35.
6. Marin VP, Landecker A, Gunter JP. Harvesting rib cartilage grafts for secondary rhinoplasty. Plast Reconstr Surg 2008;121(4):1442–8.
7. Wolfe SA. Lengthening the nose: a lesson from craniofacial surgery applied to post-traumatic and congenital deformities. Plast Reconstr Surg 1994; 94(1):78–87.

Revision Rhinoplasty

Myriam Loyo, MD, Tom D. Wang, MD*

KEYWORDS

- Revision • Rhinoplasty • Facial plastic surgery

KEY POINTS

- Revision rhinoplasty is a challenging surgical operation.
- The surgeon dedicated to mastering rhinoplasty should understand not only the technical challenges but also the psychological impact this surgery has on patients.
- Communication with patients is key to a successful surgery.
- Listening to patients ultimately leads to more satisfactory outcomes. We can learn much from listening to our patients.
- Remember function is as important as aesthetics in rhinoplasty.

INTRODUCTION

Revision rhinoplasty is one of the most challenging operations the facial plastic surgeon performs given the complex 3-dimensional anatomy of the nose and the psychological impact it has on patients. The intricate interplay of cartilages, bone, and soft tissue in the nose gives it its aesthetic and function. Facial harmony and attractiveness depends greatly on the nose given its central position in the face. In the following article, the authors review common motivations and anatomic findings for patients seeking revision rhinoplasty based on the senior author's 30-year experience with rhinoplasty and a review of the literature.

ASSESSMENT OF PATIENTS WITH REVISION RHINOPLASTY

Every rhinoplasty surgery is performed with the intent of improving appearance and nasal breathing and achieving a satisfactory outcome. Despite our best efforts, rhinoplasty revision ranges in the literature from 5.0% to 15.5%.[1] At a certain level, all patients who are seeking revision surgery experience disappointment with their original surgery. The possibility of a dissatisfied patient is very real. Being prepared to treat patients seeking revision rhinoplasty is part of the facial plastic surgeon's practice. Additionally, as a surgeon becomes more experienced and established in the community, more patients seeking revision rhinoplasty will come to his or her practice. A facial plastic surgeon should prepare thoughtfully for these challenging cases.

Analyzing a nose preoperatively to prevent the need for revision requires careful assessment of the anatomy. Surgical maneuvers should be planned to produce the desired effects in a durable fashion that will remain satisfactory through the long process of healing and many years after the initial surgery. Surgeons should take into account that subcutaneous fat of the nose thins with aging and grafts placed in the nose of a teenager may show in later adult years. Modern rhinoplasty has shifted away from reduction rhinoplasty to techniques that reshape and support the nose. In reduction rhinoplasty, weakened cartilages collapse and twist under the strong forces of scar contraction that over time, sometimes decades later, gives an unappealing external appearance to the nose and cripple breathing. Support is particularly important in revision rhinoplasty where strong scar contractions are present. Experience will help the rhinoplasty surgeon with these

Division of Facial Plastic and Reconstructive Surgery, Department of Otolaryngology-Head and Neck Surgery, Oregon Health and Science University, Portland, OR, USA
* Corresponding author. Division of Facial Plastic and Reconstructive Surgery, Department of Otolaryngology–Head and Neck Surgery, Oregon Health and Science University, 3303 SW Bond Avenue, Mail Code CH5E, Portland, OR 97239.
E-mail address: wangt@ohsu.edu

Clin Plastic Surg 43 (2016) 177–185
http://dx.doi.org/10.1016/j.cps.2015.09.009
0094-1298/16/$ – see front matter © 2016 Elsevier Inc. All rights reserved.

intraoperative decisions to establish the size and shape of cartilages and grafts that will provide the desired outcome.

In a recent retrospective review of an established rhinoplasty practice, Dr VanderWoude and colleagues identified risk factors for postoperative dissatisfaction and need for revision rhinoplasty. Postoperative complications, a history of nasal fracture, and lack of anatomic correlation were risk factors for dissatisfaction.[1] Postoperative infections, displaced nasal stents or casts, and scarring led to poor healing and negatively impacted the patients' outcomes. Traumatic crooked noses are well recognized as a technically challenging rhinoplasty group. In a prospective study by Cingi and Eskiizmir[2] in Turkey, patients with deviated noses undergoing rhinoplasty experienced decreased satisfaction and worse postoperative quality of life as compared with patients with straight noses. Technical and, perhaps more importantly, psychological aspects impact these differences. In the study, the outcomes of patients with deviated noses were judged equally successful to the nondeviated noses by peers and surgeons. The patients did not agree with other examiners.

Psychological aspects are often quoted as the most difficult aspect of revision rhinoplasty by experienced surgeons.[3] In order to have a successful surgery, the surgeon must understand what motivates patients to seek revision. Specific alterations to the nose or concerns with nasal obstruction and nasal breathing should be discussed. Accurate and open communication will help define the operative goal. Communication is crucial for the doctor and patients to have a satisfactory outcome. It is important to note that often the patients and the surgeon differ in their evaluation of the nose. Studies have shown rhinoplasty surgeons will identify many more abnormalities than what the patients themselves point out. Rhinoplasty surgeons are trained to look at noses critically. In a recent study, the surgeon identified approximately 40% more nasal deformities than the patients.[4] The surgeon must recognize the patients' concerns and make it a priority to address them. Gaining the patients' trust depends on the physician being able to understand the patients' concerns and expectations and project realistic outcomes. Evaluating the nose together, with the use of a mirror or photography, facilitates communication. Consider using computer simulations, either 2-dimensional or 3-dimensioal, if it will improve communication.

Establishing realistic goals for surgery is key in achieving satisfaction. It is necessary to differentiate and recognize patients' perceived and truly inadequate results. A quest for a perfect nose can have high risks with minimal benefits and should be addressed before moving forward with surgery. The anatomy of the particular nose and face might have limitations that preclude a specific outcome. Every patient has a unique facial structure and nose with certain traits, such as cartilage shape, strength, and skin thickness and quality. With each trait come certain advantages and disadvantages that will require different handling in surgery. Patients with thick skin that requires more grafting and increased projection to enhance definition are often hesitant to choose this option for fear of a big nose. Successful surgeons are able to discuss these issues with their patients and manage expectation. Finally, identifying patients with depression and body dysmorphic disorder (BDD) can help prevent unhappy patients. The incidence of BDD can be as high as 13% of the patients seeking cosmetic surgery.[5] Do not be afraid to turn patients down or refer them to another surgeon.

COMMON MOTIVATION FOR PATIENTS SEEKING REVISION RHINOPLASTY

Rhinoplasty surgeons continue to try to understand the type of defect that leads to revision rhinoplasty. In the following section, the authors review studies that have looked at common complaints and findings in patients with revision rhinoplasty. Patients seeking revision rhinoplasty often have different concerns than those of patients seeking primary rhinoplasty. Adamson and colleagues performed a retrospective review of primary (308 surgeries) versus revision (92 patients) rhinoplasty during 9 years of their practice.[6] The most common concerns for patients with primary rhinoplasty were a dorsal hump (50%), large nose (44%), bulbous tip (44%), and nasal obstruction (33%). In contrast, patients with revision rhinoplasty complain of persistent deviation (38%), nasal obstruction (36%), bulbous tip (33%), and large nose (25%). Complaints that had a dramatic increase in revision surgeries compared with primary surgery were tip asymmetry (22%), dorsal sloop (11%), wide nostrils (19%), columellar show (11%), and alar retraction (4%). Stigmata of prior rhinoplasty leading to unnatural results, such as those discussed earlier, were often mentioned as causes for revision surgery. In a different study, Guyron and colleagues analyzed 100 consecutive revision rhinoplasties to identify the most common causes of revision.[4] The most common causes for revision were nasal obstruction (65%), dorsum asymmetry (33%), nostril asymmetry (18%), and tip asymmetry (14%). In the study, septoplasty was performed in 71% of patients. Other maneuvers commonly performed were alar rim graft (67%), dorsal graft (63%), osteotomies (60%), and dorsal hump removal (46%). The final study in the literature assessing the motivations for patients to undergo revision rhinoplasty is by Constantian,[7] who interviewed 150 patients in his practice.[7] Commonly, patient motivation was a new deformity after rhinoplasty (40%). Other common motivations were failure to correct the original deformity (33%) and loss of a familial or ethnic trait (15%). The importance of understanding different ethnic and cultural backgrounds will continue to grow as the population in the United States and the world continues to diversify. Interestingly, 10% of patients found their initial results to be good but were seeking rhinoplasty for further improvement.

The relatively high degree of nasal obstruction in patients seeking revision rhinoplasty in these studies is striking.[4,6–8] These findings highlight function is as important as appearance in rhinoplasty. Surgeons must address the septum and internal nasal valve to prevent nasal obstruction in patients with rhinoplasty. A recent study of patients with primary and revision rhinoplasty using rhinomanometry found that nasal valve obstruction and lateral wall collapse were equal or surpassed the degree of obstruction caused by a septal deviation.[8] Additionally, patients who have procedures to address their nasal valve have the same degree of improvement as patients who had procedures to address the nasal valve and the septum. The importance of the internal nasal valve should not be underestimated.

An encouraging finding for both patients and surgeon embarking on revision rhinoplasty is the high success rate of this surgery in adequately selected patients. In the study by Constantian,[7] self-reported patient satisfaction was 97%. A study from Netherlands reported 88% of patients had significant improvement 2 years after revision rhinoplasty using a validated questionnaire and 79% of patients would undergo surgery again.[9]

Preoperative and 1-year postoperative pictures of a case of revision septorhinoplasty are shown in **Fig. 1**.

PREPARING FOR REVISION RHINOPLASTY

Preparing for the revision surgery requires performing a detailed examination and constructing a mental plan for surgery. After discussing with patients and reviewing old photographs and operative notes, surgeons should take time to analyze the photographs and construct a plan. Although flexibility is still required during surgery,

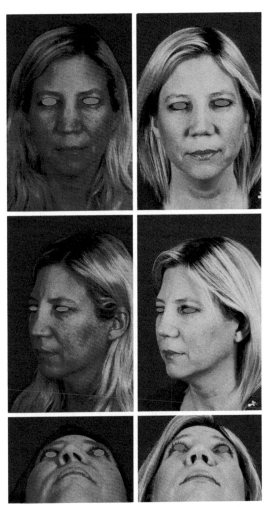

Fig. 1. Preoperative and 1-year postoperative photographs of a patient with revision rhinoplasty.

anticipating challenges will minimize improvisation. Tailor your treatment to your goal minimizing any majorly disruptive maneuvers. The authors recommend following a reconstructive ladder. The spectrum in revision surgery ranges from minimally invasive filler augmentation for small contour depressions to more extensive reconstruction with rib cartilage grafting. Complete deconstruction of the nose is not necessary in all cases. A word of caution is warranted for the use of filler for augmentation rhinoplasty. The risk of vascular occlusion leading to skin necrosis is real, and the correct plane of injection should be within deep to the superficial musculoaponeurotic system (SMAS). Infection is another known complication of filler injection. Different surgeons can be very opinionated as to advocate for or against the use of nasal filler. Current available evidence shows that complications do occur with nasal fillers, but the incidence is rare. Webster and colleagues[10] published their results with 347 patients who had silicone injected in the nose, establishing a safety profile for this material. More modern fillers have the advantage of being temporary. The largest series of temporary filler augmentation of the nose comes from Dr Rivkin. In the calcium hydroxyapatite (Radiesse, Merz Aesthetic, Frankfurt, Germany) study, 385 patients underwent injections with satisfactory outcomes. There were 2 cases of partial skin necrosis that required wound care. Of note, 46% of patients required reinjection.[11]

When planning for a revision surgery, expect a revision case to take longer than a primary case. Revision surgeries are often more complex because of the scar tissue and the changes to the anatomic components of the nose. Revision might seem deceptively simple but often take longer as tedious and delicate dissection is necessary. Be prepared to take the time needed in surgery to restore and refine the intricate anatomy of the nose. Nasal bones and cartilages are often collapsed, weak, twisted, or nearly absent. Restoring all of the components while maintaining a natural external appearance requires precision and surgical proficiency. Waiting 1 year for optimal healing before attempting revision has long been customary. The authors adhere to this rule, with some exceptions. When there is an abnormality that will not improve with time and decreased swelling, the authors will proceed with revision earlier. In a recent survey of the Rhinoplasty Society members, most surgeons reported using open rhinoplasty in most of their revision cases instead of an endonasal approach and at increased frequency when compared with primary rhinoplasty.[12]

Planning for revision rhinoplasty also requires the surgeon to discuss with patients the materials that will be used. Commonly, septal cartilage and even auricular cartilage may be depleted. Autologous costal cartilage can be considered.

A recent meta-analysis reports the rate of warping at 3.0%, reabsorption at 0.2%, infection at 0.5%, migration at 0.3%, unfavorable chest scar at 3.0%, and pneumothorax at 0% (range 0%–0.32%).[13] Irradiated rib is also a convenient option given the lack of donor-site morbidity. This option has long been criticized for its risk of reabsorption; however, in the authors' experience, reabsorption has been rare. The largest available case series to date in irradiated rib graft for rhinoplasty is by Kridel and colleagues,[14] which evaluated 1025 grafts and describes a rate of warping at 3.25%, infection at 0.9%, and reabsorption at 1.2%. Some of the patients in the study had follow-up of longer than 10 years.

Alloplast is also an option for rhinoplasty. The most commonly used alloplastic materials for rhinoplasty are silicone, expanded polytetrafluoroethylene (e-PTFE, Gore-Tex WL Gore and Associates, Flagstaff, AZ) and porous polyethylene (Medpor, Porex Surgical, Newnan, GA). Historically, alloplastic grafting materials have been considered less desirable than autologous materials because of reports of infection, migration, and extrusion. However, the unlimited supply, along with no donor-site morbidity, has always made alloplastic material an attractive option. Recent case series and meta-analysis place the risk of infection as high as 12.6% and extrusion at 16.0%.[15] Extrusion can occur many years after implantation, and cases of extrusion decades after implantation are not uncommon in the literature. The available studies on alloplasts have the limitations of being retrospective and subject to recall bias likely underestimating the rates of complications. Additionally, different locations might exhibit different rates of complications. The nasal dorsum might have a lower risk of complications and the nasal tip an increased risk.[16]

COMMON SURGICAL DEFORMITIES AND CORRECTIVE PROCEDURES

Surgical maneuvers used to address the nose during revision surgery are not much different from the maneuvers used in primary rhinoplasty. More extensive reconstruction of previously resected or manipulated cartilages is not uncommon. Tedious dissection through scar and prior grafts may be necessary. But the maneuvers and principles in primary and revision rhinoplasty stay congruent. The first step, and perhaps the most important step, is correctly identifying the deformity to address. The following section briefly describes common deformities and the techniques used to correct them during revision rhinoplasty. This section is meant to provide a general guideline. Detailed surgical steps for the techniques are beyond the scope of this article.

Upper Third of the Nose

Assessment of the dorsum and hump removal becomes more difficult later in the case as swelling begins affecting the soft tissue envelope sometimes leading to postoperative asymmetries that were not identified during surgery. The most common defects on the nasal dorsum are under-resection, over-resection, and persistent deviations. Under-resection of the bony nasal dorsum can be addressed by repeat hump removal with osteotomes or raspatories. An over-resected dorsum or scooped dorsum can be addressed with dorsal grafting. Diced cartilage graft or carved onlay dorsal struts may be used to augment the dorsum. The authors prefer using a long piece of cartilage from the septum or rib as a dorsal onlay, given that they feel a more predictable outcome is possible in their hands. Careful contouring to allow transition from the onlay to the bony pyramid is necessary. Disadvantages of using a single piece of cartilage as a dorsal onlay are the need for a relatively long straight piece of cartilage (usually measuring 3.5 cm) and the risk of warping.[17] Advocates of the diced cartilage highlight the ease of preparation, the ability to use small remnant pieces of cartilage, the ability of the grafts to contour to the nose, and the lack of any possibility of warping. Structural stability is not obtained with diced cartilage grafting.

Straightening rhinoplasty is one of the hardest technical surgeries in rhinoplasty, and it requires overcoming not only the bony and cartilaginous deviations but also the tissue memory and soft tissue. Persistent crookedness is often attributed to failure to straighten the nose.[18,19] The septum constitutes the foundation of the nose, and residual septal deviation should be addressed during revision. Guyron and colleagues[4] describe using revision septoplasty in 71% of their revision rhinoplasties. If necessary, complete septal replacement with extracorporeal septoplasty can be performed.[20] Dorsal asymmetries with rates as high as 15% have been reported, in experienced hands.[21] After complete septal replacements, the authors prefer, when possible, to preserve a dorsal strut to prevent dorsal asymmetries, facilitate reconstruction, and preserve dorsal support. Incomplete osteotomies can also lead to inadequate mobilization of the nasal dorsum. Bilateral lateral osteotomies with either an intermediate osteotomy on the longer side or bilateral medial osteotomies with sequential open book can be used to straighten the nose.[22] The authors favor the use of the intermediate osteotomy, given that this preserves the dorsal support at the rhinion and prevents asymmetries on the area of the nose with the thinnest skin. On severe deviations, a transverse osteotomy to separate the perpendicular plate of the ethmoid from the base of skull might be necessary. Both techniques, intermediate or bilateral medial osteotomies, can be used equally successfully. Camouflage grafts are important in addressing residual dorsal asymmetries or deviations.

Middle Third

Nasal obstruction due to persistent asymmetries in the middle third of the nose is a common finding in revision surgery. Revision septoplasty will often address high septal deviations that were not previously addressed. Spreader grafts can be used to treat internal nasal valve stenosis and/or treat inverted V deformities. **Fig. 2** shows a preoperative and postoperative patient with inverted V deformity requiring revision septorhinoplasty. Spreader flaps, also referred to as auto-spreader grafts, are rarely available during revision surgery.[23] The authors favor the use of the butterfly graft to strength and support the internal nasal valve.[24]

Pollybeak deformity with supratip prominence can result from inadequate lowering of the cartilage and/or soft tissue scarring. The combination of a relatively high anterior septal angle and weak tip support is a set up for postoperative pollybeak as scarring leads to contraction and deprojection of the nasal tip. Pollybeak might not be initially evident in the operating room. A case of revision septorhinoplasty for pollybeak deformity is shown in **Fig. 3**. Correction of the cartilaginous pollybeak involves lowering the anterior septal angles and projecting and supporting the nasal tip. Soft tissue pollybeak is often the results of scarring when an excessive supratip break has been created. Disruption of the subdermal plexus can predispose patients to have this complication. Steroid injections in the supratip area can be effective in treating soft tissue pollybeak deformity in the early postoperative period.

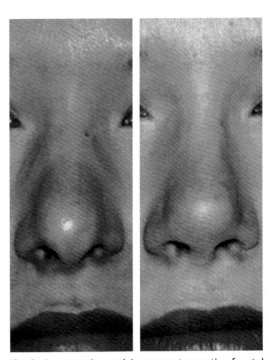

Fig. 2. Preoperative and 1-year postoperative frontal view of a patient with revision rhinoplasty treated for inverted V deformity.

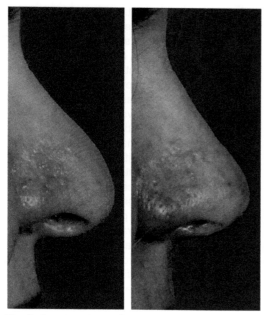

Fig. 3. Preoperative and 6-month postoperative profile view of a patient with revision rhinoplasty with a pollybeak deformity.

Lower Third

In the authors' opinion, revision of the nasal tip is often the most complex portion of revision rhinoplasty. Their approach to the nasal tip begins by establishing support and a solid foundation for the central complex of the nasal tip with a columellar strut, tongue-in-groove, or caudal septal extension graft.[25,26] Tip rotation is established at this point. Many of the tip support mechanism are disrupted during rhinoplasty, and restoring the support to allow for results that will endure the stress of healing and time are necessary. The authors routinely secure the medial crura to the central stabilizing graft and to each other. Medial crura division and overlap can be done at this point, although the authors rarely use this maneuver. Short and over-rotated noses require lengthening at this point. The authors favor the use of a caudal septal extension graft or extended spreader graft to a strong columellar strut for lengthening of the nose. For the opposite cases whereby long and ptotic noses are being treated, trimming of the nasal septum is done before establishing the position of the nasal tip.

The authors subsequently address the orientation and symmetry of the lower lateral crura. Technical steps to improve the lower lateral crura include cephalic turn-in flaps, lateral crural struts, and if necessary lateral crura repositioning.[27–29] The butterfly graft can be used to support and flatten the lower lateral crura. A patient with

primary septorhinoplasty treated with a butterfly graft is shown in **Fig. 4**. The authors routinely perform posterior transdomal binding to ensure symmetry. Although some investigators have successfully used suture modification techniques for the lower lateral crura, such as mattress sutures with the lateral crura or alar spanning sutures, the authors tend not to use them and instead prefer structural grafting.[30–32]

The final step is assessing whether tip and dome projection is adequate. If the nasal tip is overprojected, a dome division can be considered. Lateral crura overlaps can also be used at this point. Because of changes in the shape and volume of the lateral crura, the authors tend not to perform lateral crura overlap and instead prefer dome division. If the nasal tip is underprojected, additional projection is necessary and they will consider a

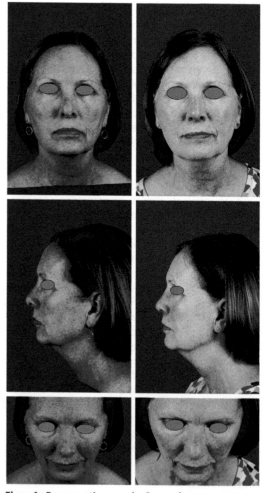

Fig. 4. Preoperative and 6-month postoperative pictures of a patient with primary septorhinoplasty treated with a butterfly graft. Frontal, profile, and frontal oblique views included.

well-camouflaged cap or shield tip graft. Tip grafts have to be carefully contoured to prevent visibility particularly in thin-skinned individuals. Patients with strong cartilages and thin skin are at an increased risk for bossae formation. A case of revision rhinoplasty for tip asymmetries is shown in **Fig. 5**.

Alar retraction, either congenital or as a postrhinoplasty deformity, is very noticeable and distracting. The evaluation of patients with alar retraction should first establish if the nose is over-rotated and shortened and should differentiate between excessive columellar show and true alar retraction. Aggressive and overzealous cephalic resection and cephalic malposition of the lower lateral crura decreases alar support and predisposes patients to postoperative alar retraction. Techniques used to correct and prevent alar retraction include alar rim graft, lateral crura repositioning, and composite auricular grafts to the vestibule. Alar rim grafts will support the ala and maintain a smooth transition from the dome region to the caudal margin of the ala. Lateral crura can be detached from the pyriform aperture and repositioned from a cephalic position to a more favorable caudal position. If there is a significant deficiency of the vestibular skin, composite auricular grafts caudal to the lower lateral crura can be helpful to treat alar retraction. **Fig. 6** shows preoperative and postoperative photographs of a patient treated for alar retraction with composite grafts.

Alar base widening can occur after deprojection on a reduction rhinoplasty. After significant deprojection, the alar base should be assessed for excess alar flare, increased nostril size, or a

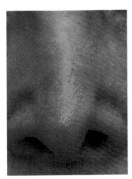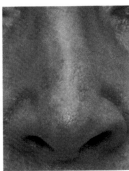

Fig. 6. Frontal preoperative and 1-year postoperative view of a patient with alar retraction treated with composite grafts.

combination of these.[33] Alar base reduction can be performed in the office under local anesthetic.

Soft Tissue

Soft tissue scarring and contracture is perhaps the most difficult deformity to address in rhinoplasty. The skin can be compromised as a result of infection or vascular injury. Dissection in the sub-SMAS plane prevents disruption of the vessels and lymphatics of the nose. Severe alar notching from a soft tissue injury can often only be addressed by expanding the soft tissue envelope, and composite grafts are helpful in these scenarios.

Poorly placed incisions are difficult to correct. Incisions placed in the alar rim and soft tissue triangle instead of marginal incisions often lead to visible scars that alter the shape of the nostril. If the soft tissue triangle has been scarred, it can be augmented with composite grafts. Alar base reduction incisions that efface the alar-facial sulcus will create an unnatural appearance. Revision of alar base reduction can be done with V-to-Y advancements to help restore the previously effaced alar-facial sulcus. Finally, skin resurfacing with laser or dermabrasion can be beneficial to treat external scars.

SUMMARY

Revision rhinoplasty is a challenging surgical operation. The surgeon dedicated to mastering rhinoplasty should understand not only the technical challenges but also the psychological impact this surgery has on patients. Communication with our patients is key to a successful surgery. The authors firmly think listening to our patients ultimately leads to more satisfactory outcomes. Functional outcome is as important as aesthetics in rhinoplasty. Nasal breathing should not be

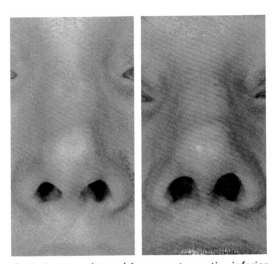

Fig. 5. Preoperative and 1-year postoperative inferior oblique view of a patient with revision rhinoplasty treated for tip asymmetry.

sacrificed toward the goal of a perfect or smaller nose. Structure, shape, and support are more important principles than reduction in rhinoplasty. The internal nasal valve is as important as the septum for nasal breathing.

A successful surgeon anticipates the long-term results over time. The technical maneuvers in secondary rhinoplasty are not dramatically different from primary rhinoplasty; however, revision surgery will always be more challenging. Prepare for a longer dissection when tackling scar and deficient anatomy is necessary. Surgeons are not born with an innate ability but continuously work toward improvement. Remember anything worth doing, is worth doing right! and mediocre is never better than best. The authors hope this review of revision rhinoplasty is helpful to the surgeons in the community performing this formidable operation.

REFERENCES

1. Neaman KC, Boettcher AK, Do VH, et al. Cosmetic rhinoplasty: revision rates revisited. Aesthet Surg J 2013;33(1):31–7.
2. Cingi C, Eskiizmir G. Deviated nose attenuates the degree of patient satisfaction and quality of life in rhinoplasty: a prospective controlled study. Clin Otolaryngol 2013;38(2):136–41.
3. Adamson PA, Warner J, Becker D, et al. Revision rhinoplasty: panel discussion, controversies, and techniques. Facial Plast Surg Clin North Am 2014; 22(1):57–96.
4. Lee M, Zwiebel S, Guyuron B. Frequency of the preoperative flaws and commonly required maneuvers to correct them: a guide to reducing the revision rhinoplasty rate. Plast Reconstr Surg 2013;132(4): 769–76.
5. Dey JK, Ishii M, Phillis M, et al. Body dysmorphic disorder in a facial plastic and reconstructive surgery clinic: measuring prevalence, assessing comorbidities, and validating a feasible screening instrument. JAMA Facial Plast Surg 2015;17(2):137–43.
6. Chauhan N, Alexander AJ, Sepehr A, et al. Patient complaints with primary versus revision rhinoplasty: analysis and practice implications. Aesthet Surg J 2011;31(7):775–80.
7. Constantian MB. What motivates secondary rhinoplasty? A study of 150 consecutive patients. Plast Reconstr Surg 2012;130(3):667–78.
8. Constantian MB, Clardy RB. The relative importance of septal and nasal valvular surgery in correcting airway obstruction in primary and secondary rhinoplasty. Plast Reconstr Surg 1996;98(1):38–54 [discussion: 5–8].
9. Hellings PW, Nolst Trenite GJ. Long-term patient satisfaction after revision rhinoplasty. Laryngoscope 2007;117(6):985–9.
10. Webster RC, Hamdan US, Gaunt JM, et al. Rhinoplastic revisions with injectable silicone. Arch Otolaryngol Head Neck Surg 1986;112(3):269–76.
11. Rivkin A. Nonsurgical rhinoplasty with calcium hydroxyapatite (Radiesse). Cosmet Dematol 2009; 12:619–24.
12. Lee M, Unger JG, Gryskiewicz J, et al. Current clinical practices of the Rhinoplasty Society members. Ann Plast Surg 2013;71(5):453–5.
13. Wee JH, Park MH, Oh S, et al. Complications associated with autologous rib cartilage use in rhinoplasty: a meta-analysis. JAMA Facial Plast Surg 2015;17(1):49–55.
14. Kridel RW, Ashoori F, Liu ES, et al. Long-term use and follow-up of irradiated homologous costal cartilage grafts in the nose. Arch Facial Plast Surg 2009; 11(6):378–94.
15. Loyo M, Ishii LE. Safety of alloplastic materials in rhinoplasty. JAMA Facial Plast Surg 2013;15(3):162–3.
16. Winkler AA, Soler ZM, Leong PL, et al. Complications associated with alloplastic implants in rhinoplasty. Arch Facial Plast Surg 2012;14(6):437–41.
17. Daniel RK. Diced cartilage grafts in rhinoplasty surgery: current techniques and applications. Plast Reconstr Surg 2008;122(6):1883–91.
18. Kim DW, Toriumi DM. Management of posttraumatic nasal deformities: the crooked nose and the saddle nose. Facial Plast Surg Clin North Am 2004;12(1): 111–32.
19. Foda HM. The role of septal surgery in management of the deviated nose. Plast Reconstr Surg 2005; 115(2):406–15.
20. Gubisch W. Twenty-five years experience with extracorporeal septoplasty. Facial Plast Surg 2006;22(4): 230–9.
21. Gubisch W. Extracorporeal septoplasty for the markedly deviated septum. Arch Facial Plast Surg 2005; 7(4):218–26.
22. Most SP, Murakami CS. A modern approach to nasal osteotomies. Facial Plast Surg Clin North Am 2005; 13(1):85–92.
23. Gruber RP, Park E, Newman J, et al. The spreader flap in primary rhinoplasty. Plast Reconstr Surg 2007;119(6):1903–10.
24. Clark JM, Cook TA. The 'butterfly' graft in functional secondary rhinoplasty. Laryngoscope 2002;112(11): 1917–25.
25. Kridel RW, Scott BA, Foda HM. The tongue-in-groove technique in septorhinoplasty. A 10-year experience. Arch Facial Plast Surg 1999;1(4):246–56 [discussion: 57–8].
26. Caughlin BP, Been MJ, Rashan AR, et al. The effect of polydioxanone absorbable plates in septorhinoplasty for stabilizing caudal septal extension grafts. JAMA Facial Plast Surg 2015;17(2):120–5.
27. Murakami CS, Barrera JE, Most SP. Preserving structural integrity of the alar cartilage in aesthetic

rhinoplasty using a cephalic turn-in flap. Arch Facial Plast Surg 2009;11(2):126–8.

28. Gunter JP, Friedman RM. Lateral crural strut graft: technique and clinical applications in rhinoplasty. Plast Reconstr Surg 1997;99(4):943–52 [discussion: 53–5].

29. Toriumi DM, Asher SA. Lateral crural repositioning for treatment of cephalic malposition. Facial Plast Surg Clin North Am 2015;23(1):55–71.

30. Gruber RP, Peled A, Talley J. Mattress sutures to remove unwanted convexity and concavity of the nasal tip: 12-year follow-up. Aesthet Surg J 2015; 35(1):20–7.

31. Robinson JK. Placement of the tension-bearing suture in repairing the alar facial junction. J Am Acad Dermatol 1997;36(3 Pt 1):440–3.

32. Lang PG, Retief CR. The use of a suspension suture in lieu of a cartilage strut for deep alar defects. Dermatol Surg 2000;26(6):597–8.

33. Foda HM. Nasal base narrowing: the combined alar base excision technique. Arch Facial Plast Surg 2007;9(1):30–4.

Pyriform Aperture Augmentation as An Adjunct to Rhinoplasty

Michael J. Yaremchuk, MD*, Dev Vibhakar, DO

KEYWORDS

- Pyriform aperture augmentation • Paranasal implants • Adjunct to rhinoplasty
- Treatment of lower midface deficiency

KEY POINTS

- Pyriform aperture augmentation increases the convexity of the lower midface.
- Increasing the convexity of the midface makes the nose seem less prominent.
- Pyriform aperture augmentation increases the projection of the nasal base and nasal tip.
- Pyriform aperture augmentation opens the nasolabial angle and effaces the nasolabial fold.
- Avoid making the intraoral incision directly over the area to be augmented.

Skeletal deficiency in the central midface impacts nasal aesthetics.[1] This lack of lower face projection can be corrected by alloplastic augmentation of the pyriform aperture. Creating convexity in the deficient midface will make the nose seem less prominent. Augmentation of the pyriform aperture is often a useful adjunct during the rhinoplasty procedure. Augmenting the skeleton in this area can alter the projection of the nasal base, the nasolabial angle, and the vertical plane of the lip.

The implant design and surgical techniques described here are extensions of others' previous efforts to improve paranasal aesthetics. Severe cases of the nasomaxillary deficiency, seen with Binder syndrome, have been treated with bone and cartilage grafts alone or together with ostesotomies.[2–8] Lower midface deficiency has also been treated with cartilage grafts or silicone implants as adjuncts to aesthetic rhinoplasty.[9–12]

PREOPERATIVE EVALUATION
Anthropometric Data

Midface concavity is often considered less attractive. Augmentation of the pyriform aperture area is usually performed to move a flat or concave lower midface profile to relative convexity.

When used as an adjunct to rhinoplasty, augmentation later to the pyriform aperture will increase the projection of the nasal base. Augmentation of the maxillary alveolus below the pyriform aperture will increase the nasolabial angle and the vertical plane of the lip (**Fig. 1**).

Pearl

Pyriform aperture augmentation increases the convexity of the lower midface and improves the projection of the nasal base, thereby opening the nasolabial angle.

Disclosure Statement: The authors have nothing to disclose.
Division of Plastic and Reconstructive Surgery, Massachusetts General Hospital, Harvard Medical School, 55 Fruit Street, WACC 435, Boston, MA 02114, USA
* Corresponding author. 170 Commonwealth Avenue, Suite 101, Boston, MA 02116.
E-mail address: dr.y@dryaremchuk.com

Clin Plastic Surg 43 (2016) 187–193
http://dx.doi.org/10.1016/j.cps.2015.09.012

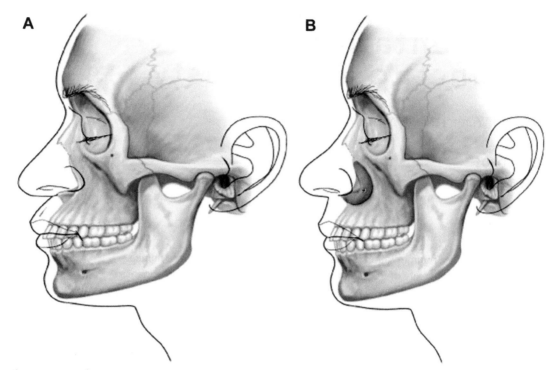

Fig. 1. Impact of implant relative to profile including midface, nasolabial angle, and nasal tip. (*A*) Before pyriform aperture augmentation. (*B*) After pyriform aperture augmentation.

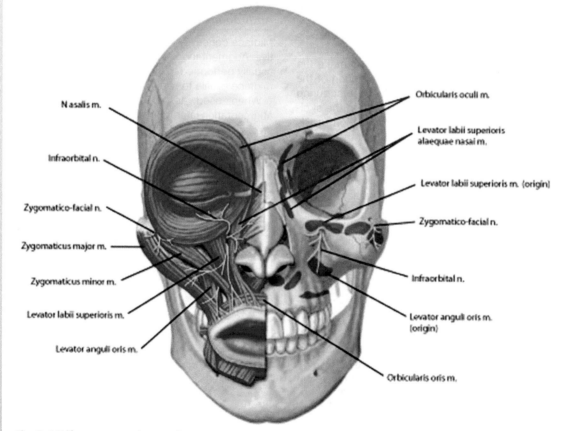

Fig. 2. Midface anatomy (see text).

SURGICAL ANATOMY

The anterior or facial surface of the maxilla is very irregular (**Fig. 2**). Inferiorly, this is due to a series of eminences and corresponding depressions reflecting the apices of the teeth. The incisive fossa is the depression above the prominent incisors. This depression gives rise to the origin of the depressor septi. The canine tooth forms a vertical ridge that separates the incisive fossa from the canine fossa, which is deeper and larger than the incisive fossa. The canine fossa gives rise to the levator anguli oris. The infraorbital foramen is located just above the canine fossa. It allows exit of the infraorbital nerve and vessels. They travel beneath the levator superioris and above the levator anguli oris. The infraorbital nerve supplies the skin of the lower lid, the side of the nose, most of the cheek, and upper lip. Medial to the infraorbital foramen is the nasal notch, which is a concavity whose margin gives rise to the dilator naris as it ends below as the anterior nasal spine.

The deeply located levator anguli oris (caninus), dilator naris, and depressor septi as well as portions of the maxillary origins of the buccinator are separated from the maxilla during implant placement. The lip elevators and the infraorbital nerve are retracted to provide exposure. As a result of these manipulations there is usually temporary dysfunction of these structures postoperatively.

THE IMPLANT

Pyriform aperture (or paranasal) implants are available from Stryker Medical (Kalamazoo, MI) and MatrixSurgical (Atlanta, GA). Implant material consists of porous polyethylene. It is easily carved with a scalpel and is conformable and able to be contoured with a high-speed burr. They are designed as right and left crescents and come in 2

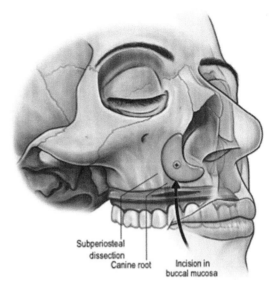

Subperiosteal dissection

Canine root   Incision in buccal mucosa

Fig. 4. Paranasal implant surgery. An incisions is made on the labial side of the buccal sulcus. The green area indicates the area of subperiosteal dissection. Note proximity of infraorbital nerve. Note that the root of the canine tooth lies below the area to be augmented. It must be avoided during screw immobilization of the implant.

sizes. The smaller implant is 27 mm long by 25 mm high and provides 4.5 mm of projection. The larger implant, which is 30 mm long by 28 mm high, provides 7 mm of projection. These implants are designed to be tailored to the patients' particular aesthetic needs. The implant is positioned to sit flush on the bone. The patients' anatomy will determine whether the entire crescent or just the horizontal or vertical limb of the crescent will be used (**Fig. 3**).

OPERATIVE TECHNIQUE

Paranasal augmentation can be done under local or general anesthesia. After sterile preoperative

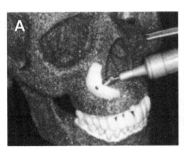
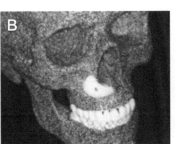
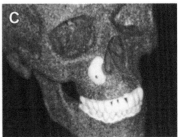

Fig. 3. Porous polyethylene paranasal implants are designed to augment both the lateral and inferior aspects of the pyriform aperture. Implants can be carved to allow selective augmentation. Screw fixation prevents movement of the implant and allows in-place contouring. (*A*) Screw fixed implant. (*B*) Implant contoured and positioned to selectively augment alveolus. (*C*) Implant contoured and positioned to selectively augment maxilla lateral to the pyriform aperture.

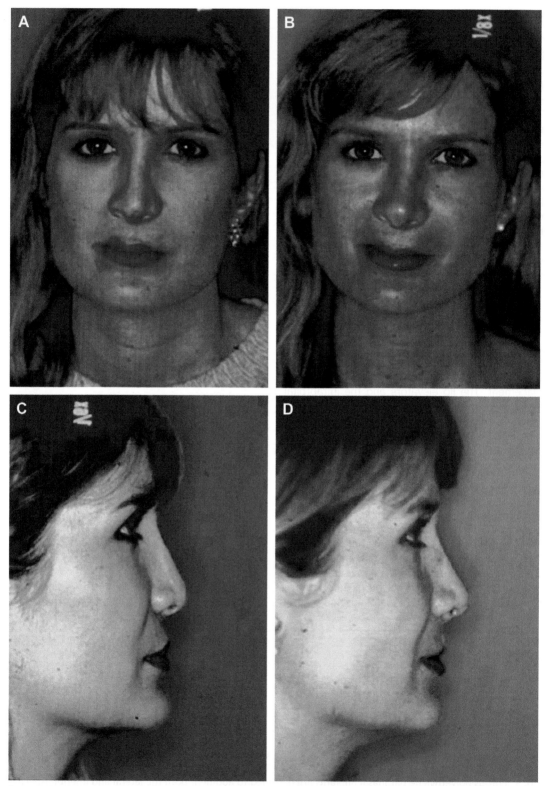

Fig. 5. A 31-year-old woman, after remote cleft lip repair, cleft palate repair, and 2 rhinoplasties. She underwent rhinoplasty with a tip graft, alar base repositioning, and a paranasal augmentation. A larger implant was placed on the cleft side. (*A*) Preoperative frontal view. (*B*) Postoperative frontal view. (*C*) Preoperative lateral view. (*D*) Postoperative lateral view.

preparation and draping, a local anesthetic with 1:200,000 epinephrine is infiltrated at the surgical site. An upper gingivobuccal sulcus incision is made just lateral to the pyriform aperture to avoid placing incisions directly over the implant (**Fig. 4**). The incision is made at least 1 cm above the sulcus to provide an adequate cuff of mucosa inferiorly to allow layered closure. The lip elevators

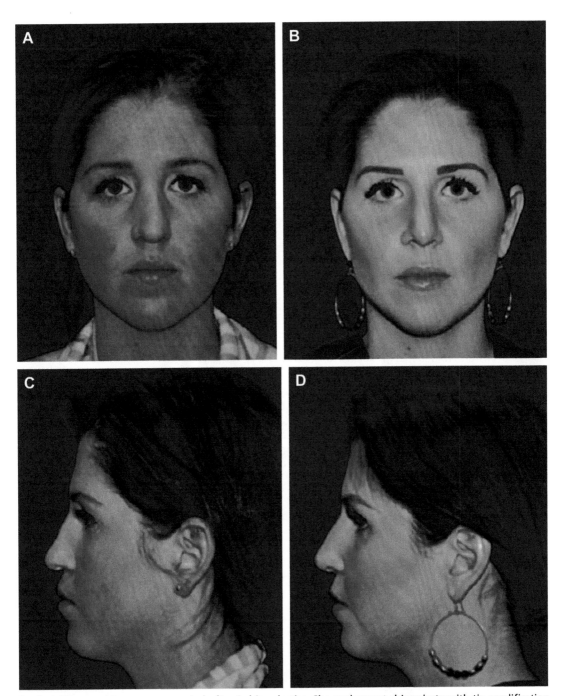

Fig. 6. A 28-year-old woman presented after 2 rhinoplasties. She underwent rhinoplasty with tip modification, placement of spreader grafts, osteotomies, and paranasal augmentation. (*A*) Preoperative frontal view. (*B*) Postoperative frontal view. (*C*) Preoperative lateral view. (*D*) Postoperative lateral view.

can be seen after the mucosa is incised. These muscles are not divided but, rather, retracted during the exposure of the maxilla.

> **Pearl**
>
> Avoid making the incision directly over the area to be augmented.

Subperiosteal dissection exposes the area to be augmented. The levator anguli oris (caninus) and maxillary origins of the buccinator are separated from the maxilla during implant placement. The lip elevators and the infraorbital nerve are retracted to provide exposure. The borders of the pyriform aperture, the infraorbital nerve, and the root of the canine tooth should be identified during surgery. Defining the bony edges of the pyriform aperture provides bony landmarks facilitating precise and

symmetric implant placement. The implant may compromise the nasal airway if positioned beyond the bony edge of the aperture. Identification of the nerve avoids inadvertent retractor or implant damage to the structure. The root of the canine tooth will be visible as a distinct bulge just lateral to the pyriform aperture. The implant will, in part, lie directly over it. The surgeon must avoid damaging these structures if screw fixation is used.

The incision is closed in layers. Because of the relatively small area of dissection, no drains are used.

> **Pearl**
>
> The implant may compromise the nasal airway if malpositioned. The subperiosteal plane is preferred for implant placement. The surgeon should avoid the root of the canine tooth during screw fixation of the implant.

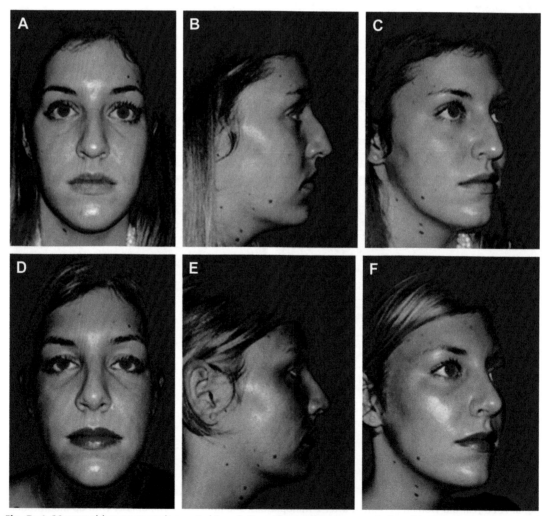

Fig. 7. A 20-year-old woman underwent rhinoplasty and paranasal augmentation. (*A–C*) Preoperative frontal, lateral, and oblique views. (*D–F*) Postoperative frontal, lateral, and oblique views after 1 year.

CLINICAL EXAMPLES

Many, if not most, patients with lower midface sagittal deficiency will benefit from pyriform aperture augmentation as an adjunctive procedure during rhinoplasty. Transforming a flat or concave midface to one of relative convexity will make a large nose seem smaller or less projecting. Improving the balance of a face in this way is not dissimilar to the impact of increasing the projection of a deficient chin during rhinoplasty.

A deficiency in lower midface projection is common in patients with surgically corrected clefts. Both the alteration of soft tissue skeletal relationships during surgical repair and the growth-retarding forces of scarring are thought to restrict palatal and maxillary growth in cleft patients. As shown in **Fig. 5**, selective augmentation of the cleft alveolus and lower lateral paranasal area will improve lip and nasal relationships and overall facial balance.

Fig. 6 represents a patient who underwent primary aesthetic rhinoplasty and augmentation of the pyriform aperture. Augmentation of the vertical aspect of the pyriform aperture created convexity of the midface and lessened the apparent size of the nose relative to its midface platform. This allowed a more conservative nasal reduction. Note how augmentation of the horizontal aspect of the pyriform aperture increased the nasolabial angle and projection of the nasal tip.

Fig. 7 shows a 28-year-old woman who had undergone 2 previous rhinoplasty procedures. She has obvious midface deficiency as seen by her sunken base-to-nose appearance on lateral view. Her procedure involved revision rhinoplasty with tip modification, placement of spreader grafts, osteotomies, and paranasal augmentation. This skeletal augmentation created a more pleasing midface profile, opened the nasolabial angle, and increased the projection of the nasal tip.

SUMMARY

Alloplastic implants selectively augment the pyriform aperture. This procedure can transform the flat or concave lower midface to one of relative convexity. Skeletal augmentation of the nasal platform can decrease the apparent size of the nose and increase the nasolabial angle and projection of the nasal tip. This relatively simple skeletal augmentation can have powerful effects on midface and nasal aesthetics. It has shown to be an important adjunct during rhinoplasty in patients with a deficient sagittal midface morphology.

REFERENCES

1. Yaremchuk MJ, Israeli D. Paranasal implants for correction of midface concavity. Plast Reconstr Surg 1998;102:1676.
2. Converse JM. Techniques of bone grafting for contour restoration of the face. Plast Reconstr Surg 1954;14:332.
3. Converse JM, Horowitz SL, Valauri AJ, et al. Treatment of nasomaxillary hypoplasia. Plast Reconstr Surg 1970;45:427.
4. Jackson IT, Moos KF, Sharpe DT. Total surgical management of Binder's syndrome. Ann Plast Surg 1981;7:25.
5. Obwegeser HL. Surgical correction of small or retrodisplaced maxillae. Plast Reconstr Surg 1969;43:351.
6. Ortiz-Monasterio F, Molina F, McClintock JS. Nasal correction in Binder's syndrome: the evolution of a treatment plan. Aesthetic Plast Surg 1997;21:299.
7. Psillakis JM, Lapa F, Spina V. Surgical correction of mid-facial retrusion (nasomaxillary hypoplasia) in the presence of normal dental occlusion. Plast Reconstr Surg 1973;51:67.
8. Ragnell A. A simple method of reconstruction in some cases of dish-face deformity. Plast Reconstr Surg 1952;10:227.
9. Caronni E. A new method to correct the nasolabial angle in rhinoplasty. Plast Reconstr Surg 1972;50:338.
10. Guerrerosantos J. Nose and paranasal augmentation: autogenous fascia and cartilage. Clin Plast Surg 1991;18:65.
11. Hinderer UT. Nasal base, maxillary, and infraorbital implants-alloplastic. Clin Plast Surg 1991;18:87.
12. Farkas LG, Hreczko TA, Katic MJ. Craniofacial norms in North American Caucasians from birth (one year) to adulthood. In: Farkas LG, editor. Anthropometry of the head and face second edition. New York: Raven Press; 1994.

Harvesting Rib Cartilage in Primary and Secondary Rhinoplasty

Christopher Spencer Cochran, MD*

KEYWORDS

- Rib cartilage graft • Costal cartilage • Rhinoplasty • Secondary rhinoplasty • Technique

KEY POINTS

- The rib offers an abundant supply of cartilage for use in virtually every aspect of rhinoplasty and is the preferred donor site when rigid support is necessary.
- The most significant advantage of rib cartilage is that grafts can be produced with considerable versatility with respect to shape, length, and width.
- Rib cartilage allows reconstruction of the nasal framework in patients with virtually all types of functional and aesthetic requirements.

INTRODUCTION

Satisfactory and consistent long-term results in primary and secondary rhinoplasty rely on adequately supporting or reconstructing the nasal osseocartilagenous framework. Septal cartilage is generally considered the preferred grafting material in rhinoplasty; however, severe deformities or a paucity of available septal cartilage often requires an alternative source of grafting material. This is particularly true in secondary rhinoplasty when structural deformities result from overresection of the osseocartilaginous framework during previous procedures.[1–3]

Alloplastic materials have the advantages of being easy to use, readily available, and having an unlimited supply. Unfortunately, many of these alloplastic materials are fraught with long-term complications, such as infection, migration, extrusion, and palpability.[4–7] Thus, autogenous tissue continues to be our preferred source of grafts.

Autogenous rib cartilage has been our graft material of choice for major nasal reconstruction when sufficient septal cartilage is not available.

Rib provides the most abundant source of cartilage for graft fabrication and is the most reliable when structural support is needed.[1,3] To avoid warping of smaller grafts, we follow the principle of carving balanced cross-sections originally described by Gibson and later substantiated by Kim and colleagues.[8,9] The use of internal K-wire stabilization in columellar struts and dorsal onlay grafts should be avoided owing to the increased risk of late complications such as infection, broken or bent K-wires, and extrusion of the K-wires.

TREATMENT GOALS AND PLANNED OUTCOMES

The rib offers an abundant supply of cartilage for use in virtually every aspect of rhinoplasty and is the preferred donor site when rigid support is necessary. Dorsal augmentation with rib cartilage grafts has proven useful in the secondary rhinoplasty patient. It is also useful in patients with congenital deformities, posttraumatic deformities, or in primary rhinoplasty patients who require a

Disclosure Statement: None.
Department of Otolaryngology-Head & Neck Surgery, University of Texas Southwestern Medical Center at Dallas, Dallas, TX, USA
* Dallas Rhinoplasty Center, 8144 Walnut Hill Lane, Suite 170, Dallas, TX 75231.
E-mail address: drcochran@dallas-rhinoplasty.com

Clin Plastic Surg 43 (2016) 195–200
http://dx.doi.org/10.1016/j.cps.2015.09.018

significant amount of structural support. The most significant advantage of rib cartilage is that grafts can be produced with considerable versatility with respect to shape, length, and width. This facilitates reconstruction of the nasal framework in patients with virtually all types of functional and aesthetic requirements.

PREOPERATIVE PLANNING AND PREPARATION

The choice of rib to harvest depends on the planned use because the amount of cartilage required dictates whether the cartilaginous segment needs to be harvested from 1 rib, 1 rib and a portion of another, or the entire cartilage segments of 2 ribs. In general, the surgeon should choose the cartilaginous portion of a rib that provides a straight segment because it is often possible to construct all required grafts from a single rib. For augmentation with dorsal onlay grafts, we harvest the cartilage from the fifth, sixth or, on occasion, the seventh rib, depending on which rib feels the longest and straightest. If additional grafts are needed, a part or the entire cartilaginous portion of an adjacent rib may be harvested.

In older patients, ossification of the cartilaginous rib is a significant concern, and a limited computed tomography scan of the sternum and ribs with coronal reconstructions is recommended in those patients where there is a high index of suspicion. Despite appropriate preoperative screening, occasionally patients will present with premature calcification of the cartilaginous rib. Frequently, this is limited and occurs commonly at the junction of the osseous and cartilaginous portions of the rib. Small foci of calcification may also be found within the body of the rib cartilage itself. This can impair the preparation of individual grafts as well as act as a site of weakness often having a tendency to fracture during graft harvest. We have found that the use of a smooth diamond burr can also prove useful in contouring areas of calcification to salvage these uncommon circumstances.

PATIENT POSITIONING

Rib cartilage harvesting is performed with the patient in the supine position under general anesthesia. The rib cartilage graft may be harvested from either the patient's left or right side.

PROCEDURAL APPROACH

In female patients, the incision is marked approximately 5 mm above the inframammary fold and measures 3 to 5 cm in length (**Fig. 1**). The incision should not extend beyond the medial extent of the

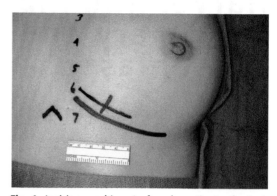

Fig. 1. Incision marking. In female patients, the incision is marked approximately 5 mm above the inframammary fold and measures 3 to 5 cm in length.

inframammary fold. This avoids postoperative visibility of the incision if the patient wears low-cut clothing. In males, placement of the incision is not as important, and the incision is usually placed directly over the chosen rib to facilitate the dissection.

The skin is incised with a scalpel, and the subcutaneous tissue is divided with electrocautery. Once the muscle fascia has been reached, the surgeon palpates the underlying ribs and divides the muscle and fascia with electrocautery directly over the chosen rib (**Fig. 2**). The dissection should be carried medially until the junction of the rib cartilage and sternum can be palpated. The most lateral extent of the dissection is demarcated by the costochondral junction. Identification of the junction is facilitated by the subtle change in color at the interface; the cartilaginous portion is generally off-white in color, whereas the bone demonstrates a distinct reddish-grey hue.

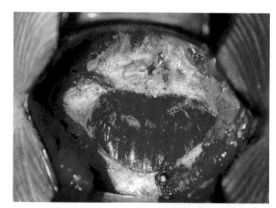

Fig. 2. Dividing fascia. Once the muscle fascia has been reached, the surgeon palpates the underlying ribs and divides the muscle and fascia with electrocautery directly over the chosen rib.

After exposing the selected rib, a longitudinal incision is made with electrocautery through the perichondrium along the length of the central axis of the rib (**Fig. 3**). Perpendicular cuts are also made at the most medial and lateral aspects of the cartilaginous rib to facilitate reflection of the perichondrium.

A periosteal elevator is then used to elevate the perichondrium superiorly and inferiorly from the cartilaginous rib. The subperichondrial dissection is then continued circumferentially along the length of the cartilaginous portion of the rib until the posterior aspect of the rib is exposed. During elevation, the perichondrium may become tight and limit further dissection. If this occurs, it is useful to perform additional perpendicular "back-cuts" on the anterior surface of the perichondrial flap to release tension. Perichondrial elevators are then used to release the posterior adherence between the cartilage and perichondrium as far as possible (**Fig. 4**). A curved rib stripper completes the posterior dissection (**Fig. 5**). We have found it useful to pass the tip of the rib stripper with gentle upward force to stay within the subperichondrial space. However, care must be taken to not enter the body of the cartilaginous rib or cause a fracture, which may limit graft fabrication.

The remainder of the subperichondrial dissection is generally straightforward and bloodless as long as the perichondrium is not violated and the correct plane is maintained. The curved rib stripper is slid back and forth along the rib, taking care to stay between the cartilage and perichondrium until the undermining is complete. Perichondrial tears should be avoided so that a tight postoperative closure can later be accomplished to help "splint" the wound, which aids in relieving postoperative pain.

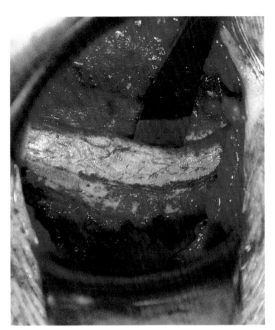

Fig. 4. Perichondrial elevation. Perichondrial elevators are used to release the posterior adherence between the cartilage and perichondrium as far as possible.

The final step involves separating the cartilaginous rib from its medial attachment near the sternum and laterally at the bony rib. This is performed by making a partial thickness incision perpendicular to the long axis of the rib using a number 15 blade at the aforementioned junctions. The cartilaginous incision can then be completed with the end of a Freer elevator using gentle side-to-side movement (**Fig. 6**). Once the cartilage segment is released both medially and laterally, the graft is removed easily from the wound and placed in

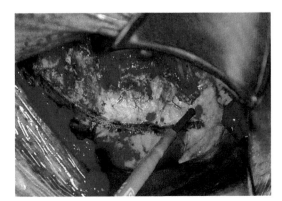

Fig. 3. Exposing the selected rib. A longitudinal incision is made with electrocautery through the perichondrium along the length of the central axis of the rib.

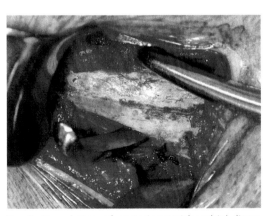

Fig. 5. Completion of posterior perichondrial dissection. A curved rib stripper completes the posterior dissection.

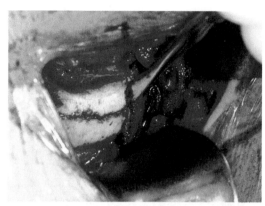

Fig. 6. Separating cartilaginous rib. The cartilaginous rib is cut free using the end of a Freer elevator with a gentle side-to-side movement.

sterile saline until the surgeon is ready for graft fabrication. If more grafting material is required, a portion of cartilage or the entire cartilaginous part of another rib should then be harvested. After choosing an adjacent donor rib, access to the perichondrium is obtained by undermining deep to the existing muscle to avoid an additional incision through the fascia and muscle. This prevents the creation of a "bridge" of denervated and devascularized muscle between adjacent ribs, which may result in delayed healing at the donor site. The adjacent rib is then harvested in a similar fashion.

After hemostasis is achieved, the donor site is checked to ensure that no pneumothorax has occurred. The wound is filled with saline solution and the anesthesiologist applies positive pressure into the lungs. If no air leak is detected, a pneumothorax can be excluded. A 16-gauge angiocatheter is inserted through the skin and placed in the subperichondrial space to allow instillation of a long acting local anesthetic at the conclusion of the procedure. The wound may then be closed in layers using 2-0 Vicryl sutures. Particular attention should be directed at reapproximating the perichondrium. It is important to close the perichondrium, muscle, and muscle fascia layers tightly to prevent a palpable or visible chest wall deformity. A tight closure also helps to "splint" the wound and reduce postoperative pain. Skin closure is carried out using deep dermal and subcuticular 4-0 Monocryl sutures.

POTENTIAL COMPLICATIONS AND MANAGEMENT OF THEM

The use of rib cartilage also has several disadvantages. First, an additional incision at a distant donor site is required to harvest the cartilage. Fortunately, the resulting scar is relatively short

(approximately 5 cm) and is generally inconspicuous in women owing to its placement under the breast (**Fig. 7**). Additional concerns include postoperative pain, the risk of pneumothorax, excessive calcification of rib cartilage, and the potential of rib cartilage to warp. Hypertrophic scarring and keloiding of the incision can be treated conservatively with steroid injections and silicone sheeting. Persistent or recurrent unsightly scars can be excised and the wound reapproximated.

If a pneumothorax has been diagnosed, this usually represents an injury only to the parietal pleura and not to the lung parenchyma itself. As such, this does not mandate chest tube placement. Rather, a red rubber catheter can be inserted through the parietal pleural tear into the thoracic cavity. The incision should then be closed, as previously described, in layers around the catheter. Positive pressure is then applied and the catheter is clamped with a hemostat until the surgeon is prepared for removal. At the end of the operation, the anesthesiologist applies maximal positive pressure into the lungs and holds

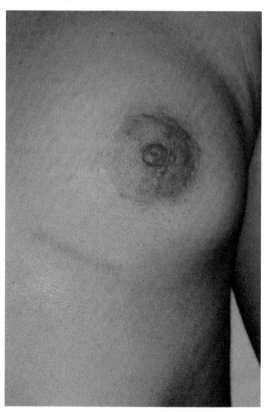

Fig. 7. Incisions site at 1 year postoperatively. The resulting scar is relatively short (approximately 5 cm) and is generally inconspicuous in women owing to its placement under the breast.

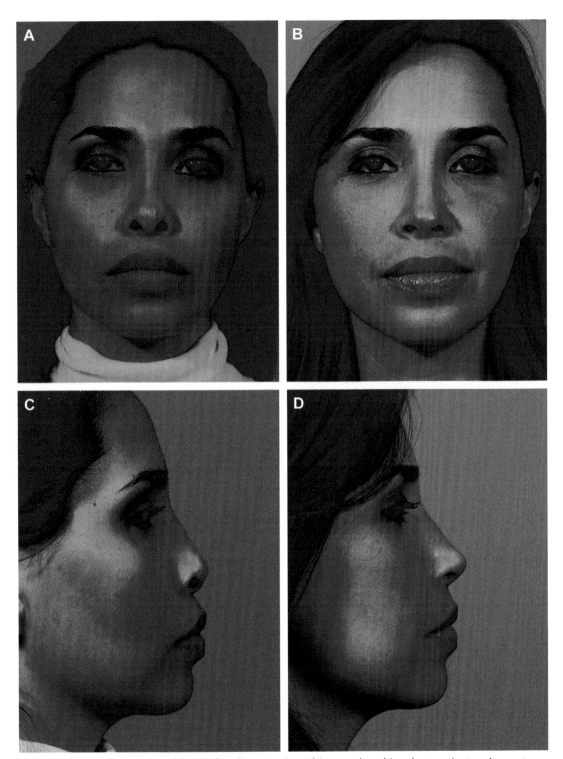

Fig. 8. (*A, C*) One year before and (*B, D*) after the operation. This secondary rhinoplasty patient underwent open secondary rhinoplasty with rib cartilage grafts to reconstruct her overresected nasal framework resulting from a prior surgery by another surgeon.

this as the catheter is placed on suction and removed. A postoperative chest radiograph should be taken if there is any concern about the effectiveness of reestablishing negative pressure within the pleural space.

POSTPROCEDURAL CARE

At the conclusion of the procedure, a long-acting local anesthetic such as bupivacaine is injected through the angiocathether that was placed at the end of the procedure to minimize postoperative pain. Patients may be discharged home or kept in our overnight surgical facility for 23-hour observation and released the following day. Patients are encouraged to ambulate and to also perform incentive spirometry and deep breathing exercises to minimize the change of atelectasis resulting from shallow breathing related to pain with deep respiration.

REHABILITATION AND RECOVERY

Patients are instructed to gradually return to daily activities. Patients are instructed to refrain from exercise or other strenuous activity for 2 to 3 weeks after surgery and are and instructed not to lift objects heavier than 10 to 15 pounds for 6 to 8 weeks after surgery.

OUTCOMES

Rib cartilage grafts are often necessary to reconstruct the nose during secondary rhinoplasty for patients in whom the original osseocartilaginous framework was overly resected in prior surgeries. For example, this secondary rhinoplasty patient required extended spreader grafts, caudal septum replacement graft, and lateral crural strut grafts (**Fig. 8**).

SUMMARY

Rib cartilage harvest can be performed safely and can yield reliable, reproducible results. Our technique has proven useful not only in secondary rhinoplasty, but also in primary rhinoplasty and in correcting posttraumatic deformities.

REFERENCES

1. Gunter JP, Rohrich RJ. Augmentation rhinoplasty: dorsal onlay grafting using shaped autogenous septal cartilage. Plast Reconstr Surg 1990;86:39.
2. Sheen JH, Sheen AP. Aesthetic rhinoplasty. 2nd edition. St. Louis (MO): Quality Medical Publishing; 1998 (reprint of 1987 ed.).
3. Gunter JP, Rohrich RJ. External approach to secondary rhinoplasty. Plast Reconstr Surg 1987;80:161.
4. Hiraga Y. Complications of augmentation rhinoplasty in the Japanese. Ann Plast Surg 1980;4:495.
5. Davis PKB, Jones SM. The complications of silastic implants: experience with 137 consecutive cases. Br J Plast Surg 1971;24:405.
6. Godin MS, Waldman R, Johnson CM. The use of expanded polytetrafluoroethylene (Gore-Tex) in rhinoplasty. Arch Otolaryngol Head Neck Surg 1995;121: 1131.
7. Raghavan U, Jones NS, Romo R III. Immediate autogenous cartilage grafts in rhinoplasty after alloplastic implant rejection. Arch Facial Plast Surg 2004;6: 192–6.
8. Gibson T. Cartilage grafts. Br Med Bull 1965;21:153.
9. Kim DW, Shah AR, Toriumi DM. Concentric and eccentric carved costal cartilage: a comparison of warping. Arch Facial Plast Surg 2006;8(1):42–6.

Costal Cartilage Grafts in Rhinoplasty

Fred G. Fedok, MD[a,b],*

KEYWORDS

- Costal cartilage • Rib • Rhinoplasty • Revision rhinoplasty • Grafting in rhinoplasty • Augmentation
- Saddle nose • Spreader grafts

KEY POINTS

- The use of costal cartilage in rhinoplasty carries with it a risk of both donor site and rhinoplasty complications. The decision to use costal cartilage should be made after considering the alternative sources of cartilage grafts.
- After cartilage is harvested, the integrity of the chest wall and the absence of pneumothorax should be confirmed.
- Costal cartilage has a significant risk of warping. Various technical considerations allow the surgeon to take advantage of or to minimize the warping of grafts.
- Pain will be reduced if a muscle-sparing technique is used during the exposure of the rib cartilage segment.
- The intended incision on a female chest wall should be marked with them in an upright position and the incision placed a few millimeters inferior to the inframammary crease.

INTRODUCTION

Rhinoplasty has become increasingly popular and is more frequently performed than in any time in the past. The reasons for this are several. Rhinoplasty was at one time a somewhat secret craft that the most famous practitioners were reticent to share. It has now become the focus of numerous teaching venues with the willing sharing of ideas and techniques. The number of practitioners doing rhinoplasty has therefore increased. The procedure is also being performed on a larger segment of the population. What was initially a procedure that was performed for the generally well-to-do or the significantly afflicted has now become accessible to a larger segment of population.

It is a changing world where rhinoplasty is being performed across many different ethnicities and in many different countries. What was formerly a discipline directed at a western Caucasian population is now is frequently performed for multitudes of patients with varied ethnic derivations.[1,2] Within this spectrum of ethnicities, some patients possess noses that are relatively devoid of firm cartilaginous structure, as in the Asian population, so that grafting materials are frequently necessary even in primary cases.[3,4]

With a greater understanding of the anatomy and dynamics of rhinoplasty, there has been the introduction of technically more sophisticated corrective maneuvers. The open rhinoplasty technique has made it possible to better recognize abnormalities and deficiencies in structure and as a

No pertinent disclosures.
[a] Department of Surgery, University of South Alabama Medical Center, 2451 Fillingim Street, Mobile, AL, USA;
[b] Facial Plastic and Reconstructive Surgery, Otolaryngology/Head & Neck Surgery, Hershey Medical Center, Pennsylvania State University, 500 University Drive, Hershey, PA 17033, USA
* The McCollough Plastic Surgery Clinic, 350 Cypress Bend Drive, Gulf Shores, AL 36542.
E-mail address: drfredfedok@me.com

result has ushered in a need for grafting materials to restore and create structure.[5,6] It has been realized that the application of structure will produce rhinoplasty results that are more enduring. Finally, with this increased surgical activity, there is also an increase in the number of revision surgeries that may require grafting materials.

TREATMENT GOALS AND PLANNED OUTCOMES

Every rhinoplasty procedure has multiple goals. Foremost is the resolution of all the concerns of the patient. The procedure should be safe with a minimal risk of complications. Patient satisfaction with an achievement of the desired esthetic and functional goals is central to a good outcome. Technically, the procedure should be based on sound principles of surgery, healing, and esthetics.

In rhinoplasty, favorable outcomes are achieved as a result of careful analysis, diagnosis, communication, planning, and execution. The assessment of the final result after the use of costal cartilage as a grafting material for the rhinoplasty is not primarily dependent on the desired outcome of the execution of the rib cartilage harvesting but largely on the outcome of the rhinoplasty. The two processes, however, go hand in hand, and thus, both must be executed satisfactorily. The major planning involved is primarily the planning for the rhinoplasty. The harvesting of the rib cartilage is done as an integral step in achieving the rhinoplasty goals. The decision on whether costal cartilage is to be used will depend on several factors. These factors include the availability of alternative donor sites and other patient factors as well as an assessment of the relative morbidity.

Preoperative Planning and Preparation

Through careful preoperative planning, the rhinoplasty surgeon determines which surgical maneuvers are necessary to achieve the desired goals of the surgery. When the restoration or creation of an improved nasal skeletal structure is intended, then the surgeon must determine what may be the optimal cartilage to use and what donor site is to be taken advantage of. Even in the situation of a primary rhinoplasty, there may be inadequate septal cartilage available to do the necessary grafting. Frequently those of Asian and African descent possess noses with a lesser amount of septal cartilage. In the case of revision surgery, when there has been a previous rhinoplasty performed, the paucity of available septal cartilage may be even further compounded. Auricular

cartilage is available in most patients but has limitations regarding elasticity and curvature. Although some authors use cadaver rib cartilage, many will not.[7-10]

The preoperative planning for the use of cartilage grafts in rhinoplasty is centered around the goals of the rhinoplasty. If cartilaginous grafting materials are needed, then a donor site will have to be considered. The reasonably available donor sites are the nasal septum, the ear, and the ribs. The amount of auricular cartilage available to be harvested without causing distortion of the ear is also limited compared with that which might be harvested from the rib cage. In addition, many surgeons are reticent to use auricular cartilage because of its unfavorable biomechanical properties and firm curvatures. The edges of auricular cartilage grafts are also more likely to show dorsal irregularities through an overlying thin skin envelope compared with septal cartilage and rib cartilage grafts.

The large amount of available costal cartilage makes it an attractive source for patients who have a deficient amount of septal or auricular cartilage to be used for grafting. If it is decided to use a costal donor site, several considerations will have to be made. There will have to be a determination about how much cartilage will be needed and what other components of the rib should be included, such as the perichondrium or bone. If it is decided to use costal cartilage, then the procedure will have to be described to the patient. There are some patients who will decline the harvesting of costal cartilage either because of the concern about pain or the remote risk of pneumothorax. The relative risk and benefits will have to be weighed.

When it is determined that costal cartilage will be used, the chest wall should be examined for pre-existing deformity or previous surgery and scarring. The patient's age will have some bearing on whether costal cartilage will be used. In the younger patient, the cartilage may be more prone to warping. On the other hand, in the case of the older patient, there may be calcification of the cartilage, making carving more difficult.[11,12] Their cartilage however will be less prone to warping.

Gender differences also will potentially come into play as female patients may be more resistant to having a chest wall scar. In the case of the female patient, the scar can be strategically placed just inferior to the inframammary crease, thus camouflaging it. A scar inferior to the inframammary crease will change the location of what rib may be used. In general, the costal cartilage grafts used for rhinoplasty will be harvested from the sixth or seventh ribs, although lower rib segments could be used. In female patients, the location of the incision and therefore the selection of which rib will be used are guided by the level of the inframammary crease. To avoid dissecting through a thick pectoralis muscle in an athletic male patient, a similar location can used (**Fig. 1**).

The location of the proposed incision on the patient's chest wall may be marked preoperatively. The incision is usually planned at a location medial to the midclavicular line in both male and female patients. In the female patient, it is recommended that the incision is made 2 to 3 mm below the inframammary crease. The position of the incision is marked with the female patient in the upright position so that the crease and the position of the dependent breast tissue can be reliably ascertained. It is recommended that the incision be placed in that location to avoid making the incision over breast tissue (**Fig. 2**). In addition to the decision of what rib to harvest and the incision placement, postoperative pain management is another important consideration.

Patient Positioning

The patient positioning for the harvesting of rib cartilage in the setting of rhinoplasty is relatively simple. The two surgical sites may be draped separately or in the same field. The patient is placed in the supine position with the back elevated at about 10° in a lawn-chair position.

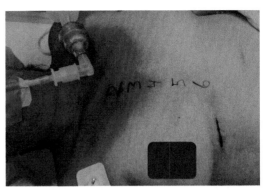

Fig. 2. Female patient marked for rib graft harvest. The location of the ribs has been marked. The placement of the incision was marked when she was in the upright position.

The neck is slightly extended (see **Fig. 2**). The costal cartilage is harvested either before the nasal procedure or simultaneously by a second surgeon. One should avoid the transfer of instruments from the nasal procedure to the chest wall procedure to lessen the risk of infection. The procedure is usually performed with the patient under general anesthesia, intubated, and receiving positive pressure ventilation.

Procedural Approach

In the operating room, local anesthetic solution (1% lidocaine with 1:100,000 epinephrine) is injected into the donor site to aid hemostasis. The anesthetic agent can be injected down to the rib perichondrium through the overlying musculature. One has to be careful at the time of the initial injection that the intercostal space is not violated or a pneumothorax can occur.

An incision of 2.5 cm or less in length usually suffices (**Fig. 3**). The size of the incision will depend on the technique for rib harvest used by the surgeon and by the habitus of the patient. The heavier the patient, the more subcutaneous adipose can be

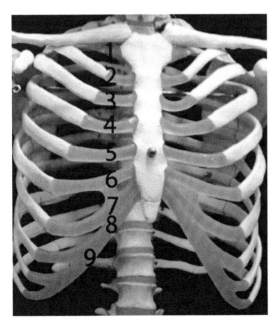

Fig. 1. Skeletal representation of the rib cage. Note the first rib articulates with the manubrium.

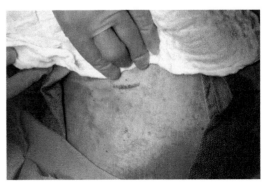

Fig. 3. Typical incision size and location.

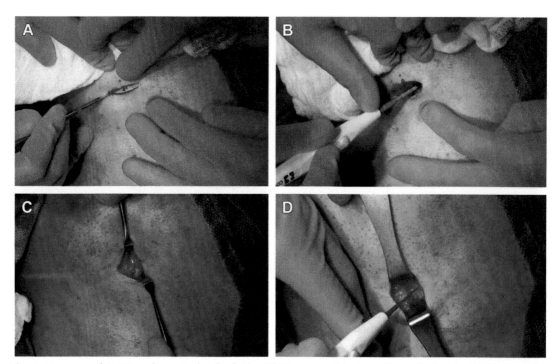

Fig. 4. Progress of incision down to level of rib. (*A*) Progress of incision through dermis. (*B–D*) Dissection continuing through superficial adipose to expose the deep fascia. Cautery is used to control small bleeding vessels.

anticipated and a greater depth of tissue will have to be dissected; therefore, a larger incision may be necessary to provide sufficient exposure of the rib. On the other hand, a thin patient with very little underlying adipose tissue may have suitable exposure obtained with a smaller incision.

The initial incision is taken down to the muscular fascia. After the skin incision is made, the subcutaneous fat can be incised with electrocautery and blunt dissection. When the deep muscular fascia is encountered, it is divided in the direction of the underlying muscle fibers with blunt but firm dissection with a hemostat. If the fascia is particularly thick, a number 15 scalpel can be used to incise the fascia. The muscle itself is not cut or cut through with cautery but instead it is divided by bluntly spreading in the direction of the muscle fibers with a hemostat. It should be noted that since using this particular muscle-sparing technique and avoiding electrocautery of the muscle, the pain after costal graft harvesting has been significantly reduced (**Figs. 4** and **5**).

This dissection is then carried down to the level of the rib perichondrium. The desired rib segment is exposed by further elevating the muscle off of the perichondrium with the use of a Freer (Anthony Products, Indianapolis, IN, USA) or Adson elevator (**Fig. 6**).

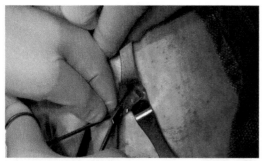

Fig. 5. Exposure of external oblique muscle and bluntly spreading through it with hemostat.

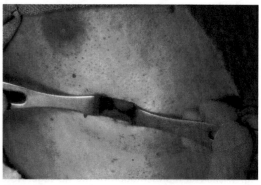

Fig. 6. Exposure of rib with overlying perichondrium.

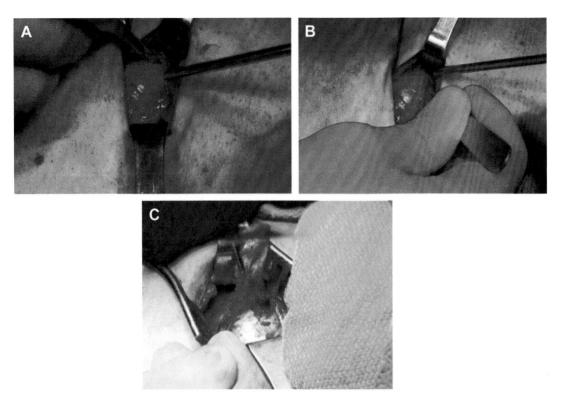

Fig. 7. Clinical intraoperative images showing method of costal perichondrium graft harvest. (*A, B*) Images depicting the outlining of the perichondrium graft with a scalpel and (*C*) Intraoperative image depicting perichondrium graft being elevated from rib with a freer elevator.

The anterior rib perichondrium can be removed as a separate graft and later used as a cushioning graft over the nasal dorsum or other nasal areas; this is especially helpful in the patient with thin skin. The periosteum is removed by first incising an outline of the desired dimensions of the perichondrium graft over the rib with a scalpel (**Fig. 7**). The perichondrium can then be elevated off of the rib with one of the previously mentioned elevators (**Fig. 8**).

Next, the location and dimensions of the segment of rib to be removed are sharply outlined with a scalpel. The medial and lateral extents of the intended graft to be removed are incised with a number 15 scalpel blade (**Fig. 9**). The segment of rib routinely harvested can be up to 3.5 to 4 cm in length and be delivered though a 2.5-cm incision. The completion of the medial and lateral rib cartilage incisions can be completed with a scalpel or by using a Freer elevator. The segment of rib is

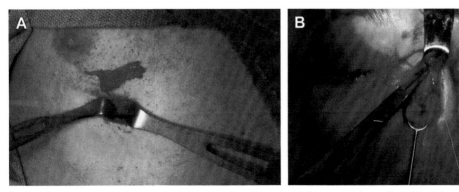

Fig. 8. (*A*) Intraoperative image depicting perichondrium graft harvested from rib. (*B*) Perichondrium graft being guided with sutures over patient's dorsum.

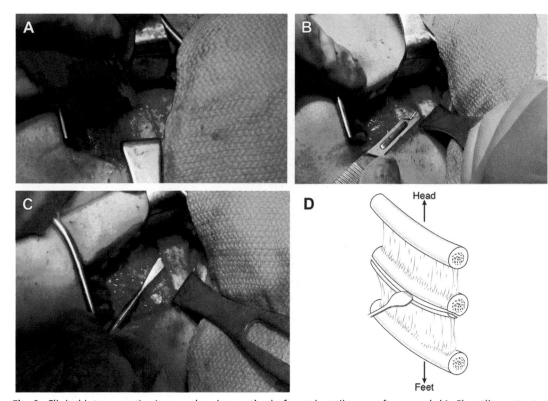

Fig. 9. Clinical intraoperative images showing method of costal cartilage graft removal, (*A, B*) outline extent of graft to be harvested from cartilage segment is deeply scored with scalpel, (*C*) with use of scalpel and freer the scoring is progressively deepened until the cartilage is mobilized from the deep perichondrium and retracted away from chest, (*D*) drawing depicting the described method of harvesting of the rib graft in which a small inferior segment of the rib is initially left attached to the perichondrium thus improving the angle of approach and reducing the risk of pneumothorax.

removed with the intention of optionally leaving a few millimeters of the inferior border of the rib intact. Mechanically, this allows for a more suitable angle of approach to the rib to accomplish an inferior-to-superior dissection and with a lesser risk of penetrating the parietal pleura. The rib segment is usually dissected while leaving the posterior perichondrium on the wound bed. The rib is cut parallel to its inferior edge with the Freer elevator. A 3- to 5-mm segment of the inferior border of the rib may be left in the wound bed. The dissection and rib cuts are completed at the previously determined medial and lateral dimensions of the rib segment. The cuts are carefully deepened until the rib segment can be mobilized. The mobilized segment is retracted away from the chest. In the course of the dissection, the rib can be grasped with either forceps or an Allis clamp (Anthony Products, Indianapolis, IN, USA) and retracted away from the wound bed. In this manner, the rib is retracted away from the chest cavity rather than having the force of the dissection directed toward the chest cavity. This

retraction will minimize the risk of pneumothorax and also facilitate the removal of the rib. After the segment of rib is removed, the remainder of the inferior portion of the rib can be removed for additional grafting material (**Fig. 10**).

After the rib segment is removed, hemostasis is accomplished with the use of electrocautery. The

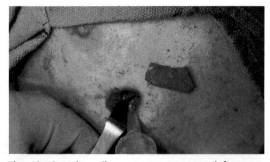

Fig. 10. Costal cartilage segment removed from patient's rib. Note the wound is being flooded with saline in order to test for any air leaks or chest wall defects.

wound is inspected for bubbling or any suggestion of a pleural leak. To further verify the integrity of the parietal pleura and confirm the absence of a pneumothorax, the wound bed is further tested for leaks. Testing for leaks is performed by flooding the wound bed with saline solution and asking the anesthesiologist or anesthetist to "Valsalva" (hold positive pressure through the ventilation circuit) the patient for 30 seconds. If the saline solution seems to drain into the chest or bubbles are visible during the Valsalva maneuver, a pleural tear should be suspected. If there is no evidence of a leak and the integrity of the chest wall is confirmed, the wound can be closed (**Fig. 10**).

The wound is closed in layers. The remaining perichondrium and muscular and subcutaneous layers are closed using absorbable suture. These deeper layers may be injected with bupivacaine to aid with pain management in the early postoperative period. The skin can be closed with a permanent suture such as polypropylene or with a buried running subcuticular absorbable suture. In the patient in which the dissection and closure have resulted in minimal dead space that has been successfully eliminated, a drain may not be necessary. In patients where there has been a significant amount of dead space created, that is, in the heavier patient, a drain may be necessary.

The harvested rib is prepared for use in the following ways. The remaining perichondrium and a small amount of adjacent cartilage are sharply removed from the harvested cartilage graft. The cartilage may be preliminarily divided into segments to be later carved into specific grafts (**Fig. 11**). There are principles of rib cartilage management and various carving methods used by investigators to lessen the risk of warping.[11–15] The cartilage is set on the back table and kept moist in sterile saline while the chest wall is closed and while the rhinoplasty procedure proceeds. By allowing some time to pass before the cartilage is used for the final graft creation, it will show its tendency to warp and in which direction. This knowledge will be used to determine which segments to be used for what grafts and to decide on the best placement.

POTENTIAL COMPLICATIONS AND MANAGEMENT

Potential donor site complications include infection, pneumothorax, bleeding, hematoma, and pain. Recipient site complications include graft sizing issues, graft malposition, graft mobility, and warping. The donor site complications are relatively uncommon, but include persistent pain, seroma, and wound issues.[16,17]

Among the most significant risk during the execution of costal cartilage harvesting is pneumothorax. Pneumothorax has been stated to occur in more than 20% of the time during costal cartilage graft harvests for microtia reconstruction,[18] but is significantly less common with the small rib segments harvested for rhinoplasty. If in the course of the operation a leak in the chest wall is detected, the following method has proved to be reliable to identify and repair the chest wall rent. If there has been an appropriate dissection, the problem will be a hole in the chest wall and the parietal pleura, not a tear in the visceral pleura or lung. The exact location of the leak in the wound bed should be identified as described above. The surgeon should confirm with the aid of the anesthesiologist or anesthetist that the patient is hemodynamically stable and the patient is being optimally ventilated. If the above conditions are met, then a red rubber catheter should be placed through the rent in the chest wall and advanced a few centimeters into the pleural space. A 2-0 or 3-0 polyglactin pursestring suture should be placed through the adjacent perichondrium and muscle and around the red rubber catheter. The suture is then tightened as the anesthesiologist "Valsalvas" the patient so that the lung is inflated and forces the air out of the pleural space and out through the red rubber catheter. While the Valsalva is maintained, the pursestring suture is tightened and the red rubber catheter is withdrawn from the wound by an assistant. If performed successfully, this maneuver should eliminate the air inside the pleural cavity and the pneumothorax. After this maneuver is completed, the wound bed should again be examined for the presence of a leak as described above, that is, flooding the wound with saline and having a Valsalva maneuver performed. If the technique has been successful, the results of this second maneuver should be normal. If the clinical situation appears different from that described above and it appears that the patient is unstable, appropriate intraoperative consultation should be obtained.

If the patient is stable after the repair of a presumably small leak in the chest wall, the rest of the operation can proceed as originally planned. If a significant pneumothorax is discovered on a postoperative chest radiograph, the management may include conservative management, aspiration, the placement of a chest tube, and consultation with a thoracic surgeon. If there is any question in regard to the management or the patient's condition, appropriate consultation should be obtained.

Other complications, such as infection, bleeding, and hematoma, are relatively uncommon and should be managed in a manner consistent with good principles of surgical care.

208

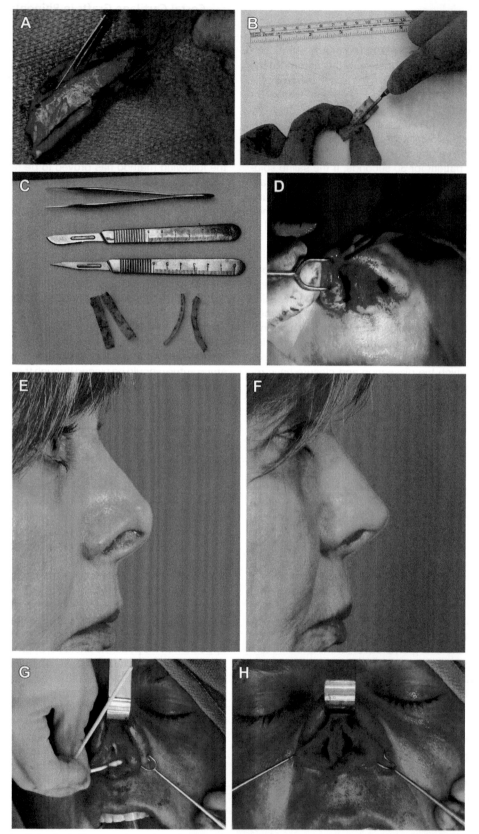

Fig. 11. (*A, B*) Carving of harvested costal cartilage into large segments devoid of perichondrium. (*C*) Prospective grafts showing tendency to warp, thus noting magnitude and direction. (*D*) Curved graft used as right alar contour graft inserted through open rhinoplasty approach. (*E*) Before and (*F*) after images of patient after insertion of the contour graft. (*G, H*) Costal cartilage–derived graft used to correct foreshortened septum with septal caudal extension graft.

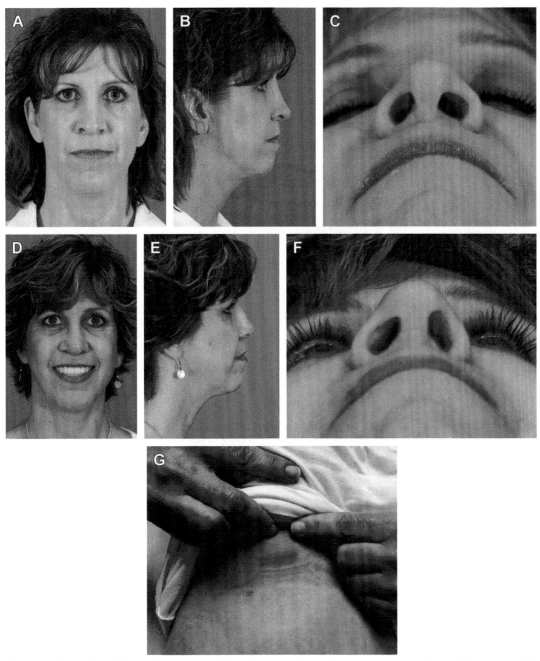

Fig. 12. Patient with a history of trauma and 2 previous nasal surgeries who presented for revision surgery. She had both esthetic and functional concerns. Anatomic problems included a crooked nose, a complex septal deformity with vertical fracture, intranasal scarring, right nasal sidewall collapse, mild saddling, tip ptosis, and bilateral alar retraction. Because of her trauma and previous surgeries, there was inadequate septal cartilage to be used for grafting material, and it was determined her surgery would require more cartilage than what would be reasonably available from the ear. Using costal cartilage, the patient underwent the reconstruction of an L-strut incorporating a small caudal septal extension graft and bilateral spreader grafts, medial and lateral osteotomies, dorsal augmentation, a left lateral crural batten graft, alar contour grafts, a small tip graft, and intradomal and interdomal tip sutures. The dorsum was covered with a blanket of rib perichondrium. (*A–C*) Preoperative clinical images. (*D–F*) Postoperative clinical images. (*G*) Rib harvest wound at 9 months.

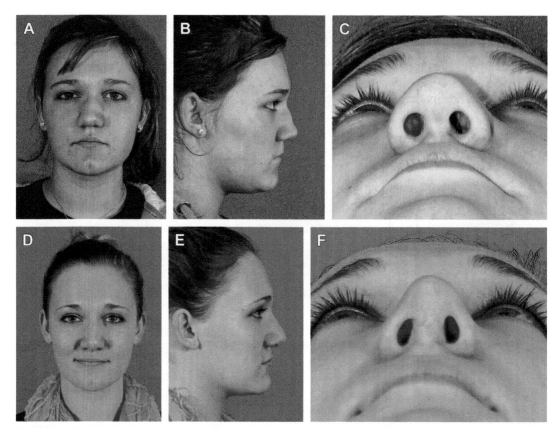

Fig. 13. (*A–C*) Preoperative photographs of patient who presented a decade after a severe playground accident. Examination revealed saddling of the bony and cartilaginous dorsum with a foreshortened nose, thickening and contraction of the soft tissue envelope, severe septal deviation, and left middle vault collapse. (*D–F*) Postoperative photographs of patient after repair was performed via an open approach, with septoplasty, application of bilateral extended spreader grafts articulated with a caudal septal extension graft creating a new L-strut constructed from a costal cartilage donor site. She also underwent medial and lateral osteotomies. After the initial reconstructive procedure, she underwent a secondary procedure to take down a small dorsal convexity and further augment the columella.

Postprocedural Care

Pain in the chest wall is common. Using previous more aggressive harvesting methods, patients experienced significant discomfort for several weeks. Formerly, patients required significant pain medication and would be managed as if they had had a significant local rib injury. In the author's patients, severe postprocedure pain has essentially been eliminated by the muscle-sparing cartilage-harvesting technique described above. Within a week, many patients are able to demonstrate they are able to rotate their torso with little to no discomfort and have a lessened need for pain control medications.

Rehabilitation and Recovery

Patients are instructed to avoid doing heavy lifting, significant exertion, Valsalva maneuvers, and strenuous activity for 4 to 6 weeks. Women are cautioned to wear a dressing over the inframammary incision while wearing bras to minimize irritation of the incision.

Outcomes

The general morbidity of the use of costal cartilage in rhinoplasty has been studied and reported.[16,17,19] In general, the outcomes have been exceedingly good in the author's practice, and no significant short-term or long-term sequelae have occurred with respect to the chest wall procedure. The vast majority of the rhinoplasty cases in the author's practice in which it was elected to use rib cartilage have been secondary cases after trauma or complicated revision rhinoplasty cases, which inherently have a higher need for further revision. Problems encountered have included inadequate dorsal graft fixation resulting in mobility, asymmetries secondary to prior

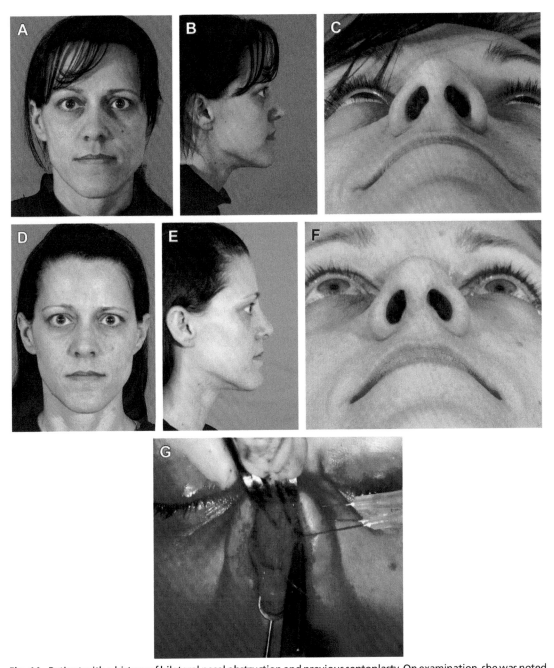

Fig. 14. Patient with a history of bilateral nasal obstruction and previous septoplasty. On examination, she was noted to have bilateral middle vault collapse and thin weak upper lateral cartilages. There was an inadequate amount of remaining septal cartilage. The patient underwent restructuring of her middle vault via an open approach. Costal cartilage was used to create bilateral spreader grafts. A columellar strut was also placed followed by intradomal and interdomal sutures. The rib perichondrium was placed over the dorsum. (*A–C*) Preoperative clinical images. (*D–F*) Postoperative clinical images. (*G*) Intraoperative images depicting the placement of the spreader grafts.

severe scarring of the soft tissue envelope, dorsal convexities, and prolonged swelling.

The patients in **Figs. 12–14** presented with clinical situations that warranted the use of costal cartilage.

SUMMARY

The limitations of available septal and auricular cartilage may compromise the results of a rhinoplasty procedure when restricted to the use of those 2 donor sites. The rib cage provides an enormous reserve of costal cartilage that can be carved into a variety of grafts necessary for the successful execution of several rhinoplasty techniques. In many circumstances, the available volume and characteristics of costal cartilage are optimal for a successful rhinoplasty operation. As with every medical interaction, there are risks of harvesting costal cartilage. There are also recipient site risks associated with the use of costal cartilage in rhinoplasty. These risks can be minimized through detailed planning and the successful adherence to recommended techniques. The use of costal cartilage for appropriate candidates is a valuable addition to the toolbox of the rhinoplasty surgeon.

REFERENCES

1. Nolst Trenite GJ. Considerations in ethnic rhinoplasty. Facial Plast Surg 2003;19(3):239–45.
2. Rohrich RJ, Bolden K. Ethnic rhinoplasty. Clin Plast Surg 2010;37(2):353–70.
3. Park JH, Jin HR. Use of autologous costal cartilage in Asian rhinoplasty. Plast Reconstr Surg 2012; 130(6):1338–48.
4. Toriumi DM. Discussion: use of autologous costal cartilage in Asian rhinoplasty. Plast Reconstr Surg 2012;130(6):1349–50.
5. Whitaker EG, Johnson CM Jr. The evolution of open structure rhinoplasty. Arch Facial Plast Surg 2003; 5(4):291–300.
6. Zijlker TD, Adamson PA. Open structure rhinoplasty. Clin Otolaryngol Allied Sci 1993;18(2): 125–34.
7. Burke AJ, Wang TD, Cook TA. Irradiated homograft rib cartilage in facial reconstruction. Arch Facial Plast Surg 2004;6(5):334–41.
8. Lefkovits G. Irradiated homologous costal cartilage for augmentation rhinoplasty. Ann Plast Surg 1990; 25(4):317–27.
9. Demirkan F, Arslan E, Unal S, et al. Irradiated homologous costal cartilage: versatile grafting material for rhinoplasty. Aesthetic Plast Surg 2003;27(3):213–20.
10. Kridel RW, Ashoori F, Liu ES, et al. Long-term use and follow-up of irradiated homologous costal cartilage grafts in the nose. Arch Facial Plast Surg 2009; 11(6):378–94.
11. Daniel RK. Rhinoplasty and rib grafts: evolving a flexible operative technique. Plast Reconstr Surg 1994;94(5):597–609 [discussion: 610–1].
12. Gunter JP, Clark CP, Friedman RM. Internal stabilization of autogenous rib cartilage grafts in rhinoplasty: a barrier to cartilage warping. Plast Reconstr Surg 1997;100(1):161–9.
13. Balaji SM. Costal cartilage nasal augmentation rhinoplasty: study on warping. Ann Maxillofac Surg 2013;3(1):20–4.
14. Lee M, Inman J, Ducic Y. Central segment harvest of costal cartilage in rhinoplasty. Laryngoscope 2011; 121(10):2155–8.
15. Toriumi DM, Pero CD. Asian rhinoplasty. Clin Plast Surg 2010;37(2):335–52.
16. Moon BJ, Lee HJ, Jang YJ. Outcomes following rhinoplasty using autologous costal cartilage. Arch Facial Plast Surg 2012;14(3):175–80.
17. Wee JH, Park MH, Oh S, et al. Complications associated with autologous rib cartilage use in rhinoplasty: a meta-analysis. JAMA Facial Plast Surg 2015;17(1):49–55.
18. Romo T, Baratelli R, Raunig H. Avoiding complications of microtia and otoplasty. Facial Plast Surg 2012;28(3):333–9.
19. Wee JH, Park MH, Jin HR. Post-rib harvesting pain should be considered as a potential significant morbidity in reconstructive rhinoplasty-reply. JAMA Facial Plast Surg 2015;17(3):226.

The Cleft Lip Nose
Primary and Secondary Treatment

Stephen Anthony Wolfe, MD, FACS, FAAP, Nirmal R. Nathan, MD,
Ian R. MacArthur, MD, FRCSC*

KEYWORDS

- Cleft rhinoplasty • Cleft lip nose • Cleft secondary correction

KEY POINTS

- The nasal deformity in cleft patients is complex, and includes malpositioning and hypoplasia of the lower lateral cartilages.
- Nasoalveolar molding helps to facilitate correction of the cleft lip nasal deformity with repositioning of the cleft side ala at the time of primary lip repair.
- During primary repair, the nasal correction is completed before closure of the lip and nasal floor to avoid tethering forces.
- The staging of bilateral cleft lip repairs can provide a longer columella and sufficient lobule and tip projection.
- Secondary correction of the cleft nasal deformity uses cartilage grafts to create a new alar structure; it is not generally possible to achieve adequate elevation of the ipsilateral alar cartilage.

CLEFT ANATOMY

Discussion of the cleft lip nasal deformity must take into account the treatment of the adjacent structures: the maxilla, the alveolus, and the lip. The cleft nasal deformity in a unilateral complete cleft has been well described by Ha and colleagues.[1] To paraphrase, the characteristic features of a unilateral cleft nasal deformity include:

1. Disruption of the muscle ring across the nasal sill;
2. A splayed cleft-sided medial crus;
3. Malposition and hypoplasia of the lower lateral cartilage;
4. A flattened nasal dome;
5. Pathologic tethering of the accessory chain of the lower lateral cartilage to the pyriform aperture; and
6. Soft tissue deficiency of the nasal floor.

Other structural deformities on the cleft side include:

7. A retrusive maxillary segment;
8. A septum that deviates posteriorly (and toward the noncleft side);
9. Abnormal insertions of the lip and cheek musculature to the alar base; and
10. A vestibular lining deficiency.

Malfunction of the cleft ala external nasal valve results from:

11. Alar base malposition;
12. An imbalanced muscular pull; and
13. Abnormal attachment of the cheek muscles to the lateral crus.

Tip projection is further compromised by a foreshortened columella, which lies obliquely with its base directed toward the noncleft side (as does

Disclosures: None.
Funding Sources: None.
Plastic and Reconstructive Surgery, Nicklaus Children's Hospital, 3100 Southwest 62nd Avenue, Miami, FL 33155, USA
* Corresponding author.
E-mail address: macarthurplastics@gmail.com

Clin Plastic Surg 43 (2016) 213–221
http://dx.doi.org/10.1016/j.cps.2015.09.008
0094-1298/16/$ – see front matter

the caudal septum). The tip deviates to the non-cleft side, there is an obtuse angle between the middle and lateral crura, and the alar base is displaced posteriorly (**Fig. 1**).

Cleft Lip Repair

Numerous authors[2,3] have shown that preoperative nasoalveolar molding (in Millard's words "to get the base right") helps to facilitate rotation advancement closure of the cleft lip. Among the many benefits, this technique lengthens the lip on the cleft side, places the scar to match the contralateral philtrum column, achieves muscle reconstitution, allows for a gingivoperiosteoplasty (and closure of the anterior palate performed by some), as well as primary repositioning of the cleft side ala by the McComb technique or other (**Fig. 2**). As such, an excellent result can be obtained that may not require further nasal surgery. Some surgeons may also choose to reposition the septum at this primary operation, and others wait.

The lip and nose are corrected at the first operation, usually completed at 6 months of age. The remainder of the palate is closed (if needed) at around 18 months, along with an extensive retropositioning of the soft palatal musculature using either a Furlow[4] or Sommerlad[5] technique. Alveolar bone grafting may still be required. If the soft tissue clefts of the alveolus and anterior palate are closed, however, this is an exceedingly easy procedure with a high success rate. Bone grafting can be performed at 5 or 6 years of age to provide bone for the eruption of the lateral incisor, if present.

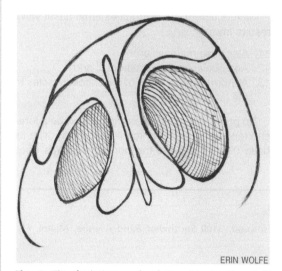

Fig. 1. Tip deviation and relationship to the cleft lower lateral cartilages.

Despite muscle repositioning, some patients may still develop velopharyngeal dysfunction. Of the available surgical treatments, the sphincter pharyngoplasty seems to be the most physiologic procedure for correction.[6]

The Incomplete Bilateral Cleft

A bilateral cleft lip may have a complete cleft lip on one side with an incomplete cleft on the other, or may be 2 incomplete clefts. These can also be symmetric or asymmetric. This deformity is essentially 2 unilateral clefts with the previously mentioned deformities. We prefer to treat them as such,[7] and repair the complete cleft first with a gingivoperiosteoplasty after nasoalveolar molding. The alveolar and anterior palate closure, as well as the nasal correction, are treated as described. A full, tension-free lip is obtained with a natural white roll and often a philtral dimple. After second stage closure, there will be reconstituted orbicularis oris muscle present in the prolabium.

Complete Bilateral Clefts

Most authors advocate a 1-stage procedure.[8] Some discard significant portions of the prolabium to obtain a philtrum that is anthropometrically correct. Nothing is done to lengthen the lip, as is done in a unilateral cleft. Millard advocated delayed columellar lengthening with forked flaps, but most of the authors mentioned have been able to obtain adequate columellar length without them.

Almost all of the 1-stage procedures that we have seen, including our own, have the following characteristics:

1. Short upper lip height (often 5–6 mm);
2. A tight upper lip that lays posterior to the lower lip on lateral view;
3. Inadequate upper buccal sulcus despite a turndown of the prolabial vermillion;
4. A missing or abnormal white roll; and
5. A nasal deformity consisting of inadequate lobule and inadequate tip projection.

Because we were pleased with the results obtained with incomplete bilateral clefts, we began applying this staged technique for complete bilateral clefts. Because we feel that a bilateral cleft is no more than 2 unilateral clefts (with the single exception that there is no native muscle present in the prolabial segment), we treat a complete bilateral exactly as we do a unilateral: nasoalveolar molding and gingivoperiosteoplasty when permitted, followed by anterior palate closure, McComb nasal correction, and rotation advancement. The wider cleft side is repaired first, followed by the second stage 3 months later (**Fig. 3**).

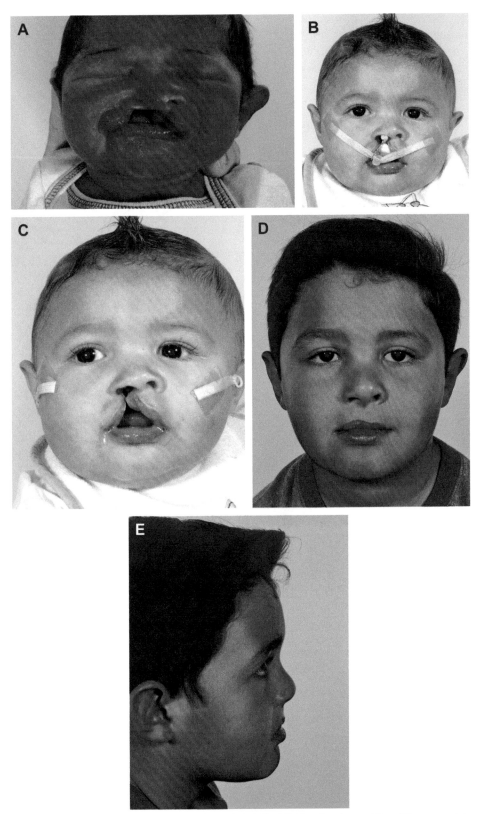

Fig. 2. A male patient born with a complete unilateral cleft lip (*A*). Nasalveolar molding (*B*) was used to prepare for surgery (*C*). Postoperative results (*D*, *E*).

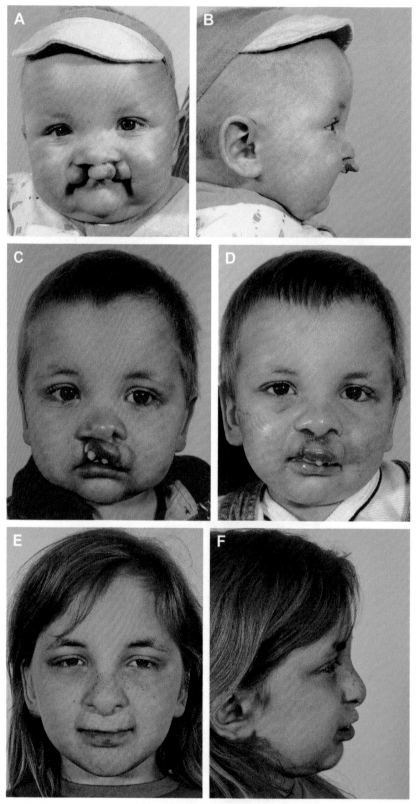

Fig. 3. A male patient born with a complete bilateral cleft lip (*A, B*). He was treated in staged fashion, first undergoing repair of the left cleft lip (*C*), followed later by the right (*D*). Postoperative results (*E, F*).

With the staged technique of bilateral cleft lip correction, we found the noses to be essentially normal. There was adequate columellar length and sufficient lobule and tip projection. The nasolabial angles were also found to be normal. In addition, the presence of a laxer, fuller upper lip allows maxillary development to proceed impeded.

Technique of Primary Nasal Correction

As indicated, the technique is the same whether one is dealing with a unilateral or bilateral cleft. We prefer to operate at 6 months of age.

The lip is marked for a rotation advancement repair, marking the high point of Cupid's bow and measuring the distance from commissure to high point of the Cupid's bow on the noncleft side. This measurement is transposed to the cleft side and marked. Nordhoff's point (the last robust portion of the white roll) is marked, and may result in a slightly shorter transverse dimension of the lip on the cleft side. The rotation segment is incised with an adequate cutback directed toward but not across the contralateral philtral column. The advancement segment is incised, with a transverse incision extending across the nostril sill as far as, but not around, the alar base. The muscle is dissected extensively from the skin of the

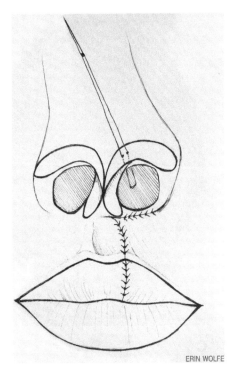

Fig. 5. Postoperative relationship of nasal correction to cleft lip closure.

advancement segment, and only for a few millimeters on the rotation segment.

If nasoalveolar molding has been performed and the maxillary segments are 2 to 3 mm apart, a

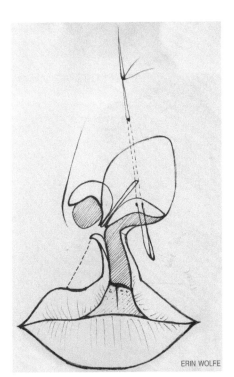

Fig. 4. Before closure of the lip, the ipsilateral lower lateral cartilage is dissected freely and sutured to the contralateral nasion using a McComb suture.

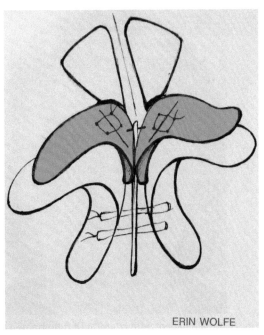

Fig. 6. "Golden arch" technique.

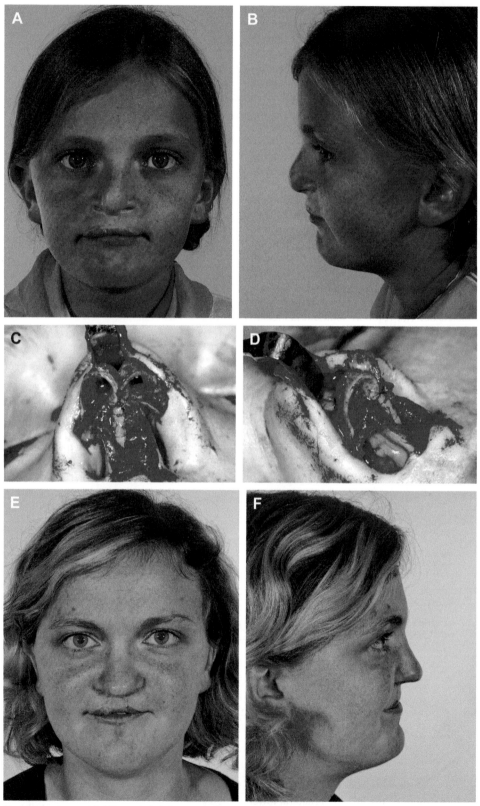

Fig. 7. Female patient with bilateral cleft lip treated at another center (*A*, *B*). A cleft rhinoplasty was created using "Golden arch" technique (*C*, *D*). Postoperative results (*E*, *F*).

gingivoperiosteoplasty (in reality the dissection is supraperiosteal) is performed with turndown flaps from the alveolar segment extended back into an anterior vomer flap. This is completed so that the palatal surface of the alveolus and first 10 mm or so of the anterior palate are closed.

The next step in sequence, as advised by McComb[9] is important: the nose is corrected before closure of the lip and the nostril floor. If the nose is done last, the lip closure may tether down the slumped alar cartilage.

The ipsilateral lower lateral cartilage and a portion of the contralateral are dissected completely from overlying skin with small, blunt-tipped Iris scissors. This is done through the incision at the base of the columella and at the alar margin. This dissection is carried up to the nasion and to the ipsilateral nasofacial junction. A Keith needle with a 4 to 0 Vicryl suture is passed through the desired position of the crus of the alar cartilage, usually about 3 mm lateral to the columella, and brought out through the skin at the contralateral nasion (**Fig. 4**). This suture may need to repeated several times until it provides the exact slight overcorrection desired. When this has been accomplished, the correction is "locked-in" with vestibular effacement sutures that begin intranasally, pass through the alar crease, and then pass back through the same hole in the skin at a different angulation. Three to 4 of these sutures are passed to obliterate the vestibular web and provide a corrected ala and defined alar crease.

Once the alar cartilage has been corrected, a superiorly based mucosal flap is dissected from the vomer and septum using the same incision used to turn down the vomer flap. The septum is exposed at this point and can be straightened if required. The inner surface of the advancement flap is now dissected back to the turbinate and freed from the pyriform rim. These medial and lateral flaps can now be sutured together to close the nostril floor, with care being taken to maintain an adequate nostril caliber. This closure is brought all the way to the transverse nostril sill, using the Millard C flap to constitute a medial foot plate (it is not needed to lengthen the hemicolumella). Symmetry of the alar bases should be present. The buccal mucosa is then closed. Transverse suturing of the orbicularis muscle is performed, the white roll tattoo marks are sewn together, and the vermillion is closed in eversion. Finally, skin closure is carried out with 7-0 Vicryl after any required trimming is completed to have the incision perfectly match the contralateral philtral column. Lengthening of the lip is provided by an adequate cutback, and no triangular flaps should be required for lengthening (**Fig. 5**).

Nostril stents are then placed, using the caliber of the normal nostril as a guide. This prevents the cleft-sided nostril from becoming "overclosed," which is not uncommon if a Millard "alar cinch" suture had been used. Steri-strips are placed to hold the McComb suture to the forehead in slight tension, and are also placed over the nasal dorsum.

One-stage bilateral cleft lip procedures usually result in an inadequate lobule; 2-stage procedures do not. The reason for this may be that bilateral McComb sutures placed at the same time contend for the same space and therefore interfere with each other's elevation. A 1-stage procedure can place the crus freely where desired, and after it has healed, will bring the contralateral side up to its height.

Secondary Correction of the Cleft Nasal Deformity

This procedure is necessary when the nose has not been corrected primarily. In unilateral cases, one may see an uncorrected slump of the alar cartilage, septal deviations (often complex), nostril size aberrations, poor lip scars, oronasal fistulae, and underlying retromaxillism. Even after an excellent correction of the nose, there often can be a persistent vestibular web that was not corrected at the primary operation. In bilateral cases, there may be a short or absent columella, alar collapse, and inadequate lobule and tip projection.

One should correct any malocclusion first with a Le Fort–type advancement. Usually this is done

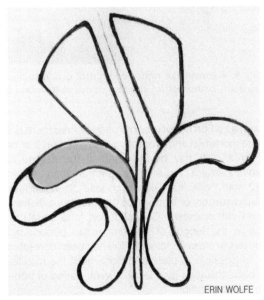

Fig. 8. Secondary alar correction in the unilateral cleft nasal deformity.

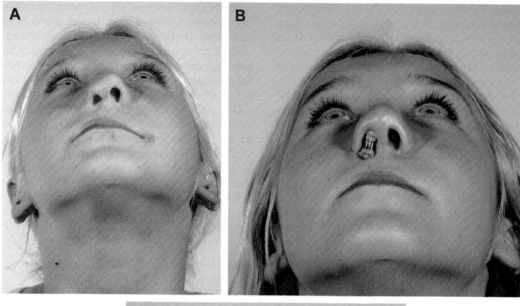

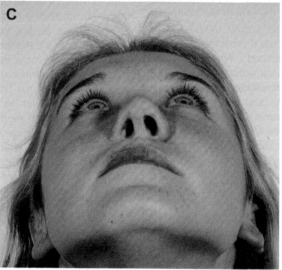

Fig. 9. A constricted right-sided nostril owing to a previous alar cinch suture (*A*). After rhinoplasty, the patient used an "orthonostric" stenting device to maintain patency (*B*). Long-term postoperative result (*C*).

with a Le Fort 1, but in some cases where there is a foreshortened and proptotic nose, a Le Fort 3 or Le Fort 3 + 1 may be indicated. If the degree of advancement required is greater than 10 to 12 mm, one can either choose to undertake 2-jaw surgery or to advance the maxilla via distraction osteogenesis. Consolidation time usually is twice the length of the distraction period, but once the class 3 malocclusion has been corrected it is possible to plate and bone graft the maxilla. This is followed by a 2- to 3-week period of inter-maxillary fixation.

Combining orthognathic surgery and nasal surgery is possible, and although we have done it

on occasion, it is generally ill advised. This is owing to the airway risk associated with the intraoperative need to change from a nasal to an oral intubation. Alveolar bone grafting, however, can be performed easily with the nasal correction.

An open rhinoplasty approach facilitates nasal correction. When choosing incision location, the use of the usual staggered midcolumellar incision does not make sense. This is because a scar is already present from the cleft lip repair located several millimeters below at the base of the columella. The alar cartilages are separated, the septal angle identified, and a thorough submucoperichondrial dissection of the septum performed.

The upper lateral cartilages are then separated from the septum.

Generally, one cannot adequately elevate the ipsilateral alar cartilage no matter how extensive the dissection of the nostril floor, giving credence to McComb's advice to correct the nose first. The dorsum is lowered if required by component reduction and a harvest of septum carried out, maintaining an L-shaped strut of at least 10 mm. If displaced from the vomer, the base of the L-shaped strut is freed and sutured to the midline. Spreader grafts or flaps are used as required, and a long columellar strut is placed that extends well above the alar domes.

At this point, a whole new alar structure is created using septal or conchal cartilage. It is sutured to the tip of the columellar strut and folded over to make a new ala, ignoring the native cartilage still tethered below. The new ala should be directed toward the lateral canthus. We call this the "Golden Arch" procedure, because it is reminiscent of the logo of a well-known fast food franchise (**Figs. 6** and **7**). In unilateral cases, one-half of the arch can be made instead (**Fig. 8**). Once the new alar construct has been sutured to the columellar strut and the underlying native ala, any number of suture techniques (eg, interdomal, transdomal, subdomal, mattress) can be used with the new ala. The skin may be thick and fatty, particularly in bilateral cases, and can be judiciously thinned. The columella is then sutured to the lip first with deep 6-0 Vicryl then 7-0 Vicryl in the skin. The intranasal incisions are closed with 6-0 monocryl, and a number (4 or more) of vestibular effacement sutures of 4-0 plain catgut are taken to elevate the lining, define the alar crease,

and prevent supratip fullness. Appropriately sized nostril stents (Porex R) are sutured in and maintained for a week. Further "orthonostric" nasal stenting is continued as required, which in the case of a stenotic nostril may be up to 3 months (**Fig. 9**).

REFERENCES

1. Ha RY, Cone JD, Byrd HS. Cleft rhinoplasty. In: Rohrich RJ, Adams WP Jr, Ahmad J, et al, editors. Dallas rhinoplasty: nasal surgery by the masters. 3rd edition. St. Louis (MO): QMP/CRC Press; 2014. p. 1306.
2. Millard DR Jr, Lathan RA. Improved primary surgical and dental treatment of clefts. Plast Reconstr Surg 1990;86(5):856–71.
3. Barillas I, Dec W, Warren SM, et al. Nasoalveolar molding improves long-term nasal symmetry in complete unilateral cleft lip-cleft palate patients. Plast Reconstr Surg 2009;123(3):1002–6.
4. Furlow LT Jr. Cleft palate repair by double opposing Z-plasty. Plast Reconstr Surg 1986;78(6):724–38.
5. Sommerlad BC. A technique for cleft palate repair. Plast Reconstr Surg 2003;112(6):1542–8.
6. Jackson IT. Sphincter pharyngoplasty. Clin Plast Surg 1985;12(4):711–7.
7. Wolfe SA, Mejia ML. Staged rotation advancements provide improved nasal results compared to 1-stage repairs in patients with complete bilateral cleft lip and palate. Ann Plast Surg 2014;72(3):307–11.
8. Tan SP, Greene AK, Mulliken JB. Current surgical management of bilateral cleft lip in North America. Plast Reconstr Surg 2012;129(6):1347–55.
9. McComb H. Treatment of the unilateral cleft lip nose. Plast Reconstr Surg 1975;55(5):596–601.

Cleft Lip Nose

Jonathan M. Sykes, MD[a],*, Abel-Jan Tasman, MD[b], Gustavo A. Suárez, MD[c]

KEYWORDS

- Cleft lip rhinoplasty • Secondary rhinoplasty • Surgical techniques • Open rhinoplasty technique
- Closed rhinoplasty technique

KEY POINTS

- A three-dimensional understanding of the anatomy of the cleft nose aids surgeons in selecting the proper technique for repair.
- Advantages of early surgical intervention include minimizing the deformity as the child grows and lessening asymmetries to allow optimal nasal growth.
- Analysis and performance of orthognathic surgery should be done before nasal surgery to optimize the overall result.
- Goals of the secondary rhinoplasty include relief of nasal obstruction, creation of symmetry and definition of the nasal base and tip, and management of nasal scarring and webbing.
- Septal reconstruction in the cleft nose is a key maneuver in cleft rhinoplasty.

INTRODUCTION

The nasal deformity associated with congenital cleft lip is a complex defect that results in significant aesthetic and functional problems. The defect involves all tissue layers, including the bony platform of the nose, the inner nasal lining, the cartilaginous infrastructure, and the external skin. The extent of the deformity varies with the degree of lip abnormality; it may be unilateral or bilateral and subtle or complete.[1]

In many patients with congenital clefts, the secondary nasal deformity is minimal. However, the appearance of the nose in some patients with clefts is often the feature that is the most noticeable to the observer. The variability of the secondary cleft nasal deformity is related to the original deformity, scarring from previous surgeries on the lip and nose, and changes related to growth.[2] In addition, many patients with clefts have significant nasal obstruction and functional problems.[3]

The goal of complete care of the cleft nasal deformity is to minimize functional problems and to maximize the appearance of the nose. This goal requires the surgeon to have an understanding of the pathophysiology of clefting, and the three-dimensional nature of the cleft nasal deformity. This article discusses the anatomy and pathophysiology of the cleft lip nasal deformity and the timing of the various repairs needed, and provides a philosophic understanding of a selection of techniques currently used to repair the cleft nasal deformity.

ANATOMY AND EMBRYOLOGY OF THE CLEFT NASAL DEFORMITY

During normal development, the paired median nasal processes fuse to form the premaxilla, philtrum, columella, and nasal tip. The bilateral maxillary processes form the lateral aspects of the upper lip.[4,5] Cleft lip deformities result from a failure of the fusion of the median nasal processes

Disclosures: Neither author has any financial or other disclosures with regard to this article.
[a] Division of Facial Plastic and Reconstructive Surgery, Department of Otolaryngology, University of California Davis, 2521 Stockton Boulevard, Suite 6203, Sacramento, CA 95817, USA; [b] Rhinology and Facial Plastic Surgery, Department of Otolaryngology-Head and Neck Surgery, Cantonal Hospital, Rorschacher Strasse 95, St. Gallen 9000, Switzerland; [c] Department of Otolaryngology - Head and Neck Surgery, Bellvitge University Hospital, Feixa Llarga s/n, L'Hospitalet de Llobregat, Barcelona 08097, Spain
* Corresponding author. 2521 Stockton Boulevard, Suite 6200, Sacramento, CA 95817.
E-mail address: jmsykes@ucdavis.edu

with the maxillary processes. Interruption of this embryonic process creates malformation of some or all of the upper lip, central alveolus, and primary palate. The extent of the associated cleft nasal deformity is related to the extent of the interruption of the normal developmental fusion process.

The characteristic unilateral and bilateral cleft nasal deformities can occur along a spectrum of severity. In patients with incomplete cleft lips, these nasal deformities are less pronounced.[6,7] Even though the nasal defects may be subtle, there is always a nasal abnormality associated with cleft lips.

Unilateral Cleft Lip Nose Deformity

In patients with complete, unilateral cleft lip, the maxilla on the cleft side is deficient. Because of this, the alar base on the cleft side does not fuse in the midline and is positioned more posterior, lateral, and inferior than the alar base on the noncleft side.[5] Consequently, the lateral crus of the lower lateral cartilage (LLC) on the cleft side is lengthened and the medial crura is shortened in relation to the LLC on the noncleft side. The septum is attached to the noncleft maxilla inferiorly, which causes the septum to be deviated to the noncleft side caudally, and bowing dorsally toward the cleft side. The attachment of the upper lateral cartilage to the LLC is affected by the change in position of the LLC, which effectively weakens the scroll region and causes compromise of the internal nasal valve. In addition, the abnormal insertion of the orbicularis oris muscle causes an asymmetric pull on the caudal septum. This pull also adds to the characteristic anterior septal deflection to the noncleft side (**Fig. 1**).

Bilateral Cleft Lip Nose Deformity

In patients with complete, bilateral cleft lip, the maxilla is deficient bilaterally, which allows the prolabium to have unopposed anterior growth. The alar bases are displaced in a more posterior, lateral, and inferior position than occurs without clefting. The deficient skeletal base leads to longer lateral crura of the LLC bilaterally and short, splayed medial crura.[8] This creates an underprojected, broad, and flat nasal tip. The columella is short because of the malposition of the prolabium and the shortening of the medial crura. The short columella makes the broad and snubbed nasal tip even more pronounced. Insertion of the septopremaxillary ligament is usually symmetric, thereby causing no alteration in the anterior septum/columella unit. Bilateral insertion of the orbicularis oris musculature into the alar base

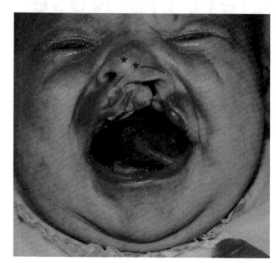

Fig. 1. Basal view of the primary unilateral cleft lip deformity showing deviation of the columella toward the noncleft side, widening of the nasal floor, displacement of the alar base, and flattening of the LLC (stars represent the domes, lines depict caudal septum [midline] and lateral crus [most lateral]).

contributes to the widening of the nose and flattening of the LLC (**Fig. 2**).

TREATMENT
Timing of the Cleft Nasal Repair

The decision to perform early nasal surgery on children with clefts is based on several factors. These factors include the extent of the deformity and the potential scarring and impact of the procedure on nasal growth. Advantages of early surgical intervention include minimizing the deformity as the child grows, lessening asymmetries to allow optimal nasal growth, and creating favorable conditions for future surgery.

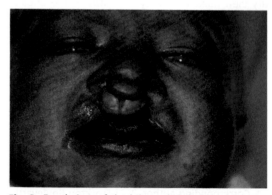

Fig. 2. Basal view of the bilateral cleft deformity. The columella is usually deviated toward the less complete side of the deformity.

Historically, controversy has existed as to whether primary tip rhinoplasty was a positive influence on the eventual appearance of the nose in patients with clefts. Major septal work and cartilaginous dissection has been thought to negatively affect nasal growth.[9] However, no experimental or clinical studies have ever proved that minor manipulations (without resection) of the nasal tip or nasal base interfere with future nasal growth.[10] For these reasons, most contemporary surgeons agree that the ideal repair of a cleft nasal deformity is performed in 2 stages. The first includes alteration in the nose at the time of lip repair (primary rhinoplasty), delaying a definitive repair until the patient has completed facial growth (secondary rhinoplasty). In female patients, secondary rhinoplasty is generally performed around 15 to 17 years of age, and in male patients at approximately 16 to 18 years of age.[5]

Presurgical Nasoalveolar Molding

Presurgical nasoalveolar molding (PNAM) can be used in patients with wide or very asymmetric clefts to (1) reposition the malaligned alveolar segments, (2) narrow the cleft gap, (3) improve nasal tip symmetry in unilateral clefts, (4) elongate the columella, and (5) expand the nasal soft tissues in bilateral clefts (**Fig. 3**). PNAM uses an intraoral alveolar molding device with nasal molding prongs. This technique requires a dedicated orthodontist and a motivated family that understands the treatment goals. If properly used, PNAM can lessen the tension across the lip wound and lessen the nasal deformity.[11] Primary rhinoplasty can then be performed to improve nasal appearance and optimize nasal growth.

Primary Rhinoplasty

The purpose of primary rhinoplasty is to close the anterior nasal floor, to relocate the displaced alar base, and to bring early symmetry to the nasal base and tip.[5] This approach allows for both a functional and aesthetic improvement without jeopardizing nasal and facial growth.

After the cleft lip incisions are made and the primary lip dissection is completed, the muscle and soft tissues of the alar base are separated from their maxillary attachments. The malpositioned alar base is freed by creating an internal alotomy at the anterior head of the inferior turbinate. If adequate soft tissue dissection of the alar base is performed, the cleft alar base can be

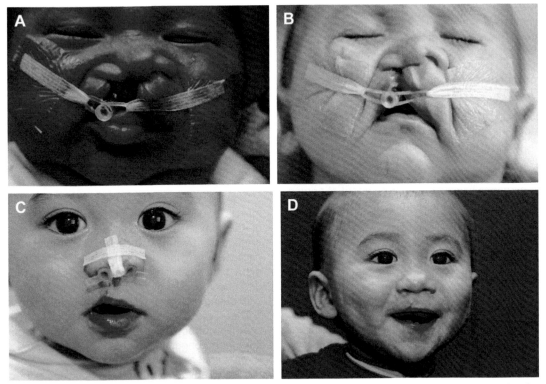

Fig. 3. (A) Initial placement of PNAM in a child with a right complete cleft lip and palate. (B) Four months after initial placement of PNAM. Note the narrowed cleft gap, narrowed lip gap, and improved overall symmetry of lip and nasal base. (C) Five months after surgery. (D) Five years after surgery.

repositioned (during closure) in the optimal three-dimensional position.

The LLC on the cleft side is then dissected from its cutaneous attachments by creating a medial and a lateral tunnel just superficial to the LLCs. These subcutaneous tunnels are connected and allow the cleft LLC to be repositioned in a more symmetric fashion. Care is taken not to violate the vestibular skin, avoiding the complication of secondary adhesions and nostril stenosis.

Primary cleft rhinoplasty begins with closure of the nasal floor and sill. This closure is first started with reapproximation of the musculature of the nasal base, which allows the cleft alar base to be reconstructed in a manner that mirrors the non-cleft alar base. Closure of the nasal sill is performed with 5-0 chromic catgut sutures. It is important not to narrow the sill too much. A nasal base that is too wide is easy to narrow secondarily, whereas a stenotic sill is difficult to widen later.

The other component of primary cleft rhinoplasty is to reposition the cleft nasal tip into a more projected, symmetric position. After the nasal sill is reestablished and the lip is repaired in a layered fashion, the cleft LLC is repositioned.[12] This step is achieved with internal mattress or tie-over external bolsters. The new dome has a lengthened medial crus and a shortened lateral crus. The resulting nasal tip is more symmetric, defined, and projected (**Fig. 4**).

Intermediate Rhinoplasty

Intermediate rhinoplasty is defined as any nasal surgery performed between the time of initial lip repair and the time of definitive rhinoplasty when the patient reaches facial skeletal maturity. The use of intermediate rhinoplasty in patients with unilateral cleft nasal deformities has decreased as surgeons have become more adept at primary rhinoplasty. However, many patients have significant nasal deformities that have not been adequately repaired after their initial cleft lip procedures. In these cases, performing intermediate rhinoplasty minimizes the social stigmata associated with a more noticeable nasal deformity.[3]

Orthognathic Surgery

In cleft patients with significant dentofacial deformities, surgery to correct the skeletal abnormalities and to optimize the dental occlusion is often necessary. Orthognathic surgery has the advantage of maximizing the skeletal profile, enhancing nasal appearance, and improving the malocclusion that commonly accompanies

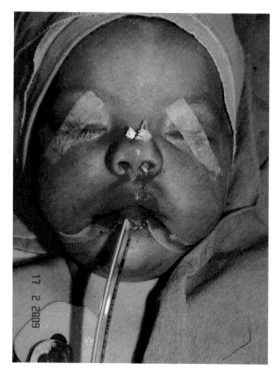

Fig. 4. After completion of primary cleft lip rhinoplasty. Note that the suture securing the bolsters is tightened until a slight blanch is seen.

oral clefting. Therefore, analysis of the facial skeleton should be done before nasal surgery to determine whether skeletal repositioning is necessary. Studies have shown that it is the cleft palatoplasty that is responsible for restriction of maxillary growth in an anteroposterior and a transverse dimension. This condition often results in maxillary hypoplasia (with a resulting underjet) and transverse maxillary width restriction (with a resulting buccal crossbite)[13] (**Fig. 5**A).

Skeletal correction of the hypoplastic cleft maxilla requires advancement, and often widening, of the maxilla. In most instances, preoperative orthodontic treatment (usually 12–18 months) is necessary to align the dental arches. This treatment can minimize the occlusal deformity and often decreases the amount of movement necessary during orthognathic surgery (**Fig. 5**B).

There are 2 basic approaches that can be used to correct the skeletal deformities associated with congenital clefting. The first approach is conventional orthognathic surgery, including maxillary advancement and widening with or without mandibular setback. The other approach is to perform a standard Le Fort I maxillary osteotomy and placement of distraction

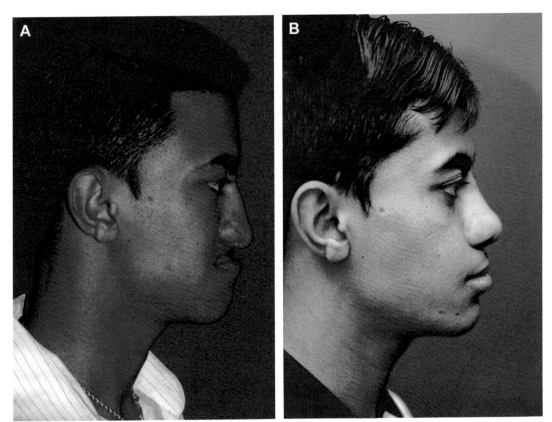

Fig. 5. (*A*) Lateral view of a patient with a cleft lip deformity. Note the class III malocclusion as a result of the maxillary hypoplasia (underjet). (*B*) After the use of distraction osteogenesis and secondary septorhinoplasty.

osteogenesis (DO) devices. If conventional orthognathic surgery is planned, upper and lower jaw surgery is often required for adequate skeletal correction.[13] The maxilla is often scarred from prior palatal surgery, precluding a large advancement to adequately correct the underjet. Operating on both jaws allows the surgeon to maximize the skeletal relationship and correct the class III malocclusion.

The DO approach uses either an internal distractor or a rigid external distractor (RED) device (**Fig. 6**). Use of DO allows the surgeon to progressively advance the maxilla. This method is often necessary to correct significant cleft jaw discrepancies. After completing the maxillary osteotomy and placing the distraction device, a waiting (latency) period is allowed before distraction begins. The maxilla is then distracted over period of 4 to 6 weeks before bony consolidation. DO grows both bone and soft tissue and improves the skeletal base that supports the nose (**Fig. 7**). Orthognathic surgery may delay the timing of the definitive septorhinoplasty, but has rewarding effects on the overall result.

Secondary (Definitive) Rhinoplasty

Once the patient has reached facial skeletal maturity, definitive septorhinoplasty can be performed. Structural reconstruction of the cleft nose often requires cartilage grafting material from the rib or septum to achieve adequate support. The goals of the secondary rhinoplasty are the creation of symmetry and definition of the nasal base and tip, relief of nasal obstruction, and management of nasal scarring and webbing. The extent of the secondary nasal deformity varies according to several factors, including the extent of the original lip and nose defect, any surgery performed between birth and definitive rhinoplasty, and the specific nasal growth.

SURGICAL TECHNIQUES
Approaches

The approach to definitive cleft septorhinoplasty varies according to surgeon preference and the requirements of the reconstruction. It is important to clearly identify the key factors contributing to the

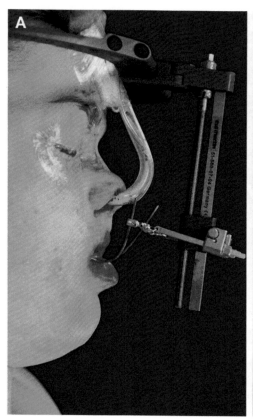
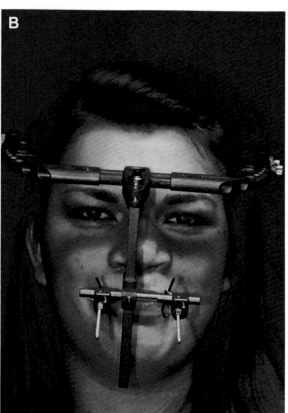

Fig. 6. (*A*) After placement of the RED device. (*B*) Four weeks after placement of the RED device.

nasal deformity and select the most appropriate approach to achieve the surgical goals. These goals include septal reconstruction and treatment of the nasal tip, alar rim, alar base, columella, and nasal sill. In most instances, all these goals can be corrected by using either the external or endonasal approach.

The preference of one of the senior authors (JMS) is to use an open or external approach. In most instances, the traditional inverted-V columellar incision is used. When there is significant lack of columellar soft tissue in unilateral clefting, the incision can be modified onto the cleft lip with a V-to-Y closure to increase columellar soft tissue (**Fig. 8**). Techniques have been described that recruit tissue from the lip repair with a sliding chondrocutaneous flap. This flap provides additional tissue to augment the vestibular lining and reduce the alar-columellar web, and, when combined with the open rhinoplasty, the chondrocutaneous flap can permit tip stability and lip refinement.[14]

The preference of the other senior author (AJT) is to use a closed or endonasal approach in secondary cleft rhinoplasty. Several incisions may be used to access the nasal infrastructure while obviating a transcolumellar incision. The advantages of the endonasal approach include maintaining an intact skin–soft tissue envelope. When cartilaginous grafts are placed under an intact envelope, the surgeon is better able to immediately visualize the impact of the graft on the eventual nasal contour. Another potential advantage of the endonasal approach is maintenance of vascular supply to the skin, allowing increased tension when placing structural grafts. With the open approach, lengthening or projecting grafts can make eventual wound closure difficult. Multiple endonasal incisions (transfixion, infracartilaginous, and intercartilaginous) are often used to obtain adequate exposure to correct the deformity (**Figs. 9** and **10**).

Septal Reconstruction

In the unilateral cleft deformity, the asymmetric unopposed pull of the orbicularis oris muscles and the deficient bony maxilla causes the septum to deviate to the noncleft side anteriorly. In the bilateral cleft lip deformity, the nasal septum is usually midline, being deviated caudally to the less involved side if asymmetry of the lip exists.[15]

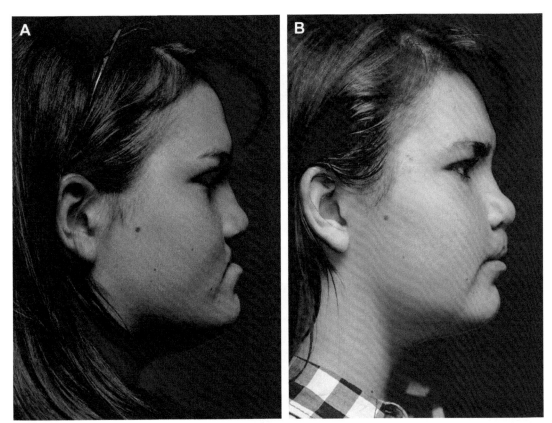

Fig. 7. (A) Preoperative lateral view of the patient shown in Fig. 6. (B) Lateral view after DO and secondary rhinoplasty.

Repair of the cleft septum is challenging and is the foundation of the rhinoplasty. Complete septal reconstruction requires adequate exposure and complete breakdown of the ligamentous attachments that contribute to the septal deviation. The septum can be approached by either an open or endonasal approach. If the external approach is used, the anterior septum is exposed

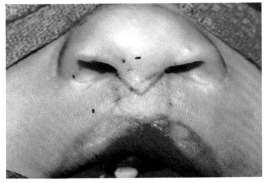

Fig. 8. Bilateral cleft lip rhinoplasty approached with a V incision to recruit skin from the lip into the columella.

by separating the ligaments that connect the 2 medial crura. If the endonasal approach is used, a complete transfixion incision is joined to bilateral intercartilaginous incisions to obtain the exposure necessary for reconstruction. In either case, adequate caudal and dorsal struts should be preserved while deviations in the cartilage and bone are corrected. To return the caudal septum to the midline, the surgeon often must remove a strip of cartilage inferiorly, allowing the septum to swing over the nasal spine (Fig. 11). This position can be maintained by suturing the cartilage to the spine with a 5-0 long-acting absorbable monofilament suture.

If the septal support is not sufficient after resection of the deviated segments, reconstruction with cartilage grafts is needed to maintain adequate central segment support. Septal support can be achieved with a variety of grafting methods. The septum can be supported with a caudal septal extension graft (SEG) or a caudal batten graft (Figs. 12 and 13). These grafts can be fashioned from different autologous materials (septal cartilage, costal cartilage, ethmoid plate bone). The SEG can be sutured to the caudal

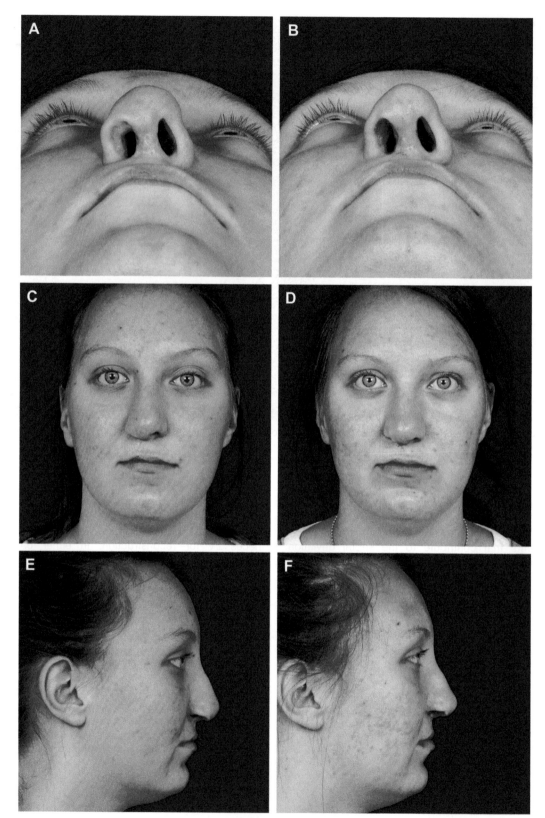

Fig. 9. A 24-year-old patient with unilateral cleft lip nose deformity who underwent revision rhinoplasty: scar tissue resection, caudal septal reconstruction, LLC reconstruction. Preoperative (*A–C*). Early postoperative (*D–F*).

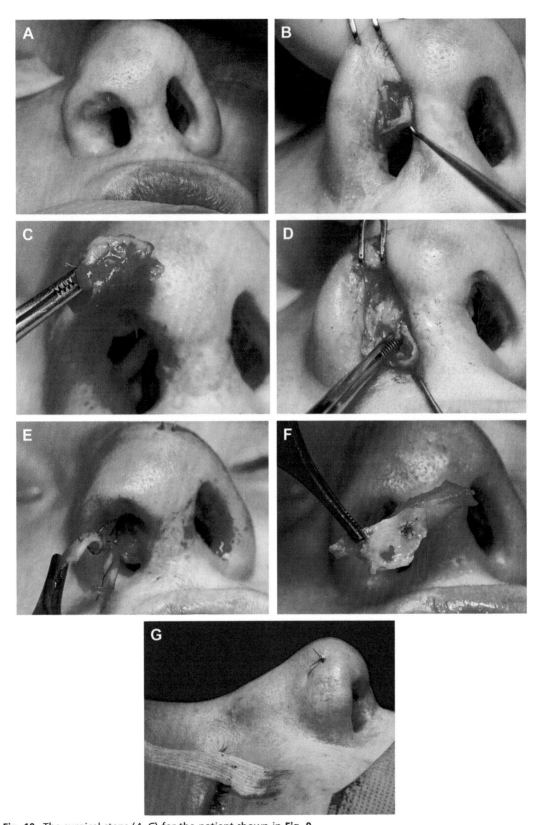

Fig. 10. The surgical steps (*A–G*) for the patient shown in **Fig. 9**.

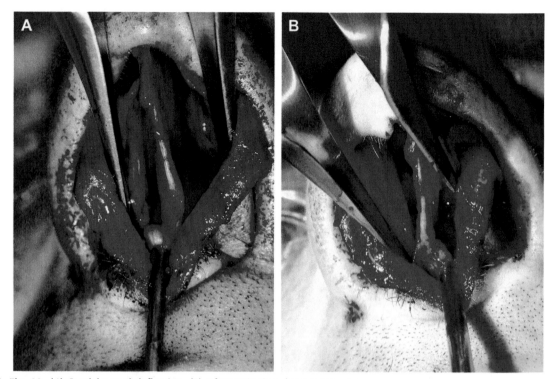

Fig. 11. (*A*) Caudal septal deflection. (*B*) After swinging-door maneuver.

end of the existing septum in an end-to-end or end-to-side technique. The important concept is that, at the conclusion of grafting and repositioning of the septum, the caudal aspect of the septum is straight and well supported. Another graft that aids in support of the caudal and dorsal septum is the extended spreader graft. Spreader grafts are thin, long pieces of cartilage placed between the septum and the upper lateral cartilage and can improve the cross-sectional airway of the internal nasal valve. These grafts can also help correct dorsal external deviations.[16]

In patients who have severe nasal septal deviation (in which resection, repositioning, and cartilage grafting are inadequate), an extracorporeal septoplasty may be required. This technique involves explantation of the septal cartilage, reshaping of this cartilage on the operative field (out of the patient), and reimplantation of the septum with fixation both caudally and dorsally.[17] Often, this technique is combined with cartilage

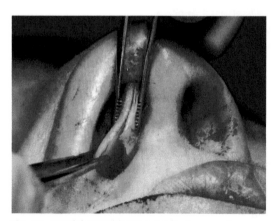

Fig. 12. Caudal septal batten graft placement.

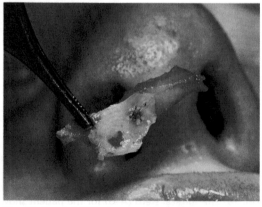

Fig. 13. Caudal SEG placement.

grafting for support and strength of the reimplanted septum. Regardless of the technique used, at the end of the septoplasty, the septum should be straight and well supported to maximize the cleft airway and to allow adequate tip resuspension.

Treatment of the Nasal Tip

The nasal tip in patients with congenital clefting of the lip is poorly supported. In the unilateral deformity, the tip is asymmetric secondary to the short medial crus on the cleft side (**Fig. 14**). In the bilateral deformity, the tip is usually underprojected and the columella is short. Tip techniques are therefore designed to improve tip symmetry, definition, and projection.

After the nasal septum is straightened and supported, the nasal tip can be resuspended on the septum to improve tip support and projection. This technique, termed the tongue-in-groove (TIG) technique, allows the tip to be projected, deprojected, lengthened, or shortened.[18] In most clefts, the cleft side nasal tip needs projection and rotation, because the secondary nasal deformity usually has underprojection and hooding of the cleft tip. The TIG technique involves suture fixation of the medial crura of the LLCs to the caudal end of the nasal septum. Typically, the cleft side alar cartilage has to be advanced more than the noncleft side to improve the flattening of the cleft LLC and enhance overall tip symmetry.

Another method used to improve support and projection is the columellar strut cartilage graft. The columellar strut graft is a sturdy piece of cartilage that is placed between the medial crura of the LLCs. The medial crura can be advanced on this graft and suture fixated to enhance projection and support.

The LLC may also be vertically divided. On the cleft side, this maneuver is usually performed lateral to the existing dome. Division of the cartilages lateral to the dome increases the medial crural element and projection of the nasal tip. After division of the LLC is performed, the cartilages are reconstituted with suture. After the central tip segment is supported with one of these maneuvers, a cartilaginous tip graft can be added to camouflage irregularities and improve tip definition. These tip grafts are typically suture fixated with 6-0 permanent monofilament suture.

Treatment of the Cleft Alar Rim

The cleft side lateral crus of the LLC is usually concave. This concavity is often associated with alar malposition, with the cartilage often being inferiorly displaced in relation to the position of the noncleft side LLC. The concavity of the alar rim often causes external nasal valve collapse and a functional nasal deformity.

Treatment of the malpositioned alar rim can be accomplished with a variety of techniques, including cartilage grafting and/or suture repositioning. The cleft side lateral crus can be supported with (1) an alar rim graft, (2) an alar strut graft, (3) an alar turn-in flap, (4) excision and turnover of the entire lateral crus of the LLC with resuturing of the segment (the so-called flip-flop of the LLC)[19] (**Fig. 15**). The alar rim graft is placed inferior to the existing cartilage in a nonanatomic position and helps to support and strengthen the LLC. The alar strut graft, also known as the lateral crural strut graft, is placed on the deep surface of the LLC, with the graft being sutured to the undersurface of the cartilage. The lateral extent of this graft is typically placed in a pocket at the pyriform aperture. Both of these grafts aid in supporting the alar rim, elevating the level of the alar rim and repositioning the rim laterally.

The LLC turn-in flap uses the cephalic portion of the LLC. In most rhinoplasty procedures, the cephalic portion of the LLC is resected and discarded. In the turn-in flap technique, this previously resected cartilage is transposed on a pedicle and sutured to the undersurface of the remaining LLC in order to strengthen and support the LLC and to flatten the preexisting concavity. The flip-flop technique involves dissecting the lateral crura of the LLC off the underlying vestibular skin, excising this portion, turning it over, and resuturing it to the vestibular lining. This procedure changes the shape of the alar rim from concave to convex. All of these maneuvers are designed to strengthen and reposition the malformed alar rim cartilage. If there is still significant malposition of the cleft LLC after these maneuvers are

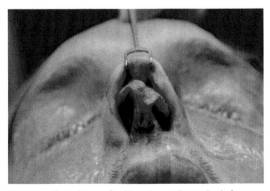

Fig. 14. The classic finding in unilateral cleft nose deformity.

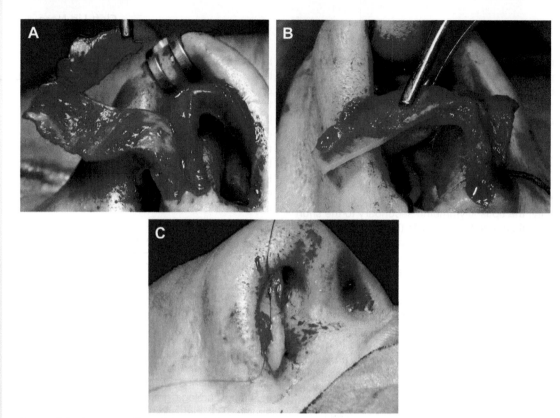

Fig. 15. (*A*) Alar turn-in flap of the cephalic aspect of LLC. (*B*) Lateral crural strut graft. (*C*) Alar batten graft.

completed, the lower LLC can be sutured to the upper lateral cartilage or to the nasal septum to reposition the alar rim more superiorly.

Treatment of the Alar Base

The alar base is often asymmetric and abnormal in shape. The cause of this deformity is related to the poorly supported skeletal nasal base, and to any surgery performed before the definitive rhinoplasty. In many cases, the insertion of the lateral alar rim (the alar-facial junction) is malpositioned as a result of the original cleft lip repair. A small malposition during the cleft lip repair can result in a larger disparity with growth. For this reason, the cleft alar-facial junction often needs to be repositioned to create alar base symmetry.

Another common secondary deformity that is a result of the original cleft lip repair is a lack of complete closure of the sill of the nose. This defect occurs when the superior portion of the orbicularis oris muscle is incompletely closed. This defect causes a lack of symmetry of the alar base at the level of the nasal sill. This deformity is often obvious to the observer and creates a noticeable abnormal shape to the inferior aspect of the nostril (**Fig. 16**). Reconstruction of this deformity requires reopening of the superior aspect of the lip and realignment of the muscle. Although sill deformity

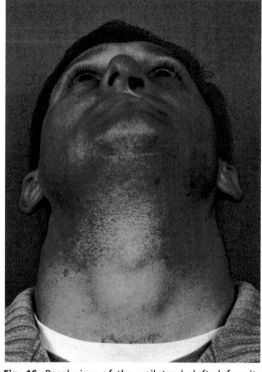

Fig. 16. Basal view of the unilateral cleft deformity showing the volume deficit in the nasal sill area along with the classic associated deformity.

is most commonly corrected with muscle dissection and closure, a dermal flap can be added to augment the base of the nose at the nasal sill. If the patient has a small deficiency at the nasal sill and does not want surgery, augmentation with injectable fillers can help with nasal base symmetry.

SUMMARY

The nose in patients with congenital cleft malformations is often the facial feature that is most noticeable to the observer. The secondary nasal deformity is variable and is affected by the extent of the original cleft, growth, and by any intervening surgery to correct the lip or nose.

Repair of secondary cleft nasal deformities is challenging. Successful reconstruction requires an understanding of the pathologic anatomy, adequate exposure to perform techniques, and attention to structural grafting to overcome scarring and provide support. Often, graft material from the septum, rib, and/or ear is required. Attention must be paid to both function and appearance.

REFERENCES

1. Sykes JM, Senders CW. Pathologic anatomy of cleft lip, palate, and nasal deformities. In: Meyers AD, editor. Biological basis of facial plastic surgery. New York: Thieme Medical Publishers; 1993. p. 57–71.
2. Sykes JM, Senders CW. Surgical management of the difficult nose. Oper Tech Otolaryngol Head Neck Surg 1990;1(4):219–24.
3. Shih CW, Sykes JM. Correction of the cleft-lip nasal deformity. Facial Plast Surg 2002;18(4):253–62.
4. Capone R, Sykes J. Evaluation and management of cleft lip and palate disorders. In: Papel ID, editor. Facial plastic and reconstructive surgery. 3rd edition. Stuttgart (NY): Thieme; 2009. p. 1059–60.
5. Sykes JM, Jang YJ. Cleft lip rhinoplasty. Facial Plast Surg Clin North Am 2009;17(1):133–44, vii.
6. Blair VP. Nasal deformities associated with congenital cleft of the lip. JAMA 1925;84:185–7.
7. Huffman WC, Lierle DM. Studies on the pathologic anatomy of the unilateral hare-lip nose. Plast Reconstr Surg 1949;4:225–34.
8. Coleman J, Sykes J. Cleft lip rhinoplasty. In: Papel ID, editor. Facial plastic and reconstructive surgery. 3rd edition. Stuttgart (NY): Thieme; 2009. p. 1082.
9. Sarnat BG, Wexler MR. Growth of the face and jaws after resection of the septal cartilage in the rabbit. Am J Anat 1966;118:755–67.
10. McComb HK, Coghlan BA. Primary repair of the unilateral cleft lip nose: completion of a longitudinal study. Cleft Palate Craniofac J 1996;33:23–31.
11. Grayson BH, Maull D. Nasoalveolar molding for infants born with clefts of the lip, alveolus, and palate. Clin Plast Surg 2004;31(2):149–58, vii.
12. Mulliken JB, Martinez-Perez D. The principle of rotation advancement for the repair of unilateral complete cleft lip and nasal deformity: technical variations and analysis of results. Plast Reconstr Surg 1999;104:1247–9.
13. Sykes J, Rotas N. 3rd edition. Orthognathic surgery in cleft lip and palate patient. FPS Cln NA, vol. 4. Philadelphia: WB Saunders; 1996. p. 351–75.
14. Wang TD, Madorsky SJ. Secondary rhinoplasty in nasal deformity associated with the unilateral cleft lip. Arch Facial Plast Surg 1999;1:40–5.
15. Crockett D, Bumstead R. Nasal airway, otologic, and audiologic problems associated with cleft lip and palate. In: Bardach J, Morris HL, editors. Multidisciplinary management of cleft lip and palate. Philadelphia: WB Saunders; 1990.
16. Haack J, Papel ID. Caudal septal deviation. Otolaryngol Clin North Am 2009;42(3):427–36.
17. Most SP. Anterior septal reconstruction: outcomes after a modified extracorporeal septoplasty technique. Arch Facial Plast Surg 2006;8(3):202–7.
18. Kridel RW, Scott BA, Foda HM. The tongue-in-groove technique in septorhinoplasty. A 10-year experience. Arch Facial Plast Surg 1999;1(4):246–56.
19. Murakami CS, Barrera JE, Most SP. Preserving structural integrity of the alar cartilage in aesthetic rhinoplasty using a cephalic turn-in flap. Arch Facial Plast Surg 2009;11(2):126–8.

Rhinoplasty in Latino Patients

Roxana Cobo, MD

KEYWORDS

- Ethnic rhinoplasty • Latino patient • Bulbous nasal tip • Thick skin • Mestizo rhinoplasty
- Hispanic patient • Mesorrhine nose

KEY POINTS

- Rhinoplasty is the main facial plastic procedure that is performed in Latin America in all age groups independent of gender.
- Latino or Mestizo patients have noses with thick skin–soft tissue envelope; tips that are bulbous, undefined, and flimsy; and a poor underlying osteocartilaginous structure.
- A structural approach is used in which conservative tissue excision is performed and structural grafting is used to reinforce the support structures of the nose.
- A gradual approach is used to work on the nasal tip. Sutures and grafts are used to reshape cartilaginous structures by creating tips with greater refinement and definition without making them look bigger.

 Videos of placement of intercrural and septoclumellar sutures accompany this article at http://www.plasticsurgery.theclinics.com/

INTRODUCTION

In Latin America, rhinoplasty is the most frequently performed facial plastic procedure in both men and women of all age groups.[1] All facial plastic surgeons should be able to perform this surgery properly.

Latin American patients are mixed-race patients commonly known as mestizo, Hispanic, or Latino people.[2] Because of the intermixing of races, noses can have important structural deficiencies. This article shows how, by using a structural approach using sutures and grafts, consistent satisfactory functional and cosmetic long-term results can be achieved.

Concepts of Beauty and Mestizo Patients

Mestizo was a term used originally in Spain and in Latin America to describe a person of mixed European and Indian descent. Over time, and because of migration of different ethnic groups over the years to Latin America, pure races became less distinct and the mixing of ethnic groups more evident. This intermixing now comprises all the different racial groups that exist in Latin America and for this reason mestizo patients are considered mixed-race patients.[2,3] Migration patterns have also changed, and in the last 50 years many people have migrated from Latin American countries to developed countries like the United States, Canada, and European countries (mainly Spain) looking for better job opportunities or for political reasons. In United States the biggest minority ethnic group is the Latin group. This group is commonly referred to as Hispanic or Latino people."[4]

There is now an increased awareness of cosmetic procedures that are being performed

Disclosure: The author has no disclosures.
Department of Otolaryngology, Centro Médico Imbanaco, Carrera 38 A #5A-100 Cons, Cali 231A, Colombia
E-mail address: rcobo@imbanaco.com.co

Clin Plastic Surg 43 (2016) 237–254
http://dx.doi.org/10.1016/j.cps.2015.09.003

worldwide. Cosmetic surgery is no longer a privilege of the few and has become available to patients of all social groups and economic levels, independent of their race or ethnic group. Beauty standards have changed and patients usually want to fit in and be part of their social and cultural groups. Beauty is defined by what the models, sport icons, actors and actresses, and favorite rock stars look like. Most Latin patients consider their noses too broad and too big for their faces. Patients usually want noses that look more defined, with greater definition but without looking bigger[5]

Mestizo Nasal Characteristics

Nasal characteristics in mestizo or Latino patients are those of mixed-race patients. Because of the intermixing of races it can be difficult to define predominant racial characteristics and it is crucial to

be able to make an accurate anatomic diagnosis of the patient's nasal findings. In general, mestizo noses have a tendency to have a thick skin–soft tissue envelope (S-STE), and a weak underlying bony and cartilaginous framework. Bones tend to be small and cartilages thin and flimsy. Tips have a tendency to be bulbous, undefined, with poor projection and rotation (**Fig. 1**).[5]

THE CONSULTATION

The consultation is probably the most important step when planning a rhinoplasty. A solid relationship needs to be established with the patient because clinicians need to understand each patient's desires and expectations to decide whether, depending on their clinical history and physical examination, treatment options can objectively be offered that will fulfill their desired goals. A systematic checklist is performed in

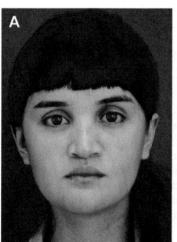
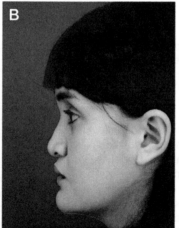
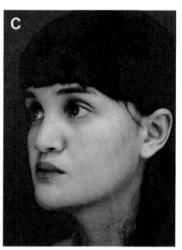
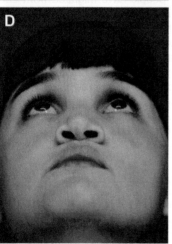

Fig. 1. Nasal characteristics of Latino patients. Latino patients are mixed-race patients. Also known as mestizo patients. Noses have S-STE that can be normal to thick with weak underlying bony and cartilaginous structures. (*A*) Frontal view showing bones that can be small, slightly wide, and flattened. The upper lateral cartilages frequently are weak and collapsed and tips show cartilages that are weak and flimsy with little support. (*B, C*) Lateral and oblique views can show a low radix with a small hump or pseudohump. Nasolabial angles can be acute with retrusive caudal septa and short nasal spines. (*D*) Base view can show normal to short columellas with poor support, wide nasal base, and flaring ala

which the following items need to be clearly defined:

- Definition of the patient's desires and expectations
- Previous clinical and surgical history
- Physical examination
- Photographic documentation/digital imaging
- Definition of surgical options

As mentioned earlier, mestizo patients are mixed-race patients. Trying to define the ethnic or racial background is often impossible. What is important is to make adequate anatomic diagnoses so that real surgical solutions can be offered. Most of the noses have a thick S-STE with a poor bony and cartilaginous framework. These patients want noses that have more definition and projection. For surgeons, the challenge is to create noses that have a strong underlying structural framework with greater definition but without looking big or overprojected. This challenge necessarily means using sutures and grafts to be able to obtain these results.

STRUCTURAL APPROACH TO THE MESTIZO OR LATINO NOSE

A structural approach in which conservative tissue excision and preservation and reinforcement of support structures of the nose using structural grafts has been used by the author for more than

20 years. Grafts and sutures are used to shape and give additional definition to the nasal tip.[5]

To help organize surgery in an efficient manner, the nose is divided into anatomic thirds and techniques are defined for each area depending on the needs of each patient:

- Upper third of the nose (bony dorsum)
- Middle third of the nose (cartilaginous dorsum)
- Lower third of the nose (nasal tip)

SURGICAL TECHNIQUE

All surgeries are done under general anesthesia. The nose is infiltrated using 1% to 2% Xylocaine with 1:100,000 epinephrine. The author performs most Latino rhinoplasties using an external approach. Material for grafting must be defined and harvested at the beginning of surgery. Septal cartilage is the first and best choice for cartilage grafting. In the absence of septal cartilage, additional choices are conchal or rib cartilage (**Fig. 2**).

Mestizo patients commonly have noses with a mesorrhine configuration in which the quadrangular cartilage that is available is modest and not very thick (usually 2–3 mm). Septal cartilage should be harvested en-bloc leaving an inverted-L strip of cartilage of at least 1.0 to 1.5 cm dorsally and caudally. This inverted L becomes an important support to the nose postsurgically. Septal deviations are corrected and the caudal edge

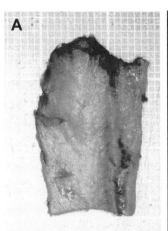
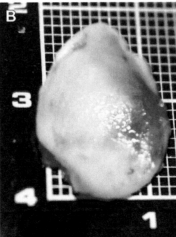
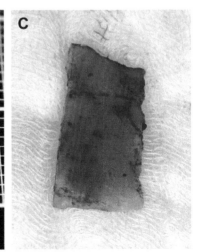

Fig. 2. Types of cartilage for nasal grafting. (*A*) Septal cartilage is the cartilage of choice for most grafts in rhinoplasty. It is mainly used for struts, extension grafts, augmentation grafts, and in any graft that requires a straight piece of cartilage. (*B*) Conchal cartilage can be used for grafts in the nasal tip. It does not give the support that the septal cartilage has. (*C*) Rib cartilage is used when large quantities of grafting material are needed, and is ideal in areas that require strong support. It is hard to carve and can warp if not carved properly.

should be perfectly centered over the nasal spine. When necessary, additional fixation of the caudal edge to the nasal spine is performed. Septal mucosa is closed using absorbable 5-0 mattress sutures. Usually no packing is left inside the nose (**Fig. 3**).

Once the nose is opened and the underlying structures exposed, work is performed by dividing the nose into anatomic thirds. Work is done starting from the upper bony third and finishing with the lower third or nasal tip area. It is the author's preference to set the height of the dorsum before doing any work on the nasal tip area.

THE UPPER THIRD OF THE NOSE (BONY DORSUM)

Nasal bones tend to be short, slightly flattened, and wide. A small convexity or pseudohump can frequently be seen with a normal to low radix on the side view.

Problems encountered:

1. Short, wide nasal bones without hump
2. Low radix with pseudohump or dorsal convexity
3. Low nasal dorsum

Surgical Solutions

1. Medial and/or lateral osteotomies
2. Radix graft

Placement of a radix graft is usually preferred to any reduction of dorsal convexities of the nasal bones. When necessary, conservative rasping of bone with trimming of cartilage excess can be done before placement of radix grafts. These grafts are fashioned from gently morselized cartilage and placed in a small pocket over the bone (**Fig. 4**).[6]

3. Low nasal dorsum

When dorsal augmentation is needed, cartilage is the material of choice. Septal cartilage is preferred to auricular cartilage. The following options can be used:

Slight augmentation
Septal cartilage is preferred. Edges are usually crushed and cartilage can be wrapped in fascia to camouflage edges (**Fig. 5**A).

Moderate augmentation
Diced cartilage wrapped in fascia is the method of choice. Conchal or rib cartilage is frequently used. Septal cartilage is usually used as grafting material in other areas of the nose. The cartilage should be diced so that the tiny pieces can fit through a 1-mL tuberculin syringe without plugging the embolus (**Fig. 5**B, C).[7]

Marked augmentation
Rib cartilage or, when not available, implants can be used (**Fig. 5**D–F). The author's preference is expanded polytetrafluoroethylene (Gore-Tex) sheeting. The complication rate is low and the results are excellent if the patients are chosen

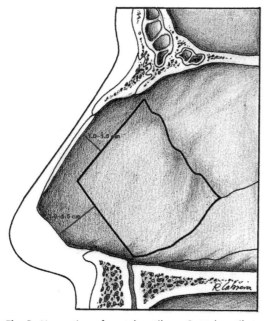

Fig. 3. Harvesting of septal cartilage. Septal cartilage is harvested leaving an inverted L of at least 10 to 15 mm dorsally and caudally, making sure the caudal edge is centered securely over the nasal spine. The cartilage is harvested en-bloc so grafts can be designed properly (see **Fig. 2**A).

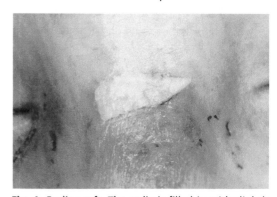

Fig. 4. Radix graft. The radix is filled in with slightly crushed cartilage, ideally harvested from the nasal septum and placed in a small pocket in the nasion. It is usually not fixed to skin externally. Crushing the cartilage prevents visibility.

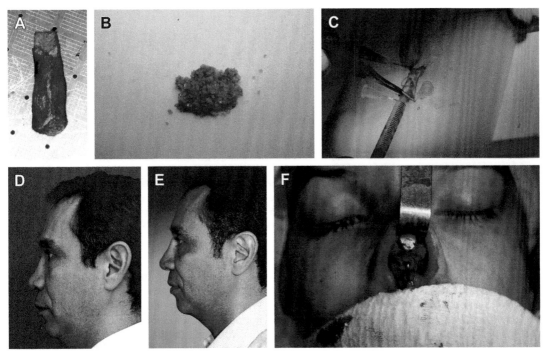

Fig. 5. Techniques for dorsal augmentation. (*A*) Augmentation ideally should be done with cartilage, and septum is the cartilage of choice. Edges should be beveled so no irregularities become visible over time. (*B*) The Turkish graft is diced cartilage wrapped in fascia inserted over the dorsum. The fascia is sewn together so it looks like a sac that posteriorly is filled in with cartilage. It has the advantage that once inside the patient it can be molded depending on patients needs (*C*). In cases of marked augmentation, the cartilage of choice becomes the rib. If handled and carved properly the risk of warping is diminished (*D*, *E*). If an implant is going to be used, polytetrafluoroethylene (Gore-Tex) is the implant of choice by the author. Implant is carved according to patients needs and placed in a precise pocket over the dorsum. If possible it should be sutured in place (*F*).

properly. These implants are placed using an external approach because the risk of infection is lower. The implant is carved, soaked in antibiotic solution, and placed in a precise pocket over the dorsum. When possible, the implant is fixed in place with sutures to the cartilaginous middle third of the nose.[8,9]

THE MIDDLE THIRD OF THE NOSE (CARTILAGINOUS DORSUM)

Upper lateral cartilages tend to be weak in mestizo patients. If any work is going to be done in the middle third of the nose, the cartilages should be reinforced to prevent functional and structural deformities. If no work is going to be done but cartilaginous structures have deformities or are naturally weak, these can be reinforced to improve final surgical outcomes.

Problems encountered:

1. Weak and flattened upper lateral cartilages (ULC)
2. Narrow middle third of nose

Surgical Solutions

Spreader grafts
Rectangular pieces of cartilage measuring 18 to 25 mm (length) by 3 to 5 mm (width) by 1 to 3 mm (thick) that are placed in a pocket between the dorsal edge of the septal cartilage and the ULC. Spreader grafts can be placed in only 1 or both sides of the septum and either as single or multiple grafts. They are sutured in place using absorbable Vicryl or polydioxanone (PDS) sutures (**Fig. 6**).

Uses:
- Correct weak or buckling ULC
- Widen a narrow middle third of the nose
- Correct inverted V deformities and internal nasal valve collapses, and help align a crooked dorsal edge of the nasal septum

Flaring mattress sutures
Mattress sutures using a 4-0 PDS or a nonabsorbable suture can be used to open up naturally weak ULC, widen a slightly narrow middle third of the nose, or help align slight dorsal deviations.

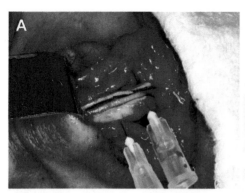
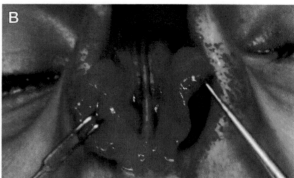

Fig. 6. Spreader grafts. (*A*) Rectangular pieces of cartilage are placed in a pocket between the ULC and the dorsal septum. They are sutured in place with 5-0 Vicryl or PDS using a 27-gauge to 30-gauge needle. (*B*) The middle cartilaginous vault is closed leaving ULC at the same level of the spreader grafts and the dorsal edge of the septum.

Onlay grafts/crushed cartilage

Onlay grafts and/or crushed cartilage can be used to fill in and smooth out irregularities over the middle nasal vault. Grafts should be placed in precise pockets or fixed in place if possible.

LOWER THIRD OF THE NOSE (NASAL TIP)

The nasal tip is formed by the pedestal and nasal tripod. The pedestal is formed by the caudal edge of the septum and the nasal spine and the tripod is a more flexible structure that is formed by the 2 conjoined medial crura and the diverging lateral crura.[10] These 2 structures and its covering, the S-STE, give shape and support to the nasal tip.

If our structural approach is followed, the pedestal should be strengthened before any tip work is done because it is the more stable structure. In this way, changes done on the tripod will not be lost because of loss of support of the underlying pedestal.

The Pedestal

Latino or mestizo patients tend to have noses with mesorrhine characteristics. Their septum can be modest in size with a retrusive caudal edge and a small nasal spine.

Problems encountered:

1. Normal caudal septum, small nasal spine, poor tip recoil
2. Small nasal spine, short and weak caudal septum, acute nasolabial angle

Surgical Solutions

Columellar strut

The columellar strut is a thin rectangular piece of cartilage measuring from 18 to 25 mm in length by 3 to 4 mm of width that is placed in a precise pocket between the medial crura and sutured in place with absorbable 5-0 Vicryl or PDS sutures. When suturing the strut in place, sutures should not be placed too far up near the domes because this would efface the natural double break of the columella.

Uses
- Aligns medial crura and gives additional strength to the pedestal
- Maintains projection and rotation of nasal tip
- Provides a stable base so sutures and grafts can be used in the nasal tip

Caudal septal extension graft

The caudal septal extension graft is indicated in patients in whom the columellar strut will not give the necessary support. A straight piece of cartilage should be used for this graft. Its shape is usually rectangular, although, depending on what needs to be done to the nasal tip, it can be left wider at the top (to produce counter-rotation) or at the bottom (to produce rotation). The graft is sutured in place slightly overlapping the caudal edge of the patient's septum. This overlapping portion is thinned so that it will not create any obstruction at the nasal valve area. Once the pedestal has been stabilized, the position of the nasal tip is defined (depending on how much rotation and projection must be obtained) and the feet of the medial crura are sutured to the caudal edge of this graft using the tongue-in-groove technique (**Fig. 7**).[11]

Uses[12,13]:
- Severely acute nasolabial angles
- Retrusive weak caudal septa/small nasal spine/short nasal septa
- Inadequate alar-columellar relationships (heavy alas with retrusive columellas)

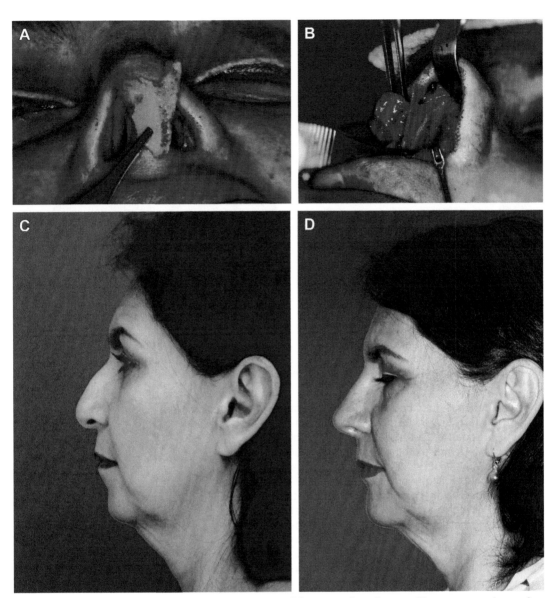

Fig. 7. Septal extension graft. (*A*)The graft ideally is carved from septal cartilage and has a rectangular configuration. It is sutured in place overlapping the existing caudal edge of the septal cartilage. (*B*) The portion of the graft that overlaps the caudal edge of the septum is thinned out before suturing in place with absorbable 5-0 Vicryl sutures. (*C, D*) Preoperative and postoperative lateral views of the patient in whom a septal extension graft was placed to correct a severely acute nasolabial angle.

The Nasal Tip

Latin or mestizo noses commonly have tips that are bulbous, undefined, and with poor support. Our Latino or ethnic patients want noses that look more refined, with greater tip definition but without looking bigger. This requirement is a challenge for the surgeon because alar cartilages can be wide and flimsy with a tendency to collapse. To be able to address this properly means using grafts and sutures to increase support and create definition but without making the nose look bigger.

The intention to use a structural approach when working with the nasal tip means little if extensive tissue has been resected. Instead, most of the tip contour, definition, and additional support are obtained by using sutures and grafts. A gradual approach to the nasal tip is used in all patients. Alar cartilages are evaluated in their vertical and horizontal components and changes are

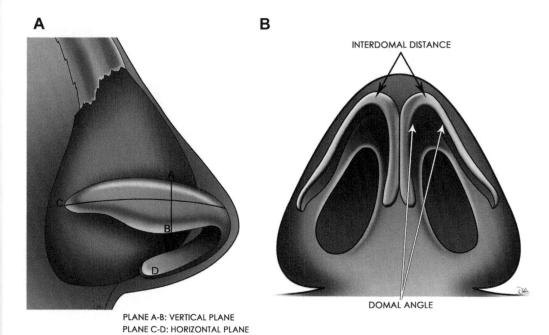

A

B

INTERDOMAL DISTANCE

DOMAL ANGLE

PLANE A-B: VERTICAL PLANE
PLANE C-D: HORIZONTAL PLANE

Fig. 8. Alar cartilages are analyzed in their vertical and horizontal dimensions. The vertical component (A–B) describes how wide the cartilage is and whether it is concave or convex (*A*). The horizontal component measures how long the cartilage is (C–D) and also measures the interdomal distance and the domal angle (*B*).

performed depending on the anatomic findings at this level (**Fig. 8**). The vertical component (A–B) indicates how wide the cartilage is. The horizontal component (C–D) indicates the length of the alar cartilage, characteristics of the domal angle (acute, obtuse, pinched or collapsed), and definition of the dome (whether it is flattened, prominent, or asymmetric compared with the contralateral side). Because the alar cartilages are paired structures, sides must be compared to obtain symmetry.

Surgical techniques that can be performed on the nasal tip are multiple. For clarity, these are divided into techniques that treat the vertical component and techniques that treat the horizontal component. Procedures done on the horizontal component can be divided into complete strip procedures and incomplete strip procedures (cartilage splitting procedures). In addition, grafts can be used in all areas of the nasal tip (**Table 1**). When deciding what technique should be used, it is recommended to start with more conservative and predictable procedures, leaving the more aggressive and less predictable techniques for nasal tips that need more dramatic changes. All procedures are done using 5-0 PDS or nonabsorbable sutures like Ethilon or Prolene.[14]

Problems encountered:

1. Thick S-STE
2. Wide, flimsy alar cartilages
3. Short columellas
4. Poor projection and rotation

Intact tip procedures
These are procedures in which the whole strip of alar cartilage is left intact. The length of the cartilage is not changed. What can be modified is the width of the alar cartilage or the shape (A–B in **Fig. 8**).

Reduction of the width of the alar cartilage The author usually preserves the entire width of the alar cartilage unless it is excessively wide. An alar width of at least 9 to 10 mm at the lateral crus and 5 to 7 mm in the domal area should be preserved. When width needs to be reduced, this can be done in 2 ways: resecting the cephalic edge of the alar cartilage or performing a lateral crural turn-in flap of the cephalic edge of the alar cartilage. A cephalic trim is only done when cartilages are strong and excessively wide.

Lateral crural turn-in flap This technique is especially useful in patients with wide cartilages that are flimsy and lack support. The amount of cartilage that otherwise would be trimmed is marked, folded under the cephalic edge, and sutured in place. This turn-in flap gives additional structural support to the lateral crural area and improves the postsurgical supra-alar pinching that is commonly seen in our patients (**Fig. 9**).[15]

Table 1
Gradual approach to the nasal tip

Anatomic Finding	Surgical Solution
Management of the Vertical Component	
	Intact strip procedures
Wide alar cartilage	• Cephalic trim of lateral crura • Lateral crural turn-in flap
	Grafts on the nasal tip
Concave or convex lateral crura of alar cartilages	• Lateral crural strut graft • Alar batten grafts
Management of the Horizontal Component	
	Intact strip procedures (Suturing techniques)
Underprojection/ under-rotation of nasal tip	• Lateral crural steal • Dome defining sutures • Septocolumellar suture
Increased interdomal distance	• Lateral crural spanning sutures
	Incomplete strip procedures (cartilage dividing techniques)
Overprojected tip/ long plunging nose	• Lateral crural over-lay technique • Medial crural over-lay technique
	Grafts on the nasal tip
Bulbous undefined nasal tip	• Shield graft • Morcelized carti-lage over nasal tip
Buckling or flaring of lateral alar sidewalls	• Alar rim grafts

Suturing techniques The list of possible suturing techniques that can be used in ethnic bulbous tips is extremely long and only the most frequently used techniques are mentioned here. Most suturing techniques used are to refine, project, and rotate the bulbous undefined nasal tip. The advantage they have is that they are predictable and, if the final result is not what was desired, the sutures can be easily undone. Sutures are done with 5-0 PDS or, if this is not available, a 5-0 nonabsorbable suture is used.

Lateral crural steal
This is the workhorse suture for most ethnic Latino patients. A new dome is created by lateralizing the existing dome. The medial crura is lengthened and the lateral crura is shortened, resulting in an increase in rotation and projection of the nasal tip (**Fig. 10**).[14,16]

Uses:
• Creates dome definition
• Increases rotation and projection

Dome-defining sutures
This is a suture whose objective is to define the patient's existing dome. A mattress suture is placed at the level of the existing dome, narrowing this area. Knots should not be tied too tight (to prevent domal pinching) and should be placed in the midline so they can be well hidden.

Uses:
• Creates dome definition and defines nasal tip
• Increases projection slightly

Alar-spanning suture
A mattress suture is placed crossing the cephalic margin of both alar cartilages directly behind the dome area and tied in the midline. This suture narrows a wide nasal tip, decreases the interdomal distance, decreases supratip bulbosity, and gives slight additional projection to the nasal tip (**Fig. 11**).[17]

Uses:
• Corrects bulbosity in lateral crus area
• Increases rotation of nasal tip
• Corrects supratip fullness

Intercrural suture
This is a loop suture that is placed between both medial crura. The needle is introduced 3 to 4 mm below the dome, exiting at the level of the foot of the medial crura; the suture is then crossed over to the contralateral side, going in through the foot of the medial crura of the contralateral alar cartilage and exiting 3 to 4 mm below the contralateral dome. The suture is tied in the midline, decreasing the interdomal distance and increasing the projection of the nasal tip (**Fig. 12**; Video 1).

Uses:
• Gives additional support to medial crura/columellar strut complex
• Increases projection of nasal tip
• Decreases interdomal distance

Septocolumellar suture
The septocolumellar suture is a loop suture that fixes the medial crura/columellar complex up

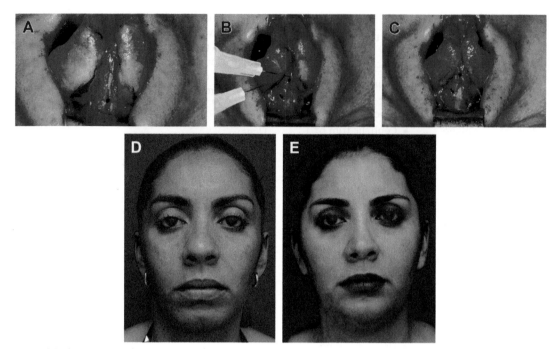

Fig. 9. (*A*) The amount of cartilage that otherwise would be resected is marked. (*B*) The marked cephalic area is folded on itself and sutured in place, giving extra strength to the cephalic margin. (*C*) The cephalic margin in both cartilages is sutured in place. (*D, E*) Preoperative and late postoperative pictures showing frontal view of the patient in whom this technique was used. Note that the patient has no supra-alar pinching.

against the caudal septum, resulting in an increase in rotation and projection of the nasal tip. The suture is usually placed after the final work on the nasal tip has been done and it requires a stable pedestal that should be firmly set in the midline (**Fig. 13**; Video 2).[14] The suture is introduced at a point low near the medial crura footplate on one side, crosses to the contralateral side at the level of the anterior septal angle, and exits near the medial crura footplate of the contralateral side. When the knot is tied in the midline, the whole medial crura complex is pulled up against the caudal septum.

Uses:
- Increases projection and rotation of nasal tip
- Fixes medial crura/columellar complex to caudal edge of nasal septum

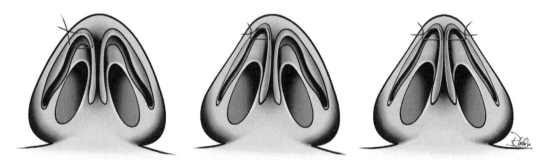

Fig. 10. The lateral crural steal. The medial crura is lengthened at the expense of the lateral crura. This lengthening results in rotation and projection of the nasal tip, pushing the tip backwards and creating a base that is more triangular.

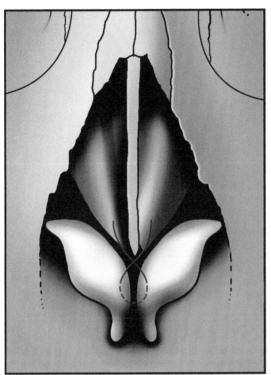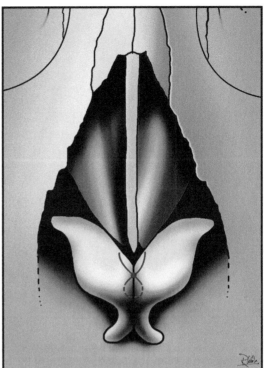

Fig. 11. The lateral spanning suture helps correct the lateral bulbosity of the nasal tip and increases rotation and projection if needed. A mattress suture is passed just posterior to the domes in the lateral crura and ties the knot in the midline. The posterior domal distance is diminished, giving increased rotation to the nasal tip.

Incomplete strip procedures (cartilage splitting techniques)

It is common to have ethnic patients with an over-developed horizontal component (overprojected noses, long plunging tips) resulting in alar cartilages that are excessively long. Instead of resecting a strip of cartilage, a lateral crural overlay and/or a medial crural overlay (MCO) technique are

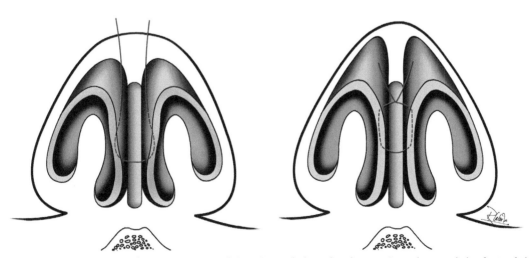

Fig. 12. Intercrural suture. The suture is passed 2 to 3 mm below the dome oriented toward the foot of the medial crura, crosses to the contralateral side, and exits 2 to 3 mm below the dome of the contralateral side. The suture is then knotted in the midline, resulting in an increase in the projection of the medial crura (Video 1).

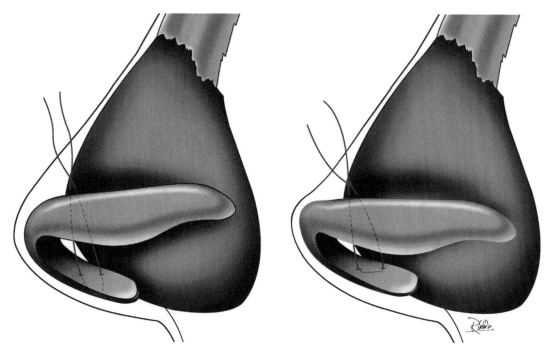

Fig. 13. Placement of a septocolumellar suture. A 5-0 nonabsorbable suture passed from a point low in the feet of the medial crura is directed upward exiting at the level of the anterior septal angle, crossing it to the contra-lateral side and exiting low at the level of the foot of the contralateral medial crura. The suture is then tied in the midline, bringing the crural/strut complex up against the caudal edge of the septum and resulting in an increase of rotation and projection of the nasal tip.

used. Depending on what area is going to be shortened, the medial or lateral crura is cut, and the edges overlapped and sutured in place. The result is a shortened, reinforced alar strip.[11,13,14]

Lateral crural overlay This is indicated in plunging tips in which the lateral crura is much longer than the medial crura. The shortening of the lateral crura produces upward rotation of the nasal tip and shortening of the nose. The incision is placed approximately 10 mm lateral to the existing dome. When cut edges are overlapped this strengthens the lateral crural area (**Fig. 14**).

Uses:
- Plunging nasal tips in which the lateral crura is much longer than the medial crura.

Medial crural overlay MCO is indicated in long noses with long medial crura. An incision is placed a few millimeters below the existing dome and incised fragments are overlapped and sutured in

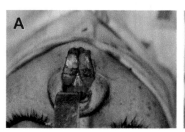
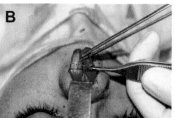
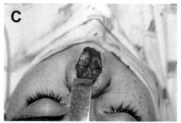

Fig. 14. Lateral crural overlay (LCO) technique. (*A*) Ten millimeters lateral to the dome the area is marked as to how much overlay is going to be done. (*B*) Alar crus is sectioned and elevated. (*C*) Segments are overlapped and sutured together. Note how the alar cartilage is shortened and rotated.

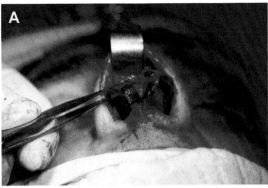

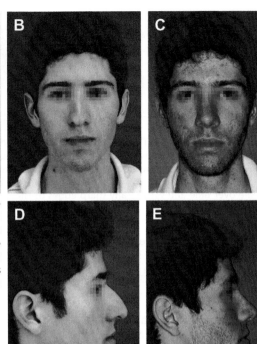

Fig. 15. MCO technique. (*A*) MCO on the right side. The dome on the right side lowered. (*B, D*) Frontal and lateral preoperative views showing the patient with large, overprojected, plunging nose. (*C, E*) Postoperative views after hump reduction, placement of bilateral spreader grafts, LCO, MCO, LCS, and suturing techniques on the nasal tip. The nose is smaller, with an increase in rotation of the nasal tip. LCS, lateral crural steal.

place. When an MCO is done alone, counter-rotation of the tip is produced. When it is combined with a lateral crural overlay, deprojection of the nasal tip is produced (**Fig. 15**).

Uses:
- Counter-rotation of nasal tip
- Deprojection of nasal tip

Grafts

Latino or Mestizo noses commonly have tips that are bulbous and undefined, with poor projection and rotation. Grafts on the nasal tip are important, should be used wisely, and are indicated for support, to create definition, to fill in concavities, and to camouflage irregularities or asymmetries.

Shield graft The shield graft is an excellent tool in bulbous, undefined nasal tips with thick S-STE. It should be carved from a straight piece of cartilage, ideally septal cartilage, beveling all edges. Measurements can vary: 8 to 12 mm at the leading edge, 10 to 20 mm length, 1 to 3 mm thick. The graft is sutured to the caudal edge of the medial crura/intermediate crura complex with PDS or 6-0 nonabsorbable sutures. The author generally fixes the leading edge of the shield graft at the level of the domes or 1 to 2 mm above the leading edge.

The area is then covered with crushed cartilage, fascia, or perichondrium. No sharp edges should be seen because these can become visible over time (**Fig. 16**).

Uses:
- Definition of a bulbous nasal tip
- Increase in projection
- Lengthens a short columella

Alar strut grafts Alar strut grafts are rectangular thin pieces of cartilage that are used to flatten out any concavities or convexities of the lateral crus of the alar cartilages. The lateral crus is dissected from the underlying mucosa and the piece of cartilage is placed in the undersurface and sutured in place (**Fig. 17**).

Uses:
- Give additional support to flimsy lateral crura
- Correct buckling of lateral crura
- Flatten concave or convex alar cartilage

Alar rim grafts Alar rim grafts are thin, long pieces of cartilage that are placed in a precise pocket along the alar rim in from of the caudal edge of the alar cartilage. With sharp-pointed scissors a pocket is created following the alar rim. The

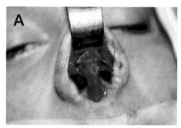
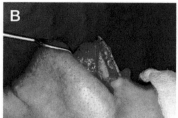
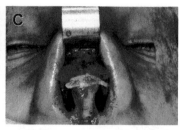

Fig. 16. Shield graft. (*A*) The shield graft ideally should be carved from a straight piece of septal cartilage. The graft is fixed in place in front of the caudal edge of the medial/intermediate/strut complex with 6-0 nonabsorbable suture. (*B*) On the side view the leading edge of the graft is left 1 to 2 mm above the existing domes. (*C*) This leading edge is covered with morcelized cartilage or perichondrium, which makes the edge of the graft less visible over time and softens any sharp edges of the graft.

graft is inserted and fixed in place. The superior leading edge of the graft should be gently crushed so that it will not become visible over time (**Fig. 18**).

Uses:
- Correct flaring of ala
- Correct buckling of ala
- Give additional support to ala

Morselized cartilage/crushed cartilage Morselized cartilage is a piece of cartilage that is carefully crushed using a cartilage crusher without disintegrating it into small fragments. The result should be a consistent piece of cartilage that is soft, pliable, can be manipulated, and looks like a rug. It can be used anywhere in the nose to soften edges, hide irregularities, and fill in defects. The ideal material to morselize is septal cartilage. Conchal cartilage has a tendency to break up into pieces and costal cartilage can be difficult to manipulate and convert into something soft and pliable. The cartilage should be sutured delicately

in place whenever possible, and if not it should ideally be placed in precise pockets to avoid shifting (**Fig. 19**).[4,13]

Uses:
- Hide irregularities
- Fill in concavities or defects
- Soften sharp edges

THE NASAL BASE

Alar base reduction is only done if, after closing all incisions and having obtained adequate projection, rotation, and definition of the nasal tip, there is persistent alar flaring and a wide nasal base. Many times after having done all the surgical techniques for the nasal tip in a consistent fashion, the configuration of the nasal base has changed, resulting in a base that looks more triangular. If there is a need to perform alar base reduction, it is done at this point.

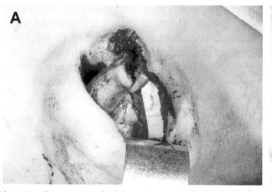
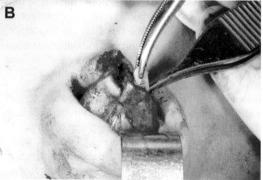

Fig. 17. Alar strut graft. (*A*) A rectangular piece of cartilage is fashioned to be placed under the alar cartilage. The length depends on what needs to be done on that cartilage. (*B*) The undersurface of the alar cartilage is dissected from the mucosa and the graft is placed in a pocket and secured with an absorbable suture. The graft can correct buckling of the lateral crus and convex and concave deformities, and gives additional strength to the lateral nasal sidewall.

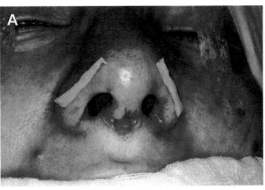
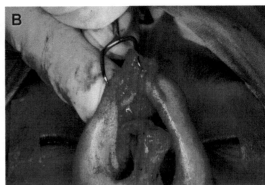

Fig. 18. (A) The alar rim grafts are thin, long pieces of cartilage that are placed following the patient's alar rim in an anatomic position in front of the caudal edge of the alar cartilages. (B) A pocket is created and the graft is introduced. The leading edge of the graft is sutured in place and crushed to avoid any visible sharp edges.

POSTSURGICAL FOLLOW-UP

Inflammation is an important issue with Latino ethnic patients. Patients are asked to sleep with their heads elevated and icing is placed over eyes and malar area on a regular basis for the first 72 hours after surgery. Tapes, stitches, and cast are removed on day 7 to 8 and the nose is taped for an additional week.

The S-STE in mestizo or Latino patients is usually thicker, oilier, and with a tendency to be acne prone. Breakouts, presence of blackheads, and marked edema of the nasal tip are frequently seen. Proper follow-up should be performed and, when necessary, steroid injections with Kenalog (0.02–0.05 mL) can be used, taking care to place them in the deep subdermal plane. These injections can be repeated every 4 to 6 weeks.[14] Our patients have a tendency to hyperpigment. Dark circles under the eyes are frequently seen and patients should be warned that they will have them but that they eventually disappear. Nasal exercises can help with lymphatic drainage and help control inflammation (see **Fig. 21**). Long-term follow-up is essential when treating ethnic patients. Good results might not be evident until the inflammation goes down, so it is important to be able to follow up patients closely. Postsurgical photographs are taken at 6 months and 1 year and, if possible, every year after surgery (**Figs. 20 and 21**).

SUMMARY

Rhinoplasty is the most frequently performed facial plastic procedure in Latino or Mestizo patients of all age groups. Latino or mestizo patients are mixed-race patients. Their noses tend to have a poor osteocartilaginous framework with a thick S-STE. Nasal tips commonly are bulbous, undefined, and with poor rotation and projection. A structural rhinoplasty approach is shown in which, with minimal tissue excision and adequate

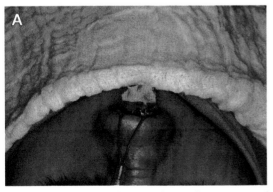
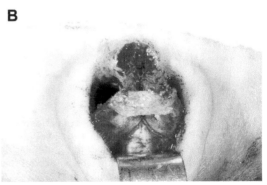

Fig. 19. Morcelized cartilage can be used in any part of the nose to fill in; hide irregularities; and, if used in the tip, give the tip a rounder look. Cartilage should not be crushed excessively because it will be reabsorbed. (A) Morcelized cartilage over the nasal tip. (B) Graft fixed in place.

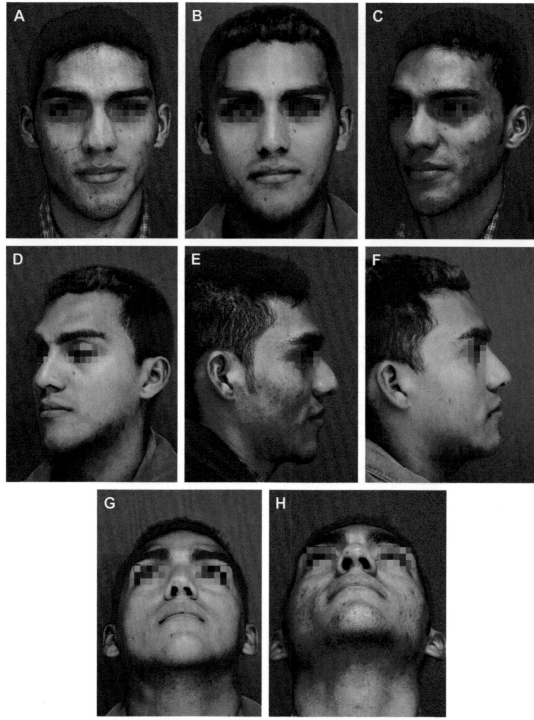

Fig. 20. (*A, C, E, H*) Preoperative images of patient with thick, acne-prone skin; bulbous tip with poor projection; and rotation and bony hump. (*B, D, F, G*) Two years after hump removal and placement of bilateral spreader grafts, septal extension graft, shield graft, and alar rim grafts. The tip was defined and rotated with a lateral crural steal, septocolumellar suture, and alar crural spanning sutures. In addition, the patient was placed on Accutane treatment of his thick acneic skin.

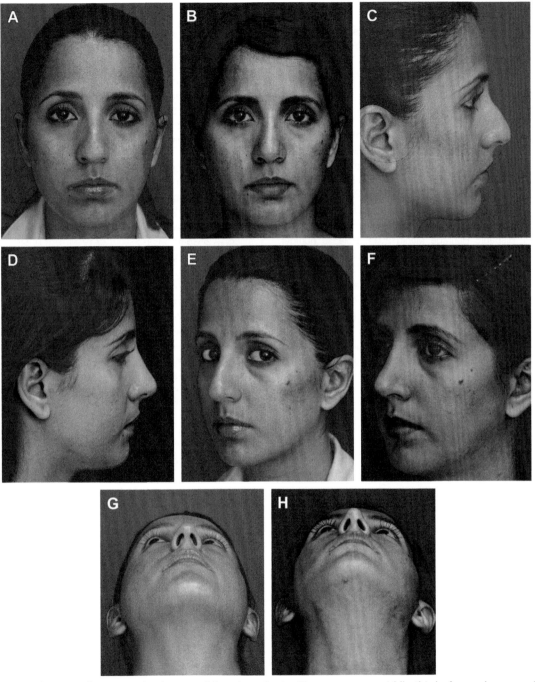

Fig. 21. (*A, C, E, G*) Preoperative images of female patient with very narrow middle third of nose, hump, and bulbous undefined nasal tip. (*B, D, F, H*) Postoperative images after lowering the hump with rasps, placement of bilateral spreader grafts, rotation of nasal tip using LCS, IC, and septocolumellar and alar crural spanning sutures. Morcelized cartilage was placed over the nasal tip and in the radix. IC, intercrural; LCS, lateral crural steal.

use of grafts and sutures, support structures of the nose are reinforced. Instead of resecting tissue, grafts and sutures are applied using a gradual approach with which refinement and definition are obtained without making the nose look bigger. The desired results are patients with noses that are very attractive but that do not lose their ethnicity.

SUPPLEMENTARY DATA

Supplementary data related to this article can be found online at http://dx.doi.org/10.1016/j.cps.2015.09.003.

REFERENCES

1. Cobo R. Trends in facial plastic surgery in Latin America. Facial Plast Surg 2013;29:149–53.
2. Fernández FL. Composición Étnica de las Tres Áreas Culturales del Continente Americano al Comienzo del Siglo XXI. Convergencia Revista de Ciencias Sociales 2005;12(38):185–232. Mayo-Agosto.
3. Ospina W. América Mestiza-El país del Futuro. Bogotá (Colombia): Villegas Editores; 2000. p. 23–38.
4. Hispanic Heritage Month 2014. Release number: CB14-FF. Available at: www.census.gov. Accessed September 22, 2014.
5. Cobo R. Structural rhinoplasty in Latin American patients. Facial Plast Surg 2013;29:171–83.
6. Becker D, Pastorek NJ. The radix graft in cosmetic rhinoplasty. Arch Facial Plast Surg 2001;3(2):115–9.
7. Daniel R, Calvert J. Diced cartilage grafts in rhinoplasty surgery. Plast Reconstr Surg 2004;113:2156.
8. Romo T III, Abraham MT. The ethnic nose. Facial Plast Surg 2003;19:269–77. #3.
9. Godin MS, Waldman SR, Johnson CM. Nasal augmentation using Gore-Tex: a 10 year experience. Arch Facial Plast Surg 1999;1(2):118–21.
10. Johnson CM, To WC. The tripod-pedestal concept. In: Johnson CM, To WC, editors. A case approach to open structure rhinoplasty. 1st edition. Philadelphia: Elsevier Saunders; 2005. p. 9–20.
11. Kridel RW, Scott BA, Foda HM. The tongue-in-groove technique in septorhinoplasty. A 10 year experience. Arch Facial Plast Surg 1999; 1:246–56.
12. Toriumi DM. New concepts in nasal tip contouring. Arch Facial Plast Surg 2006;8(3):156–85.
13. Cobo R. Rhinoplasty in the Mestizo nose. Facial Plast Surg Clin North Am 2014;22:395–415.
14. Cobo R. Nuances with the Mestizo tip. Facial Plast Surg 2012;28:202–12.
15. Murakami CS, Barrera JE, Most S. Preserving structural integrity of the alar cartilage in aesthetic rhinoplasty using a cephalic turn-in flap. Arch Facial Plast Surg 2009;11(2):126–8.
16. Konior RJ, Kridel R. Controlled nasal tip positioning via the open rhinoplasty approach. Facial Plast Surg Clin North Am 1993;1(1):53–62.
17. Perkins S, Patel A. Endonasal suture techniques in tip rhinoplasty. Facial Plast Surg Clin North Am 2009;17:41–54.

Rhinoplasty in the African American Patient
Anatomic Considerations and Technical Pearls

Grace Lee Peng, MD*, Paul S. Nassif, MD, FACS

KEYWORDS

- Ethnic rhinoplasty • African American rhinoplasty • African rhinoplasty • Augmentation rhinoplasty

KEY POINTS

- There are several anatomic considerations as well as variations in patients of African heritage.
- The goal of improvement in aesthetics and functionality must be in balance with racial preservation.
- Preoperative counseling must discuss patient expectations and surgical limitations based on patients' skin and cartilage.
- Dorsal augmentation, increased tip projection, and rotation are often needed.
- Understanding the thick, sebaceous skin often seen in African Americans assists in postoperative management of swelling.

INTRODUCTION

Rhinoplasty in African Americans has become increasingly common; thus, the challenge for facial plastic surgeons is to create a nose that improves functionality and aesthetics while embracing ethnicity. In a 2012 survey by the American Academy of Facial Plastic and Reconstructive Surgery, 27% of surgeons reported an increase in African American patients seeking facial plastic surgery. Of these patients, 80% are interested in rhinoplasty.[1,2] Currently, African American rhinoplasty presents a unique set of anatomic challenges as well as cultural considerations. As surgeons attempt to better serve patients of African descent, it is important to understand that ethnic rhinoplasty must still be approached as an individualized procedure tailored to the specific goals of each patient.

ANATOMY

In planning an African American rhinoplasty, surgeons must first understand the unique nasal anatomy. There is also variability, however, within the African American population. Ofodile and James[3,4] describe 3 groups, the first of which is an African nose—short with a wide, low, concave dorsum; less defined tip with decreased tip projection; and a short columella. There is also an Afro-Caucasian nose, a higher, more narrow nose with better tip definition and less flaring of the ala. Finally, the third group is the Afro-Indian nose, which has a high and wide dorsum and is an overall larger nose. Although there are still flared alae and lack of tip definition, there is slight increase in tip projection when compared with the purely African nose.[5] This variability requires the physician to carefully evaluate and tailor surgical planning to each patient. This article addresses the first group that represents the most typical African American patient presenting for rhinoplasty.

African American noses are thought to be more broad and flat (platyrrhine) compared with white noses, which are thought to be tall and thin (leptorrhine).

Department of Otolaryngology, Head and Neck Surgery, Keck School of Medicine, University of Southern California, Los Angeles, CA 90033, USA
* Corresponding author.
E-mail address: drpeng@spaldingplasticsurgery.com

plasticsurgery.theclinics.com

The skin–soft tissue envelope is generally thick and inelastic with abundant sebaceous glands and fibrofatty tissue, measuring up to 2 mm to 4 mm thick.[6] This is often the contributing factor to the bulbosity of the tip. This thick skin makes refining the tip difficult even with cartilage grafting.

The lower lateral cartilages are more horizontally oriented. Historically, it was thought that the lower lateral cartilages were distinctly shorter and thinner than those of whites. Cadaver studies, however, performed by Ofodile and James[3] have shown that the lower lateral cartilages of African Americans are similar in size and strength to that of whites. Despite similarities in size, the orientation leads to more flared and horizontal alae and the proportions of the width of the base in relation to the height of the medial crura may cause the appearance of the broader and wider tip.[7]

Under the skin and cartilage, the bony structure is unique as well. The pyriform aperture is described as wider and more oval in shape.[8] This causes the nasal base to become wider. The septum is often short with an underdeveloped nasal spine. This leads to a decrease in tip projection.[9,10] Because the maxilla is often retruded and hypoplastic, the combination leads to a more retracted columella, which can lead to under-rotation of the tip and an acute nasolabial angle. The nasal tip is bulbous, poorly projected, and counter-rotated, with abundant fibrous nasal superficial musculoaponeurotic system (SMAS), broad domes, and poor definition.

The nasal bones are generally short and flat.[9] Due to the lack of height of the bones, the naso-frontal angle is more obtuse (127°–133°) compared with that in whites (120°).[11,12] The radix is often deeper and more inferiorly set. Additionally, the dorsum is lower, which not only affects the appearance but also contributes to a lower and broader middle third of the nose, causing collapse of the internal nasal valve.[13]

In African Americans, the intercanthal distance is found proportionally shorter than that of the nasal base. In conjunction with the flared alae, the base view is no longer triangular but flat, with the nostrils horizontally oriented. This then also leads to obtuse soft tissue triangles.

TREATMENT GOALS AND PLANNED OUTCOMES

In a preoperative consultation, a history is performed with emphasis on the patient's nasal airway and the patient's aesthetic concerns. Patients are asked to identify the specific areas they would like to have improved. If a patient is seeking a revision rhinoplasty, the dates of the previous surgeries and the previous operative reports are obtained and reviewed to better understand the patient's surgical history. Preoperative photographs are taken from the frontal, lateral, and base views in preparation for computer morphing during the consultation with the patient.

Rohrich and Muzaffar[6] describe the goals of African American rhinoplasty as maintaining harmony and balance; a narrower, straighter dorsum; enhanced tip projection and definition; slight alar flaring; and narrower interalar distance. Although these are often the requests of the patients who come in seeking consultation, it is important to tailor each visit to the patient because the skin quality and cartilage structure as well as facial composition may not allow these to be realistic goals. Regardless of efforts at reconstructing the tip, the thick, sebaceous nature of some patients' skin may prevent a very refined tip. Additionally, due to the inelastic nature of the skin, there may be a limit on the augmentation and tip projection that is feasible for a particular patient. A clear discussion with the patient can help prevent postoperative dissatisfaction and unrealistic expectations.

PREOPERATIVE PLANNING AND PREPARATION

On physical examination, bilateral paramedian vertical light reflexes along the dorsum are analyzed for symmetry. From the frontal view, the middle vault is examined for narrowing and symmetry whereas the nasal bones are analyzed for their length, height, width, and symmetry. Careful palpation also helps determine the strength of the tip support.

The nose must then be analyzed from the lateral view to gauge the nasal starting point, shape of the dorsum, nasal length, nasal projection, nasofrontal angle, nasolabial angle, alar retraction, columellar show, depressor nasi function, and chin projection.

The nasal base is evaluated from the basal view and the frontal view to evaluate the width and shape. The ala is inspected for flaring and for its width compared with the medial canthal distance. The width of the alar base should approximate the intercanthal distance and the extension beyond this point is noted. The caudal septum is evaluated for deflection and deviation.

In a patient with nasal obstruction, its location and alleviating and exacerbating factors are documented. Anterior rhinoscopy may visualize additional sources of nasal obstruction, including the nasal septum, which is characteristically short. Due to its small size, the cartilaginous septum may be insufficient for reconstructive nasal grafting.

Computer imaging and morphing software can be useful methods of communication. They allow the surgeon and patient to communicate about aesthetic goals. It is important to communicate that imaging is not a guarantee of results and that imaging is a 2-D representation of a 3-D result. Imaging software is used to evaluate surrounding facial features, including the chin. As with all rhinoplasty patients, the chin must be evaluated and discussed. African Americans may have microgenia, in which a chin implant may be recommended. Standard preoperative rhinoplasty photographs are taken, which include (**Fig. 1**).

- Frontal view
- Right and left lateral views
- Right and left three-quarter views
- Close-up frontal view
- Base view

During preoperative planning, it is important to decide the source of structural cartilage grafting. The options include septal, conchal, and costal cartilage. Given the smaller size of the septal cartilage, however, it is generally not sufficient to use septal cartilage alone. Conchal cartilage, which can be sufficient in quantity, is often too soft for structural support for caudal septal extension grafts/columellar struts. It is the authors' preference to use rib cartilage for structural grafting. Limitations are seen in patients who are older and may have calcified rib cartilage or in others who have had injury to that area that may also lead to calcifications.

Primary goals in African American rhinoplasty often include

- Bridge: narrower on frontal view
- Dorsum: augmented height on lateral view, including radix augmentation
- Tip: improved definition, increased projection, and increased rotation
- Base: vertical-oblique nostrils, narrower and more triangular orientation
- Columella: increased columellar show and length
- Nasolabial junction: increased nasolabial angle

Should a patient decide to proceed with surgery, a second preoperative consultation is scheduled so that the plan for the rhinoplasty and patient expectations can be again reviewed and discussed.

During the preoperative visit, expectations, goals, and informed consent are discussed. A surgical plan already outlined on a nasal diagram during the consultation is reviewed. This is explained to the patient and the sheet is signed by the patient indicating agreement to the surgical plan.

SURGICAL TECHNIQUES

Dr P.N. prefers the external approach given the amount of tip work and dorsal augmentation often required for African American rhinoplasties. Through the external approach, there is sufficient exposure to allow for the techniques that may be used to create the changes that are desired. Although hypertrophic scarring and keloiding are often concerns for transcolumellar incisions in patients of African American descent, the authors have not observed any keloid formation in this area. Many other investigators' experiences have corroborated the authors'.[6,14,15] The most common goals of surgery are to augment the dorsum, increase tip projection and definition, and reduce alar base width and flare.

Initial Dissection

Local injection with 1% lidocaine with 1:100,000 epinephrine is injected in the septum and the nasal soft tissue envelope. The goals of injection include not only vasoconstriction in preparation for incisions and dissection but also hydrodissecting the skin–soft tissue envelope and vestibular tissue from the underlying cartilaginous framework. The dissection is transitioned into a subperiosteal plane over the nasal bones. The pocket of dissection is kept narrow to allow for a tighter pocket. This tight space helps keep dorsal augmentation grafts in place. During this initial dissection, the mucoperichondrium overlying the lower lateral crura can be hydrodissected and sharply excised. This slightly thins out the skin as well as acting as camouflage for subsequent cartilage grafting (**Fig. 2**).

Septoplasty and Inferior Turbinoplasty

Septoplasty is performed for either a deviated septum or for cartilage harvest. At least 10 mm to 15 mm of a caudal and dorsal strut is left for support. If hypertrophic turbinates are present, a conservative turbinate infracture and outfracture with possible additional turbinoplasty with cautery is performed.

Cartilage Grafting

Cartilage grafts are carved and secured to the native cartilage framework to improve the airway and refine the nose. This cartilage may be

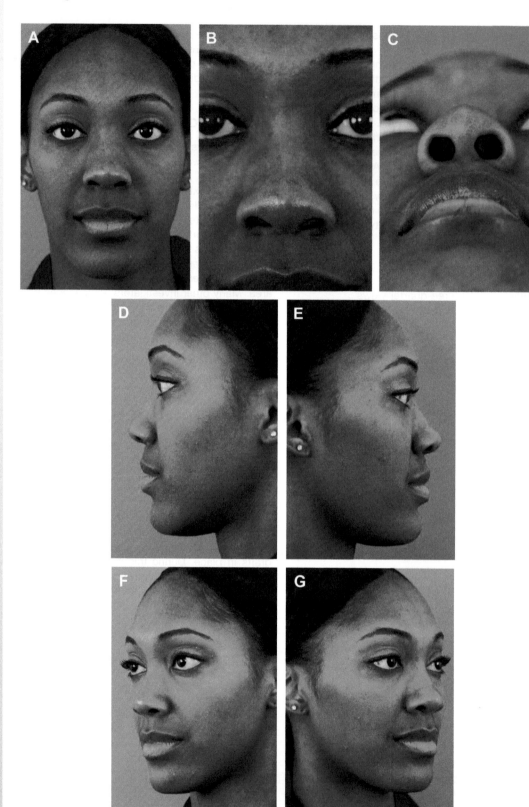

Fig. 1. Preoperative photographs showing (*A*) frontal, (*E*) right and (*D*) left lateral, (*G*) right and (*F*) left three-quarter, and (*B*) close-up frontal and (*C*) base views.

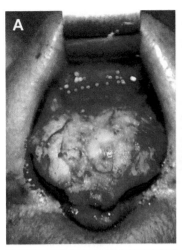

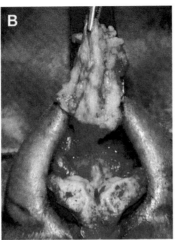

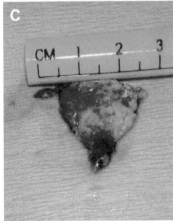

Fig. 2. (*A*) Tip mucoperichondrium just prior to dissection and removal. (*B*) Elevation of muchoperichondrium. (*C*) Piece of mucoperichondrium after excision.

harvested from the septum, ear, or rib. Often, the septal cartilage is inadequate for nasal reconstruction; therefore, additional autologous cartilage is harvested. Auricular cartilage is harvested from the cavum concha and is generally approached from the posterior surface. If a surgical plan entails extensive cartilage grafting, the authors recommend using costal cartilage. If a patient is averse to costal cartilage harvest, bilateral conchal cartilage harvest with the use of a polydioxanone (PDS) plate (Mentor Worldwide, Santa Barbara,

California) can be an alternative. A PDS plate is a thin sheet of polydioxanone that can be secured to the convex side of the conchal cartilage to straighten the cartilage. Patients must understand, however, that the strength of the grafts is not equivalent to that of costal cartilage (**Fig. 3**).

Nasal Tip Surgery

Surgery of the African American tip is challenging because structural grafting is needed to

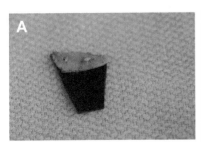

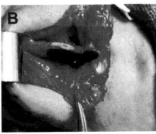

Fig. 3. (*A*) Combined septal extension/columellar strut graft can be carved from cartilage and tapered as necessary. This has been sutured to a PDS plate. (*B*) The graft with PDS plate is now sutured to the caudal septum.

compensate for the thick and inelastic nature of the skin. The nasal tip requires increased projection and definition. Judicious thinning of the nasal SMAS can be performed. Care must be taken to prevent injury to the skin vasculature in the subdermal plexus.[16]

Cephalic trim of the lower lateral crura may be performed. The authors preserve approximately 8 mm of the lower lateral cartilage to maintain nasal support. The vestibular tissue may be carefully dissected off from the undersurface of the cartilage to maintain the natural curvature of the lower lateral crura. This maneuver can help increase tip projection as it releases the constraints of the soft tissue envelope on the cartilages.

A combination septal extension graft and columellar strut is created using either costal or septal cartilage. This is then sutured to the caudal aspect of the septum using 5-0 PDS sutures. Design of this graft (either tapering superiorly or tapering inferiorly) can also allow for lengthening of the nose and rotation or counter-rotation. This can be reinforced bilaterally with pieces of PDS plate, which can help with structural support and prevent deviation.

Next, the medial crura are sutured to the combination septal extension graft/columellar strut with a 4-0 chromic gut suture to set the tip projection. Tip sutures, including intradomal sutures, transdomal sutures, three-quarters transdomal sutures, and interdomal sutures, can all be used to help with tip refinement. The authors' preferred suture is a 5-0 PDS suture with knots buried when possible. A lateral crural steal can allow for advancement of the lateral crura onto the medial crura and can increase nasal tip projection.[17]

Additional grafts may modify tip projection and rotation, including shield, domal, tip, and infratip lobular grafts. Multiple layers of grafts may be needed to compensate for the thick skin. One advantage, however, is that with thicker skin, layered grafts are more easily camouflaged. These grafts can also be effectively used to improve supratip and infratip breaks. Should the graft edges be visible, the cartilage can be morselized and, in addition, rib perichondrium, deep temporalis fascia, or previously resected nasal SMAS can be placed over the tip complex to camouflage the visibility of the graft edges (**Fig. 4**).

Osteotomies

Many African American patients have low nasal bones; therefore, osteotomies are difficult to perform. If asymmetric and indicated, high-low-low lateral osteotomies with infracturing or

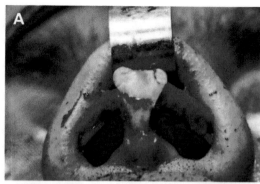
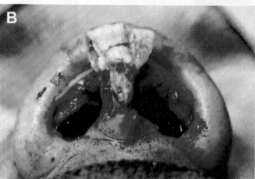

Fig. 4. (*A*) Grafts, such as shield grafts (or tip, domal, infratip lobule grafts) can be sutured in place. (*B*) Rib perichondrium is secured to the shield graft to camouflage the visibility of graft edges.

in conjunction with fading medial osteotomies are performed. Generally, dorsal augmentation rather than osteotomies are used for creating the appearance of nasal narrowing. In 5% of African Americans, there may be a hump that requires removal, and in these patients, osteotomies may be needed to close an open roof deformity.

Radix and Dorsal Augmentation

Dorsal augmentation can be achieved using a combination of septal, conchal, and costal cartilage rather than with allogenous grafts. Historically, en bloc cartilage grafts placed over the dorsum have often been used for augmentation. They may be associated, however, with an unnatural appearance or warping over time.[18]

Thus, a diced cartilage wrapped in fascia (DCF) is the authors' preferred method of dorsal augmentation.[19] It is constructed by placing finely diced cartilage within a sheath made from deep temporalis fascia. The deep temporalis fascia is first sewn around a 1-mL syringe. Subsequently a syringe filled with finely diced cartilage is inserted inside the sewn fascia and the appropriate amount, regarding the amount of dorsal augmentation desired, is injected in. The fascia is sutured with a running locking 5-0 Vicryl suture (Ethicon Inc) and greased with bacitracin to allow for easier passing of the suture. The newly created DCF can then be placed on the dorsum to check for the height of the implant and to decide whether the cartilage inside is sufficient. To allow for a supratip break, the cartilage within the DCF should not extend beyond the supratip. This can be achieved with a DCF that ends at the supratip or one that extends beyond the supratip but only filled with cartilage to the supratip and sewn across to prevent cartilage migration caudally. The draped temporalis fascia beyond the supratip can be used to help camouflage tip and domal grafts (**Fig. 5**).

To ensure proper graft placement, a precise pocket of appropriate width is created over the desired area of augmentation in the subperiosteal plane to prevent migration of the implant.

Alar Flare and Base Reduction

The alar base should be assessed at the completion of all other portions of the rhinoplasty. The alae should not extend laterally beyond a line drawn from the medial canthi. Alar base procedures can help both reduce the width of the base and correct alar flaring while orienting the nostril more vertically.

These procedures can narrow the alae with or without modifying the nostril sill and floor. Sheen and Sheen[20] describe 2 commonly encountered alar base configurations in the African American nose. Type I includes a larger than ideal alar lobule with appropriately sized nostrils, whereas type II includes a larger than ideal alar lobule with larger than ideal nostrils.[20]

Classic Weir incisions can be performed for the type I configuration, whereas a combination of Weir and sill incisions extending into the vestibular skin is required for the type II configuration. Dissection is carried down to the dilator nasalis muscle. An overlying wedge of soft tissue is excised and the amount removed on both sides are compared for symmetry. Generally, a reduction of approximately 3 mm to 5 mm provides sufficient decrease in the flare (**Fig. 6**).

Although traditional teaching places the alar incision approximately 1 mm on the nasal side of the alar-facial junction, the authors think that this may create a visible scar at the cephalad alar lobule. Thus, the authors make incisions within the alar-facial junction to camouflage the full extent of the scar. Subcutaneous buried sutures of 5-0 poliglecaprone are placed to help decrease the tension on the wound. After closure of the deeper tissues, a running 6-0 polypropylene is used for the skin closure.

Postoperative Complications and Management

At the conclusion of the rhinoplasty, the nasal dorsum is dressed with a thin piece of Gelfoam (Pfizer, NY, USA), paper tape, and a silastic nasal cast. This is removed at postoperative day 7. All sutures are also removed at this time, including those at the soft tissue triangles, to prevent any notching as the area heals. At this time, the nose is retaped for 1 week.

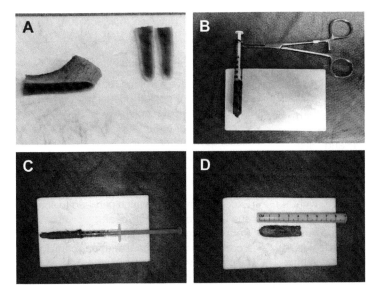

Fig. 5. (*A*) Harvested rib cartilage cut into pieces for grafting. (*B*) Suturing of a harvested piece of fascia for the DCF. (*C*) Filling the DCF with finely diced cartilage. (*D*) The DCF – an autologous dorsal implant.

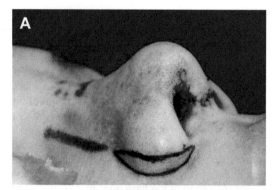

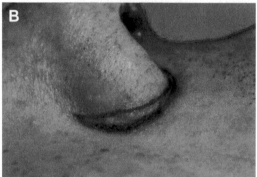

Fig. 6. (*A*) The incision does not extend into the sill for type I alar configuration. (*B*) The incision is carried into nasal sill in type II alar configuration.

Care must be taken when placing external splints and tape because even minor trauma to the skin can occasionally result in hypopigmentation or hyperpigmentation. Hyperpigmentation of the transcolumellar incision and alar base incisions themselves, however, is rarely seen. During the first week, patients are to clean incisions, use nasal saline irrigations, and place antibiotic ointment on their incisions in the same fashion as other rhinoplasty patients.

At the second week, the patients are asked to transition away from the antibiotic ointment and use Aquaphor (Eucerin) on all incisions. At the conclusion of the second week, patients are then encouraged to use a silicone scar gel with sun protection for 4 to 6 additional weeks.

Careful closure of the transcolumellar incision can alone prevent notching of the midcolumellar region. The transcolumellar incision and alar base incisions do not form keloids or hypertrophic scars. Keloid formation after auricular cartilage harvest and costal cartilage harvest, however, has been reported. This can be avoided with meticulous tension-free closure and use of silicone scar gel. These incisions should be monitored during the patients' postoperative visits to decide whether steroid injections are needed to prevent scarring.

In patients who develop prolonged swelling, nighttime taping is continued for 6 to 8 weeks. This taping is often in the location of the supratip to prevent scar buildup and a soft tissue pollybeak. To decrease early postoperative edema and prevent scar tissue buildup, subcutaneous injection of a combination of 0.3 mL of 5-fluorouracil and 0.03 mL of Kenalog (5 mg/mL) is administered; 5-fluorouracil inhibits thymidylate synthase and interferes with RNA synthesis and has been used safely in the treatment of keloids and hypertrophic scars.[21] The anti-inflammatory can prevent and treat early pollybeak deformities. This injection is commonly used for the supratip, infratip, and nasal dorsum. The injections can begin as early as 1 week after surgery and can be repeated every 1 to 2 weeks as needed.

At the first week postoperative appointment, it is important to note the position of the DCF, should that have been used for dorsal augmentation. If the DCF appears slightly deviated, it may be manipulated within the first 2 to 3 weeks and retaped. It is imperative to be extremely careful with taping and casting immediately after surgery, because this autologous implant can shift. Retaping the nose at the postoperative week 1 appointment must also be performed gently and precisely.

Postoperative photographs are taken at 3 months, 6 months, 1 year, and yearly thereafter to evaluate the nasal healing (**Fig. 7**).

PRECAUTIONS

Care must be taken prior to surgery to avoid

- Misguided expectations
- Unclear understanding of the timeline for healing
- Discrepancy between surgeon and patient goals

Care must be taken during surgery to avoid

- Overaggressive cartilage removal
- Loose implant pocket due to wide dissection in the subperiosteal plane
- Excessive alar reduction
- Nasal asymmetry
- Graft visibility at the tip

Care must be taken after surgery to avoid

- Excessive swelling, which can lead to scar tissue formation and pollybeak
- Poor healing of weir and sill incisions
- Poor healing of rib cartilage, ear cartilage, or fascia donor sites
- Sun exposure

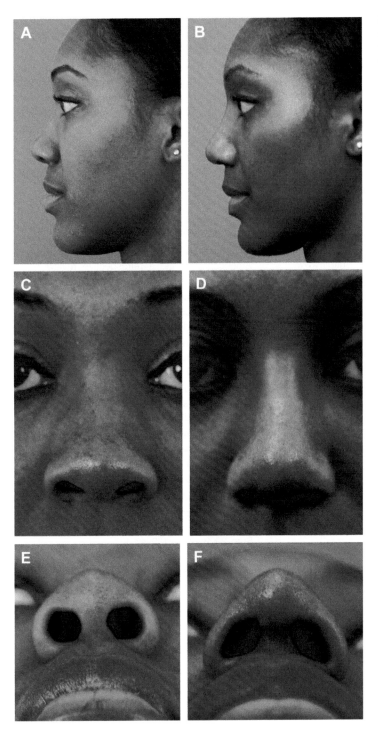

Fig. 7. Postoperative photographs (*B, D, F*) are taken and compared with preoperative photographs (*A, C, E*).

SUMMARY

To perform a rhinoplasty in African American patients, a thorough understanding of the unique anatomy and expectations of these patients is needed. In the preoperative consultation, a detailed evaluation is performed and a surgical plan is discussed with the patient. Realistic goals are established for both patient and surgeon based on a patient's cartilage structure and skin and grafts to be used. Adequate cartilage grafting can be obtained from septum, ear, or rib. The authors' preferred method for dorsal augmentation is using a DCF graft because it does not hold the risks from en bloc augmentation with cartilage, such as warping and unnatural appearance. Ultimately, African American rhinoplasty remains a challenge secondary to candidates' thick skin, weaker native nasal cartilages, and requirement for cartilage grafting to counter-rotate as well as project the nose.

REFERENCES

1. Cosmetic Surgery National Data Bank Statistics. 2012. Available at: http://www.surgery.org/sites/default/files/ASAPS-2012-Stats.pdf. Accessed June 2015.
2. American Academy of Facial Plastic Surgery 2012 membership survey. Available at: http://www.aafprs.org/wp-content/themes/aafprs/pdf/AAFPRS-2012- REPORT.pdf. Accessed May 2015.
3. Ofodile FA, James EA. Anatomy of alar cartilages in blacks. Plast Reconstr Surg 1997;100(3):699–703.
4. Ofodile FA, Bokhari F. The African-American nose: part II. Ann Plast Surg 1995;34(2):123–9.
5. Stucker FJ. Non-caucasian rhinoplasty. Trans Sect Otolaryngol Am Acad Ophthalmol Otolaryngol 1976;82(4):417–22.
6. Rohrich RJ, Muzaffar AR. Rhinoplasty in the African-American patient. Plast Reconstr Surg 2003;111(3):1322–39.
7. Berman WE. The non-caucasian (ethnic or platyrrhine) nose. Ear Nose Throat J 1995;74:747–51.
8. Ofodile FA. Nasal bones and pyriform apertures in blacks. Ann Plast Surg 1994;32(1):21–6.
9. Momoh AO, Hatef DA, Griffin A, et al. Rhinoplasty: the African American patient. Semin Plast Surg 2009;23(3):223–31.
10. Chike-Obi CJ, Boahene K, Bullocks JM, et al. Tip nuances for the nose of African descent. Facial Plast Surg 2012;28(2):194–201.
11. Porter JP. The average African American male face: an anthropometric analysis. Arch Facial Plast Surg 2004;6(2):78–81.
12. Porter JP, Olson KL. Analysis of the African American female nose. Plast Reconstr Surg 2003;111(2):620–6.
13. Boyette JR, Stucker FJ. African American rhinoplasty. Facial Plast Surg Clin North Am 2014;22:379–93.
14. Patrocinio LG, Patrocinio JA. Open rhinoplasty for African-American noses. Br J Oral Maxillofac Surg 2007;45(7):561–6.
15. Slupchynskyj O, Gieniusz M. Rhinoplasty for African American patients: a retrospective review of 75 cases. Arch Facial Plast Surg 2008;10(4):232–6.
16. Kontis TC, Papel ID. Rhinoplasty on the African-American nose. Aesthetic Plast Surg 2002;26(Suppl 1):S12.
17. Kridel RW, Konior RJ, Shumrick KA, et al. Advances in nasal tip surgery: the lateral crural steal. Arch Otolaryngol Head Neck Surg 1989;115(10):1206–12.
18. Gibson T, Davis WB. The distortion of autogenous cartilage grafts: its causes and prevention. Br J Plast Surg 1956;10:257.
19. Calvert JW, Brenner K, DaCosta-Iyer M, et al. Histological analysis of human diced cartilage grafts. Plast Reconstr Surg 2006;118(1):230–6.
20. Sheen JH, Sheen AP. Aesthetic rhinoplasty. 2nd edition. St Louis (MO): Mosby; 1978. p. 228–9.
21. Haurani M, Kenneth F, Yang JJ, et al. 5-Fluorouracil treatment of problematic scars. Plast Reconstr Surg 2009;123(1):139–48.

Rhinoplasty in the Asian Patient

Hong Ryul Jin, MD, PhD[a],*, Tae-Bin Won, MD, PhD[b]

KEYWORDS

- Rhinoplasty • Nose • Asian • Nasal tip

KEY POINTS

- For successful Asian rhinoplasty, not only specific anatomic distinctions but also cultural nuances and social framework surrounding the patient need to be considered.
- Nasal tip skin is typically thick and sebaceous, and the lower lateral cartilages and septum are paradoxically small, weak, and deficient.
- The mainstream of dorsal augmentation is using alloplast, such as silicone or expanded polytetrafluoroethylene (e-PTFE); however, tip-plasty is safely performed with autogenous cartilage.
- Septal extension graft with added onlay tip graft is the workhorse for the tip.
- Alloplast-related complications are common causes of revision rhinoplasty. Proper selection of patients, judicious use of alloplast, and the ability to manage relevant complications are important attributes in Asian rhinoplasty.

Video of an end-to-end style septal extension graft (SEG) used to modify the Asian nasal tip accompanies this article at http://www.plasticsurgery.theclinics.com/

INTRODUCTION

Rhinoplasty is one of the most common facial plastic surgeries performed in Asia. The primary objective in an Asian rhinoplasty is fundamentally the same as with all rhinoplasty patients. The goal is to sculpture a natural-looking and appealing Asian nose that goes well with the ethnic face. An attractive white nose, although maybe beautiful as a nose itself, does not harmonize with the Asian face. Anatomic characteristics of the Asian nose coupled with differences in aesthetic standards demand that they be approached in a unique way. Numerous articles have been published highlighting these different approaches and techniques.[1–4] These collectively stress that rhinoplasty among Asians includes peculiarities that distinguish the procedure from its white counterpart.

This article highlights the characteristics and techniques of different aspects of Asian rhinoplasty. Procedures performed on the nasal dorsum including dorsal augmentation and management of the nasal hump and procedures performed on the nasal tip with emphasis on tip augmentation are discussed. Finally, revision rhinoplasty in Asians is briefly addressed.

CHARACTERISTICS OF THE ASIAN NOSE AND CLINICAL IMPLICATIONS

Although there are individual variations, most Asian noses are characterized by thick skin with abundant subcutaneous fibrofatty tissue, a weak

[a] Department of Otorhinolaryngology-Head and Neck Surgery, Boramae Medical Center, Seoul National University College of Medicine, 39 Boramae Road, Dongjak-gu, Seoul 156-707, Republic of Korea; [b] Department of Otorhinolaryngology-Head and Neck Surgery, Seoul National University Hospital, Seoul, Republic of Korea
* Corresponding author.
E-mail address: doctorjin@daum.net

Clin Plastic Surg 43 (2016) 265–279
http://dx.doi.org/10.1016/j.cps.2015.09.015

cartilaginous framework, short nasal bones, underdeveloped anterior nasal spine, and small quadrilateral septal cartilage. The associated cutaneous findings include a wide and underprojected dorsum; a low radix and nasion; a nasal tip that is bulbous, lacking definition, underprojected, and either ptotic or overrotated (short nose); with a short columella and an alar base that is wide and flaring. These features are summarized in **Table 1** and depicted in **Fig. 1**.

Clinical implications of these characteristics are as follows:

- Thick skin can better tolerate alloplastic or autogenous material than thin skin. It camouflages grafts in a more natural fashion. However, it also obscures minor changes performed on the cartilaginous framework.
- Tip definition is harder to achieve in Asian noses. Delicate and weak lower lateral cartilages together with thin, weak septal cartilaginous support generally require reinforcement to obtain a desirable tip shape. Cephalic resection or pure cartilage reshaping sutures often do not work; instead, struts, grafts, and battens are needed to effectively modify the shape of the tip.
- The lack of septal cartilage frequently places the surgeon in a challenging situation because in most cases there is a need for significant amount of cartilage. Consequently, one of the primary sources of augmentation material in Asia remains alloplastic implants.
- The shorter nasal bone width with flatter nasal pyramid makes osteotomy more difficult because the path tends to follow the thicker part of the ascending process of maxilla.[5] In patients requiring large dorsal hump reductions, there is a higher chance for middle vault collapse because of short nasal bone width

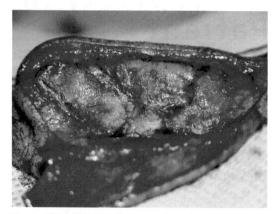

Fig. 1. The anatomy of a typical Asian nose. Note the weak cartilages, short nasal bones, and thick skin.

and length resulting in an inverted "V" deformity.[2] Because of the wide nasal valve angle and thick skin envelope, nasal obstruction caused by the internal nasal valve problems is rare in Asians.[6]

MANAGEMENT OF THE NASAL DORSUM
Dorsal Augmentation

Most Asian patients request greater dorsal height together with increase in tip projection. Prerequisites for a successful augmentation rhinoplasty include a thorough evaluation of the patient's anatomy, knowledge of the ideal shape and size of the nose within the context of cultural harmony, execution of proper surgical technique, and most importantly appropriate choice of augmentation material.

Determining the level and height of the nasion
The key in preoperative planning is determining the level and height of the nasion, which is the starting point of the nose. The difference in the starting point among different races has been extensively debated in the literature.[7] Traditionally, the supratarsal crease has been considered as the ideal starting point for whites, and the midpupillary line for Asians. However, there is a trend for contemporary Asian patients to seek a higher starting point. The authors consider the starting point in Asians to be somewhere in between the supratarsal crease and midpupillary line depending on individual preferences. The height of the nasion is usually determined by the nasofrontal angle. The ideal nasofrontal angle in Asians is around 135 for males and 140 for females.

Choice of augmentation material
The most important practical issue in dorsal augmentation is the choice of augmentation material. The amount of augmentation needed, skin thickness, and patient's age, wishes, and available

Table 1
Characteristic features of the Asian nose

Location	Characteristics
Radix	Low and inferior
Dorsum	Underprojected, short nasal bones
Tip	Underprojected, poor definition
Lower lateral cartilage	Weak, small, and pliable
Ala	Thick, flared, short columella
Skin	Thick with abundant subcutaneous fibrofatty tissue
Septum	Thinner, smaller

cartilaginous structures are a few of the factors to consider.[8–10] In addition, the surgeon should be aware of the advantages and disadvantages of each grafting material (**Table 2**). Dorsal augmentation with autologous cartilage is not dealt with in this article. However, readers are advised that the authors prefer using autologous cartilage whenever possible.

Dorsal augmentation using alloplastic implant
Although the preferred implant material in rhinoplasty is autologous cartilage, most Asian noses require substantial augmentation, which on occasion is beyond the amounts available from autologous cartilage. This realistic limitation has popularized the use of alloplastic implants in many Asian countries. The mainstay of practice is using alloplastic implant for the dorsum and autogenous grafting material for the tip. It is also the authors' personal opinion to restrict the use of alloplastic implants if needed in the nasal dorsum and use autologous materials for nasal tip to reduce the risk of extrusion or infection of the implant. When alloplastic implants are

Table 2
Advantages and disadvantages of commonly used graft materials in Asian rhinoplasty

Types of Graft Materials	Advantages	Disadvantages
Autogenous grafts		
Septal cartilage	Stable (lower absorption rates) Reliable long-term results Rare donor site morbidity Resistant to infection Ideal for various grafts	Relatively small amount in Asians Often limited in revision surgery
Conchal cartilage	Stable (low absorption rates) Resistant to infection Suitable for tip grafts, alar reconstruction	Requiring separate donor site Has curvature and pliability
Rib cartilage	Larger quantities Ideal for dorsal augmentation, septal support grafts	Risk of pneumothorax Donor site scar and pain Warping tendency
Calvarial bone	Larger quantities Useful for grafting of the upper one-third of the nose	Risk of dural or brain injury Higher rate of absorption
Temporalis fascia	Larger quantities Suitable for camouflage grafts	Requiring separate donor site
Homologous grafts		
Irradiated rib	Larger quantities Relatively biocompatible Low infection and extrusion rates	Potential disease transmission Higher rate of absorption Warping tendency
Alloderm	Larger quantities Relatively biocompatible Compensation for irregularities Suitable for covering graft edges	Potential disease transmission Higher rate of absorption
Synthetic allografts		
Expanded polytetrafluoroethylene (Gore-Tex)	Relatively biocompatible Soft/sculptable Useful for dorsal augmentation	Possible infection and rejection Not suitable for structural support
Porous high-density polyethylene	Relatively biocompatible Sculptable Useful for spreader grafts, columellar strut	Possible infection and rejection Difficult to remove Too rigid
Silicone (solid form)	Ease of use Sculptable Easily removed in revision Suitable for dorsal augmentation	Possible infection and rejection Capsule formation No tissue ingrowth

(*Adapted from* Jin HR, Won TB. Recent advances in Asian rhinoplasty. Auris Nasus Larynx 2011;38(2):157–64.)

considered, the benefits and risks should be explained to the patient before the surgery.

There is a wide array of alloplastic materials available for rhinoplastic use. These include silicone, expanded polytetrafluoroethylene (e-PTFE), and high-density porous polyethylene implant (**Fig. 2**). Thus far, which material is best remains a controversial issue.

Procedural approach

Before local infiltration, the cephalic limit of the implant or graft pocket is marked. Next, the pocket where the implant will sit is outlined. The prefabricated silicone or e-PTFE implants can be shaped with a 15-blade preoperatively and then sterilized for insertion, or can be shaped intraoperatively. In cases of isolated dorsal augmentation, an intercartilaginous incision is made and extended into a partial transfixion incision along the upper caudal end of the septal cartilage. When tip surgery is combined, an infracartilaginous incision with extension into the medial crus is used. The supraperichondrial plane over the upper lateral cartilage is dissected, exposing the nasal pyramid. The periosteum is incised and elevated to the marked new nasion level. It is important to make a pocket where the implant can fit snugly. The nasal implant is inserted into the pocket and adjusted as necessary (**Fig. 3**, Video 1).

Avoiding complications using alloplastic implants

Alloplastic implants used to augment the dorsum are associated with several complications. The most common ones include deviation of the implant, infection, extrusion, mobility of the implant, and visibility of the implant.

To avoid deviation or migration (cephalic or caudal) of the implant, it is important to raise a symmetric pocket for implant insertion. For beginners, bilateral intercartilaginous or infracartilaginous incisions and dissection is recommended to prevent unilateral deviation of the implant. It is usually helpful to make the pocket a little bigger than the implant so that the implant can snugly fit into the pocket and minimize the chances of displacement. Creation of an oversized pocket can result in shifting or displacement of the implant. It is also important to mark the starting point of the nose in the radix area and refrain from overdissection beyond this point because it can cause unwanted cephalic migration especially with silicone implants (**Fig. 4**). It is necessary to fix the implant in the desired location by suturing it to the surrounding tissue in an open approach. Making a few small holes on the implant helps to prevent caudal migration by fibrous ingrowth into the holes (**Fig. 5**).

To avoid infection, cautious handing of the implant and strict adherence to intraoperative aseptic techniques and postoperative care is essential. We usually prepare the nose with cotton balls soaked in betadine solution, and irrigate the nose frequently with antibiotic solution. The implant is handled aseptically with new gloves and inserted after soaking them in antibiotic solution. Postoperative broad-spectrum antibiotics are given for 2 weeks.

Insertion in the proper subperiosteal plane is important to avoid mobility of the implant, decrease visibility, and reduce the chance of infection because the periosteum can act as a natural barrier. The chance of extrusion is greatly enhanced if the resulting tension on the nose is increased and when the implant is located on the more mobile portion of the nose, such as the nasal tip. Therefore excessive augmentation and using implants that extend to the nasal tip should be avoided.

Management of the Dorsal Hump

Nasal hump surgery is frequently regarded as a "reduction" surgery in most Western rhinoplasty

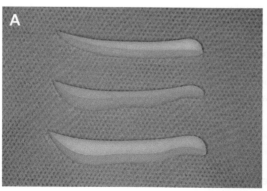
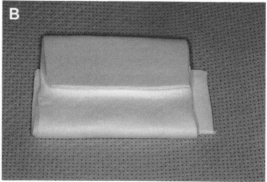

Fig. 2. The two most commonly used alloplastic implants for augmentation rhinoplasty in Asians are I-shaped silicone implant (*A*) and expanded e-PTFE implant as a sheet form (*B*).

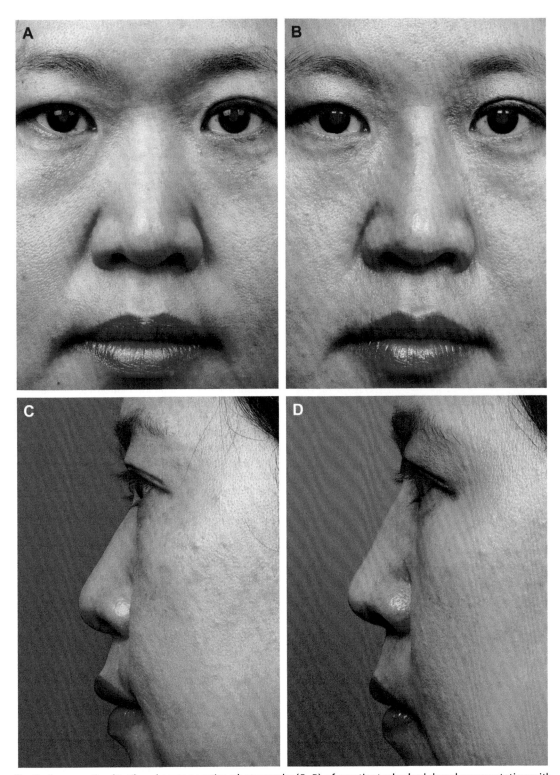

Fig. 3. Preoperative (*A, C*) and postoperative photographs (*B, D*) of a patient who had dorsal augmentation with I-shaped silicone implant. Tip augmentation was done with columellar strut and onlay grafts using septal cartilage through an endonasal approach.

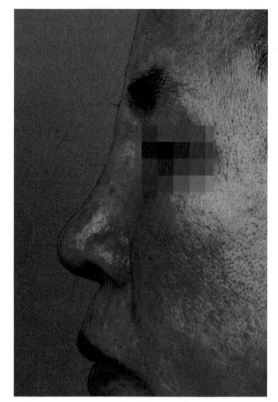

Fig. 4. Cephalic migration of a silicone implant resulted in a flat nasofrontal angle.

textbooks and is also referred as "reduction rhinoplasty." The common goal of treating a dorsal hump is to obtain a natural contour of the nasal dorsum through adequate dorsal reduction while dealing with the issues of an open roof. Although there are Asian patients who have large humps, most Asian dorsums differs from their Western counterpart in that the size of the nasal hump is limited, and is frequently associated with a low radix and underprojection or underrotation of the

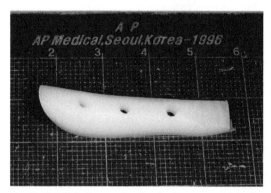

Fig. 5. Small holes on the implant were made with skin biopsy puncher. Fibrous tissue ingrowth into these holes prevents migration of the implant.

nasal tip. Naturally, correcting a nasal hump in Asians has distinct differences in concept and technique. A small hump and additional need for radix augmentation of the dorsum and the tip often minimize the amount of hump removal or sometimes obviate resection itself. Therefore "profiloplasty" instead of "reduction rhinoplasty" might be a more suitable word when dealing with Asian dorsal humps.

Many techniques have been introduced including en bloc resection, component resection, and Skoog dorsal resection.[11–14] In the classic "composite en-bloc" resection of the hump, components of the hump (bone, dorsal septum, and both upper lateral cartilages) are removed all together (en bloc) leaving an open roof. The use of bilateral spreader grafts after removal of substantial amount of hump cannot be stressed enough. Supporting and reinforcing the rhinion (keystone) with spreader grafts to prevent an inverted V deformity is specially important in Asians who have short nasal bones.[15]

For the relatively small dorsal hump, simple bony rasping with minor trimming of the dorsal septal cartilage is usually sufficient to achieve the desired dorsal height or obtain the platform for further dorsal augmentation. Using a small straight osteotome instead of the larger Rubin osteotome followed by incremental rasping with a small or powered rasp under direct visualization is helpful. Bony humpectomy reveals the overlapping cartilaginous vault underneath and precise reduction of the cartilaginous vault can follow. The author uses the term "conservative" humpectomy, and it is used in most small or isolated dorsal humps in Asian patients. Subsequent dorsal augmentation with onlay grafts cephalic and/or caudal to the hump in combination with tip surgery contributes to the successful use of conservative hump removal (**Fig. 6**).

Although the overlapping upper lateral cartilage is visible underneath the nasal bones in the rhinion, there is rarely an open roof deformity obviating lateral osteotomies. Another reason that lateral osteotomy is not frequently performed is because further radix and dorsal augmentation camouflage the wide nasal base. Small amount of resection of the cartilaginous hump decreases the need for spreader grafts and rarely violates the nasal mucosa, which can reduce the risk of infection when using alloplastic implants for dorsal augmentation.

The final touch of Asian hump rhinoplasty is dorsal augmentation. Dorsal augmentation is performed to achieve the desired height of the dorsum and camouflage any remaining irregularities. This can be in the form of radix augmentation or radix and dorsal augmentation (**Fig. 7**). The latter has

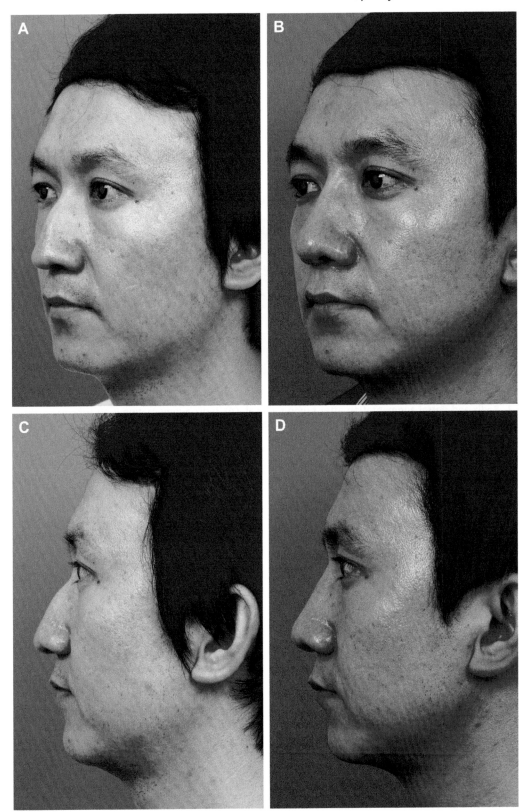

Fig. 6. Conservative humpectomy with radix and tip augmentation. (*A, C*) Preoperatively photographs show a mild hump, low radix, and slightly underprojected tip. (*B, D*) One-year postoperative photographs show smooth dorsal profile, elevated radix, and more harmonious tip shape.

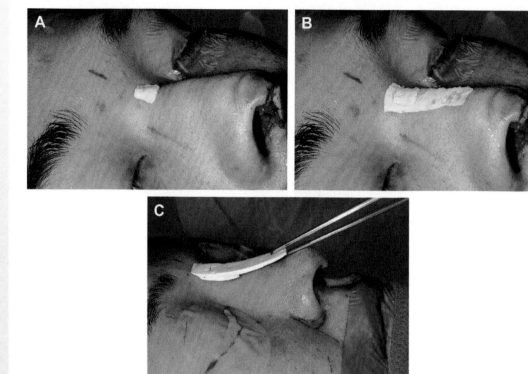

Fig. 7. Radix and dorsal augmentation after hump removal. (*A*) Radix augmentation with soft tissue. (*B*) Radix and dorsal augmentation with perichondrium. (*C*) Dorsal augmentation with e-PTFE.

the advantage of a smooth and gapless transition in the thin-skinned rhinion area. Careful palpation with wet gloves is important for detecting irregularities after humpectomy. When performing radix augmentation, we try to avoid using solid cartilage grafts because they are prone to be visible. We prefer soft tissue grafting material, such as fascia (autologous or homologous) or e-PTFE. When more augmentation is needed, crushed cartilage is inserted below the soft tissue graft.

When the desired dorsal height exceeds the height of the hump there is a choice of leaving it alone or augmentation performed on top of it. The author prefers to perform hump reduction to smoothen the dorsum before augmentation. The amount of resection in this situation depends on the material used for dorsal augmentation. When silicone is used, the undersurface of the implant corresponding to the rhinion area can be carved away thereby camouflaging small residual convexity. For other grafting materials, such as cartilage, e-PTFE, and homologous fascia, complete humpectomy is performed to reduce the chance of an irregular dorsum and/or residual convexity.

MANAGEMENT OF THE NASAL TIP

Projection, rotation, and volume are the three most important factors to consider in tip rhinoplasty in

Asian patients. The projection of the nasal tip must be in harmony with the augmented dorsum. Furthermore, a gentle round shape is preferable to a well-defined, angulated tip.

The main goal of tip rhinoplasty in the Asian patient is to obtain better projection, rotation, definition, aesthetically pleasing width, and minimal flare at the nostrils while maintaining symmetry. One important point that should be kept in mind is that many Asian patients request an increase in tip projection while maintaining or even decreasing tip rotation. The amount of projection and rotation differ according to personal preference, age, sex, occupation, and overall facial features. In general, because the dorsum of Asians is low most undergo augmentation; therefore, the amount of tip projection should be balanced accordingly. Nasal tip width should always be evaluated in the context of other facial anatomy and not as an isolated feature. If the face is relatively wide, a narrow tip can appear conspicuous and operated.

Tip Augmentation (Controlling Projection and Rotation)

Augmenting the Asian nasal tip is more challenging because the fragile cartilage has to be stabilized to a degree that it can withstand the gravitational and contractile forces of the thick skin soft tissue envelope (SSTE). Therefore, common tip surgery techniques, such as cartilage reshaping sutures or cephalic resection, often yield inconsistent and incomplete results.[16] Instead, tip projection and rotation are more effectively modified using structural grafts. The choice of maneuvers to augment the nasal tip depends on two factors: degree of tip support and amount of projection needed to achieve the final outcome.[3]

For the typical Asian patient with weak tip support, augmentation is usually accomplished in two steps. The first step is stabilization of the nasal tip. This step is the most important and key step in Asian tip rhinoplasty. The objective is to establish a firm foundation on which further grafting can be performed. Stabilization of the nasal tip is achieved either by a columellar strut or a septal extension graft (SEG). Of the two, the SEG is by far the more powerful tool that can be used reliably in patients who have very weak tip support and/or need substantial increase in tip projection. It can alter projection and control rotation simultaneously. The second step is fine sculpturing of the nasal tip. This is done by combining sutures and a variety of grafts to obtain the desired outcome (**Fig. 8**).

The septal extension graft

We emphasize the SEG because we believe that it is a workhorse for tip rhinoplasty in the Asian nose. Not only does it provide a firm foundation on which the lower lateral cartilages can be repositioned, but it can control tip projection, rotation, and nasal length simultaneously. By varying its shape and location, it is efficiently used to augment, rotate/counterrotate, lengthen the nose, and/or correct the nasolabial angle.[4]

There are different ways of executing the SEG and it depends on the underlying deformity, desired outcome, surgeon's preference, strength

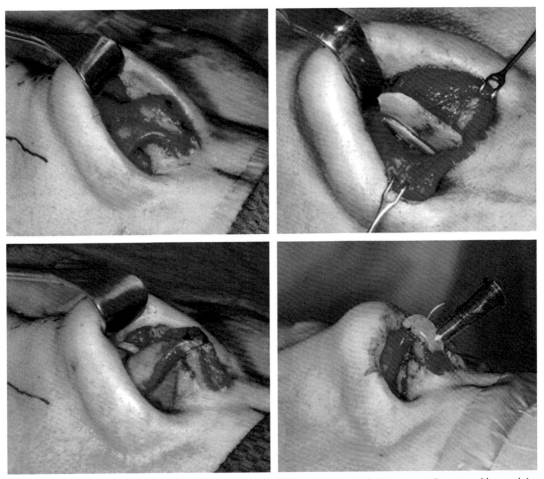

Fig. 8. Asian tip rhinoplasty using septal extension graft (clockwise rotation). Tip support is restored by applying a septal extension graft and repositioning the lower lateral cartilages. Fine sculpting is done with additional onlay tip grafts. (*From* Won TB, Jin HR. Nuances with the Asian tip. Facial Plast Surg 2012;28(2):187–93.)

of the cartilage, integrity of the caudal septum, and the amount of available grafting material.[17–19] It can be placed on the anterior nasal spine, integrated to an extended columellar strut, overlapped to the caudal septum (unilaterally or bilaterally), or secured in an end-to-end fashion to the caudal septum. It can also be sculpted in different shapes and sizes, depending on the desired changes of the tip. The septal cartilage is the preferred grafting material but in depleted cases the costal cartilage can be used as an alternative source.

Procedural approach

Usually the SEG is performed unilaterally overlapping the caudal septum by at least 5 mm or more (see Video 1). Care is taken to bevel or thin this portion of the graft overlapping the septal cartilage because nasal obstruction can occur postoperatively from increased thickness in this area. If the caudal septum is deviated, it is important to straighten it first so that the extended portion of the graft lies in the midline. Occasionally, the SEG is used as a batten to straighten the deviated caudal septum and augment the tip projection simultaneously. The caudal septum to which the SEG is fixed must be stable and strong enough to withstand the pressure exerted by the thick overlying SSTE characteristic of the Asian nose and predictably maintain projection. Deviation of the SEG can lead to the deviation of the nasal tip especially if the caudal septal support is weak. In cases where the caudal septum is weak, the SEG can be also secured to the anterior nasal spine, batten grafts, and/or extended spreader grafts (**Fig. 9**).

Once the SEG is securely positioned in the midline, the lower lateral cartilages are repositioned by suturing it to the SEG. In cases where

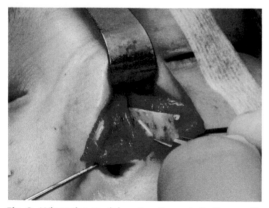

Fig. 9. When the caudal septum is weak, batten grafts with septal cartilage or bone can further stabilize the septal extension graft.

substantial augmentation is needed or when lengthening of the nose is involved, it is important to release the lower lateral cartilages as much as possible to reduce the tension exerted on the SEG–caudal septum complex and minimize distortion of the lower lateral cartilages. This is achieved by thorough dissection of the lower lateral cartilages laterally to the pyriform aperture and cephalically releasing the scroll area adjacent to the upper lateral cartilages.

When the SEG is applied, the nasal tip tends to become stiff and even though it softens with time, it can be a source of postoperative complaint. We consider this added stiffness an acceptable trade-off for achieving desirable tip projection and patients should be warned of this change preoperatively if a SEG is considered.

Managing the Bulbous Asian Tip (Decreasing Volume and Increasing Definition)

Bulbous nose is a term used to describe the shape of the nasal tip where it resembles a ball. The common features of a bulbous tip include rounded shape, broad or absent tip defining point, poor definition, and increased sense of volume. Although the final shape of the nose is similar, the causative factor that gives rise to this peculiar shape of the tip is not uniform. Thick SSTE and the character of the alar cartilages, namely the size, shape, strength, and orientation, are the principal causative factors. The contribution of each varies within individual patients. Because of this diversity, there have been limited attempts to try to classify the bulbous nose.[20] Techniques to manage a bulbous nose are targeted to correct the underlying causative factors.[21] Procedures targeted to the alar cartilage include reorientation and volume reduction of alar cartilages. Diverse suture techniques and/or grafts are used for the reorientation, and excision techniques are used for the volume reduction. Managing the thick skin is challenging and has limitations. Soft tissue trimming is the most commonly performed procedure (**Fig. 10**). We usually limit our soft tissue trimming to the deep fatty layer, taking care not to include the superficial musculoaponeurotic system layer because this can lead to excessive scar contracture and adhesions that can cause noticeable irregularities. The limitations of tissue excision are overcome or supplemented by expanding the skin envelope.

Because most Asian noses need dorsal and tip augmentation, a tip may appear less bulbous and more balanced without any modification if the dorsum and tip are augmented. An algorithm

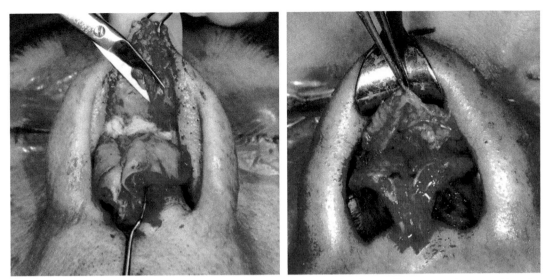

Fig. 10. Soft tissue excision can be done in situ (*left*) or after subsuperficial musculoaponeurotic system dissection (*right*). (*From* Won TB, Jin HR. Nuances with the Asian tip. Facial Plast Surg 2012;28(2):187–93.)

for the management of the bulbous nose in Asians should include all these considerations and the strategy needs to be personalized (**Fig. 11**).

REVISION RHINOPLASTY IN ASIANS

The main reasons for revision rhinoplasty in Asians often involve alloplastic implant.[22] Common indications for unsatisfactory primary rhinoplasty

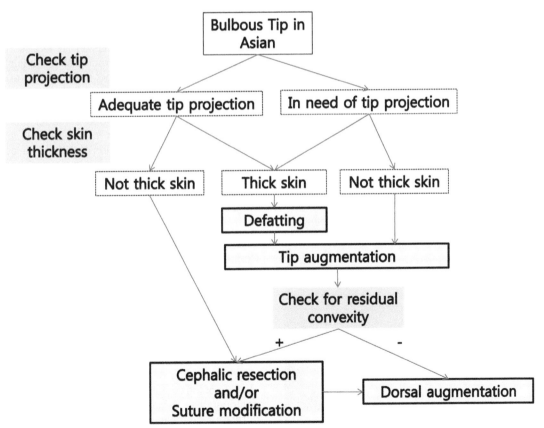

Fig. 11. A simplified algorithm for the management of the bulbous nose in Asians. (*From* Won TB, Jin HR. Nuances with the Asian tip. Facial Plast Surg 2012;28(2):187–93.)

outcome are as follows: alloplast-related complications, such as deviation, extrusion, and infection; short, contracted nose after multiple surgeries; dorsal deviation/irregularity; and tip problems related with SEG.

Alloplast-Related Complication

Although alloplast-related complications are endless, typical examples are deviation, extrusion, infection, foreign body reactions, unnatural or operated appearance, and compromised SSTE. Proper selection of patients, adherence to operative techniques that help avoid common complications associated with alloplastic implants (discussed previously), and the ability to manage complications when they occur are important attributes in Asian rhinoplasty.

Infections with alloplastic implants may occur immediately or even years after surgery (**Fig. 12**).[23–26] Although aggressive antibiotic therapy is always initiated, the implant almost always needs to be removed, especially in cases of e-PTFE.[24,26] The major dilemma in cases of an infected implant is the timing of the definitive revision rhinoplasty after its removal. Currently, the mainstay of treatment in most clinics in Asia is a staged approach with removal of the alloplast and subsequent revision operation after

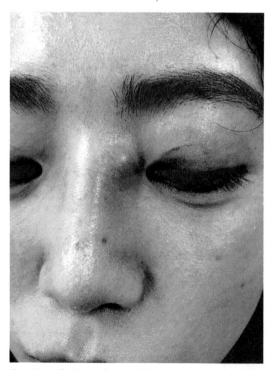

Fig. 12. Infection after e-PTFE augmentation of the dorsum. Purulence is seen at the left sidewall near the radix.

the inflammation has subsided. Although this staged approach can provide a more sterile environment for the subsequent revision surgery, delaying surgery in a patient with nasal disfigurement is a cause of frustration for the already unhappy patient. Furthermore, contracture of the overlying skin can occur, which is a greater challenge in correction.[27] In a recent study, we have shown that immediate reconstruction using autologous cartilage after removal of an infected alloplast is associated with a favorable outcome with minimal chances of infection and resoprtion.[28]

Short, Contracted Nose

A short, contracted nose is also a common complication. It is a devastating complication usually associated with repeated surgeries and alloplastic material in dorsal and tip augmentation. The pathogenesis is unknown but capsular contraction around the implant, lower lateral cartilage necrosis by long-term pressure from implants, chronic inflammation, and scar contraction from multiple rhinoplasties are thought to be possible etiologies. As the contraction progresses, the soft nasal tip gets constricted and a so-called snub nose develops (**Fig. 13**).

For correction, caudal rotation of the tip with superior movement of the nasion is necessary. Wide undermining of the contracted skin, readjusting the lower lateral cartilage on the SEG, and additional onlay tip grafts are key technical points for caudal rotation of the tip. A firm structural support of the SEG using extended spreader grafts and conchal composite graft in the vestibule are needed to overcome the tension of stiff and inelastic skin with deficient vestibular mucosa. Dorsal onlay graft to fill the dorsal defect after removal of the alloplast also helps to make the nose appear longer (**Fig. 14**).

Dorsal Deviation and Irregularity

Common postoperative dorsal problems include residual/iatrogenic deviations of the nasal dorsum, dorsal irregularity or depression, and a visible cartilaginous or alloplastic graft. Postoperative residual dorsal deviation is mostly caused by failure to recognize or correct the pre-existing deviation. Improper osteotomy with or without adequate correction of septal deviation is the most common cause. Deviation of the dorsal graft/implant and warping of the costal cartilage graft can also cause postoperative deviation. Complete realignment or restoration measures of the bone and cartilaginous structures is required to create more symmetry. If residual deviation remains after all these

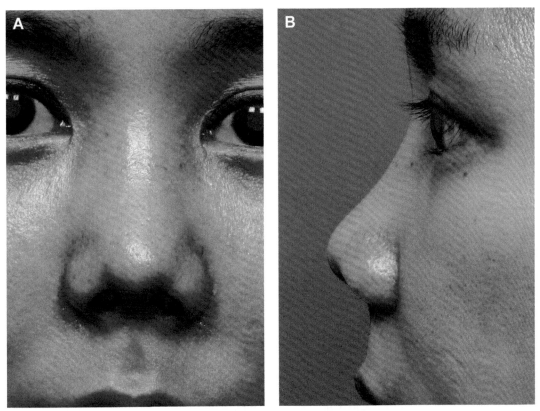

Fig. 13. (*A, B*) Severely short and contracted nose after multiple rhinoplasties.

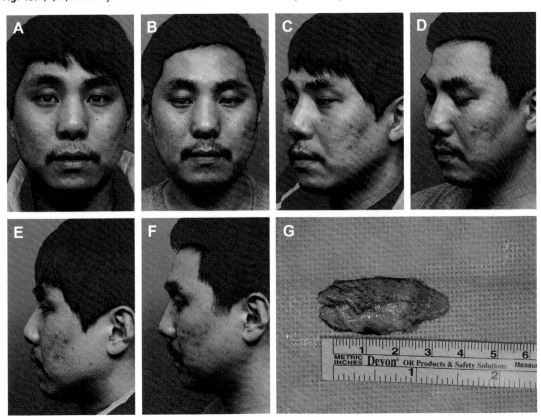

Fig. 14. Preoperative (*A, C, E*) views of a short and contracted nose following augmentation rhinoplasty with porous high-density polyethylene (*G*). One-year postoperative photographs (*B, D, F*) showing improved nasal shape.

measures, camouflage grafts are applied to make the nose look symmetric and straight.

A supratip depression or fullness after alloplastic dorsal augmentation is not uncommon. Careful design of the implant and fine adjustment with soft tissue or cartilage onlay graft at the supratip area may be necessary. Radix irregularity after hump removal is more common when the radix is augmented with cartilage rather than alloplast. To avoid this, radix graft should be bruised and/or placed with soft tissue coverage in a small pocket. Mastoid periosteum provides a good material to smoothly elevate the radix area.

Tip Problems Related with Septal Extension Graft

Tip problems include underprojection (or loss of) or overprojection, overrotated tip, visible or protruding grafts, tip deviation/asymmetry, and pain or severe pressure sensation. Recent increase of SEG for tip surgery in Asian rhinoplasty has resulted in many complications, such as overly aggressive tip projection (Pinocchio nose), pain/dullness, deviated/asymmetric tip, and nasal obstruction caused by caudal septal deviation. Overly aggressive tip projection using septal bone or Medpor beyond tissue's acceptance is the main cause for continuous pain, tenderness, and pressure sense of the tip. Careful history

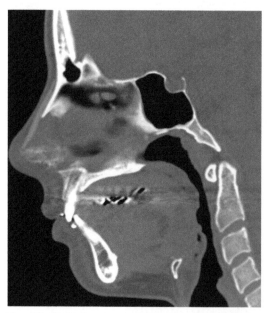

Fig. 15. Sagittal computed tomography scan of a patient complaining of nasal tip pain, tenderness, and hardness. Dorsal silicone implant and suspicious bone at the caudal septal area used as septal extension graft are observed.

taking and detailed examination including computed tomography scan often reveal excessive projection of the tip by the septal bone or Medpor as the possible cause (**Fig. 15**). Removing the stiff materials and reconstructing proper projection with cartilage is the best solution.

Inadequate stabilization of the overlapping SEG in the midline is the main reason for tip deviation, nostril asymmetry, and deviation of the caudal septum with nasal obstruction. Stable fixation of the SEG in the midline and symmetric restoration of the lower lateral cartilage on the new dome is most important to prevent these complications. This often requires securely suturing the graft to the anterior nasal spine and positioning the end into the midline in overlapping type of SEG. In end-to-end-type SEG, it needs reinforcement with the extended spreader graft.

SUMMARY

Although the main principles of various rhinoplasty techniques apply equally to the Asian nose, some modifications are inevitable caused by anatomic and aesthetic differences. Understanding these differences and mastering the techniques unique to the Asian nose based on the general principles of rhinoplasty lead to a successful outcome. These differences can only be recognized with continuous exposure to Asian rhinoplasty and sustained efforts to compare the differences between the two practices.

SUPPLEMENTARY DATA

Supplementary data related to this article are found online at http://dx.doi.org/10.1016/j.cps.2015.09.015.

REFERENCES

1. Toriumi DM, Swartout B. Asian rhinoplasty. Facial Plast Surg Clin North Am 2007;15:293–307.
2. Jin HR, Won TB. Nasal hump removal in Asians. Acta Otolaryngol Suppl 2007;558:95–101.
3. Jin HR, Won TB. Nasal tip augmentation in Asians using autogenous cartilage. Otolaryngol Head Neck Surg 2009;140:526–30.
4. Won TB, Jin HR. Nuances with the Asian tip. Facial Plast Surg 2012;28(2):187–93.
5. Lee HM, Kang HJ, Choi JH, et al. Rationale for osteotome selection in rhinoplasty. J Laryngol Otol 2002;116(12):1005–8.
6. Suh MW, Jin HR, Kim JW. Computed tomography versus nasal endoscopy for the measurement of the nasal valve angle in Asians. Acta Otolaryngol 2008;128(6):675–9.

7. Jin HR, Won TB. Recent advances in Asian rhinoplasty. Auris Nasus Larynx 2011;38(2):157–64.

8. Ahn JM, Honrado C, Horn C. Combined silicone and cartilage implants: augmentation rhinoplasty in Asian patients. Arch Facial Plast Surg 2004;6(2): 120–3.

9. Ahn JM. The current trend in augmentation rhinoplasty. Facial Plast Surg 2006;22(1):61–9.

10. McCurdy JA Jr. Considerations in Asian cosmetic surgery. Facial Plast Surg Clin North Am 2007; 15(3):387–97.

11. Ishida J, Ishida LC, Ishida LH, et al. Treatment of the nasal hump with preservation of the cartilaginous framework. Plast Reconstr Surg 1999;103(6): 1729–33.

12. Rohrich RJ, Muzaffar AR, Janis JE. Component dorsal hump reduction: the importance of maintaining dorsal aesthetic lines in rhinoplasty. Plast Reconstr Surg 2004;114(5):1298–308.

13. Skoog T. A method of hump reduction in rhinoplasty: a technique for preservation of the nasal roof. Arch Otolaryngol 1966;83:283–7.

14. Hall JA, Peters MD, Hilger PA. Modification of the Skoog dorsal reduction for preservation of the middle nasal vault. Arch Facial Plast Surg 2004;6: 105–10.

15. Sheen JH. Spreader graft: a method of reconstructing the roof of the middle nasal vault following rhinoplasty. Plast Reconstr Surg 1984; 73:230–9.

16. Jang TY, Choi YS, Jung YG, et al. Effect of nasal tip surgery on Asian noses using the transdomal suture technique. Aesthetic Plast Surg 2007;31: 174–8.

17. Ha RY, Byrd HS. Septal extension grafts revisited: 6-year experience in controlling nasal tip projection and shape. Plast Reconstr Surg 2003;112: 1929–35.

18. Toriumi DM. New concepts in nasal tip contouring. Arch Facial Plast Surg 2006;8:156–85.

19. Kang JG, Ryu J. Nasal tip surgery using a modified septal extension graft by means of extended marginal incision. Plast Reconstr Surg 2009;123: 343–52.

20. Rohrich RJ, Adams WP Jr. The boxy nasal tip: classification and management based on alar cartilage suturing techniques. Plast Reconstr Surg 2001;107: 1849–63.

21. Constantian MB. The boxy nasal tip, the ball tip, and alar cartilage malposition: variations on a theme-a study in 200 consecutive primary and secondary rhinoplasty patients. Plast Reconstr Surg 2005;116: 268–81.

22. Won TB, Jin HR. Revision rhinoplasty in Asians. Ann Plast Surg 2010;65(4):379.

23. Endo T, Nakayama Y, Ito Y. Augmentation rhinoplasty: observations on 1,200 cases. Plast Reconstr Surg 1991;87:54–9.

24. Mendelsohn M, Dunlop G. Gore-Tex augmentation grafting in rhinoplasty-is it safe? J Otolaryngol 1998;27:337–41.

25. Rothstein SG, Jacobs JB. The use of Gore-Tex implants in nasal augmentation operations. Entechnology 1989;68:40–5.

26. Jin HR, Lee JY, Yeon JY, et al. A multicenter evaluation of the safety of Gore-Tex as an implant in Asian rhinoplasty. Am J Rhinol 2006;20(6):615–9.

27. Jung DH, Moon HJ, Choi SH, et al. Secondary rhinoplasty of the Asian nose: correction of the contracted nose. Aesthetic Plast Surg 2004;28: 1–7.

28. Won TB, Jin HR. Immediate reconstruction with autologous cartilage after removal of infected alloplast in revision rhinoplasty. Otolaryngol Head Neck Surg 2012;147(6):1054–9.

Rhinoplasty in Middle Eastern Patients

Ali Sajjadian, MD

KEYWORDS

- Middle Eastern rhinoplasty • Rhinoplasty • Ethnic rhinoplasty • Nasal tip contouring

KEY POINTS

- Facial and racial congruity should be preserved by recognizing the features that are common in Middle Eastern rhinoplasty patients. Understanding of the maneuvers and techniques that lead to predictable result can prevent unnatural or an overoperated nose.
- For every Middle Eastern patient undergoing rhinoplasty, the measure of success is the ability to shape the nose into more pleasing proportions while maintaining the structure and improving nasal function.
- Detailed analysis and knowledge of structural differences among various ethnic groups within Middle Eastern patients are required to ensure predictable and harmonious results.
- Racial congruity and symmetry are achieved by conservative dorsal hump reduction, modest alar base and nasal tip narrowing, and avoiding overrotation of the nasolabial angle. In addition, the visible grafts should be reserved for patients with thicker skin.

INTRODUCTION

The recent upward socioeconomic movement of ethnic (nonwhite) minorities in the United States has provided many with the opportunity to seek elective plastic surgery, and many desire rhinoplasty. Mainstreaming has also helped erase the social stigma once associated with plastic surgery procedures.

Most ethnic patients have the aesthetic goal of preserving their ethnic heritage and cultural identity. However, most wish to improve their nasal features so that their nose is more harmonious with the rest of their face. Middle Eastern patients generally do not want to lose the important facial features that show their racial character and congruity.

Comprehensive knowledge of the nasal anatomy and familiarity with the nasal and facial features common in the Middle Eastern nose allow the surgeon to anticipate and prepare for the challenges. Properly choosing the surgical techniques, along with a realistic appreciation of the limits imposed by the particular ethnic skin quality and the underlying framework architecture, should allow the surgeon to achieve a predictably favorable outcome and a satisfied patient.

"Middle Eastern" often refers to individuals of Persian, Arabic, Turkish, and North African descent. One can consider broad categories to be (1) the Gulf countries (Iran, Saudi Arabia, Kuwait, Qatar, Bahrain, and United Arab Emirates), (2) the North African countries (Egypt, Libya, Algeria, and Morocco), (3) regional groups (Lebanon, Afghanistan, Syria, Turkey, Greece, and Armenia), and (4) the near Asia countries (India and Pakistan).

Rhinoplasty is the most difficult of all plastic surgery procedures, and there are particular challenges when treating the Middle Eastern or any "ethnic" nose, as opposed to the white nose.

Disclosures: None.
Funding Sources: None.
Conflict of Interest: None.
Department of Plastic Surgery, Hoag Hospital, 496 Old Newport Boulevard, Newport Beach, CA 92663, USA
E-mail address: drsajjadian@gmail.com

Clin Plastic Surg 43 (2016) 281–294
http://dx.doi.org/10.1016/j.cps.2015.09.020

Although there is a large spectrum of variability in the Middle Eastern nose, there are some common characteristics and features, which are reviewed in detail. This article also specifically addresses the challenges presented by Middle Eastern noses and the treatment options that can lead to successful outcome.

TREATMENT GOALS AND PLANNED OUTCOMES

In addition to extensive training in rhinoplasty, it is imperative that the plastic surgeon has additional training and experience in performing ethnic rhinoplasty to address the unique characteristics of the ethnic nasal anatomy. Rhinoplasty for Middle Eastern patients is a specialization. It requires great surgical skill, sensitivity, and proven results to achieve a cosmetic result that improves the nose and face while respecting and preserving the patient's ethnicity.

Many plastic surgeons have experience operating primarily on white noses and may not have experience to perform "ethnic rhinoplasty." Occasionally the standard has been for surgeons to perform rhinoplasty on all patients in exactly the same way regardless of their ethnicity. This is probably because communications media have popularized the Western look and thus it became the goal in rhinoplasty. However, this has produced noses for some ethnic patients that appear unnatural and unbalanced when compared with their other facial features and physical characteristics (racial incongruity).

The important fact to be aware of for ethnic rhinoplasty is that there is no universal standard of beauty. It is best to avoid "westernizing" the ethnic nose; one should not try to create something based on the European ideal. Every attempt should be made to create a nose that is harmonious with the individual's face and honor the cultural differences in the concept of beauty (also known as "ethnically consistent improvement").

Ideally the surgeon should fully appreciate ethnic preservation and use an ethnosensitive approach, because it is no longer a foregone conclusion that ethnic nasal features must be eliminated. Rhinoplasty in ethnic patients often requires a different approach than in white patients.

The nasal and facial proportion guidelines that plastic surgeons in North America are taught have not, traditionally, taken different ethnicities into account. When altering a white nose, rhinoplasty often removes cartilage and bone because the nose is too long, too big, or too overprojected and refinement of the nasal bridge, the tip, and possibly modification of the alar base may be needed. Although similar procedures may be used in Middle Eastern rhinoplasty, the surgeon should cultivate deep understanding of the ethnic nasal structure to provide the best possible result.

As with all groups, patients with an ethnic background have specific characteristics typical of their nasal structure and architecture. However, each patient may also require a highly individualized approach because each nose can vary dramatically. Because of the variability of soft tissue thickness and cartilage resiliency, rhinoplasty in a Middle Eastern patient may require significant alteration of the nasal framework to change the external appearance. These factors make Middle Eastern rhinoplasty challenging because they must be addressed to achieve an optimal result.

The task is to artistically sculpt the Middle Eastern nose (ideally with subtle changes when possible) to achieve facial balance and enhance each patient's natural beauty. The "triangle of beauty" around the patient's nose should blend seamlessly into the rest of the patient's facial structure. The desired result is a refined and aesthetically balanced nose, overall facial harmony, and a patient that feels more confident in their appearance. A successful surgery draws attention to a person's eyes, not nose.

The internal and nasal framework changes to the Middle Eastern nose have an impact on the function of the nose. The surgeon must take great care in maintaining open nasal airways for optimal postsurgical breathing. Nasal function should never be compromised in the interest of beauty and should always be a primary goal.

Common aesthetic deformities and areas of concern of the Middle Eastern rhinoplasty patient include the following: prominent arching dorsum; wide bony vault; long and drooping tip with narrow nasolabial angle; bulbous, large, and ill-defined tip; and nostril asymmetry.

PREOPERATIVE PLANNING AND PREPARATION

The most important part of preoperative planning and preparation for successful Middle Eastern rhinoplasty is effective communication with the patient.

Race is the genetic heritage one is born with, regardless of location; ethnicity is the learned cultural behavior of a particular group (behavior, beliefs, and values). How a person perceives their place within each of these groups affects his or her self-image and approach to cosmetic surgery. Even within the same race and culture, facial characteristics are appreciated differently. For example, a recent immigrant may have different cosmetic surgery goals than a third-generation transplant or foreign national (typically, a Middle Eastern patient born in the United States wishes to have more drastic change to the appearance of their nose). The surgeon must determine the patient's wishes before surgery and never make assumptions; it is inappropriate to assume that all of any racial/ethnic group would want a "standard" nose. It has been the author's experience that the younger Middle Eastern patients usually desire a more significant change to the appearance of their nose following rhinoplasty.

When interacting with patients of Middle Eastern origin, surgeons should provide culturally competent care, communicating without letting cultural differences hinder the conversation, but rather enhance it. This sometimes can pose a challenge because patient and surgeon bring individual patterns of language and culture to the meeting and both must be transcended to communicate effectively. The surgeon should learn about the particular ethnic culture and its approach to health care. Also, English may be a second language for these patients and an interpreter may be needed to ensure that patient-surgeon communication is accurate.

Surgeons are additionally cautioned not to impose their own aesthetic ideals, perceptions, or expectations on the patient. These conflicts with patient desires may not become apparent until after the surgery is completed, hence making the preoperative understanding of the patient's goals and desires extremely important.

Patient satisfaction is the primary goal; however, that goal must also be aesthetically and surgically realistic. In addition, the patient's desires should not result in an "operated" look. Computer imaging is useful for communicating this information and for educating the patient; it can provide examples for the patient to choose from, and a digital picture can be morphed from before to after showing the patient what is realistically possible. Computer imaging can also promote discussion of the specifics (eg, "I want a nose like this picture"), rather than generalities (eg, "I want a narrower nose"), and may prevent misunderstandings.

Some of the most challenging rhinoplasty cases are found among individuals of Middle Eastern origin. Common nasal anatomic features of the Middle Eastern nose include thick or regionally variable skin/soft tissue envelope, overprojecting osseocartilaginous vault, facial and nasal asymmetry and deviation, airway compromise, weak and asymmetric alar cartilages, and short medial crura. These can result in the following facial malformations and clinical findings: deviated, asymmetric nose; large bulbous nose; high arching dorsum; elongated nose; poorly defined drooping tip; broad bony middle vault; obtuse nasolabial and columellar-labial angle; and overall nasal asymmetry (**Figs. 1** and **2**). Schematic diagram of the typical and ideal aesthetic proportions and ratios for Middle Eastern patients is found in **Figs. 3** and **4**.

Additionally, some of the most difficult nasal tip anomalies are seen in a subgroup of Middle Eastern patients as a result of weak and nonresilient lower lateral cartilages and heavy skin–soft tissue envelope (**Figs. 5** and **6**).

Procedural Approach to Middle Eastern Rhinoplasty

It is essential that surgeons have a good understanding of the unique nasal anatomy and the effective techniques used with this group of patients. Difficulties intrinsic to the nasal anatomy among the Middle Eastern population can make surgical results less predictable and less enduring. Additionally, anatomic variations ensure that no single or standardized surgical approach works for all cases. Thus, the importance of a thorough anatomic facial and nasal analysis cannot be overstated.

Common features of the Middle Eastern nose include variable skin, asymmetric face, asymmetric nose, deviated dorsum, long upper lateral cartilages, long nasal bones, wide and asymmetric nasal vault, ptotic and asymmetric tip, and base asymmetry. On profile view these group of patients have high or normal radix, large hump, inadequate tip projection, and dependent tip and columella. On basilar view the common features of the Middle Eastern nose include tip asymmetry, tip deviation, nostril asymmetry, weak soft triangle, and short columella.

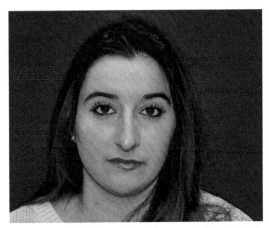

Fig. 1. Common features and characteristics of Middle Eastern nose in frontal view.

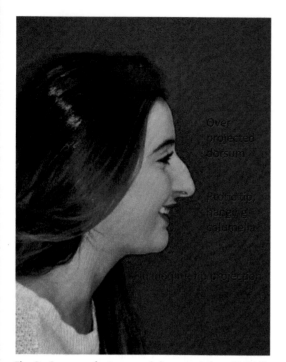

Fig. 2. Common features and characteristics of Middle Eastern nose in lateral view.

The usual treatment goals include moderate dorsum reduction as needed, narrowing of wide nasal bones, preserving and improving nasal airway, correction of alar flaring, straightening of the midvault and septum, correction of nasal asymmetry, addressing nostril-tip imbalance, and

conservative debulking of fibrofatty tissues as needed.

The common features of Middle Eastern nose and recommended surgical techniques and maneuvers are summarized in **Table 1**.

Surgical Correction

Typically the open approach rhinoplasty is used and dissection is done in a complete subperiosteal/subperichondrial plane. Minimal and conservative trimming of cephalic rim of the lower lateral cartilages is done. Component reduction of the hump is performed as needed after separating the septum from upper lateral cartilages (which are always saved and used as spreader flaps). Dorsal reduction necessitates use of spreader grafts and/or spreader flaps to close the open roof, to protect the nasal airway and internal nasal valves, and prevent inverted V deformity (see **Table 1**).

Nasal bone reshaping using lateralized medial oblique osteotomies, intermediate osteotomies (in cases of excessive width, convexity, or asymmetry of nasal bones), and lateral osteotomies are needed in most patients.

Heavy skin–soft tissue envelope is thinned judiciously and conservatively deep to the subdermal plexus layer. In addition, nasal tip should be supported and/or projected with the use of either approximation of footplates, placement of columellar graft, and/or tailored tip grafts.

Destructive excisional techniques are never used; instead, multiple suturing techniques are

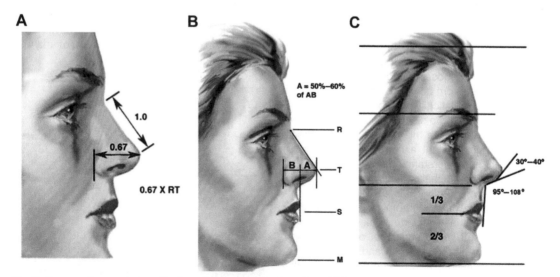

Fig. 3. Commonly accepted aesthetic ratios and proportions for Middle Eastern patients. (*A*) On lateral view the nasal tip projection should be typically 67% of the nasal length. (*B*) The segment from the upper lip to the nasal tip should commonly be equivalent to the distance from the facial-alar crease to the nasal tip. (*C*) The columellar-labial and nasolabial angles should ideally be 90° to 95°. M, menton; R, rhinion; S, stomion; T, nasal tip.

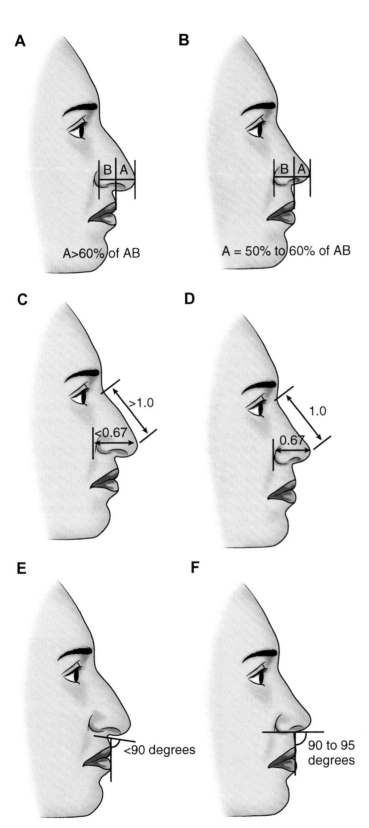

A

A>60% of AB

B

A = 50% to 60% of AB

C

>1.0
<0.67

D

1.0
0.67

E

<90 degrees

F

90 to 95 degrees

Fig. 4. Commonly found anomalies of ratios and proportions in Middle Eastern nose that need correction include: (*A*) On lateral view the nasal length is disproportionately long compared to the nasal tip projection. (*C*) The segment from the upper lip to the nasal tip is frequently greater than the distance from the facialalar crease to the nasal tip. (*E*) The colu-mellar-labial and nasolabial angles are commonly less than 90 degrees. Post-Opertatively, the improved ratios and proporations include: (*B*) On lateral view the nasal projection is corrected to be 60% of nasal length. (*D*) The segment from the upper lip to the nasal tip is frequently corrected to be equal to the distance from the facialalar crease to the nasal tip. (*F*) The columellar-labial and nasolabial angles are commonly improved to 90–95 degrees.

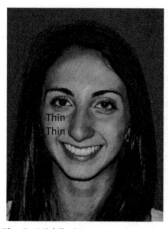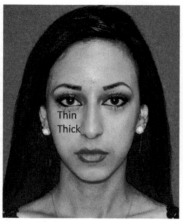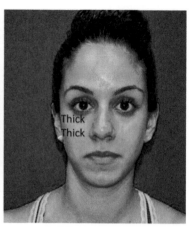

Fig. 5. Middle Eastern patients could have variable thickness of skin in different portions of the nose. It is important to closely evaluate the thickness of the skin in different regions of the nose because it dictates the techniques and determines the use of visible and invisible grafts used to obtain predictably favorable aesthetic outcome.

used to reshape the lower lateral cartilages reliably and predictably. The commonly used tip reshaping sutures include transdomal, hemitransdomal, interdomal, dome equalizing, intercrural, and lateral convexity mattress sutures.

When additional rotation of the tip is needed, depending on the anatomy and the degree of correction needed, a combination of techniques may be used. These include the previously mentioned sutures and medial crura–septal anchor sutures. In addition, removal of a triangular piece of caudal septum and occasionally reduction of membranous septum are indicated in cases of elongated nose and/or excessive columellar show.

Although intercrural sutures can improve the strength of the medial leg of the "tip tripod complex," columellar strut is used when additional support is needed. Extended columellar graft is

used commonly in cases of obtuse nasolabial angle with deficient premaxilla.

When the nasal spine is deficient, placement of columellar strut can correct the deformity. Alar rim grafts, lateral crural strut grafts, or lateral crura mattress sutures may be needed to support and improve the tip and lower lateral cartilages morphology.

Asymmetry of the lower lateral cartilages is common and requires transection and overlapping. This maneuver done unilaterally or bilaterally promotes symmetry and allows creation of more stable tripod, which permits favorable rotation of the nasal tip when indicated.

To correct the deviated nose and improve nasal function, typically a combination of a through septoplasty/septal reconstruction and individualized osteotomies are performed. When tilting of the lower part of the septum is noted, relocation of

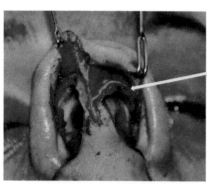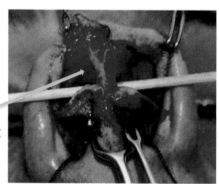

- Pliable, Non-resilient LLC
- Excess subdermal Fat

Fig. 6. Intraoperative finding in heavy skin patients revealing pliable nonresilient lower lateral cartilage (LLC) that requires grafting and suturing to increase support and strength. In addition, excessive subcutaneous fibrofatty tissues may need reduction deep to subdermal plexus to improve outcome.

Table 1
Anatomic characteristics and recommended procedures for Middle Eastern rhinoplasty

	Common Anatomic Features/Characteristics	Surgical Techniques and Maneuvers
Skin and soft tissue	Normal to thick envelope	Selective thinning of soft tissues deep to dermal plexus, use of cartilage grafts
Nostrils	Wide sills, usually asymmetric	
Septum	Usually deviated	
Nasal vault	Usually wide, sometimes normal, usually deviated	Alar base and sill modification
Radix	Normal to high, rarely low	Correct septal and nasal deviation
Dorsal hump	Commonly osteocartilagenous	Individualized ostotomies, correction of deviation, asymmetric spreader grafts
Tip morphology	Underprojected/underrotated	
Alar orientation	± Cephalic malposition	Selective reduction or augmentation
Nasal length	Excessive causing downward rotation of ala	Reduction of bony cap and creation of spreader flaps
Depressive septi	Sometimes hyperdynamic	Improve rotation and projection
Lower lateral cartilage length	Usually asymmetric and size asymmetry	Correct alar malposition
Airway compromise, septal deviation, turbinate hypertrophy, and nasal valve compromise		Caudal septal shortening
		Muscle modification
		Correct lower lateral cartilage asymmetry
		Septoplasty/septal reconstruction, submucuous turbinate reduction, and nasal valve preservation and reconstruction

From Sajjadian A. Middle eastern rhinoplasty. In: Shiffman M, Di Giuseppe A, editors. Advanced aesthetic rhinoplasty. Art, science, and new clinical techniques. Berlin; Heidelberg (Germany): Springer-Verlag; 2013. p. 188; with permission.

the septum to midline or anterior nasal spine is required. Additionally, modification and submucous reduction of concha of the enlarged inferior turbinates are performed as needed to improve the patency of the nasal airway (**Fig. 7**).

Avoiding Potential Complications in Middle Eastern Rhinoplasty

Difficulties intrinsic to the nasal anatomy among the Middle Eastern population can make surgical results less predictable and less enduring. Additionally, anatomic variations ensure that no single or standardized surgical approach works for all cases. Thus, the importance of a thorough anatomic analysis cannot be overstated.

Assumptions persist that Middle Eastern skin is thick and highly sebaceous. However, this is not true of all Middle Eastern patients; there is a great deal of variability of skin thickness depending on the origin of these patients. Those from the more northern areas (Northern Iran, Armenia, and Turkey) often have thinner lighter skin. Those from North African and Arabian ethnic groups have thicker skin, which can contribute to a bulbous appearance. Clearly, surgical plans have to take this variability into account because

treatment of patients with thick versus thinner skin is different. In thinner-skin patients invisible or soft tissue grafts are preferred to avoid visibility and bossae formation. In thicker-skin patients, columellar strut or a carefully carved tip graft is helpful in contouring of the nasal tip. Every attempt should be made to avoid reduction of the cartilaginous framework in thicker-skin patients. Instead grafts and sutures should be used to increase support and resiliency of the tip-tripod complex.

Nasal airway compromise needs to be addressed to prevent postoperative nasal obstruction. Reconstruction of the keystone area is necessary to avoid postoperative cosmetic and functional deficits, such as inverted V deformity and nasal valve incompetence. Significant deviation of the caudal septum is often observed in Middle Eastern noses contributing to the generalized asymmetry within the face causing malformations in other features. If asymmetry of the lower lateral cartilage is not corrected, persistent deviation and asymmetry may present itself postoperatively.

Additionally, there may be limitations to correction that patients must understand and accept. Significant nasal and facial asymmetry should be reviewed with patients preoperatively. Along with this, patients must also understand aesthetic

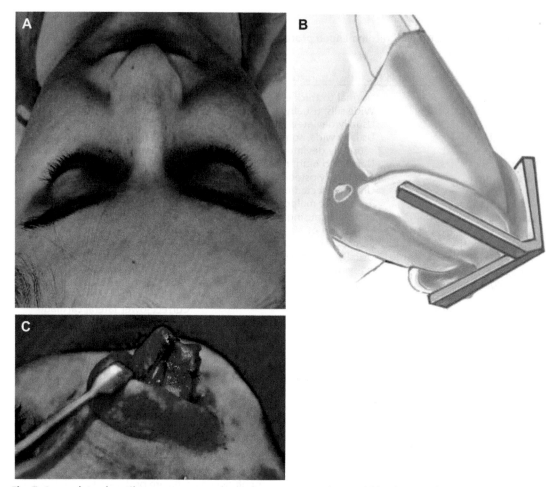

Fig. 7. Lower lateral cartilages can commonly display asymmetry that could lead to nasal tip asymmetry. (*A*) The right lower lateral cartilage was noted to have excessive length. (*B*) Using the tripod concept the right lower lateral cartilage was overlapped by 2 mm. (*C*) Intraoperative view after correction.

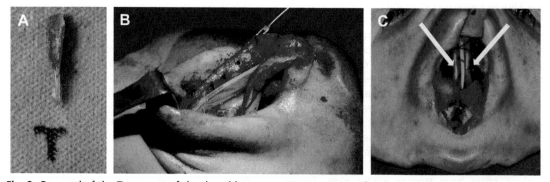

Fig. 8. Removal of the T segment of the dorsal hump creates an open roof deformity. Closure of the open roof necessitates the use of spreader grafts or spreader flaps. (*A*) Removal of the T segment of the dorsal septum. (*B*) Creation of the spreader flap on the right side with mattress sutures. (*C*) Bilateral spreader flaps (*arrows*) used in closing the open roof. In addition, the use of bilateral transdomal sutures, dome equalization sutures, and intercrural sutures is seen in this view.

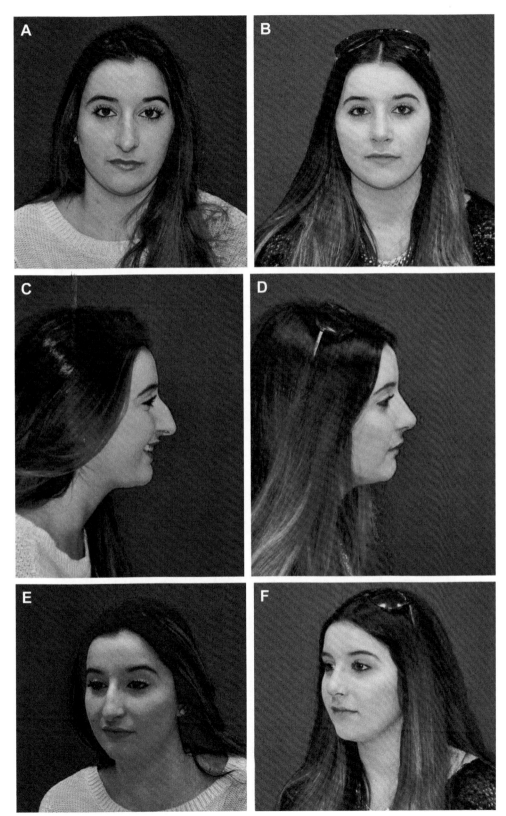

Fig. 9. Middle Eastern rhinoplasty in a thin-skinned patient, preoperative views (*A, C* and *E*) and postoperative views (*B, D,* and *F*).

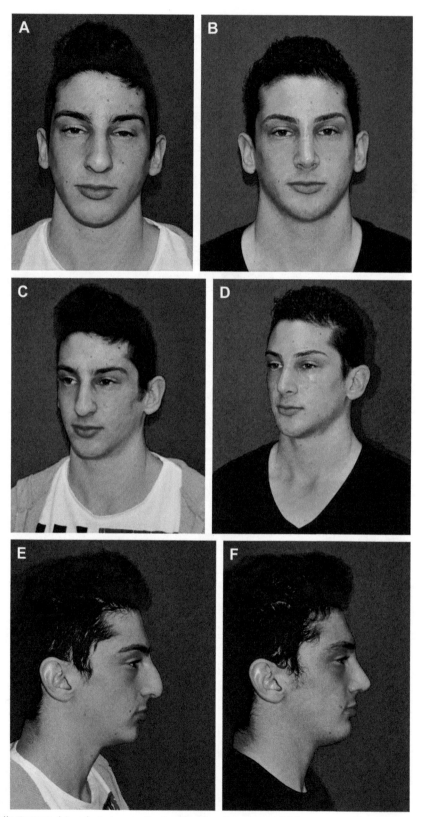

Fig. 10. Middle Eastern rhinoplasty in a patient with skin of moderate thickness, preoperative views (*A*, *C* and *E*) and postoperative views (*B*, *D*, and *F*).

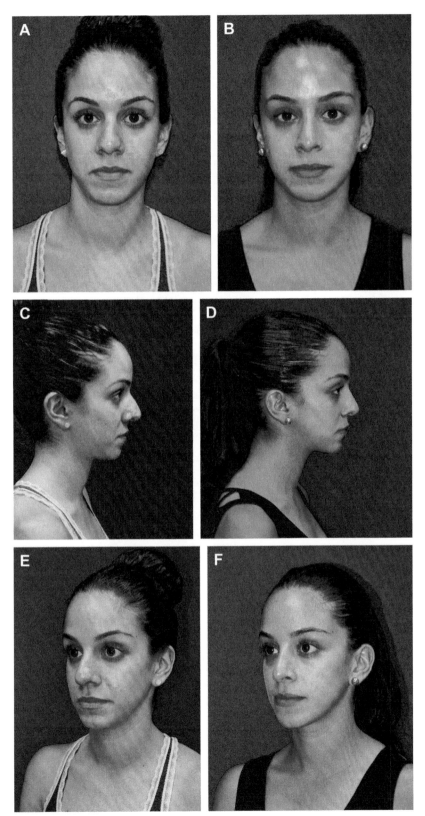

Fig. 11. Middle Eastern rhinoplasty in thick-skinned patient, preoperative views (*A, C* and *E*) and postoperative views (*B, D,* and *F*).

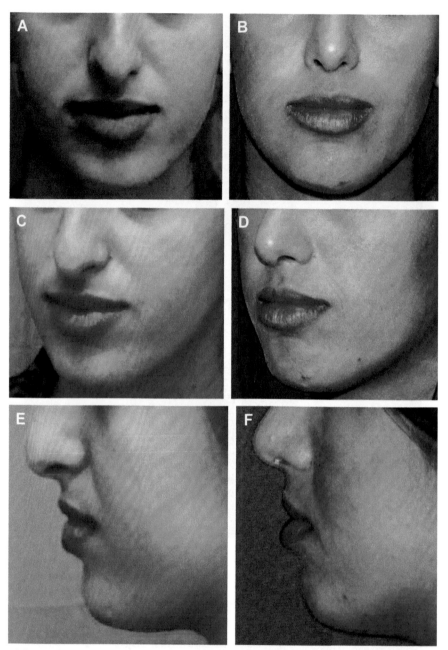

Fig. 12. Middle Eastern rhinoplasty in a patient with underdeveloped radix, dorsal pseduohump, and tip underrotation and underprojection. Preoperative views (*A, C* and *E*) and postoperative views (*B, D,* and *F*).

limitations; a small nose of white dimensions and proportion is not aesthetically or functionally appropriate or racially congruent for a Middle Eastern face.

SUMMARY

For every Middle Eastern patient undergoing rhinoplasty, the measure of success is the ability of the surgeon to shape the nose into more

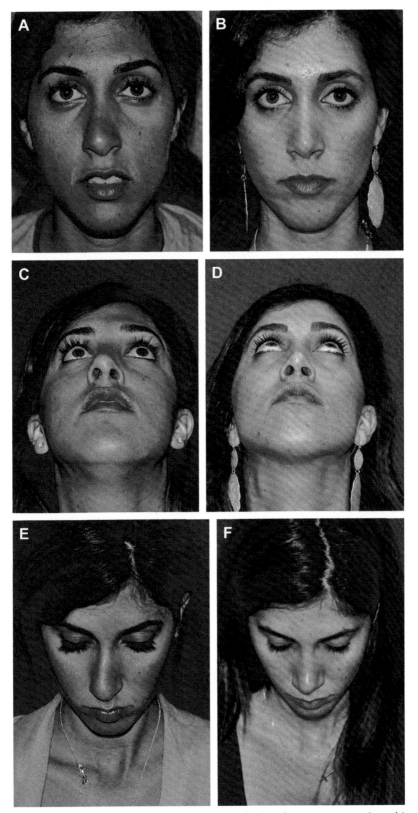

Fig. 13. Revision Middle Eastern rhinoplasty in a patient who had undergone two previous rhinoplasty procedures and was referred for correction of persistent nasal deviation, nasal valve collapse, and airway compromise. Correction included septal reconstruction, septoplasty, spreader grafts, and lateral crural strut grafts. Preoperative views (*A*, *C* and *E*) and postoperative views (*B*, *D*, and *F*).

pleasing proportions and maintain the structure and functionality that enables the patient to breathe efficiently and comfortably. In general, patients of Middle Eastern origin undergoing rhinoplasty require a greater degree of perfection because they are keenly aware of any flaws. Experience and detailed analysis and knowledge of structural differences among various ethnic groups within Middle Eastern patients are required to ensure predictable results. Correction of different deformities in a conservative fashion can lead to achievement of balance of beauty and function in Middle Eastern rhinoplasty patients.

Figs. 8–13 provide before and after pictures showing successful outcomes of Middle Eastern rhinoplasty in patients with different morphology and skin thickness.

Chin Advancement, Augmentation, and Reduction as Adjuncts to Rhinoplasty

Jonathan M. Sykes, MD[a],*, Gustavo A. Suárez, MD[b]

KEYWORDS

- Chin deformities • Microgenia • Macrogenia • Chin implant • Genioplasty • Mentoplasty
- Rhinoplasty

KEY POINTS

- Chin retrusion is of importance for facial plastic surgeons because it is a commonly encountered defect in patients seeking rhinoplasty.
- The chin should be evaluated as it relates to other adjacent structures, such as the lips, nose, and teeth. It is crucial to evaluate the chin in 3 dimensions: horizontal (anteroposterior), vertical, and transverse.
- Horizontal chin deficiency may be camouflaged by an alloplast implant or filler injection.
- Bony osteotomy of the mentum (genioplasty) can correct vertical and transverse chin deformities.
- Injectable fillers, although often not permanent, give the advantage of three-dimensional chin augmentation, with the added benefit of allowing precise chin shaping.

Videos of chin augmentation and osseous genioplasty accompany this article at http://www.plasticsurgery.theclinics.com/

INTRODUCTION

Commonly recognized features of facial beauty include symmetry and harmonious proportions.[1] Chin deformities may detract from an otherwise aesthetically pleasant facial profile. The chin projection and shape are generally regarded as important characteristics of facial attractiveness, especially in men.[2] Some evidence suggests that men with broad chins are viewed as socially dominant across cultures.[3,4] Broad-chinned men attain higher ranks in the military,[5] are regarded as more masculine and attractive,[6–8] and have greater reproductive success in some societies than do men with narrower and less projecting chins.[9] Because cortical bone growth is stimulated by testosterone, and testosterone is immunosuppressive in high concentrations, the ability to have a broad chin and still be healthy is hypothesized to show high mate quality.

In studies analyzing female attractiveness, it is commonly reported that a small or narrow chin is associated with a more feminine appearance,[7,8] which reinforces the notion that a broad chin is a

Disclosures: Neither author has any financial or other disclosures with regard to this article.
[a] Division of Facial Plastic and Reconstructive Surgery, Department of Otolaryngology, UC Davis, 2521 Stockton Boulevard, Suite 6203, Sacramento, CA 95817, USA; [b] Department of Otolaryngology - Head and Neck Surgery, Bellvitge University Hospital, Feixa Llarga s/n, L'Hospitalet de Llobregat, Barcelona 08097, Spain
* Corresponding author. 2521 Stockton Boulevard, Suite 6200, Sacramento, CA 95817.
E-mail address: jmsykes@ucdavis.edu

Clin Plastic Surg 43 (2016) 295–306
http://dx.doi.org/10.1016/j.cps.2015.09.021
0094-1298/16/$ – see front matter © 2016 Elsevier Inc. All rights reserved.

signal of masculinity and suggests that chin size may have opposite effects in men versus women regarding selection. Recent studies have found significant geographic differences in male and female chin shapes. This finding is consistent with region-specific sexual selection and/or random genetic drift and thus challenges the universal sexual selection theory.[10]

Retrusion of the chin is a condition that is commonly encountered in patients seeking rhinoplasty. Moreover, it is striking that most patients seeking rhinoplasty who have a retruded chin are often unaware of their microgenia, and the impact that their chin size has on their nasal and facial appearance. This lack of awareness is compounded by most patients seeing themselves in the mirror directly, rather than obliquely or laterally. Viewing only from a frontal perspective minimizes the impact that chin projection has on facial appearance. However, failure to address chin deformities is a common omission in patients having rhinoplasty. In patients with deficient projection of the chin (horizontal microgenia), the nose appears to project a large amount, even though nasal projection may be appropriate for the face. Several methods have been proposed for defining horizontal projection of the chin.[11,12] None of these analyses is ideal. An appreciation of facial proportions, measurements, and relationships of the bony structures and soft tissues of the face assists surgeons in preoperative planning and establishing the goals of surgery.

When properly indicated and performed, a simultaneous rhinoplasty and chin augmentation, advancement or reduction, can produce a significant improvement in facial appearance. This article outlines the methods to analyze the chin, and discusses the treatment options available for correction of microgenia and macrogenia. These treatments can be important adjuncts to achieving a more harmonic profile in patients requesting rhinoplasty.

PREOPERATIVE PLANNING AND PREPARATION

To precisely correct any chin deformity, careful preoperative analysis is essential.[13,14] Specifically, the chin should be evaluated as it relates to other skeletal and soft tissue structures, including the lips, teeth, nose, and soft tissues of the neck. A detailed history of past trauma, orthodontic treatment, temporomandibular joint dysfunction, or prior oral surgery is important because many patients with dental malocclusion and underlying facial skeletal abnormalities are treated initially with orthodontics. This method of dental

compensation may correct the malocclusion, but fails to improve the underlying skeletal deformity. It is therefore important to discuss prior therapy and the effects of chin shape and position on the facial profile with the patient.

Physical examination should include inspection and palpation of the chin, lips, nose, and teeth. The entire face should be observed at rest and during animation to evaluate the mentalis soft tissue mound and its support. With aging, patients may develop ptosis of the soft tissue pad of the chin. In patients with open bite deformities and lip incompetence, hyperactivity of the mentalis muscles (mentalis strain) can occur. For this reason, the dental occlusion should be carefully examined to determine whether orthodontics or orthognathic surgery is needed.

The evaluation of all patients for possible chin surgery should include consistent and reproducible clinical photographs in at least 3 views: anterior-posterior (AP; frontal), lateral (profile), and oblique. These photographs allow analysis of the contour and projection of the chin as it relates to other structures of the face and neck. If the physical evaluation and clinical photographs show a minor deformity requiring augmentation with an alloplast, radiographs of the chin are usually not necessary. However, if the deformity is more complex, (eg, vertical chin excess with horizontal deficiency or transverse bony asymmetry), radiographic analysis is usually obtained.

Radiographic evaluation of the chin routinely includes a panoramic radiograph (Panorex) and cephalometric radiographs in the AP and lateral views. The Panorex shows the cortical outline of the mandible and the vertical mandibular height. Also, this radiograph delineates the position of the tooth roots and the inferior alveolar or mandibular canals and mental foramina (**Fig. 1**). This information aids in avoiding damage to the mental nerve during surgery. The inferior alveolar nerve, a branch of the third division of the fifth (V_3) cranial nerve, travels through the mandibular canal and exits the mental foramen as the mental nerve (**Fig. 2**). The mental nerve supplies sensation to the skin and mucous membranes of the lower lip and chin. The mandibular canal is often located 2 to 3 mm below the level of the mental foramen.[15] Bony osteotomies should therefore be performed at least 5 mm below the mental foramen.

If bony genioplasty is considered, AP and lateral cephalometric radiographs should be obtained. AP radiographs allow detection and evaluation of transverse skeletal asymmetries of the chin. Chin asymmetries are common in patients with oculoauricular vertebral spectrum or hemifacial microsomia, but they are also commonly seen in

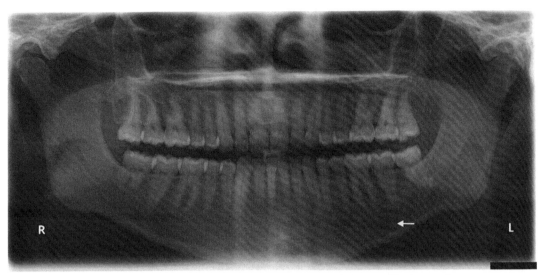

Fig. 1. Panorex radiograph. The white arrow indicates the position of the mandibular canal.

nonsyndromic patients considering aesthetic surgery. When transverse bony or soft tissue asymmetries are overlooked preoperatively in patients with microgenia, augmentation of the chin with an alloplast can accentuate the deformity.[14] Lateral cephalometric radiographs allow detailed analysis of both the facial soft tissues and the facial skeleton. The cephalogram should be obtained at a standard distance with the head positioned so that the Frankfurt horizontal line is parallel to the floor.[16] From this standardized lateral radiograph, a series of soft tissue and skeletal points can be identified (**Fig. 3**), which allows various analyses of the chin, as described by Ricketts,[17] Steiner,[18] Burstone,[19] Gonzalez-Ulloa and Stevens,[11] and others (**Figs. 4** and **5**).

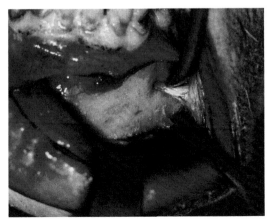

Fig. 2. Cadaveric dissection showing the position of the left inferior alveolar nerve.

The most frequently used evaluation of the chin drops a perpendicular line from the vermillion border of the lower lip and compares the AP position of this line with the soft tissue pogonion (the anteriormost projecting chin point). As a general guide, the pogonion in a male patient should ideally be at the level of this vertical line, whereas in women the pogonion should be positioned just posterior to this line. When class I occlusion is present and the position of the soft tissue pogonion is anterior to the proposed line, horizontal macrogenia is diagnosed, whereas microgenia is present if the chin is positioned posterior to the ideal line. Although this evaluation is effective for horizontal deformities (microgenia or macrogenia), it does not account for vertical or transverse discrepancies. Because many surgeons primarily use this evaluation method, vertical or transverse chin problems are often overlooked.

Analysis of vertical plane is also essential in determining the appropriate heights of the lower facial third and the chin. The simplest technique involves division of the face into 3 equal thirds (**Fig. 6**). Because the frontal hairline can vary significantly between individuals, an alternate method described by Powell and Humphreys[15] more accurately analyzes the vertical heights of the lower 2 thirds of the face. This method describes the middle portion of the face as the distance from the nasion to the subnasale and the lower portion as the distance from the subnasale to the menton. Other important analyses include inspection of the face in repose, when the maxillary incisor teeth should show 0 to 3 mm. If more than 3 mm of the maxillary incisors are visible at rest, excessive facial length, usually in the midface, may be present. Additional

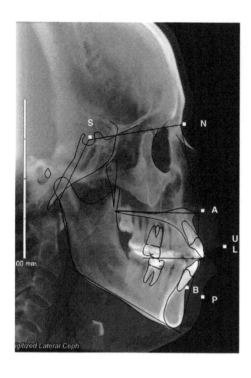

FH - SN (°)	6.5	6.0
SNA (°)	97.6	82.0
A-N Perpendicular (mm)	12.7	0.0
SNB (°)	86.7	80.9
Pog-N Perpendicular (mm)	10.4	4.0
Facial Angle (FH-NPo) (°)	95.8	89.6
ANB (°)	10.9	1.6
Wits Appraisal (mm)	1.2	-1.0
Convexity (A-NPo) (mm)	7.5	0.1
U1 - Palatal Plane (°)	101.4	110.0
U1 - NA (°)	-0.6	22.8
U1 - NA (mm)	-3.4	4.3
U1 - SN (°)	97.0	103.1
IMPA (L1-MP) (°)	108.1	95.0
L1 - NB (°)	39.8	25.3
L1 - NB (mm)	9.0	4.0
L1 Protrusion (L1-APo) (mm)	1.2	2.7
Holdaway Ratio (L1-NB:Pg-NB) (%)	1.9	2.0
Interincisal Angle (U1-L1) (°)	129.8	130.0
Overbite (mm)	1.9	2.5
Overjet (mm)	2.3	2.5
Occ Plane to SN (°)	16.5	14.4
FMA (MP-FH) (°)	18.5	22.9
MP - SN (°)	25.0	33.0
Y-Axis (SGn-SN) (°)	53.9	67.0
Facial Axis-Ricketts (NaBa-PtGn)(°)	97.4	90.0
Lower Face Height (ANS-Xi-Pm)(°)	36.4	45.0
Saddle/Sella Angle (SN-Ar) (°)	97.2	124.0
P-A Face Height (S-Go/N-Me) (%)	66.4	65.0
Upper Gonial Angle (Ar-Go-Na) (°)	50.0	49.0
Lower Gonial Angle (Na-Go-Me) (°)	65.5	72.0
Posterior Cranial Base (S-Ar) (mm)	22.2	37.0
Ramus Height (Ar-Go) (mm)	50.8	53.0
S-Ar/Ar-Go (%)	43.7	75.0
Mandibular Body Length (Go-Me) (mm)	83.1	71.0
Anterior Cranial Base (SN) (mm)	82.9	77.3

Fig. 3. Lateral cephalogram. A, anterior nasal spine; B, supramentale, N, nasion; P, soft tissue pogonion; S, sella; UL, upper lip.

analysis of the lower face includes subdividing the lower third of the face. All of these analyses relate the height of the chin and lower face to the total facial height. In complex chin deformities, a vertical discrepancy, as well as a horizontal deficiency or excess, is often present.[20]

Another parameter of the chin that should be assessed is chin width and symmetry in the sagittal plane. Transverse asymmetries of the chin exist in many patients with congenital anomalies and in patients who have had significant skeletal facial trauma. However, many patients with only aesthetic concerns have minor but definite asymmetries of the chin. In patients with horizontal microgenia and chin asymmetry, augmentation with an implant may correct the horizontal deficiency but accentuate the skeletal asymmetry. AP cephalometric radiographs allow a comparison of the bony midline of the chin with the dental midlines of the maxilla and mandible. If the skeletal and soft tissue midlines of the chin are not aligned with the dental midlines and with the upper facial skeletal midline (eg, nasion), an asymmetric bony genioplasty or chin implant can be performed to eliminate or reduce the chin asymmetry.

Analysis of the labiomental fold is crucial to determine the appropriate treatment of horizontal deformities. The labiomental fold is analyzed to determine its height, depth, and distinctness. A key point is to determine the percentage of lower facial height that is related to the lip-to-menton chin pad height versus lip-to-labiomental-fold height. If the labiomental fold is high or close to the lower lip, the pad percentage is high, and vice versa (**Fig. 7**). In patients with a high chin pad percentage (deep labiodental sulcus), an alloplastic chin augmentation can be aesthetically unpleasant.

No single method provides comprehensive evaluation of the chin, but each allows a reference for assessing the bony and soft tissues of the chin and lower face. Using a variety of methods, a thorough analysis of chin deformities can be achieved.

Chin Deformities

Deformities of the chin and lower face may be related to either bony abnormalities or to soft tissue malposition. The chin should be analyzed in

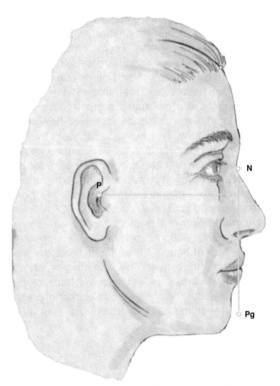

Fig. 4. The method described by Gonzales-Ulloa and Stevens. Pg, pogonion. (*Data from* Gonzales-Ulloa M, Stevens E. The role of chin correction in profileplasty. Plast Reconstr Surg 1966;41:477–86.)

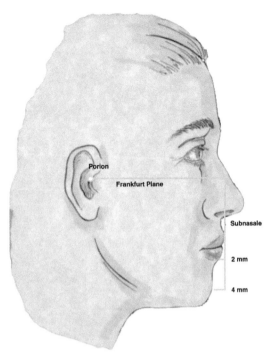

Fig. 5. The horizontal relationships of the chin and upper and lower lips as they relate to the nasal perpendicular line.

all 3 planes: horizontal (AP), vertical (superior-inferior), and sagittal (transverse). The horizontal and vertical dimensions can each be deficient, normal, or excessive. Simple deformities such as mild horizontal chin deficiency (microgenia) are easily corrected using either an implant or bony advancement. More complex deformities, such as in patients with horizontal deficiency and vertical excess, usually require horizontal osteotomy for adequate correction.[13]

Soft tissue deformities of the chin and submental region also exist. Ptosis of the soft tissues of the chin often accompanies other signs of facial aging. This condition, commonly called witch's chin or senile chin deformity, is caused by a weakening of the muscular attachments of the mentalis and depressor labii inferioris muscles. In this deformity, the soft tissue pad of the chin descends below the mandibular line, and a deep horizontal crease develops in the submental region. Descent of the soft tissue chin pad is accentuated with smiling. This deformity can be inadvertently created or worsened surgically if the mentalis muscles are not reapproximated while inserting a chin implant.

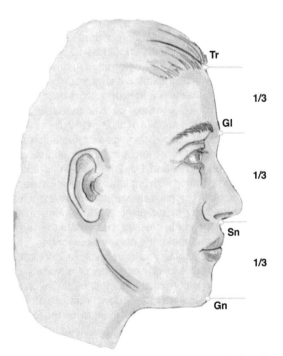

Fig. 6. Division of the face into 3 equal thirds. Gl, glabella; Gn, gnathion; Sn, subnasale; Tr, trichion.

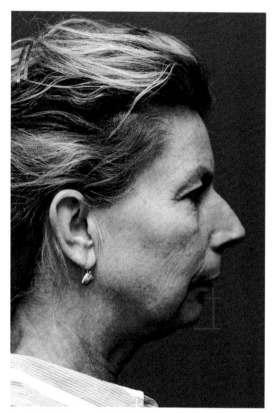

Fig. 7. A patient with deep labial sulcus (high chin pad percentage).

PROCEDURAL APPROACH

Selection of the best procedure to correct aesthetic chin problems should be based on the type and extent of the deformity. Augmentation of the chin with an implant is a simple and effective method of correcting a horizontal chin deficiency. This technique is limited by the availability of various sizes and shapes of alloplast implants (**Table 1**). Several shapes and sizes of implants may be required, but most implants are manufactured in only 3 or 4 sizes and 1 or 2 shapes. In addition, chin augmentation with implants is less effective in patients with significant vertical discrepancies (vertical excess or deficiency). Placement of an implant in such patients may exacerbate the vertical excess and make the chin appear longer.

Osseus genioplasty is a versatile and reliable procedure that allows correction of a variety of skeletal chin deformities. This technique involves horizontal osteotomy and downfracture of the chin with repositioning and fixation of the distal bony chin segment. Osseous genioplasty allows advancement or retrusion of the chin in the AP direction, lengthening or shortening in the vertical direction, and correction of transverse asymmetries

of the chin. Although customized chin implants can be made to correct chin asymmetries, preformed implants are usually symmetric.

Correction of soft tissue ptosis has been described by Peterson[21] and other investigators. This technique involves the removal of an ellipse of submental skin, creation of a flap of chin soft tissue, and advancement and plication of the soft tissue flap inferiorly. This technique tightens the soft tissue pad and obliterates the horizontal submental crease. However, this procedure may move the soft tissue pogonion posteriorly, and some form of simultaneous augmentation (implant or bony advancement) is usually required.

Augmentation of the chin can also be accomplished with injection of soft tissue fillers or autologous fat. Although these techniques are not permanent, they have the advantages of not needing the incisions and scarring that are the inevitable result of surgery, and enabling practitioners to shape and augment the chin in 3 dimensions.

SURGICAL TECHNIQUE
Chin Implant

To ensure precise midline placement of the chin implant, the midlines of the chin, lower lip, and neck (thyroid cartilage) are marked externally before the infiltration of local anesthesia (Video 1). A mental nerve block is then performed using Xylocaine 1% with epinephrine 1:100,000. Additional infiltration of anesthesia into the submental region, gingivolabial sulcus, and central portion of the lower lip and chin is performed to ensure adequate anesthesia and vasoconstriction. Either an intraoral or extraoral (submental) approach can be used to place a chin implant, although the authors prefer the submental approach.

The external approach uses a 2-m to 3-cm incision made 2 mm behind the submental crease, which is carried through the dermis and subcutaneous fat. The mentalis muscle is then divided to enter a dissection plane just superficial to the periosteum of the anterior face of the mandible. The chin implant can be placed in either the subperiosteal or the supraperiosteal plane. The advantage of placing an implant beneath the periosteum is improved fixation of the implant; however, subperiosteal placement has been shown to result in some erosion of the anterior mandible. For these reasons, most surgeons advocate dissection in the supraperiosteal plane centrally with subperiosteal placement laterally. This method theoretically minimizes mandibular erosion while maximally fixing the implant. Many types of implants have been used for chin

Table 1
Implant characteristics

Material	Trade Name	Tissue Interface	Pros	Cons	Complications	Common Sites for Use
Polydimethylsiloxane	Silastic (silicone rubber; Dow Corning, Midland, MI)	Fibrous capsule	Can be carved and removed	Bone resorption, exposure	Malposition, extrusion, infection	Chin, malar, nasal
Fibrillated expanded polytetrafluoroethylene	Gore-Tex (WL Gore, Flagstaff, AZ)	Limited tissue ingrowth	Sheets or tubular (lips)	Palpable	Malposition, extrusion, infection	Lips, nose
High-density polyethylene	MEDPOR (Porex Surgical, Newnan, GA)	Limited tissue ingrowth	Versatile, resistant to infection	Difficult to remove	Malposition, extrusion	Malar, orbit, chin, nasal
Hydroxyapatite/ carbonated apatite	BoneSource (Stryker Leibinger, Flint, MI) and Norion CRS (Synthes-Stratec, Paoli, PA)	Osseointegration	Paste consistency; can be molded	Exposure or infection	Exposure, infection (ie, frontal sinus)	Craniofacial, forehand

augmentation. In general, the 2 shapes of implants are the central button implant and the extended anatomic implant. Two advantages of longer, tapered implants are that they can be placed in the subperiosteal plane laterally, and they allow for lateral mandibular augmentation.

During the lateral subperiosteal dissection, the mental nerves should be identified and preserved. The implant should be placed along the inferior border of the mandible; if the implant extends laterally beyond the mental foramina, it should be positioned below the exit of the mental nerve. After placement and fixation of the implant, the mentalis muscles should be reapproximated in order to avoid postoperative chin ptosis,[22] and the soft tissue should be meticulously resuspended. The wound is then closed in layers with attention being given to carefully reapproximating the mentalis muscle. A secure chin-strap dressing is placed for 3 days to ensure immobility of the implant.

If an intraoral approach is used, the gingivolabial incision can be either horizontal or vertical. In either case, dissection through the mentalis muscles again occurs with placement of the implant in a supraperiosteal plane centrally and a subperiosteal pocket laterally. Closure is accomplished in 2 layers with the muscle closure achieving soft tissue resuspension (**Figs. 8** and **9**).

Fixation of alloplast chin implants

Fixation of alloplast chin implants can be performed with either screw or suture fixation to the underlying bone. Alternately, the implant can be placed through a precise pocket with a subperiosteal dissection (as described earlier). Various screw fixation methods can also be used to affix the implant directly to the underlying bone; titanium screws are typically used, with the screw going through the implant and entering the anterior face of the mandible by about 4 to 5 mm (monocortical fixation).

Osseous Genioplasty

Horizontal bony osteotomy of the chin, or osseous genioplasty, can be performed under general anesthesia or intravenous sedation with a mentalis nerve block (Video 2). If general anesthesia is used, nasotracheal intubation is preferred; however, if simultaneous rhinoplasty is also performed, orotracheal intubation should be used.

An incision is made on the labial side of the gingivolabial sulcus, from one canine tooth to the other. This incision creates an adequate mucoperiosteal soft tissue cuff for later closure. Dissection is then carried through the soft tissues and mandibular periosteum. A subperiosteal dissection is performed

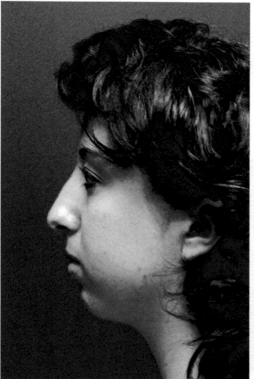
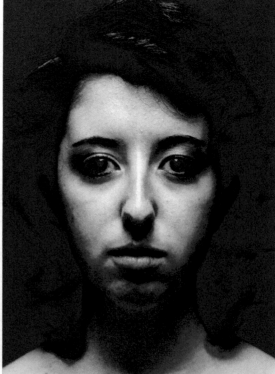

Fig. 8. A patient about to undergo septorhinoplasty and chin augmentation with an alloplast implant.

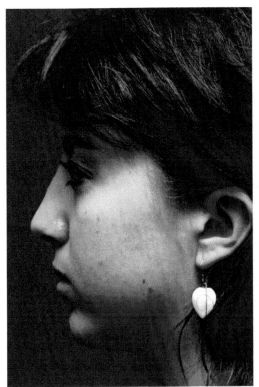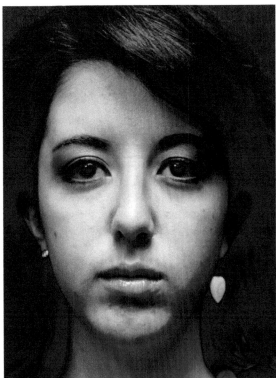

Fig. 9. A patient after undergoing septorhinoplasty and chin augmentation with an alloplast implant.

laterally with identification and preservation of both mental nerves. A small inferior segment of soft tissue is preserved over the central segment (bony mentum) to provide vascular supply to the distal bony segment after osteotomy.[23] Once the lateral subperiosteal dissection is completed, the proposed osteotomy is carefully measured and marked with calipers, to ensure a symmetric osteotomy (Video 2).

The bony midline is vertically inscribed with a side-cutting burr to allow proper alignment and repositioning after osteotomy (**Fig. 10**). In order to prevent dental injury, the horizontal osteotomy should be placed below the level of the tooth roots. During the preoperative assessment, a decision is made on the three-dimensional movement of the chin that will be required. This treatment plan will affect the orientation of the osteotomy as well as the chin movement after the osteotomy.

Osteotomies

If only horizontal (AP) advancement is needed, the osteotomy is made with a horizontal orientation. If vertical movement (shortening) is also needed, the osteotomy is made in a more oblique orientation. An oblique osteotomy allows some vertical

shortening, because the distal segment is advanced. If the chin length is excessive, and significant shortening is planned, 2 oblique osteotomies are made, and the intervening bone is removed.

After the osteotomy is marked, a reciprocating saw blade is used in a lateral-to-medial direction. The lateral extent of the osteotomy should be made at least 5 mm below the mental foramen to

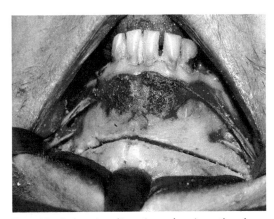

Fig. 10. Cadaveric dissection showing the bony midline vertically inscribed with a side-cutting burr.

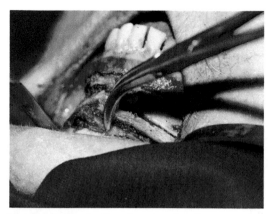

Fig. 11. Cadaveric dissection showing the osteotomy for the correction of a vertical macrogenia.

avoid injuring the mental nerve. Gentle digital pressure is used to downfracture the bony segment, and a small amount of soft tissue must usually be separated from the posterior aspect of the distal segment to facilitate movement. Repositioning of the distal segment is performed according to the preoperative plan.

If vertical lengthening is required, grafts are placed using autogenous or allogenic bone. If vertical shortening is planned, a second parallel osteotomy is made above the first one, or the intervening bone is burred away. After the distal bony segment is repositioned, fixation is performed using adaptation plates, positional screws, or interosseous wires (Video 2).

If macrogenia exists and chin reduction is desired, this is usually performed using an oblique osteotomy of the mentum. It is important to diagnose whether the macrogenia is horizontal or vertical. If the chin projects too much in the horizontal plane the inner segments are drilled down with a cutting bur and setback and fixation of the segments is accomplished. If vertical macrogenia exists, a second parallel osteotomy is performed with intervening ostectomy (**Fig. 11**). It is important to discuss with the patient that the soft tissue changes after bony chin reduction are less predictable than the changes after augmentation.

At the end of the procedure the soft tissues of the chin and lips are replaced, and the new contour is assessed. The wound is closed in 2 layers with care taken to resuspend the soft tissues of the chin (**Figs. 12** and **13**).

Soft Tissue Fillers

Many patients with microgenia are reluctant to undergo surgery or placement of an alloplast.

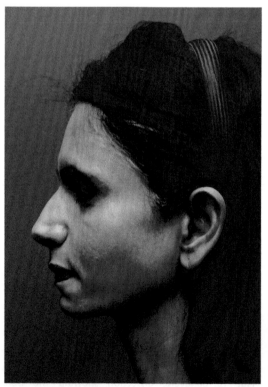
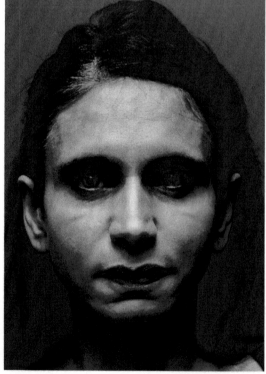

Fig. 12. A patient before undergoing septorhinoplasty and genioplasty with advancement and lengthening.

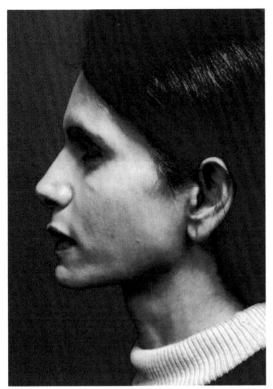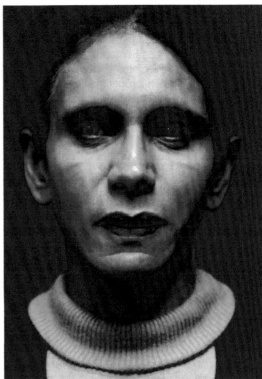

Fig. 13. A patient after undergoing septorhinoplasty and genioplasty with advancement and lengthening.

For these individuals, injection of soft tissue fillers, or autologous fat, can provide chin augmentation. The advantages of this procedure are no surgical incision or division of the mentalis muscles, and reversibility of the outcome, allowing surgically anxious patients to visualize the desired results.

Filler injections into the chin are performed in a layer deep to the mentalis muscle centrally. This procedure is usually done with bolus technique. A filler with a high G prime is usually used. If lateral augmentation is desired, this can be performed in a supraperiosteal plane. Filler or fat injections allow three-dimensional augmentation and shaping of the chin.

Postoperative care

At the conclusion of a chin augmentation with an implant or a bony genioplasty, a chin-strap dressing is placed in order to minimize dead space and improve soft tissue adhesion. A soft diet is indicated in patients with chin implants for 1 to 3 days and in bony genioplasty surgeries for 5 to 7 days. In 10% to 15% of cases, mentalist muscle dyskinesis occurs. This dyskinesis is usually treated with injection of 2 to 5 units of botulin toxin.

Complications

Complications after mentoplasty are uncommon. Chin implants can become malpositioned and occasionally are bothersome to patients with a thin overlying soft tissue pad. Infections with both the intraoral and submental approaches are infrequent. Anterior mandible resorption has been reported with subperiosteal implant placement, occasionally causing secondary chin deformities.[24] Although bony resorption often occurs, this condition is rarely clinically significant. Complications after genioplasty include mental nerve injury and malunion or nonunion of the bony segments. Nerve damage during genioplasty is extremely uncommon with careful dissection. Malunion of the bone segments can occur, but the excellent vascularity and lack of directional force on the osteotomy site make this an infrequent problem.

SUMMARY

The chin plays an important role in overall facial appearance, and aesthetic surgery of the chin is extremely rewarding when performed in carefully selected patients. Chin augmentation may improve facial balance and proportion, and may also require less reduction of the nose.

Simultaneous nose-chin correction is a powerful combination and obviates a second surgical session, thus reducing postoperative discomfort and overall cost.[25] Chin augmentation with alloplasts is a simple and effective means to correct mild to moderate horizontal microgenia. Horizontal osteotomy of the bony mentum (osseous genioplasty) is a more flexible and versatile procedure that can correct chin deformities in all 3 planes of space. When properly planned and executed, both procedures provide important adjuncts for the facial plastic surgeon.

SUPPLEMENTARY DATA

Supplementary data related to this article can be found online at http://dx.doi.org/10.1016/j.cps.2015.09.021.

REFERENCES

1. Tolleth H. Concepts for the plastic surgeon from art and sculpture. Clin Plast Surg 1987;14:585–98.
2. Grammer K, Fink B, Møller AP, et al. Darwinian aesthetics: sexual selection and the biology of beauty. Biol Rev Camb Philos Soc 2003;78:385–407.
3. Rhodes G, Yoshikawa S, Clark A, et al. Attractiveness of facial averageness and symmetry in non-Western cultures: in search of biologically based standards of beauty. Perception 2001;30:611–25.
4. Keating CF, Mazur A, Segall MH. A cross-cultural exploration of physiognomic traits of dominance and happiness. Ethol Sociobiol 1981;2:41–8.
5. Mazur A, Mazur J, Keating C. Military rank attainment of a West Point class: effects of cadets' physical features. Am J Sociol 1984;90(1):125–50.
6. Rhodes G, Chan J, Zebrowitz L, et al. Does sexual dimorphism in human faces signal health? Proc Biol Sci 2003;270:S93–5.
7. Keating CF. Gender and the physiognomy of dominance and attractiveness. Social Psychology 1985; 48(1):61–70.
8. Perrett D, Lee K, Penton-Voak I, et al. Effects of sexual dimorphism on facial attractiveness. Nature 1998;394:884–7.
9. Mueller U, Mazur A. Facial dominance in *Homo sapiens* as honest signaling of male quality. Behav Ecol 1997;8:569–79.
10. Thayer ZM, Dobson SD. Geographic variation in chin shape challenges the universal facial attractiveness hypothesis. PLoS One 2013;8(4):e60681.
11. Gonzales-Ulloa M, Stevens E. The role of chin correction in profileplasty. Plast Reconstr Surg 1966;41:477–86.
12. Simons RL. Adjunctive measures in rhinoplasty. Otolaryngol Clin North Am 1975;8:717–42.
13. Sykes JM. Orthognathic surgery. In: Papel I, editor. Facial plastic and reconstructive surgery. 3rd edition. New York: Thieme; 2009. p. 1095–118.
14. Sykes J, Frodel JL. Genioplasty. Op Tech Otolaryngol 1995;6(4):319–23.
15. Powell N, Humphreys B. Proportions of the aesthetic face. New York: Thieme-Stratton; 1984.
16. Rakosi T. An atlas and manual of cephalometry radiography. Philadelphia: Lea & Febiger; 1982.
17. Ricketts RM. Esthetics, environment and the law of lip relation. Am J Orthod 1968;54:272.
18. Steiner CC. Cephalometrics in clinical practice. Angle Orthod 1959;29:8.
19. Burstone CJ. Lip posture and its significance in treatment planning. Am J Orthod 1967;53:262.
20. Precious DS, Delaire J. Correction of anterior mandibular vertical excess: the functional genioplasty. Oral Surg Oral Med Oral Pathol 1985;59:229.
21. Peterson RA. Correction of the senile chin deformity in face lift. Clin Plast Surg 1992;19:433.
22. Bell WH, Gallagher DM. The versatility of genioplasty using a broad pedicle. J Oral Maxillofac Surg 1983;41:763.
23. Chaushu G, Blinder D, Taicher S, et al. The effect of precise reattachment of the mentalis muscle on the soft tissue response to genioplasty. J Oral Maxillofac Surg 2001;59(5):510–7.
24. Li K, Cheny M. The use of sliding genioplasty for treatment of failed chin implants. Laryngoscope 1996;106:363.
25. Nocini PF, Chiarini L, Bertossi D. Cosmetic procedures in orthognathic surgery. J Oral Maxillofac Surg 2011;69(3):716–23.

Use of Fillers in Rhinoplasty

Hyoung Jin Moon, MD

KEYWORDS

- Rhinoplastly • Filler • Injectables • Nose • Nonsurgical rhinoplasty • Injection rhinoplasty
- Botulinum toxin

KEY POINTS

- The nose is the area in which most people make enquiries for procedures – especially filler augmentation, and the most important thing is to make the shape of nose that fits each person's image.
- The nonsurgical nose augmentation procedure with filler is classified in 2 categories: the dorsum of the nose and the tip of the nose.
- After comparing and analyzing the ideal nose shape and the patient's nose shape, decide which part is to be raised and by how much.
- The most common report of dissatisfaction of nonsurgical nose augmentation with filler is asymmetry. To prevent this, the tip of the needle should be located in the center line during the procedure.
- Filler must be injected to the deep fatty layer (between the perichondrium or periosteum and muscle layer) where important blood vessels are not located. That helps avoid severe side effects, such as skin necrosis.

INTRODUCTION

Rhinoplasty is one of the most common procedures in the field of aesthetic surgery. Asians, in particular, often have a flat nose and a wide nasal tip; hence, augmentation rhinoplasty is frequently performed in Asian countries. Existing techniques for rhinoplasty using implants and autologous cartilage are associated, however, with a long recovery time, high cost, and implant-related problems, so there often is a psychological barrier for patients considering surgery.[1] Also, it is well recognized that there is a steep learning curve for rhinoplasty. As such, many patients prefer not to undergo a surgical rhinoplasty. This has led to an increase in popularity of rhinoplasty using fillers (**Fig. 1**).[2] The goal of this article is not to endorse the use of fillers but rather to provide education and guidance to improve outcome and reduce complications for the many physicians who do perform these procedures.

A filler is any material that can augment volume when injected into the body and is usually an injectable material. Well-known fillers include hyaluronic acid (HA) products, collagen, paraffin, liquid silicon. Fillers are usually classified by their components.

Fillers also are classified by their longevity. Fillers with duration of less than 2 years are called temporary fillers; those with duration of 2 to 5 years are called semipermanent fillers; and those lasting no less than 5 years after injection are called permanent fillers. Fillers can also be divided based on the mechanism of action, such as volumizing fillers and stimulatory fillers. Collagen and hyaluronic fillers, in which the injected material itself constitutes the augmented volume, are classified as volumizing fillers, and those that augment

Disclosure Statement: The authors have nothing to disclose.
Dr Moon's Aesthetic Plastic Surgery Clinic, B-2010 Acrovista 188 Seocho Joongang-Ro Seochogu, Seoul 06600, Republic of Korea
E-mail address: Beautymoon@hotmail.co.kr

Clin Plastic Surg 43 (2016) 307–317
http://dx.doi.org/10.1016/j.cps.2015.08.003

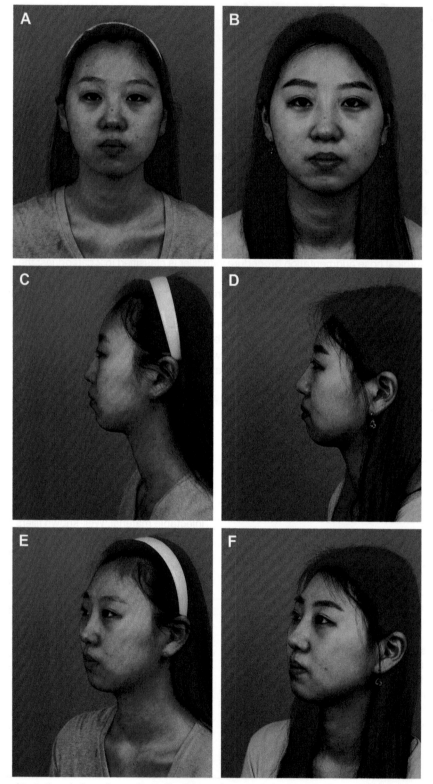

Fig. 1. Before (*A*, *C*, *E*) and after photos (*B*, *D*, *F*) of rhinoplasty performed with fillers. This procedure is becoming more widely performed because the shape of the nose can be improved almost instantly with minimal complications.

volume by stimulating fibroblasts to synthesize collagen or depositing fibrous tissues through inflammatory response are called stimulatory fillers.

Most fillers have a good safety profile. Serious side effects, however, such as granuloma formation and inflammation due to tissue reaction, have been reported with several filler products, so it is necessary to select a desirable filler by understanding the characteristics of each product. An ideal filler should have no tissue reaction, be long-lasting, be safe and easy to use, and have no intratissue migration or allergic reaction.

Restricting the paranasal muscular movement using botulinum toxin shows better and longer-lasting results than using filler alone.

ANATOMY FOR RHINOPLASTY USING FILLER

Rhinoplasty using filler can only be successfully performed if the surgeon has a good understanding of nasal anatomy. Rhinoplasty using filler is a procedure of reshaping the nose by injecting filler into the space between the bony–cartilaginous structure of the nose and the skin. The solid frame of the nose functions as the supporting structure to maintain the shape of the injected filler and to achieve an aesthetic result. Therefore, a satisfactory result cannot be expected after the procedure if the frame of the nose is deformed or weakened. Rhinoplasty using filler is said to reflect the personal ability of the surgeon, the anatomic characteristics of the patient's nose, and the surgeon's recognition of such individual variation. When performing rhinoplasty using filler, all structures of the nose, including the thickness and properties of the skin and the soft tissue and the size, shape, and strength of the cartilage and bone, must be taken into consideration.

Soft Tissue of the Nose

It is important to assess the skin of the nose before performing filler rhinoplasty. In general, Asians have thicker skin than white people with rich and oily subcutaneous tissue. The soft tissue of the nasal bridge is the thickest at the nasion and the thinnest at the rhinion, which is the junction of the upper lateral cartilages and the nasal bones.[3] There are 4 layers between the skin and the bony–cartilaginous framework: superficial fatty layer, fibromuscular layer, deep fatty layer, and periosteum or perichondrium.[4]

It may be more difficult to perform filler rhinoplasty on patients with thick, oily skin because they may experience severe postprocedure edema more often, and creating a pleasing 3-D shape is challenging. On the other hand, in such patients, minute irregularities or asymmetry is camouflaged more easily compared with patients with thin skin. Major blood vessels of the external nose are located in the superficial muscular aponeurotic system (SMAS) layer or the superficial fatty layer.[5] Therefore, the ideal layer for filler injection is the deep fatty layer located between the SMAS and the perichondrium or periosteum, to minimize damage to the vessels (**Fig. 2**).

Understanding the location, size, and function of the muscles of the nose is essential because some of them are sometimes paralyzed using botulinum toxin to enhance the effect of rhinoplasty using filler. The depressor septi nasi muscle originates from the orbicularis oris and terminates at the medial crura of the lower lateral cartilage. This muscle lowers the nasal tip when smiling or making a facial expression, and it is often paralyzed by injecting botulinum toxin to inhibit the function.[6] It is better to paralyze the procerus muscle located at the glabella with botulinum toxin beforehand because filler injected at the glabella may move when the procerus muscle contracts intensely. The levator labii superioris alaeque nasi muscle causes flaring of the nasal ala and nasal tip ptosis when smiling; hence, it is also often paralyzed using botulinum toxin in patients who have dynamic nasal tip ptosis or alar flaring. The dilator naris muscle can be paralyzed if the nasal ala is too wide.

Vascular Supply of the External Nose

The most feared complications of filler injection are intra-arterial embolization into the blood vessel and dermal necrosis due to vascular compression. The surgeon must be familiar with the vascular supply of the external nose to prevent such consequences.

Both the internal carotid artery and the external carotid artery supply blood to the external nose via the ophthalmic artery and the facial artery, respectively. The ophthalmic artery mainly supplies blood to the upper part of the nose via the external nasal branch of the anterior ethmoid artery and the dorsal nasal artery; the facial artery gives rise to the angular and superior labial arteries, which supply the lower part of the nose. Each of these branches out to the lateral nasal artery and the columellar artery. The nasal tip receives blood supply from the dorsal nasal artery superiorly and the lateral nasal artery and the columellar artery inferiorly.

SELECTION OF TARGET PATIENT

The physician must be able to select patients who are suitable for rhinoplasty using filler. This requires a thorough understanding of ideal nasal aesthetics and anatomy (described previously). If physicians have not been trained and do not

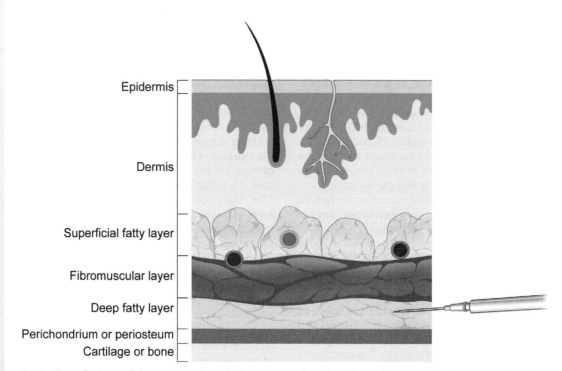

Fig. 2. The soft tissue of the nose consists of 4 layers: superficial fatty layer, fibromuscular layer, deep fatty layer, and periosteum or perichondrium. Therefore, the ideal layer for filler injection is the deep fatty layer located between the SMAS and the perichondrium or periosteum, to minimize damage to the vessels or the nerves. The deep fatty layer also has an advantage of being able to augment the filler volume sufficiently due to loose tissue compared with other layers.

have thorough knowledge, they should not embark on injecting fillers in the nose. Patients in whom good results cannot be achieved with filler should be offered surgery instead. The patient group that generally has good results includes those with mild dorsal hump, mildly deviated nose, high nasal tip with flat radix, slight imbalance from surgery. Those with moderate to severe dorsal hump, severely deviated nose, upturned nose, and bulbous nose are not expected to have good results from filler alone. Physicians should be cautious when offering this procedure to patients who have had nasal implants inserted or those with history of paraffin or liquid silicon injections, because skin irregularities and vascular compromise may occur.

METHOD OF PROCEDURE

Rhinoplasty using filler comprises 2 main parts: injecting over the nasal dorsum and injection the tip. The nasal dorsum has a solid and firm structure, namely, the nasal bones and the upper lateral cartilages, so it is easier to lift with filler injection. It is not easy, however, to lift or lengthen the nasal tip, especially in Asians, due to weak supporting structures.

After comparing and analyzing a patient's nose, the surgeon must decide which part is to be raised and by how much. Applying local anesthetic ointment for approximately 40 minutes is usually sufficient for anesthesia before the procedure. Using a plastic dressing can augment the effects of the local anesthetic.

The midline is marked along the nasal dorsum after anesthesia. It should be marked accurately to prevent complications, such as imbalance or intravascular injection, because mostly the blood vessels are not located in the center line of the nose. To find the ideal starting point for the nasofrontal angle is important. The nasal radix should begin at the level of supratarsal fold on lateral view in Asians, but it varies depending on the preference of the patient, height of the forehead, and the length of the nose.[7] The nasal dorsum should lie 1 mm to 2 mm below a line drawn from the nasion to the nasal tip for both Asian and white patients.[8] Some patients, however, may prefer a straight nasal bridge.

The nose is divided into 4 parts for the procedure—radix, rhinion, supratip, and tip (**Fig. 3**). Each part has different thickness of the subcutaneous tissue as well as different characteristics and strength of supporting structures, so different

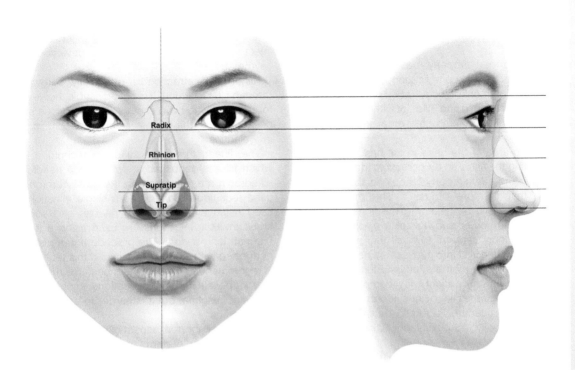

Fig. 3. Mark the midline of the nasal dorsum before the procedure. The midline line has to be marked accurately to prevent complications, such as imbalance and intravascular injection. The next step is to mark the point of the ideal radix position. In Asians, this is the supratarsal crease. The filler procedure is performed by dividing the nose into 4 sections, that is, the radix, rhinion, supratip, and tip. The reason is that each part has different thickness of the subcutaneous tissue as well as different characteristics and strength of supporting structures, so different injection methods have to be used.

injection methods have to be used. After marking the 4 sections, any defect on either side of the nose should be marked out.

The radix and the supratip regions have thick soft tissue, and the underlying structure (bone and cartilage, respectively) is concave. Therefore, a large filler volume has to be injected into these 2 regions to avoid depressions at the nasion and the supratip due to pressure from the overlying soft tissue (**Fig. 4**).

Filler is generally injected in the order of radix, rhinion, tip, and, finally, supratip area. The reason that the nasal tip is injected before the supratip area is because nasal tip support is weak, especially in Asians, making it difficult to predict the amount of projection that can be achieved. If the

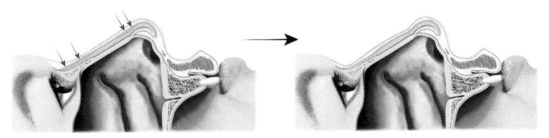

Fig. 4. The radix and the supratip regions have thick soft tissue, and the underlying structure (bone and cartilage respectively) is concave. Therefore, a large filler volume has to be injected into these 2 regions to avoid depressions at the nasion and the supratip due to pressure (*red arrow*) from the overlying soft tissue.

supratip area is injected before the nasal tip and the physician is unable to achieve adequate tip projection thereafter, a polybeak deformity may occur.

If performed properly, nasal tip injection with fillers has a low complication rate.[9] The areas that are commonly injected when performing nasal tip augmention using filler are the nasal spine, columellar space, interdomal area, and alar margin (**Fig. 5**).

Filling area of the nasal spine has the effect of elevating the nasal tip by increasing the supporting power and can alter an acute nasolabial angle to one that is more obtuse.[10] The membranous septum should be held with the fingers to keep filler in the center and not let it budge from the membranous septum toward the nasal cavity when injecting filler into the nasal spine area. If filler bulges from the membranous septum toward the nasal cavity, the patient may complain of nasal obstruction. If the filler bulges into the nasal cavity after the procedure, it should be molded to the center. Usually, approximately 0.5 mL of filler is used.

If filler is injected into the columellar space, it can function as a column to increase the support for the nasal tip and potentially correct a retracted columella. Usually, 0.2 mL to 0.3 mL of filler is used. Because the arterial vasculature of the columella is mostly located between the medial crura and the epidermis, it is best to inject filler between the medial crus to prevent vascular compromise.[11]

Injecting the tip with filler creates volume for reshaping. The volume and location of the injection depends on the desired appearance. Usually, approximately 0.2 mL is sufficient, and injection into the subfibromuscular tissue is recommended. When injecting filler into the nasal tip, it is safer to inject in the midline to minimize tip deviation and asymmetry.

Minor alar retraction is potentially corrected through filler injection. It is not advisable, however, for patients who have scarring from previous surgery due to the risk of dermal necrosis or irregularities.

The linear threading injection technique, in which filler is deposited as the syringe needle is withdrawn after insertion, is the most commonly used technique. Sometimes a single injection is used using a 2.5-inch long needle, and sometimes multiple injections are used using a small 0.5-inch long needle. The procedure can also be performed with a blunt cannula and this technique is recommended for beginners because there is a smaller possibility of complications, such as intravascular injection, but it is harder to achieve precise results.

The most important aspect of using filler in nasal reshaping is to perform the procedure without deviating from the midline. The most common complaint after any rhinoplasty is asymmetry or imbalance. This is true of rhinoplasty using filler as well. As discussed previously, the physician should always mark the midline on the nasal bridge and perform the procedure without deviating from the midline to minimize such complications.

It is strongly recommended that clinicians use both hands when using filler. While using one hand for injection, the noninjecting hand should

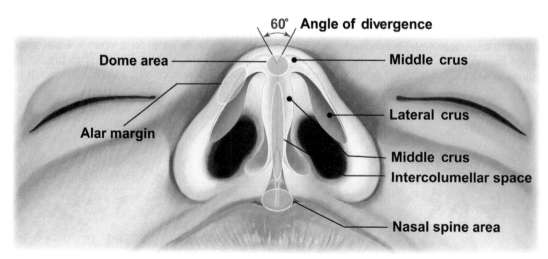

Fig. 5. The areas that are commonly injected when performing nasal tip augmention using filler are the nasal spine, columellar space, interdomal area, and alar margin. The amount of filler injected to each part is approximately 0.2 mL to 0.5 mL.

guide the needle and product in the tissue. This ensures minimal spreading or diffusion of the product.[12] After injection, gentle massage to mold and smooth out the filler is advisable. Any area with excessive filler should be pressed toward the base, and the areas that are underfilled should have additional injections. It is good to perform the touch-ups after 2 weeks because mild edema may occur after the procedure. No special dressings or antibiotics are needed.

COMPLICATIONS

Nasal reshaping with filler is safe but occasionally complications may occur. Most complications can be prevented by selecting safe products and performing the procedure in an appropriate manner.

The most common complications of filler injections are swelling, erythema, bruising, discoloration, irregularity, lump, and granuloma formation. Infections may occur, and serious complications, such as dermal necrosis due to vascular compromise, are rare but possible as well.[13]

Bruising

Bruising is a common complication of filler injections; it is caused by vascular damage by the needle. To reduce bruising, piercing of muscular layers must be minimized during filler injection, the injection site should be cleaned with an alcohol swab, and the procedure should be performed in a bright room with adequate lighting. Patients should be informed not to take blood thinners, such as aspirin, 1 week before the procedure. Applying ice packs on the injection site immediately postprocedure helps minimize bruising, and special needles or cannulae are used to minimize vascular injury. If bleeding occurs during the procedure, the injection site is covered with gauze and pressed for several minutes to avoid the formation of a hematoma. Patients should be informed that bruising is only temporary and does not affect the final therapeutic effect. It should also be explained that bruising can darken in the days after after the injection but will slowly fade over approximately 10 days.

Asymmetry

One of the most common complications of rhinoplasty using filler is asymmetry. To prevent asymmetry, the needle tip must be placed precisely in the midline, and the direction of the bevel should be toward the median plane. When injecting filler into a patient with a deviated nose, it is prudent to watch the shape of the nose closely while slowly injecting small amounts of filler.

Visible Implant

Injecting filler that is placed superficially (close to the skin surface) may result in unevenness of the injected site or visibility. To avoid this, the filler should be injected into the appropriate layer according to its characteristics.[14]

Hypersensitivity

Occasionally, there may be hypersensitivity to the filler ingredients. The main symptoms are pain and erythema, accompanied by pruritus and fever. In most cases, the symptoms subside as the causative substance disappears. In severe cases, administering corticosteroid products and warm compression may help alleviate the symptoms. Pulsed dye laser treatment can be used for persistent erythema. Many reactions that are assumed to be allergic or hypersensitivity responses are most likely caused by bacterial reactions.[15]

Lumps

Lumps can form after filler injection – these are due to either granuloma or nodule formation. A granuloma is an immune-mediated response to an injected foreign body and is formed by accumulation of immune response-related cells, such as lymphocytes, to eliminate the foreign body. Treatment is with corticosteroid injection or surgical removal. Nodules are round and solid. Their development is a common complication after the use of fillers for soft tissue augmentation and commonly categorized as inflammatory or noninflammatory in nature. Inflammatory nodules may appear anywhere from days to years after treatment, whereas noninflammatory nodules are typically seen immediately after implantation and are usually secondary to improper placement of the filler.[16] Treatment is with hyaluronidase (if the filler used is HA), corticosteroid, or surgical removal.

Vascular Compromise

The most serious complications that can occur with filler are dermal necrosis and blindness. The mechanism leading to tissue necrosis after HA filler injection is not fully understood. Vascular compromise is divided into intravascular or extravascular causes. Intravascular factors include direct obstruction of arteries by large-molecular-weight HA fillers and chemical damage of the endothelial lining by HA or impurities in the fillers.[17] Extravascular causes include external venous compression due to excessive volume of injection[18] or edema and inflammatory response caused by a component of the filler.[19] Among these suggested factors, intra-arterial obstruction is supported by many investigators.

Intra-arterial Embolism

Cause

Most cases of intra-arterial embolism after rhinoplasty using filler occur when filler is injected directly into the dorsal nasal artery or lateral nasal artery. The dorsal nasal artery, as its name suggests, runs along the dorsum of the nose, approximately 3 mm away from the midline. The needle tip can be inserted into the blood vessel if it is inserted in parallel with the blood vessel. The dorsal nasal artery

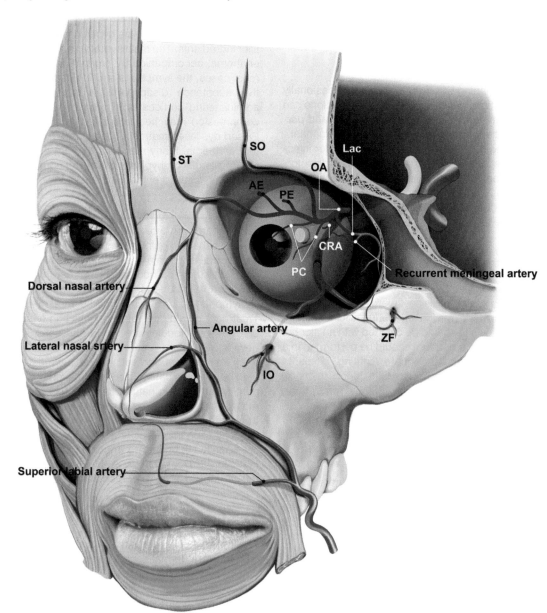

Fig. 6. The dorsal nasal artery, as its name suggests, runs along the dorsum of the nose, approximately 3 mm away from the midline. It is a fairly immobile blood vessel fixed to the surrounding tissue, and the needle tip can be inserted into the blood vessel if it is inserted in parallel with the blood vessel. The dorsal nasal artery anastomoses with the ophthalmic, infratrochlear, and angular arteries, and the widespread embolism through the connected blood vessels manifests as skin necrosis in a geographic pattern. It is also a branch of ophthalmic artery, so propagation of the filler embolus may also cause eye symptoms. AE, anterior ethmoidal artery; CRA, central retinal artery; IO, infraorbital artery; Lac, lacrimal artery; OA, ophthalmic artery; PC, posterior cilliary artery; PE, posterior ethmoidal artery; SO, supraorbital artery; ST, supratrochlear artery; ZF, zygomaticofacial artery.

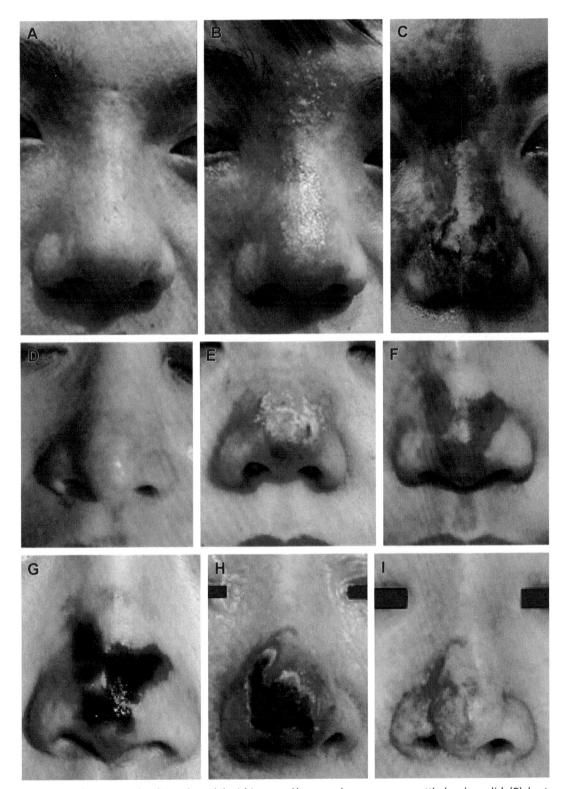

Fig. 7. The ischemic area develops edema (*A*) within several hours and soon appears mottled and purplish (*D*) due to venous congestion as a rebound phenomenon. After approximately 24 hours, multiple ulcerative lesions accompanied by erythema (*B, E*), worsening over time, resulting in desquamation of the tissue etc (*F, G*). After that, definite findings of dermal necrosis, such as eschar formation (*C, H*) occur gradually, and then the skin recovers through the wound healing process (*I*).

anastomoses with the ophthalmic, infratrochlear, and angular arteries, and the widespread embolism through the connected vaculature manifests as skin necrosis in a geographic pattern. It is also a branch of ophthalmic artery, so propagation of the filler embolus may also cause eye symptoms (**Fig. 6**).

Symptoms

Intra-arterial embolism has a low incidence, but its consequences are devastating. Once filler is injected into the arterial bloodstream, patients experience severe pain, and they sometimes complain of a sensation of something spreading out from the injection site. The area supplied by the blood vessel where filler embolism has occurred becomes pale due to ischemia. The ischemic area develops edema within several hours and soon appears mottled and purplish due to venous congestion as a rebound phenomenon. After approximately 24 hours, multiple ulcerative lesions accompanied by erythema resulting in desquamation of the tissue can occur. This typically gets worst with time. Thereafter, definite findings of dermal necrosis, such as eschar formation, may gradually occurs and then the skin recovers through the wound healing process (**Fig. 7**).

Prevention

During the procedure, the needle tip must always be located in the midline during filler injection to avoid injecting into the dorsal nasal artery because it runs in parallel with the midline, 3 mm away. If filler has to be injected into the side of the nasal dorsum, for example, for correction of deviated nose, the needle should never move in parallel with the direction of the blood vessels. After inserting the needle into the midline, the needle tip should move to the side, injecting filler at the same time to prevent injection into the blood vessel, although there may be some bleeding due to injury to the vessel (**Fig. 8**). The dorsal nasal artery is located in the superficial fatty layer and SMAS; therefore, the injection should be in the deep fatty layer to prevent embolization. Using a blunt cannula also may helpful for beginners who are not familiar with injection technique.

Treatment

If a patient complains of severe pain and blanching of the skin is observed along the area of blood vessel during the filler procedure, stop the injection immediately and aspirate as much filler as possible. If hyaluronic filler has been injected, injection of hyaluronidase is recommended because

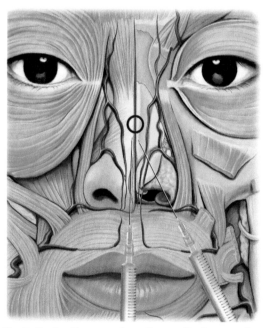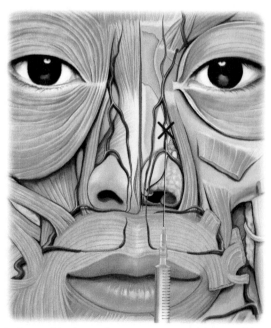

Fig. 8. During the procedure, the needle tip must always be located in the midline during filler injection (*left*) to avoid injecting into the dorsal nasal artery because it runs in parallel with the midline, 3 mm away. If filler has to be injected into the side of the nasal dorsum, for example, for correction of deviated nose, the needle should never move in parallel with the direction of the blood vessel (*right*). After inserting the needle into the midline, the needle tip should move to the side (*left*), and injecting filler at the same time to prevent injection into the blood vessel, although there may be some bleeding due to injury to the vessel.

there have been some recent reports that if hyaluronidase is injected around the artery, some of it can diffuse through the tunica intima. Some practitioners recommend injection of hyaluronidase regardless of the type injected filler because hyaluronidase is able to decrease interstitial pressure.

There are reports that low-molecular-weight heparin therapy decreases thrombosis and embolism, but it may be difficult to obtain and administer in an outpatient clinic setting. It is important to supply enough oxygen to the area of ischemia. For this purpose, hot packs and soft massage are applied, and 2% nitroglycerin paste is applied for vasodilation. Starting hyperbaric oxygen therapy is helpful if available. Administer appropriate antibiotics to prevent secondary infection.[20–23] Injection of prostaglandin E1, 10 µg a day for 5 days, is effective.[24] After approximately 1 day, appropriate dressing should be applied once desquamation and pustule formation occur. Apply wet dressing for faster wound healing, and continue to administer antibiotics.

Inflammatory Response and Edema

Sometimes, inflammatory response and edema occur due to a protein component, such as endotoxin, contained in filler and results in injury to the skin. This is caused mostly by HA filler, and symptoms, like erythematous edema, dermal hypertrophy, and pustules, may appear several days after injection.

Symptoms occur at all sites of filler injection and do well with appropriate antibiotic treatment and dressing.

REFERENCES

1. Constantinidis J, Daniilidis J. Aesthetic and functional rhinoplasty. Hosp Med 2005;66:221–6.
2. Murray CA, Zloty D, Warshawski L. The evolution of soft tissue fillers in clinical practice. Dermatol Clin 2005;23:343–63.
3. Oneal RM, Izenberg PH, Schlesinger J. Surgical anatomy of the nose. In: Daniel RK, editor. Rhinoplasty. Boston: Little Brown; 1993. p. 3–37.
4. Daniel RK, Letourneau A. Rhinoplasty: nasal anatomy. Ann Plast Surg 1998;20:5–13.
5. Jung DH, Kim HJ, Koh KS, et al. Arterial supply of the nasal tip in Asians. Laryngoscope 2000;110(2 Pt 1):308–11.
6. Tardy ME Jr. Pratical surgical anatomy. In: Tardy ME, editor. Rhinoplasty, the Art and the Science. Philadelphia: W.B. Saunders Co; 1997. p. 5–125.
7. Yun YS, Choi JC, Jung DH. External nasal appearance by Koreans, photo analysis. J Rhinol 1998; 5(2):103–7.
8. Gunter JP. Facial analysis for the rhinopalsty patient. In: Gunter JP, editor. Proceedings of the 14th Dallas Rhinoplasty Symposium. Dallas (TX): Southwestern; 1997. p. 45–55.
9. Kim P, Ahn JT. Structured nonsurgical Asian rhinoplasty. Aesthetic Plast Surg 2012;36(3):698–703.
10. Tanaka Y, Matsuo K, Yuzuriha S. Westernization of the asian nose by augmentation of the retropositioned anterior nasal spine with an injectable filler. Eplasty 2011;11:e7.
11. Lee YI, Yang HM, Pyeon HJ, et al. Anatomical and histological study of the arterial distribution in the columellar area, and the clinical implications. Surg Radiol Anat 2014;36(7):669–74.
12. Jacovella PF. Use of calcium hydroxylapatite (Radiesse®) for facial augmentation. Clin Interv Aging 2008;3(1):161–74.
13. Lemperle G, Rullan PP, Gauthier-Hazan N. Avoiding and treating dermal filler complications. Plast Reconstr Surg 2006;118(3 Suppl):92S–107S.
14. Narins RS, Jewell M, Rubin M, et al. Clinical conference: management of rare events following dermal fillers - focal necrosis and angry red bumps. Dermatol Surg 2006;32:426–34.
15. Dayan SH, Arkins JP, Brindise R. Soft tissue fillers and biofilms. Facial Plast Surg 2011;27:23–8.
16. Ledon JA, Savas JA, Yang S, et al. Inflammatory nodules following soft tissue filler use: a review of causative agents, pathology and treatment options. Am J Clin Dermatol 2013;14(5):401–11.
17. Kim DW, Yoon ES, Ji YH, et al. Vascular complications of hyaluronic acid fillers and the role of hyaluronidase in management. J Plast Reconstr Aesthet Surg 2011;64(12):1590–5.
18. Cohen JL. Understanding, avoiding, and managing dermal filler complications. Dermatol Surg 2008; 34(Suppl. 1):S92–9.
19. Weinberg MJ, Solish N. Complications of hyaluronic acid fillers. Facial Plast Surg 2009;25:324–8.
20. Grunebaum LD, Allemann IB, Dayan S, et al. The risk of alar necrosis associated with dermal filler injection. Dermatol Surg 2009;35:1635–40.
21. Glaich AS, Cohen JL, Goldberg LH. Injection necrosis of the glabella: protocol for prevention and treatment after use of dermal fillers. Dermatol Surg 2006;32:276–81.
22. Sclafani AP, Fagien S. Treatment of injectable soft tissue filler complications. Dermatol Surg 2009;35: 1672–80.
23. Hirsch RJ, Lupo M, Cohen JC, et al. Delayed presentation of impending necrosis following soft tissue augmentation with hyaluronic acid and successful management with hyaluronidase. J Drugs Dermatol 2007;6:325–8.
24. Kim SG, Kim YJ, Lee SI, et al. Salvage of nasal skin in a case of venous compromise after hyaluronic acid filler injection using prostaglandin E. Dermatol Surg 2011;37:1817–9.

Index

Note: Page numbers of article titles are in **boldface** type.

A

Aesthetics, surface, and analysis, **1–15**
African American patient, nasal anatomy of, 255–256
  rhinoplasty in, **255–264**
    preoperative planning and preparation for, 256–257, 258
    surgical techniques for, 257–262
      alar flare and base reduction in, 261, 262
      complications and management of, 261–262, 263
      initial dissection for, 257, 259
      nasal tip surgery, 259–260
      osteotomies, 260
      precautions in, 262
      radix and dorsal augmentation, 260–261
      treatment goals and planned outcomes of, 256
Alar rim deformities, **127–134**
  classification of, 127, 128
  surgical correction of, 127–133
    alar rim graft in, 129, 130
    alar rim thickness reduction in, 131, 132, 133
    cartilage graft in, 129
    secondary rhinoplasty in, 132, 133
    tissue removal in, 127–129
    V flap design in, 129–131
Asian nose, anatomy of, 266
  characteristics of, and clinical applications of, 265–266
  dorsal hump of, management of, 268–272
  nasal dorsum of, augmentation of, 266–268
    management of, 266–272
  nasal tip in, management of, 272–275, 278
  revision rhinoplasty of, 275–278
  short, contracted, as complication of revision rhinoplasty, 276, 277
Asian patient, rhinoplasty in, **265–279**
    graft materials used in, advantages and disadvantages of, 267, 268, 269, 270
    revision, 275–278

B

Barrel vault, approach to rhinoplasty, 60

C

Chin, analysis of, 297, 299
Chin deformity(ies), bony or soft tissue, 298–300
  evaluation of, 297
  lateral cephalogram in, 297, 298

  osseous genioplasty in, 302–303
  osteotomies in, 303–304, 305
  rhinoplasty in, chin advancement, augmentation, and reduction as adjuncts to, **295–306**
    implant characteristics for, 300, 301
    postoperative evaluation in, 305
    preoperative planning and preparation for, 296–299, 300
    procedural approach in, 300–301
    soft tissue fillers in, 304–305
    surgical technique in, 300–302, 303
Cleft lip nose, **213–221, 223–235**
  alar base treatment in, 233–234
  bilateral, 224
  cleft alar rim treatment in, 233–234
  cleft anatomy of, 213–214
  cleft lip repair in, 214, 215
  complete bilateral clefts in, 214–217
  incomplete bilateral cleft in, 214
  intermediate rhinoplasty in, 226
  nasal tip treatment in, 233
  orthognathic surgery in, 226–227, 228, 229
  presurgical nasoalveolar molding in, 225
  primary nasal correction in, technique of, 217–219
  primary rhinoplasty in, 225–226
  secondary cleft nasal deformity correction, 217, 218, 219–221
  secondary (definitive) rhinoplasty in, 227
  septal reconstruction in, 228–233
  surgical techniques in, approaches for, 227–228, 230, 231
  treatment of, 224–227
    timing of, 224–225
  unilateral, 224
Cleft nasal deformity, anatomy and embryology of, 223–224
Costal cartilage grafts, in rhinoplasty, complications and management of, 207–211
    patient positioning for, 203
    preoperative planning and preparation for, 202–203
    procedural approach for, 203–207, 208
    treatment goals and planned outcomes of, 202
Cottie maneuver, 31, 32

D

Dorsal hump augmentation, for underprojection, 92
Dorsal hump reduction, and osteotomies, **47–58**
  complications of, 53–54

Clin Plastic Surg 43 (2016) 319–322
http://dx.doi.org/10.1016/S0094-1298(15)00154-6
0094-1298/16/$ – see front matter © 2016 Elsevier Inc. All rights reserved.

Moving?

VOLUME NINETY TWO

ADVANCES IN
COMPUTERS

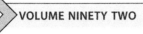

VOLUME NINETY TWO

Advances in
COMPUTERS

Edited by

ALI HURSON
Department of Computer Science
Missouri University of Science and Technology
325 Computer Science Building
Rolla, MO 65409-0350
USA
Email: hurson@mst.edu

ELSEVIER

AMSTERDAM • BOSTON • HEIDELBERG • LONDON
NEW YORK • OXFORD • PARIS • SAN DIEGO
SAN FRANCISCO • SINGAPORE • SYDNEY • TOKYO
Academic Press is an imprint of Elsevier

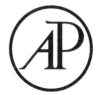

Academic Press is an imprint of Elsevier
225 Wyman Street, Waltham, MA 02451, USA
525 B Street, Suite 1800, San Diego, CA 92101-4495, USA
The Boulevard, Langford Lane, Kidlington, Oxford, OX5 1GB, UK
32 Jamestown Road, London NW1 7BY, UK
Radarweg 29, PO Box 211, 1000 AE Amsterdam, The Netherlands

First edition 2014

Notices
No responsibility is assumed by the publisher for any injury and/or damage to persons
or property as a matter of products liability, negligence or otherwise, or from any use or
operation of any methods, products, instructions or ideas contained in the material herein.

Library of Congress Cataloging-in-Publication Data
A catalog record for this book is available from the Library of Congress

British Library Cataloguing-in-Publication Data
A catalogue record for this book is available from the British Library

ISBN: 978-0-12-420232-0
ISSN: 0065-2458

For information on all Academic Press publications
visit our web site at *store.elsevier.com*

Printed and bound by CPI Group (UK) Ltd, Croydon, CR0 4YY
Transferred to digital print 2013

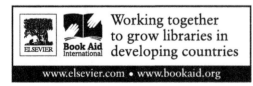

Working together
to grow libraries in
developing countries

www.elsevier.com • www.bookaid.org

CONTENTS

PREFACE

Traditionally, *Advances in Computers*, the oldest Series to chronicle the rapid evolution of computing, annually publishes several volumes, each typically comprising of five to eight chapters, describing new developments in the theory and applications of computing. The theme of this 92nd volume is inspired by the advances in information technology. Within the spectrum of information technology, this volume touches a variety of topics ranging from software to I/O devices. The volume is a collection of five chapters that were solicited from authorities in the field, each of whom brings to bear a unique perspective on the topic.

In Chapter 1, "Register-Level Communication in Speculative Chip Multiprocessors," Radulović *et al.* articulate the advantages of having register-level communication as a part of the thread-level speculation mechanism in Chip Multiprocessors. In addition, this chapter presents a case study addressing the Snoopy Inter-register Communication protocol that enables communication of the register values and synchronization between the processor cores in the CMP architecture over a shared bus. This chapter covers issues such as *thread-level speculation mechanism, thread identification, register communication,* and *misspeculation recovery.*

In Chapter 2, "Survey on System I/O Hardware Transactions and Impact on Latency, Throughput, and Other Factors," Larsen and Lee survey the current state of high-performance I/O architecture advances and explore its advantages and limitations. This chapter articulates that the proliferation of CPU multicores, multi-GB/s ports, and on-die integration of system functions requires techniques beyond the classical approaches for optimal I/O architecture performance. A survey on existing methods and advances in utilizing the I/O performance available in current systems is presented. This chapter also shows how I/O is impacted by latency and throughput constraints. Finally, an option to improve I/O performance is presented.

The concept of "Hardware and Application Profiling Tools" is the main theme of Chapter 3. In this chapter, Janjusic and Kavi describe widely acceptable hardware and application profiling tools along with a few classical tools that have advanced in the literature. A great number of references are provided to help jump-start the interested reader into the area of hardware simulation and application profiling. The discussion about application profiling is interleaved with terms that are, arguably incorrectly, used interchangeably. Thus, this chapter makes an effort to clarify and correctly classify tools based on the scope, interdependence, and operation mechanisms.

In Chapter 4, "Model Transformation Using Multiobjective Optimization," Mkaouer and Kessentini propose the application of genetic algorithm for model transformation to ensure quality and to minimize the complexity, two important conflicting parameters. Starting from the source model, randomly a set of rules are generated and applied to generate some target models. The quality of the proposed solution (rules) is evaluated by (1) calculating the number of rules and matching metamodels in each rule, and (2) assessing the quality of generated target models using a set of quality metrics. This chapter reports on the validation results using three different transformation mechanisms.

Finally, in Chapter 5, "Manual Parallelization Versus State-of-the-Art Parallelization Techniques: The SPEC CPU2006 as a Case Study," Vitorović *et al.* attempt to articulate the importance of manual parallelization of applications. This chapter studies various parallelization methods and contemporary software and hardware tools for extracting parallelism from sequential applications. It also attempts to identify typical code patterns amenable for parallelization. As a case study, the SPEC CPU2006 suite is considered as a representative collection of typical sequential applications. The automatic parallelization and vectorization of the sequential C++ applications from the CPU2006 suite are discussed, and since these potentials are generally limited, it explores the manual parallelization of these applications.

I hope that you find these articles of interest and useful in your teaching, research, and other professional activities. I welcome feedback on the volume and suggestions for topics for future volumes.

ALI R. HURSON

Missouri University of Science and Technology

Rolla, MO, USA

CHAPTER ONE

Register-Level Communication in Speculative Chip Multiprocessors

Milan B. Radulović, Milo V. Tomašević, Veljko M. Milutinović

School of Electrical Engineering, University of Belgrade, Belgrade, Serbia

Contents

Abstract

The advantage of having register-level communication as a part of the thread-level speculation (TLS) mechanism in chip multiprocessors (CMPs) has already been clearly recognized in the open literature. The first part of this chapter extensively surveys the TLS support on the register level in CMPs. After the TLS mechanism is briefly explained, the classification criteria are established, and along them, the most prominent systems of this kind are elaborated upon focusing on the details about register communication. Then, the relevant issues in these systems such as thread identification, register communication, misspeculation recovery, performance, and scalability are comparatively discussed. The second part of the chapter represents a case study that describes the snoopy interregister communication (SIC) protocol that enables communication of the register values and synchronization between the processor cores in the

Advances in Computers, Volume 92
ISSN 0065-2458
http://dx.doi.org/10.1016/B978-0-12-420232-0.00001-5

1

CMP architecture over a shared bus. The appropriate software tool, which creates and annotates the threads from a sequential binary code of the loop-intensive applications, is described. Also, the states of registers are defined and the protocol actions during producer-initiated and consumer-initiated communication among the threads. Finally, the ESIC protocol, an enhancement of the SIC protocol with more aggressive speculation on the register values, is also presented and compared to the SIC.

LIST OF ABBREVIATIONS

AMA atlas multiadaptive
CMP chip multiprocessor
CRB communication register buffer
CSC communication scoreboard
ESIC enhanced SIC
EU execution units
FOPE fork-once parallel execution
FU functional unit
FW final write
GRF global register file
HW hardware
INV invalid
INVO invalid-others
IPC instructions per cycle
IRB intermediate register buffer
LC last-copy
LRF local register file
MAJC multiprocessor architecture for Java computing
MRF multiversion register file
MUCS multiplex unified coherence and speculation
NFW nonfinal write
PE processing element
PFW possibly final write
PRO propagated
PU processing unit
RAW read after write
RC ready-CRB
RR ready-released
RVS register validation store
RVT register versioning table
SH shared high
SIC snoopy interregister communication
SISC speculation integrated with snoopy coherence
SL shared low
SM speculative multithreaded
SPEC standard performance evaluation corporation
SRB store reservation buffer

SS synchronizing scoreboard
SW software
TD$ thread descriptor cache
TLS thread-level speculation
TU thread unit
UPD updated
VLIW very-long-instruction-word
VPS valid-possibly-safe
VPSF valid-possibly-safe-forwarded
VS valid-safe
VSO valid-safe-others
VU valid-unsafe
WAR write after read
WAW write after write

1. INTRODUCTION

In the previous decade, chip multiprocessors (CMPs) have emerged as a very attractive solution in using an ever-increasing on-chip transistor count, because of some important advantages over superscalar processors (e.g., exploiting of parallelism, design simplicity, faster clock, and better use of the silicon space). Furthermore, nowadays, the memory wall, the power wall, and the instruction-level parallelism (ILP) wall have made the CMP architecture inevitable. In order to attain a wider applicability and being a viable alternative to the other processing platforms, besides running parallel workloads, CMPs also have to be efficient in executing the existing sequential applications as well. The technique of thread-level speculation (TLS) is a way to achieve this goal. In the TLS, even possibly data-dependent threads can run in parallel as long as the semantics of the sequential execution is preserved. A special hardware support monitors the actual data dependencies between threads in run time and, if they are violated, misspeculation effects must be undone. The application threads can communicate between themselves through registers or through shared memory. This kind of system is known as speculative chip multiprocessor [1–7].

The rest of this chapter is organized as follows. The short explanation of the TLS technique illustrated with appropriate examples is given in Section 2. An extensive survey of the most representative speculative commercial and academic CMPs with the TLS support on the register level is presented in Section 3 along the established classification criteria (register file organization and interconnection topology). Section 4 brings a comparative analysis of relevant issues in these systems such as thread creation and speculation scope, register communication and synchronization mechanisms, misspeculation recovery, and performance and scalability. The case study in Section 5 presents the snoopy interregister communication (SIC) protocol and its enhancement, the enhanced SIC (ESIC) protocol, that enables the communication of register values and synchronization between processor cores in a CMP over a shared bus. Some conclusions are drawn in Section 6.

2. TLS IN CMPs

Multithreading is a technique that partitions a sequential program into a number of smaller instruction streams (threads) that can be executed in parallel keeping different processor cores in a CMP simultaneously busy. If these cores are simple superscalars, the small amount of the ILP can still be exploited on top of the multithreading, since the ILP and multithreading are orthogonal to each other. The best candidates for threads are basic blocks (sequence of instructions with no transfers in or out except at the start and the end), inner- or outer-loop iterations, subprogram calls, etc.

There are two multithreading approaches: *explicit* and *implicit*. The main differences between explicit and implicit multithreading relate to thread dispatch, execution, and communication mechanisms, while the underlying processor architecture and memory hierarchy are similar.

In *explicit* (nonspeculative) multithreading, the threads can be either independent or interdependent but properly synchronized on each occurrence of data dependence, so they can be nonspeculatively executed concurrently in a correct order. The software imposes the fork primitives for thread dispatch to specify interthread control dependencies. The explicit threads in sequential applications can be identified by the advanced parallelizing compilers or manual parallelization [2,7,8]. However, the identification of explicit threads is not easy because of the problems with pointers, conditional execution, etc. Even for numerical applications, the parallelizing compilers have been successful only to a limited extent in directly explicit multithreading. The parallelizing compilers are very conservative during thread identification, because they assume the existence of interthread dependencies whenever they cannot guarantee their independence even where interthread dependencies are not very likely. As illustrated in Fig. 1.1, if the values in arrays L and K are dependent on input data, the compiler cannot determine whether or not loop iterations access distinct array elements, and hence, it marks the loop as serial.

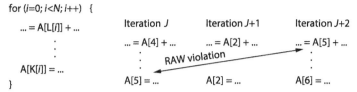

Figure 1.1 Example of the possibly dependent loop iterations. *This figure is taken from [2] with permission from the copyright holder.*

Consequently, CMPs cannot efficiently handle general-purpose sequential applications even with the sophisticated compilers in explicit multithreading. The problem can be solved by exploiting the *implicit* (speculative) multithreading. The implicit threads are identified in the application either during the compile time or during the run time with hardware support and can be (but less likely) interdependent. These threads can be executed speculatively in the CMP with some software or hardware support that can detect and correctly resolve interthread dependencies [2,7,9].

In such a system, the threads run in parallel on the different processors speculatively as long as their dependencies are not violated. If no violation occurs, the thread finishes and commits. In case of misspeculation, the thread that violates the dependence and all its successor threads are squashed and later reexecuted with correct data. The speculation hardware (thread identification, dependence prediction and detection, and data value prediction) guarantees the same result of execution as in a uniprocessor. This technique is referred to as TLS. The speculative thread architecture for mostly functional languages was first proposed in [1] where hardware is used to ensure the correct execution of parallel code with the side effects. Later on, the TLS technique was employed in a number of different CMP architectures (e.g., the Multiscalar is one the earliest tightly coupled multiprocessors fully oriented towards speculative execution [7]).

The speculative parallelism can be found in many sequential applications (e.g., [10]). The TLS provides a way to parallelize the sequential programs without a need for a complex data dependence analysis or explicit synchronization and to exploit the full potentials of CMP architecture in execution of general sequential applications. The threads are committed in the order in which they would execute sequentially, although they are actually executed in parallel. However, the TLS and synchronization are not mutually exclusive. In order to improve the performance, explicit synchronization can be used when the interthread dependencies are likely to occur.

The ideal memory system within hardware support for speculative execution should consist of the fully associative, infinite-size L1 caches intended to keep the speculative states. They should operate in write-back mode to prevent any change in the sequential state held in the L2 cache unless the thread is committed. When the speculative thread i performs a read operation, the speculative hardware must return the most recent value of data. If it is not found in the L1 cache of the processor that executes the speculative thread i, then the most recent value is read from a processor executing a thread j that is less speculative than thread i. If the value is not found in the caches of the processors executing the less speculative threads than thread i, the data are read from the L2 cache or from memory.

More precisely, an adequate hardware TLS support imposes five requirements: (a) data forwarding between parallel threads; (b) detecting read after write (RAW) hazards; (c) safe discarding of speculative state(s) after violations; (d) retiring speculative writes in the correct order, write after write (WAW) hazards; and (e) providing the memory renaming, write after read (WAR) hazards.

Firstly, in case of true data sharing between threads, when a later thread needs shared data, an earlier thread has to forward the most recent value. Sometimes, in order to minimize stalling, the producer thread sends updated data in advance on nondemand basis to the successor threads.

The RAW hazard occurs when a later thread prematurely reads data. Therefore, a situation when more speculative thread first reads a value that is later updated by some predecessor thread must be detected. It is usually resolved by squashing a thread that caused the violation and executing it again with valid data.

In case of violation, the permanent state must not be corrupted and all changes made by the violating thread must be made void. Usually, speculative state is held only in the private L1 cache and permanent state in the L2 cache, so the effects of misspeculation are easy to discard.

When a later thread writes to the same location before an earlier thread updates it (WAW hazard), this write must be seen by other threads in the correct program order. This can be achieved by allowing the threads to update the permanent state after committing strictly in the program order.

Finally, an earlier thread must never read a value produced by a later thread (the WAR hazard). This is ensured by keeping the actual data in the L1 cache that cannot be reached by earlier threads. An illustration for some of described situations is presented in Fig. 1.2.

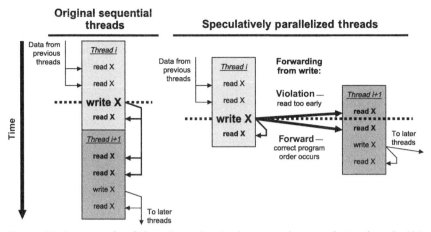

Figure 1.2 An example of data dependencies between the speculative threads. *This figure is taken from [7] with permission from the copyright holder.*

CMP with the TLS support is a high-performance and cost-effective alternative to complex superscalar processors. It has been shown that a speculative CMP of comparable die area can achieve performance on the integer applications similar to the superscalar processor [7]. However, the hardware and software support for speculative execution is not sufficient to ensure that a CMP architecture performs well for all applications. The notorious potential problems with the TLS are the following: (a) a lack of parallelism in the applications, (b) hardware overheads (a large amount of hardware remains unutilized when CMP runs a fully parallel application or a multiprogrammed workload), (c) software overheads in managing speculative threads, (d) an increased latency of interthread communication through memory, and (e) a wasted work that must be reexecuted in case a violation occurred.

Although the speculative parallelism can be exploited by software means only (e.g., [11–13]), most of the TLS systems employ the hardware support usually combined with the software support. There are three major approaches in the design of the speculative CMPs with the TLS hardware support.

The first one is related to the CMP architectures completely oriented towards exploiting speculative parallelism, for example, Multiscalar [14], Multiplex [8], Trace [15], speculative multithreaded (SM) [16], Multiprocessor Architecture for Java Computing (MAJC) [17], MP98 (Merlot) [18], and Mitosis [19]. These systems support interthread communication through both registers and shared memory and they usually have significant and effective hardware and software support for efficient speculative execution. However, when these CMPs run a true parallel application or a multiprogrammed workload, a large amount of that speculative support remains ineffective.

The second approach is oriented towards generic CMP architectures with a minimal added support for speculative execution, for example, Hydra [7] or STAMPede [20]. Such a system achieves the interthread communication through shared memory only. The limited hardware support in these CMPs is sufficient for correct speculative execution since they rely on compiler support and software speculation handlers to adapt the sequential codes for speculative execution. However, the necessity of source code recompilation can be a serious problem, especially when the source code is not available.

IACOMA [9], Atlas [21], NEKO [22], and Pinot [23] belong to the third approach that tries to combine the best of previous two approaches. They still enable the threads to communicate through both registers and memory as in the first approach, but they have mainly generic CMP architectures with modest hardware (HW)/SW support for speculative execution as in the second approach. Consequently, they can be considered as more cost-effective in running the true parallel or multiprogramming workloads.

Some studies about the impact of communication latency on the overall performance of the speculative CMP argued that a fast communication scheme between the processor cores may not be required and that interthread communication through the memory is fast enough to minimize the performance impact of the communication delays [7,9,24,25]. The limitation of the interthread communication through the memory simplifies the overall design but the need for source code recompilation is still a disadvantage for this group of CMPs.

The support for register-level communication introduces an additional complexity in the system (fast interconnect for exchanging the values, relatively complex logic, etc.). However, earlier studies have shown that register-level communication pays back by avoiding overhead of memory-level communication that requires the instructions to (a) explicitly store and load the communicated values to and from memory and (b) synchronize the communicating threads. It was concluded in [26] that register-based communication is $10 \times$ faster and synchronization is $60 \times$ faster than corresponding memory counterpart mechanism. The impact of having memory-level communication only on the overall performance degradation is evaluated in [27]. It was demonstrated that the communication through L2 cache (and not through registers) in a CMP with four superscalar cores (up to four-issue) incurs performance degradation of up to 50%. This is a strong support for employment of interregister communication mechanisms in the most of representative CMPs.

3. REGISTER COMMUNICATION MECHANISMS IN SPECULATIVE CMPs

The main goal of this chapter is to present an overview of the various CMP systems with TLS support on register level found in the open literature. There is a variety of issues in reviewing the hardware and software support for interthread register communication such as organization and implementation of the register file, interconnection topology, register communication protocol, thread identification, recovery from misspeculation, and compiler and other software tool support. The organization of register file(s) has a profound impact on the mechanisms of synchronization and communication of the register values between on–chip processor cores in speculative CMPs. Therefore, it is adopted as the main classification criterion for this presentation. Three different approaches can be recognized: distributed (local) register files, unified shared (global) register file, and hybrid design that combines both local register files (LRFs) and a global register file (GRF) (Fig. 1.3).

Traditional microprocessors have been mostly designed with a GRF shared by multiple functional units (FUs), which in turn increases the

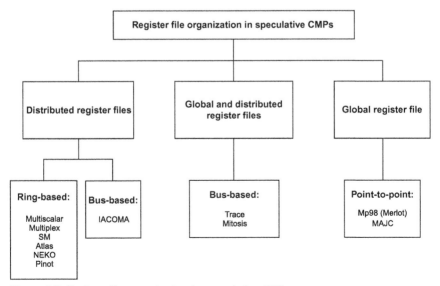

Figure 1.3 Register file organization in speculative CMPs.

number of register file read/write ports and, hence, leads to complex wiring, affects the cycle time, and increases latencies. In order to support higher degrees of instruction-level parallelism (ILP) and thread-level parallelism (TLP), the hardware implementation cost of a design with a central register file and a large and complex operand bypass network grows rapidly. In extremely small feature sizes and highly parallel processor designs like a CMP, a shared register file must be replaced with distributed file structures with local communication paths to alleviate the problems with a large number of long interconnects between the register file and operand bypass structure. This is the reason why the exclusive use of shared register file is scarce. Distributed register organizations scale efficiently compared to the traditional shared register file organization since they significantly reduce area, delay, and power dissipation. Consequently, almost all systems either employ distributed approach only or combine it with small shared register file [28–31].

Another influential design parameter is interconnection topology between cores on register level and it is adopted as a secondary classification criteria. The ring is a main design choice for the operand bypass network on register level in Multiscalar, Multiplex, SM, Atlas, NEKO, and Pinot (see Fig. 1.3). It is a natural choice for interconnection since processor cores during speculative execution primarily communicate with their two nearest neighbors—produced register values are sent to the more speculative core and consumed register values come from the less speculative core. The bus is another choice that is employed in Trace, IACOMA, and Mitosis. The simple bus architecture would be sufficient to handle a small number (4–8) of processor cores, but more cores or faster ones would require higher bandwidth, which in turn demands either more buses or hierarchy of local and global buses. Finally, in systems with GRF, MP98 (Merlot), and MAJC, the point-to-point networks are used as an operand bypass network for register value communication.

General data, architecture details, and register communication mechanisms of the speculative CMPs with the support for register-level communication, grouped by organization of register files and interconnection topology, are presented in this section.

3.1. Speculative CMPs with Distributed Register File

In almost all systems of this kind, LRFs are interconnected by a unidirectional or bidirectional ring except IACOMA, which uses shared bus for register communication.

3.1.1 Ring-Based Distributed Register File Approaches
3.1.1.1 Multiscalar

3.1.1.1.1 General Data The Multiscalar is one of the first efforts towards an architecture completely oriented to speculative execution as it performs an aggressive control and data speculation using the dedicated hardware and complex forwarding mechanisms. A program is broken into a collection of threads during compilation and the threads are distributed to the parallel processing units (PUs) under the control of a single hardware sequencer.

3.1.1.1.2 Architecture Details The PUs in Multiscalar share a common register namespace, which appears as a logically centralized register file although it consists of the physically decentralized register files, queues, and control logic with a set of control bit masks in different PUs. A fast unidirectional ring interconnects the PUs and forwards the register values to the next unit (Fig. 1.4). In this way, Multiscalar is able to exploit the communication locality and to recover the precise architectural register state among multiple PUs efficiently [14].

3.1.1.1.3 Register Communication The basic components of the register file in a Multiscalar are the modified register storage, a register queue, and a collection of the register control bit masks connected to a pipeline core (Fig. 1.5). The register storage physically consists of two register banks, one (bank 0) maintains the past while another (bank 1) maintains the present register state. While the present register set is used for execution of the current thread, the register state from previous threads is needed for recovery in case of incorrect speculation. The pointers in a form of bit masks (*past* and *present*; see storage block in Fig. 1.5) help in reducing the overhead of housekeeping operations in case of either thread committing or squashing. The queue component accepts the register values necessary for successor threads. The register control block coordinates the communication and synchronization in the register file by means of simple logic operations on a collection of bit masks: *create* mask, *sent* mask, *recv* mask, *accum* mask, *recover* mask, and *squash* mask [32].

The register values produced by previous units are communicated to the next units via the ring using queues. The propagation of the correct values is controlled by *create*, *recv*, and *sent* masks in the register control block (Fig. 1.5). The *create* mask of a thread identifies the registers in which values might be created by this thread. The *recv* and *sent* masks record the flow of register values between units, that is, when a register has been received by

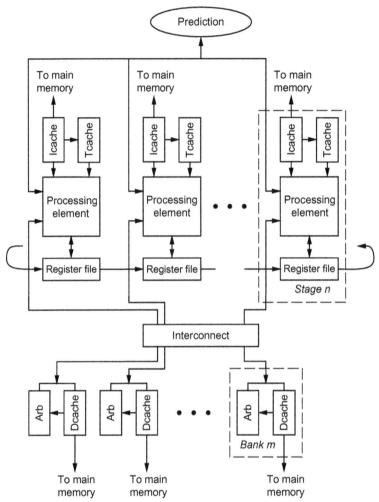

Figure 1.4 The block structure of Multiscalar. *This figure is taken from [32] with permission from the copyright holder.*

the current thread, the appropriate bit is set in *recv* mask, while the appropriate bit is set in *sent* mask when the register has been sent to the next unit.

The consumption of register values in the current thread has to be synchronized with the production of register values in the previous threads. This is handled by means of the *accum* mask. Since a current thread might require the register values from all its predecessor threads, the required information can only be provided by the combined *create* masks of all predecessors. Therefore, the reservations on registers for a successor thread are given

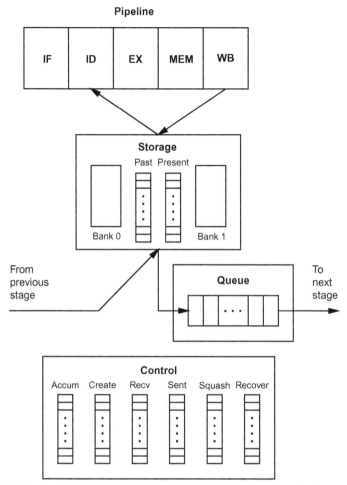

Figure 1.5 The basic components of the Multiscalar register file. *This figure is taken from [32] with permission from the copyright holder.*

in the *accum* mask that represents the union of the create masks of currently active predecessor threads.

Finally, when speculation succeeds and thread commits, the *past* mask is updated with the *present* mask indicating a safe state. In case of misspeculation, the *present* mask is updated with the *past* mask discarding the incorrect values produced in a current stage. By analyzing the control flow graph, Multiscalar compiler (a modified version of GCC 2.5.8) can help in producing the *create* register bit mask and in determining the last updates of the registers within a thread in order to further propagate their values.

3.1.1.2 Multiplex

3.1.1.2.1 General Data The Multiplex CMP [8] is the direct successor of Multiscalar. It is the first speculative CMP that unifies the explicit and implicit multithreading (see Section 2) by grouping a subset of protocol states in an implicitly threaded CMP to provide a write-invalidate protocol for explicit threads without additional hardware support. The parallelizing compiler analyzes the programs and generates the explicit threads, while the rest of the program is marked as implicit threads. Appropriate selection between two threading models at compile time helps to improve the performance. The explicit threads are used to avoid implicit threading speculation overhead, to maximize the parallelism exploited, and to minimize performance degradation in compiler-analyzable program segments, while implicit threads are used to avoid the need for serializing program segments that cannot be marked as explicit. The Multiplex can switch between implicit and explicit threading modes, but cannot execute explicit and implicit threads simultaneously.

3.1.1.2.2 Architecture Details The Multiplex has a small number of conventional cores with the private L1 data and instruction caches and shared L2 cache (Fig. 1.6). The light blocks are the components of a conventional CMP with explicit multithreading: the PUs, the L1 instruction caches, the system interconnect, and the L2 cache. The dark-gray-shaded blocks are the components that enable implicit and hybrid (implicit/explicit) threading: the thread dispatch unit, the thread descriptor cache (TD$), the L1 data caches, and the register communication queues.

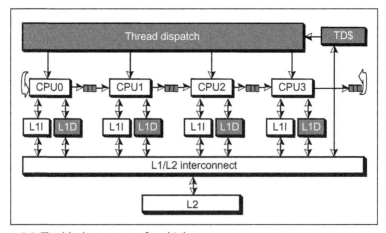

Figure 1.6 The block structure of multiplex.

3.1.1.2.3 Register Communication The multiplex unified coherence and speculation (MUCS) protocol combines the coherence and speculative versioning and both implicit and explicit threading without additional hardware. In Multiplex, like in Multiscalar, the implicit threads communicate both register and memory values whereas the explicit threads communicate memory values only as in a conventional shared memory multiprocessor. The Multiscalar's register communication mechanism [30] is applied in Multiplex for register dependencies among implicit threads.

3.1.1.3 SM

3.1.1.3.1 General Data SM processor simultaneously executes the multiple threads obtained from a sequential program using speculation techniques that do not require any compiler or user support [16,33]. It does not require any modification to the instruction-set architecture, which means that ordinary programs compiled for superscalar processors can be run on this platform. The thread identification is completely performed in hardware without affecting binary code. Multiple concurrent threads speculatively execute different iterations of the same loop while the iterations are assigned to the threads following the execution order.

The SM traces the register and memory dependencies by using an aggressive speculation on interthread data dependencies. For each new speculative thread, SM predicts its register and memory dependencies with the previous threads and values that flow through them. On the basis of predicted interthread dependencies, it executes the new speculative thread while the predicted values are used to avoid stalling because of lack of the actual data.

3.1.1.3.2 Architecture Details The SM consists of several thread units (TUs) that are connected by the ring (Fig. 1.7). Each core has its own register file partitioned into live-in registers and local registers, register map table, instruction queue, FUs, local memory, and reorder buffer for enabling out-of-order instruction execution. All TUs share the instruction cache and multivalue cache.

3.1.1.3.3 Register Communication The interthread dependencies and values that flow through them are handled using a history table called *loop iteration table* that contains two fields (register dependencies and memory dependencies). The information about the last iteration of a loop is stored in this table indexed with the loop identifier. A table entry is allocated every time a new loop execution is started. In case of replacement, the entry of

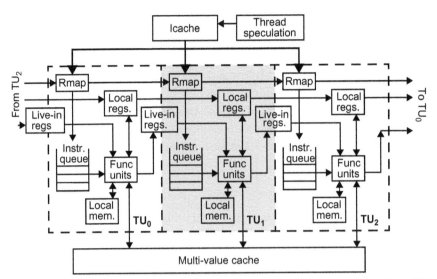

Figure 1.7 The SM block structure with three thread units. *This figure is taken from [33] with permission from the copyright holder.*

history table that corresponds to the loop with the least recently started execution is candidate for eviction [34].

As for the register dependencies, each table entry contains five fields: (a) *#write*, the number of writes for each logical register that are performed by the last iteration of the corresponding loop; (b) *live*, the indication whether the entry contained a live-in register value at the beginning of the iteration; (c) *value*, the register value at the beginning of the iteration; (d) *val_str*, the difference between the values of the last two iterations; and (e) *conf*, the indication whether the register value is predictable or not. This information is needed to detect the dependencies and to predict some register values. Each core has *Rmap* table (see Fig. 1.7), which keeps the correspondence between the logical and physical registers of current thread. When a speculative thread starts running, its LRF and its *Rmap* table are copied from its predecessor. Each register that is live and predictable can be initialized with a value predicted using a stride from history table. For nonpredictable live registers, the *Rmap* table entries are set to point to corresponding entry of the live-in register file. An additional table (*Rwrite*) keeps a predicted number of remaining writes for each register. When a write to some destination register occurs, the corresponding entry is decremented, and if it reaches 0, the register value is sent to its successor register file [16,34].

3.1.1.4 Atlas

3.1.1.4.1 General Data The support for the thread-level speculation in the Atlas CMP is characterized by an aggressive value prediction mechanism on both the register and memory levels [21]. Atlas works on unmodified sequential binaries using the MEM-slicing dynamic partitioning algorithm to identify threads. MEM slicing uses load and store instructions as the thread starting and ending points assuming that compiler allocates the variables with high temporal locality to registers and that the memory references are boundaries of data dependence chains [22,35].

3.1.1.4.2 Architecture Details The Atlas consists of eight PUs, based on the Alpha 21164, connected via bidirectional ring, while the shared L2 cache and value/control predictor are accessible via two separate shared buses. The unit architecture, with shaded new or modified structures added for thread and value speculation, is presented in the Fig. 1.8.

3.1.1.4.3 Register Communication As most of the register dependencies are expected to be short, when a thread is started, the value for a live register is always predicted rather than communicated between units. With

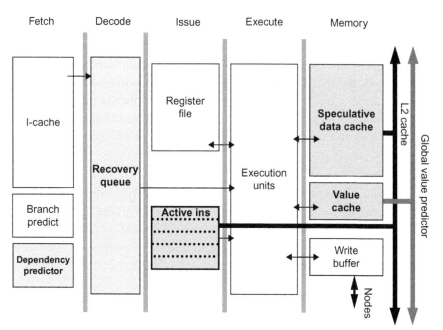

Figure 1.8 The processing unit in Atlas. *This figure is taken from [35] with permission from the copyright holder.*

this prediction, broadcasting and snooping of the register values are avoided. Atlas uses one value/control predictor for both value and control predictions. If a register value prediction is incorrect, misspeculation occurs and only instructions that depend on the incorrect predicted value will be reexecuted. Each unit has a recovery queue structure that performs fine-grained value misspeculation recovery. The *Active Ins Queue* tracks all value predictions within a unit. It is a small associative structure that keeps an in-order list of the active value predictions in the unit. Besides effective addresses of the active predictions, it also records the register number being predicted, the predicted value, the addresses of the instructions that initiated the prediction, and a few control bits. When a thread acquires the non-speculative status, the thread retirement starts with verification of register value predictions. The bit mask is sent to the previous nonspeculative node to specify the register values to be verified. The nonspeculative node in turn sends the register values further via ring to be verified.

When the verification of register values is completed, the correct values for all register value predictions on the nonspeculative unit are determined. If any predicted register value mismatches the final correct value from the previous unit, recovery from misspeculation is carried on. After recovery process is completed, the thread starts to perform two retirement tasks in parallel: the global value prediction update and write buffer flush. The global value predictor is updated with the data values from *Active Ins Queue*, while write buffer broadcasts the data to the L2 cache and all speculative units. The thread is committed when it has finished execution and write buffer and *Active Ins* are empty. The successor speculative thread acquires non-speculative status while global thread logic together with value and control predictor assigns a new speculative thread to the free unit [21,35].

3.1.1.5 NEKO

3.1.1.5.1 General Data NEKO is the SM CMP that also supports the interthread communication on both register and memory level [22,36]. Both the control and data dependencies between threads are allowed in this architecture. A program is partitioned into threads at compile time to keep the CMP hardware simple. The threads are identified from the program control graph by structural analysis [36,37].

3.1.1.5.2 Architecture Details NEKO is composed of a thread control unit, four PUs (PU1 to PU4), and a memory system (Fig. 1.9). A centralized thread control unit handles interthread control dependencies and schedules

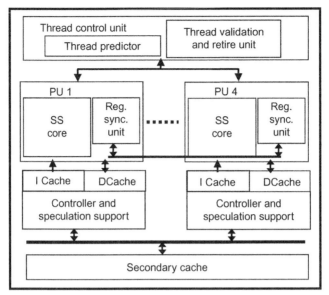

Figure 1.9 The block structure of NEKO. *This figure is taken from [36] with permission from the copyright holder.*

the threads onto PUs. It uses a thread predictor unit to predict the thread that should be executed next. Each PU has private L1 instruction and data caches, which are connected with shared bus to the unified L2 cache. The register files are distributed and the register bypass network between PUs is implemented as a one-directional ring.

3.1.1.5.3 Register Communication NEKO employs a producer-initiated register communication protocol, which sends the register values to the adjacent threads over ring datapath in order to provide low-latency transfers. A ring topology register datapath and an example of communication process are given in the Fig. 1.9. The register synchronization is supported in both software and hardware. The compiler identifies inter-thread register dependencies and inserts into binary code the information needed for safe synchronization of register values between dependent threads. The following information is generated for each statically defined thread: (a) *create mask* specifies a set of registers that might be redefined by thread; (b) *send flag*, if set, indicates that during instruction retirement, its destination register value can be safely sent to successor threads; and (c) *send instruction* that encodes the registers in the instruction that also can be safely sent to successor threads when instruction is retired.

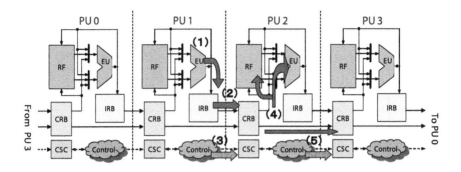

Figure 1.10 An example of communication process in NEKO. *This figure is taken from [37] with permission from the copyright holder.* (For color version of this figure, the reader is referred to the online version of this chapter.)

Hardware support in each PU consists of intermediate register buffers (IRBs), communication register buffers (CRBs), and communication scoreboards (CSCs) (see Fig. 1.10). IRB holds the produced speculative register values, while CRB holds either committed register values or values propagated by predecessor PU.

CSC keeps the status of registers involved in communication in a form of the register status bits: ready-CRB (RC) bit (indicates that a produced register value is ready in CRB), ready-released (RR) bit (indicates that a register value is released), updated (UPD) bit (indicates that a register value is locally updated), and propagated (PRO) bit (indicates that a register value is ready to be propagated to the next PU). The control of communication is performed by monitoring of register status in CSC.

In the example from Fig. 1.10, PU1 executes the instruction and generates a value for an instruction's destination register. The calculated value is written back to register file of PU1 and also to its IRB (step 1). During instruction retirement, if the *safe flag* is set, the generated register value is copied to CRB of PU2 (step 2) and RC bit of corresponding register is set in CSC of PU2 (step 3). Then, update logic of PU2 reads the corresponding register value from its CRB and updates LRF setting UPD bit of the register in its CSC (step 4). After that, if the entry of the register in PU2's *create mask* is not set, PU2 propagates the register value to CRB of PU3 and sets the RC bit in CSC of PU3 to inform it that the register value is now available in PU3's CSC (step 5). Finally, PU2 updates PRO bit for the given register in its own CSC (step 5).

This communication process is slightly different for an explicit *send instruction* if a register is redefined by a thread in PU1. In that case, it is not necessary to copy a register value from PU1's IRB to PU2's CRB since it was already copied to CRB of PU2 when the register's creating instruction in PU1 was retired. Therefore, only the RC bit of the register in CSC of PU2 has to be set.

However, if a register, which *create mask* bit is initially set, is not redefined by the thread, then the register is released by a *send instruction*. Also, if there is a value generated by a preceding PU, it is sent to the consumer or the consumer uses locally available register value for a released register [37].

3.1.1.6 Pinot

3.1.1.6.1 General Data Pinot is a multithreading architecture, which also supports the control and data speculation. Its parallelizing tool identifies threads and can extract parallelism over a wide range of granularities without modifying the source code [23].

3.1.1.6.2 Architecture Details The Pinot consists of four processing elements (PEs) with their private L1 caches connected with shared bus to the memory system. The register files are distributed and the transfer of register values between them is performed through a unidirectional ring. Besides, the ring is also used to transfer a start address of the spawned thread. The block diagram of a PE in Pinot is shown in the Fig. 1.11. The light-gray-shaded areas enclosed with dashed lines represent the speculation support logic: the decoder logic for parallelizing instructions (fork, propagate, and cancel instructions are added to existing ISA—instruction set architecture), the thread spawn control, the shadow register files, and the versioning cache for speculative multithreading. The shadow register files allow overlapping the preparation of live-in register values for the next thread with the execution of current thread.

3.1.1.6.3 Register Communication The communication of the register values in Pinot is producer-initiated since a consumer thread uses a register value that has been produced by its predecessors. The register values can be transferred without synchronization both at and after spawn time. The register numbers for the values that need to be transferred to the consumer thread are found in a register-list mask inside the fork instruction. In case of the register value transfer at spawn time, a sequencer inspects the register-list mask, fetches the required register values, and sends them via ring to the consumer thread. When the register values are transferred after spawn time,

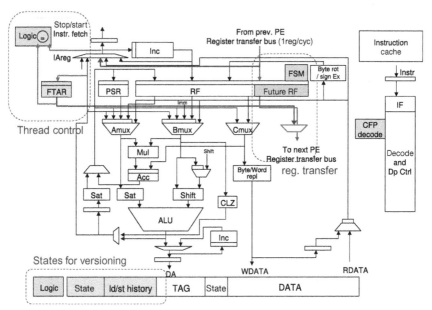

Figure 1.11 Processing element in Pinot. *This figure is taken from [23] with permission from the copyright holder.*

the requested register values are sent to the consumer thread when they are produced.

A bit field in fork instruction is intended to select the propagation modes of the register values. If its value is *after* = 1 (propagation always), the register values found in the register-list mask are transferred to the consumer thread both at and after spawn time. However, if its value is *after* = 0 (no propagation), they are transferred only at spawn time. To avoid the RAW violations, Pinot uses the propagate instructions to disable transfer of register values labeled with identical register numbers [23].

3.1.2 Bus-Based Distributed Register File Approaches
3.1.2.1 IACOMA
3.1.2.1.1 General Data It is a quite generic CMP architecture with a modest hardware support for speculative execution that supports the communication between speculative threads through both registers and memory [9,38]. A software support in the form of binary annotation tool extracts the loop-based threads from sequential binaries without the need for source recompilation.

3.1.2.1.2 Architecture Details IACOMA consists of four four-issue dynamic superscalar R10K–like cores with private L1 caches and shared on-chip L2 cache. The interthread communication is performed through registers and the shared L2 cache. To allow the register values to be communicated, IACOMA uses a simple broadcast bus between processor cores, while the distributed L1 caches are connected to the shared L2 cache through the crossbar.

3.1.2.1.3 Register Communication Binary annotator identifies the inner-loop iterations and their initiation and termination points. Then, the interthread register dependences are identified and the *loop-live* registers, which are live at loop entry/exits and may be redefined in the loop. From these loop-live reaching definitions, the binary annotator identifies the safe definitions at the points where the register value will never be overwritten and the release points for register values at the exit of the thread [9].

A modest hardware allows the interregister communication in IACOMA (Fig. 1.12). Each core has its own register file and synchronizing scoreboard (SS)—a fully decentralized directory structure with one entry per register, which enables the synchronization and communication of register values. The shared SS bus is dedicated for communicating the register values, but a distributed directory protocol is employed. The SS bus has a limited bandwidth of one word per cycle and one read and one write port for each core [9,39].

A directory entry per each register consists of the global and local parts. The global part has two 4-bit fields (1 bit per each core in each field), which

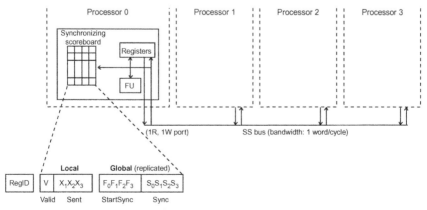

Figure 1.12 Hardware support for register communication in IACOMA. *This figure is taken from [9] with permission from the copyright holder.*

indicate whether the corresponding core is expected to produce a value in this register (F bits) and whether it is actually produced (S bits). The global part is replicated and kept consistent across the cores. A local part consists of a valid bit (V bit) and three more bits (X bits), which indicate whether a corresponding core has set the register values. The X bits are used to cope with the "last copy (LC)" problem. Although the register communication requires small additional hardware, the bus interconnect adds some latency for bus arbitration.

Register communication can be both producer- and consumer-initiated, which makes register communication protocol more complex. In consumer-initiated communication, when the consumer thread needs a register value, its SS allows a consumer to identify the corresponding producer and get the register value. When a core produces a final register value within a thread, it is sent over the SS bus, so the successors can load it. In case when a speculative thread needs some locally invalid (INV) register value, it determines the identity of the closest predecessor using F and S bits. If the requested register value is not produced yet, the consumer thread is blocked. Otherwise, the request is sent onto the SS bus and the value is obtained from the closest predecessor [9].

3.2. Speculative CMPs with GRF and Distributed Register Files

Trace and Mitosis are the speculative CMPs with a large register file shared between cores and LRFs in each core. In these systems, the register bypass network for operand communication is either a set of global and local buses as in Trace or shared bus as in Mitosis.

3.2.1 Trace
3.2.1.1 General Data
The Trace architecture is organized towards the traces—the dynamic sequences of instructions generated in run time by hardware, which embed any number of taken or not-taken branch instructions. The trace is a fundamental unit of control flow and control prediction in this system. The similarity between traces and threads is recognized in [40,41] where the traces are considered as dynamic versions of static Multiscalar threads although the threads may be arbitrarily large.

Trace reduces the complexity of all processing phases by exploiting control flow hierarchy at the trace level and within traces and the value hierarchy with global and local values. The control flow hierarchy allows sequencing through the program at the trace level instead at the level of individual instructions, which allows efficient allocation of traces to distributed processing cores. The value hierarchy involves the hierarchical register file implementation with an LRF for those register values (locals) that are produced and used within a trace and a GRF for those register values that are live between traces, on either entry (live-ins) or exit of trace (live-outs) [15].

3.2.1.2 Architecture Details

The structure of Trace is given in Fig. 1.13. It consists of four four-issue small-scale superscalar processing elements (PEs), trace cache for storing traces, and the trace dispatcher—a hardware support for dynamic thread (or trace) generation. Each PE has multiple dedicated FUs and a dedicated LRF to hold local values and a copy of the GRF (Fig. 1.14). The conventional set of logical registers is physically distributed into local and global sets resulting in smaller and faster register files. Relatively simple local and global bypass paths are used to communicate the register values between FUs within a PE [15].

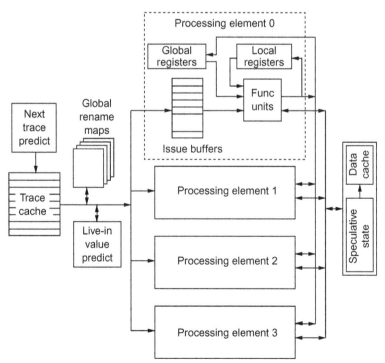

Figure 1.13 The block structure of Trace. *This figure is taken from [42] with permission from the copyright holder.*

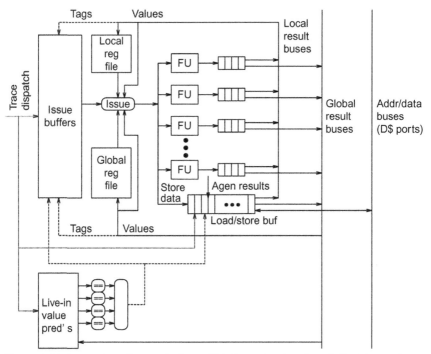

Figure 1.14 Processing element in Trace. *This figure is taken from [15] with permission from the copyright holder.*

The instruction fetch complexity is solved by predicting the trace within the next trace predictor and then storing it into the trace cache. The size of an instruction buffer in PE is large enough to hold an entire trace. The decoding, renaming, and value predictions are performed in the dispatch stage.

3.2.1.3 Register Communication

During the instruction dispatch, the local registers can be prerenamed in the trace cache since each trace is given an LRF that is not affected by other traces. This eliminates the need for dependence checking between dispatched instructions. The live-ins and live-outs are going through global renaming during trace dispatch, which reduces bandwidth to register maps. On instruction retirement, only live-outs are broadcast to all copies of the global file in each PE and mapped to physical registers. As soon as its trace is retired, the corresponding PE can be freed. Therefore, PEs are arranged in a circular queue so they are allocated and freed in a first in first out manner.

Each PE is provided with a set of registers to hold predicted live-ins together with the hardware for validating the predictions against the values received from other traces (see Fig. 1.14). When all operands are available, the instructions are ready to be issued. The live-ins may be already available in the GRF; otherwise, they may have been predicted and their values buffered with the instruction. Regardless of live-ins' availability, both local and global result buses are monitored for the operand values of new instruction. When the results are waiting for the result bus, instruction issue blocking is avoided by holding the completed results (either local register value or live-outs or both) in a queue, which is associated with each FU. The validation of live-in register predictions is performed when the computed values are written onto the global result buses. The comparator outputs that correspond to live-in predictions used by instruction buffers and store buffers are monitored in order to detect computed values. When live-in predicted values match the computed values, the instructions that used live-in predicted values will not be reissued. The local and global result buses are arbitrated separately. The local and global result buses correspond to write ports of local and GRF, respectively. The full bypassing of local register values between FUs within each PE is possible regardless of a longer latency during bypassing of global values between PEs [42].

3.2.2 Mitosis

3.2.2.1 General Data

Mitosis is a speculative CMP that uses a software approach to predict and manage the interthread data dependencies. It predicts and computes the thread input values by means of precomputation slice (p-slice)—a piece of code that is added at the beginning of each thread [19]. The compiler partitions the program into speculative threads statically by inserting the *spawning pairs*. A pair is made up of the instruction where speculative thread is spawned and the instruction where the spawned speculative thread starts its execution. The loop and subroutine boundaries, that is, any pair of basic blocks, can be considered for compiler analysis in search for potential spawning pairs in sequential program. The compiler also computes the corresponding p-slice for each spawning pair. In running the augmented binary code, when the spawn instruction is executed, an available TU is searched for to assign the p-slice of the corresponding speculative thread to it. The execution of the p-slice ends with an unconditional jump to the point where the speculative thread starts its execution [19].

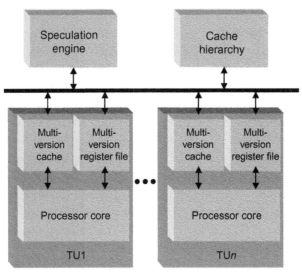

Figure 1.15 The block diagram of the Mitosis. *This figure is taken from [19] with permission from the copyright holder.*

3.2.2.2 Architecture Details

The block diagram of Mitosis is presented in Fig. 1.15. It consists of the TUs that are similar to conventional superscalar cores. Each TU has local multiversion register file (MRF) and multiversion cache, and they are connected to the global L2 cache via shared bus. The Speculation Engine handles the tasks related to the execution of the speculative thread: the allocation of free TU, the initialization of some registers, and maintaining the order among new and other active threads. Each TU in Mitosis has its own LRF while all TUs share GRF, as shown in Fig. 1.16. Also, all TUs share register versioning table (RVT) that tracks which TUs have a copy of given logical register. The number of rows in the RVT is equal to the number of logical registers, while the number of columns is equal to the number of TUs.

3.2.2.3 Register Communication

The transfer of the register values in Mitosis is both producer- and consumer-initiated. When a new speculative thread is spawned, the spawn instruction initializes the register state at LRF of the spawned thread by a mask that encodes the p-slice live-in registers. Then, the registers included in the mask are copied from the parent thread to the spawned thread.

The speculative thread stores its own produced register values into its LRF. When the first produced register value is written into the LRF, the

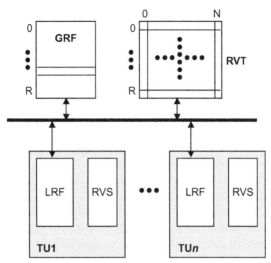

Figure 1.16 Register files in Mitosis. *This figure is taken from [19] with permission from the copyright holder.*

corresponding entry into RVT has to be set to notify TU, which owns the local copy of the given register. All the modified registers in the LRF are copied into the GRF on nonspeculative thread commit. A consumer thread that requires a register value first checks its own LRF. Then, if the value is not found in its own LRF, the RVT is checked to find the closest predecessor thread that has a copy of the requested register value. If there is no predecessor thread that has the requested register value, the GRF will be a supplier.

Each TU also has the register validation store (RVS) to store the copies of register values that are read for the first time by a speculative thread but not produced by it. The register values generated by the *p*-slice and used by the speculative thread are also stored into RVS. During the thread validation process, the register values in the RVS are compared against the actual values of the corresponding registers in the predecessor thread [19].

3.3. Speculative CMPs with GRF

3.3.1 MP98 (Merlot)

3.3.1.1 General Data

The MP98, also known as Merlot for its first prototype, is a commercial CMP that supports the control and data speculation [18,43]. Its low-power circuits and automatic parallelization software provide a high-performance and low-power computing environment for use in the smart information terminals. The creation of threads and the verification of the control speculation are supported with special instructions inserted by the compiler to fork new threads and to validate or invalidate the speculative execution.

3.3.1.2 Architecture Details

MP98 (Merlot) integrates four processing elements (PEs) on a single chip (Fig. 1.17). Each PE fetches two instructions at a time from shared instruction cache through instruction buffer and issues them to two integer-media pipelines.

For faster thread creation and data communication, four PEs share an instruction fetch unit, the global (multiport) register file that consists of four groups, each with four-read and two-write ports, and 64 KB data cache. The interconnection between a shared register file and PEs is point-to-point. Memory data are written into data cache through store reservation buffers (SRBs). Furthermore, each PE has load/store and branch pipelines for communication with GRF and SRBs. In general, MP98 (Merlot) is a very tightly coupled architecture where only the PEs are distributed, while the register file and the data cache are centralized and shared by all PEs.

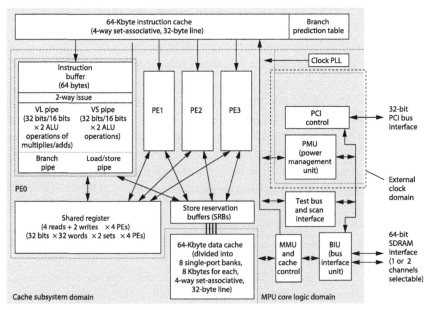

Figure 1.17 Block diagram of MP98 (Merlot). *This figure is taken from [43] with permission from the copyright holder.*

3.3.1.3 Register Communication

Data dependencies and speculation are controlled by hardware. The multi-threaded software model enables fine- to coarse-grained parallelism with the hardware-assisted low-cost thread creation. Hardware support such as fork-once parallel execution (FOPE) helps the compiler to extract parallelism from application and to manage control and data dependence speculation. FOPE simplifies the hardware support for thread management, facilitates compiler analysis for control and data dependencies among threads, and carries out efficient parallel execution.

The interthread register dependencies are not allowed in MP98 (Merlot) execution model. The fork instructions are inserted at points where all register dependencies are resolved. A new thread can inherit register values from a previous one by means of a table, which contains register-mapping information. To avoid copying all register values, MP98 (Merlot) processor employs a GRF organization shared by all PEs. Using this register file organization, MP98 (Merlot) only copies the corresponding rename map allowing a child thread to refer to the correct registers [18,42].

3.3.2 MAJC

3.3.2.1 General Data

The MAJC is a CMP especially suitable for multimedia computing [17,44]. It is designed for scalability, increased performance for applications with digital signal processing or new media computational needs, and the extremely high coherency bandwidth between multiple processors on-chip. The MAJC-5200 is the first implementation of the MAJC architecture. It is intended for networked and communication devices, client platforms, and application servers that deliver digital content and Java applications.

3.3.2.2 Architecture Details

The MAJC has three levels of hierarchy: processor cluster, processor unit, and FU. The processor cluster contains multiple processor units (CPUs) with "load–store" architecture on a single die (two in MAJC-5200). The CPU acts as the four-issue MAJC very-long-instruction-word (VLIW) engine (Fig. 1.18). Each CPU contains private instruction cache, while a coherent data cache is shared [44]. The CPUs also share few internal registers for synchronization purposes and the memory subsystem. Each CPU consists of four FUs (FU0 to FU3; see Fig. 1.18), while each of them has an LRF, local control (instruction/decode logic), and state information. This organization allows the customization to the specific application.

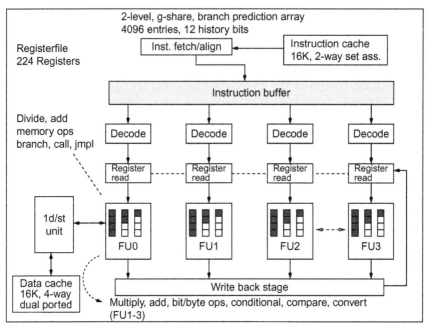

Figure 1.18 The MAJC CPU block diagram. *This figure is taken from [45] with permission from the copyright holder.*

The 32-byte aligned instruction is brought from the instruction cache during the fetch stage, and then, in the next stage, an instruction packet of 16-byte is aligned on the basis of header bits. Such aligned instructions are placed in instruction buffer for decode stage. The instructions are executed in FUs after decode stage, and the results are committed to the register file through the write-back stage.

3.3.2.3 Register Communication

Each CPU has its own set of global registers, not shared with other CPUs on the same die. This set of global registers can be accessed by any FU that belongs to the same CPU. The size of register file is implementation-specific and can vary from 32 up to 512 registers [17,44]. The registers can hold data of any type ("data agnostic"). A number of these registers can be configured as private to each FU, while the others (almost a hundred) are global and shared between all FUs within CPU in order to enable the fast communication between threads.

The MAJC speculation is based on the compiler support. The FUs have conditional instructions to increase ILP while nonfaulting loads enable speculative loading [44]. MAJC facilitates interprocessor communication and synchronization through a hardware message buffer, which includes physical channels structured as queues. In the MAJC-5200, shared register values are communicated from nonspeculative or less speculative threads to more speculative ones through *virtual channels* using the producer–consumer synchronization. The instruction that performs data transfer specifies a virtual channel within hardware message buffer to which data transfer is directed. Then, the virtual channel is translated to the physical channel within hardware message buffer on which the data transfer is performed. This mechanism could be regarded as message passing at the register level.

The virtual channels are accessible through the load and store operations and do not have direct access to the architectural registers. They also allow easy maintenance of the register dependencies between a nonspeculative thread and speculative threads and take part in recovery from misspeculation. The MAJC employs a fast interrupt mechanism in a processor cluster to allow threads to notify each other of relevant events. This mechanism reduces the overhead of thread speculation since it enables quick speculative thread creation and rollback. Both virtual channels and fast interrupt mechanism are suitable for multithreaded programs that require producer–consumer data sharing and fast communication between threads.

4. COMPARATIVE ANALYSIS OF REGISTER COMMUNICATION ISSUES IN TLS CMPs

A precise comparison between register communication techniques applied in the aforementioned speculative CMPs is difficult because of quite different architectures and design approaches. Nevertheless, some qualitative comparison is in order. This section brings a comparative analysis of register-level support in previously overviewed systems regarding the issues such as thread identification and speculation scope, register synchronization and communication, misspeculation recovery, and performance and scalability.

4.1. Thread Identification and Speculation Scope

It is necessary to identify speculative threads before an application is executed in a speculative CMP system. This can be achieved either off-line (by compiler, by some annotation or a parallelizing tool, etc.) or completely at run time with hardware support. The speculation scope (thread granularity) spans

Table 1.1 Thread Identification Support and Speculation Scope

CMP	Thread Identification Support	Speculation Scope
Multiscalar [14]	Compiler-supported	Basic block, multiple basic blocks, loop bodies, entire loops, and entire function invocations
Multiplex [8]	Compiler-supported	Basic block, multiple basic blocks, loop bodies, entire loops, and entire function invocations
SM [16]	Hardware-supported	Loops only
MP98 (Merlot) [18]	Compiler-/hardware-supported	Loops and basic blocks
MAJC [17]	Compiler-supported	Loops and method boundaries
Trace [15]	Hardware-supported	Traces (dynamic instruction sequences)
IACOMA [9]	Binary annotation tool	Loops only
Atlas [35]	Hardware-supported	Around memory references
NEKO [22]	Compiler-supported	Basic block, multiple basic blocks, loop bodies, entire loops, and entire function invocations
Pinot [23]	Binary parallelizing tool	Loops, function calls, and basic blocks
Mitosis [19]	Compiler-supported	Any pair of basic blocks

a wide spectrum from a basic block to entire subprogram call. Table 1.1 overviews the systems according to their thread identification support and speculation scope.

4.1.1 Thread Identification

Most of the approaches employ different compiler techniques to identify speculative threads from sequential application. Multiscalar and Multiplex exploit the compiler heuristics related to control flow, data dependencies, and thread size to extract more parallelism from integer and floating-point benchmarks [14]. However, besides implicit multithreading supported by both systems, Multiplex also supports explicit multithreading. It unifies Polaris compiler [46] with Multiscalar compiler [14] to provide explicit and implicit threading within a sequential application at dispatch time by including a mode bit in every thread descriptor [8].

In MP98 (Merlot), a compiler with the FOPE hardware support identifies threads from sequential applications allowing programmers to insert directives in the source code to extract explicit parallelism and to bring out the maximum performance [18,43]. The MAJC also relies on compiler to schedule instructions to FUs. Since the FUs and register files are data-type agnostic, the compiler has a flexibility in allocating data to registers to meet an application's requirements [17,44]. NEKO also uses a compiler to statically identify threads from a sequential program [22], while the Mitosis compiler statically partitions the sequential programs into speculative threads by inserting the spawning pairs into code and generates the corresponding p-slice for each spawning pair [19].

IACOMA and Pinot use dedicated software tools to identify speculative threads in sequential application. IACOMA uses a binary annotation tool to identify the units of work for each speculative thread and the register-level dependencies between them [9]. Pinot relies on a profile-guided parallelizing tool to extract thread-level parallelism at any level of granularity from sequential binaries and to convert them into SM binaries [23].

Finally, SM, Trace, and Atlas rely completely on hardware support to dynamically extract threads from sequential binaries [16,2,45]. A hardware mechanism for thread identification instead of software techniques has several advantages: (a) The compiler control flow analysis is less accurate; (b) the outcomes of data dependence profiling techniques used by compiler to enhance control flow analysis rely on concrete set of input data; (c) the use of data dependence profiling mechanisms incurs run time and memory overhead when profiling large and long-running applications; and (d) some software approaches require modification of instruction-set architecture, which does not provide backward compatibility with previous implementations.

4.1.2 Speculation Scope

Pinot is unique in extracting parallelism over a wide range of granularities from any program substructure. Its parallelizing tool can form a thread of 10 K instructions that can include entire loops or procedure calls and a fine-grained parallelism [23]. Since Multiscalar compiler ends a thread when it finds a loop head or a call, unlike in Pinot, it is not fully able to exploit coarse-grained parallelism regardless of the size of program substructures on which it speculates (one or more basic blocks, loop bodies, entire loops, and function invocations). MP98 (Merlot), MAJC, NEKO, Mitosis, and IACOMA speculate in a narrow scope (loops only, loops and basic blocks, or basic blocks).

Dynamic partitioning algorithms exploited in SM and Trace limit the threads on loop iterations and cache line boundaries, respectively. However, MEM-slicing algorithm in Atlas [47] improves on fixed interval partitioning in SM and Trace by slicing threads on memory operations making them larger and more predictable.

4.2. Register Communication Mechanisms

Most of the speculative CMPs reviewed in this chapter speculate on register values that flow between threads during execution, by using either a specific speculative register value transfer or a value prediction scheme. On the other hand, IACOMA and MP98 (Merlot) do not speculate on register values transferred between threads, but they both use synchronization mechanisms to handle the interthread communication on register level.

4.2.1 Speculative Register Value Transfer

This includes the mechanisms where an interthread-dependent instruction has to wait for the register value produced by the predecessor thread. These mechanisms impose long interprocessor communication latencies and execution stalls because of lack of the actual data. However, by exploiting different techniques, such as a direct register-to-register communication in a tightly coupled architecture, forwarding the register values from producer closer to the consumer thread whether the values are final or not, or identifying the last writer (last copy), the long latencies and execution stalls can be reduced.

Multiscalar and Multiplex use direct communication between LRFs over a unidirectional ring to reduce the interprocessor communication latencies, while the register value transfer is controlled by simple logic operations on a collection of six sets of bit masks (see Fig. 1.5). The LC problem is solved by maintaining two copies of the register file within each core. The register copies forwarded from the predecessor thread to the consumer thread are held in the past register set, while the new created register values are held in the present register set [8,14].

The NEKO register synchronization mechanism is similar to the one employed in Multiscalar but with some important differences. It heavily uses the compiler assistance in order to relax the hardware support for register synchronization by inserting into the binary code the information about registers possibly redefined in a thread and the explicit instructions for sending register values. Consequently, it requires only one additional write port of the register file and one additional port of the rename map. Also, the register values are

Table 1.2 Speculative Interthread Register Value Transfer
Parameters

CMP	Data Speculation Support	Register Communication
Multiscalar [14] Multiplex [8]	Double register sets per core Six sets of bit masks per core	Producer-initiated
NEKO [22]	IRB and CRB for buffering CSC for communication control Eagerly value forwarding Compiler support	Producer-initiated
Pinot [23]	Register-list mask inside the fork instruction	Producer-initiated
MAJC [17]	Global register file Virtual channels Fast interrupt mechanism	Producer–consumer synchronized

eagerly moved closer to the consumer thread even if they are not the final, which in turn reduces the communication latency. The IRB and CRB in each core provide register values buffering similar to the past and present register sets in Multiscalar, while the CSC, as SS in IACOMA, is used to control the communication based on the status bit values for each register [22].

Pinot transfers the register values over unidirectional ring without the need for synchronization with explicit send and receive instructions. Since the synchronous transfer would increase the dynamic count significantly, the transfer of register values is performed both at and after spawn time on the basis of the register numbers found in a register-list mask inside the fork instruction [23].

The MAJC compiler is responsible to ensure that VLIW packets must have no data, control, or resource-use interdependencies. The global shared register files in each MAJC processor unit enable fast communication of shared register values between threads by means of virtual channels and fast interrupt mechanism [17,44].

Table 1.2 summarizes the main characteristics of speculative value transfer in these systems.

4.2.2 Prediction of Register Values

The prediction of register values can be very beneficial for performance since the register values are quite predictable in comparison to memory values [9]. The register value prediction can help in providing the register values earlier than in previous systems that use different synchronization mechanisms. If the prediction is correct, the dependent threads are executed as if they were independent. However, the effectiveness of such an aggressive speculative optimization is very sensitive to the prediction accuracy. The prediction mechanisms in SM, Atlas, and Trace are hardware-based, while in Mitosis, it is software-based.

SM predicts the register dependencies for each new speculative thread relative to the predecessor thread in the control flow and the values that will flow through those dependencies. The data dependence constraints among instructions in Trace are alleviated with the use of the value prediction for live-ins of traces. Atlas uses AMA (atlas multiadaptive) predictor [48], a more aggressive correlated value prediction than SM and Trace, to avoid broadcasting and snooping of the register values. The thread identification based on loop iterations (as in SM) or on instruction traces (as in Trace) provides a good control and data predictability, but they experience severe load imbalance and coverage problems. However, extracting threads on load and store operations (as in Atlas) resolves these problems by keeping threads small and improving control predictability on fixed intervals.

Mitosis uses a software-based value prediction scheme to compute predicted register values directly from the source code, which improves prediction accuracy in comparison to hardware value prediction schemes in SM, Trace, and Atlas. Furthermore, Mitosis prediction scheme encapsulates multiple control flows that contribute to the computation of register values without using any additional hardware support for prediction of parent thread control flow like Trace.

The use of highly accurate register value prediction resolves interthread register dependencies efficiently allowing speculative thread execution to occur as early as possible. However, the validation of live-in predictions imposes a latency, which can be considered as a misprediction penalty. The characteristics and features of register value prediction schemes are summarized in Table 1.3.

4.2.3 Nonspeculative Register Value Transfer

IACOMA avoids the need for duplicated register sets while still being able to handle the sequential binaries effectively. The communication protocol is more complex than in Multiscalar and NEKO since it uses both producer- and consumer-initiated communication. The register availability and last-copy logic are maintained for each register in each core in order to support correct propagation of safe register values. The last-copy support is

Table 1.3 Prediction of Register Values
Parameters

CMP	Data Prediction Support	Register Communication
SM [16]	Hardware-based scheme Good control and data predictability Severe load imbalance Coverage problems	Producer-initiated
Atlas [35]	Hardware-based scheme Small threads Improved control predictability	Consumer-initiated verification of predicted values
Trace [15]	Hardware-based scheme Good control and data predictability Severe load imbalance Coverage problems	Producer-initiated verification of predicted values
Mitosis [19]	Software-based scheme Improved prediction accuracy Encapsulates multiple control flows	Producer- and consumer-initiated

much simpler than in Multiscalar, since each core has three extra local bits (X bits) per register only. However, using a shared bus for register value transfer between cores incurs additional arbitration latency [9].

MP98 (Merlot) exploits a register value inheritance mechanism whereby the register values of a thread that creates another thread are inherited by the new one. Instead of copying all register values, which requires a lot of bandwidth, MP98 (Merlot) exploits a global shared register file organization to copy only the corresponding rename map to allow a new forked thread to refer correct registers [18,43].

Table 1.4 summarizes the characteristics for nonspeculative register value transfer in IACOMA and MP98 (Merlot).

4.3. Misspeculation Recovery

The support for register-level communication in speculative CMPs also has to provide HW and/or SW detection of RAW violation and safe discarding of speculatively produced register values when violations occur. The misspeculation is usually resolved by squashing a violating thread and all its successors to ensure that any speculative value produced by violating thread is not forwarded to successor threads. Hence, the squashing is very costly since all speculative work will be discarded.

Table 1.4 Nonspeculative Interthread Register Value Transfer
                      Parameters

CMP	Data Synchronization Support	Register Communication
IACOMA [9]	Synchronizing scoreboard Register availability logic per core Last-copy control logic per core Check-on-store logic per core	Producer- and consumer-initiated
MP98 (Merlot) [18]	Global register file	Register inheritance mechanism

In overviewed speculative CMPs, data misspeculation may be caused either by interthread register dependence violation or by a mispredicted source register value. A misspeculation recovery support can be either entirely hardware-based (e.g., NEKO and Pinot) or hardware-/software-based (e.g., Multiscalar and Mulitplex). The misspeculation is not an issue in MP98 (Merlot) and IACOMA since they do not speculate on register values that flow between threads.

4.3.1 Dependency Violation

The Multiscalar and Multiplex use the duplicate register storage banks (bank 0 and bank 1—see Fig. 1.5) to maintain the correct register states during speculative execution. The bank 0 register storage and *past* set of bit mask are needed for recovery of the register states in case of violation. If speculation fails, the *present* mask is updated with the *past* mask discarding the incorrect values produced in a current unit and keeping the correct past register values. The more complex part of the recovery process is to discard the values propagated to other units. Any register created in a unit that is a part of incorrect execution must be recovered. This activity consults the *recover* and *squash* bit masks to identify propagated incorrect values. The *recover* mask denotes the registers for which the unit must propagate correct values to other units in order to replace the incorrect values. The *squash* mask is a combination of *recover* masks of all predecessor units that have been involved in recovery process and it is used for the synchronization of recovered register values. Although this mechanism is implemented completely in hardware, its efficiency is enhanced by a certain compiler support [14].

In case of misspeculation in NEKO, a recovery process first has to reset the status of communication and, then, to reinitiate the processes of updating and propagating register values. Each PU that needs to be restarted must

Table 1.5 Misspeculation Recovery Support

CMP	Misspeculation Recovery Support
Multiscalar [14]	Double register sets per core
Multiplex [8]	Recover and squash bit masks per core
MAJC [17]	Virtual channels
NEKO [22]	Hardware support (CSC and CRB per core)
Pinot [23]	Hardware support with modified ISA

clear UPD and PRO bits in its scoreboard (CSC) to restart updating and propagating process and RC and RR bits in the scoreboard of successor PU in order to invalidate the status of register values in CRB [22].

In case of a register RAW violation in MAJC, the nonspeculative or less speculative thread forwards the register value through the virtual channel to the speculative thread that caused a violation. This way, the violating speculative thread gets the actual register value produced by its predecessor, which allows it to maintain the sequential semantics of the original single-threaded program [17].

The original spawning thread in the Pinot checks the correctness of the speculation, and in case of misspeculation, it cancels the spawned thread and any possible successors. RAW violation is detected by hardware, which is supported with minor changes in the executing binaries by issuing either another fork instruction or a special cancel instruction when misspeculation is detected [23].

Table 1.5 summarizes the different misspeculation recovery support in speculative CMPs that speculate on interthread register dependencies.

4.3.2 Misprediction

Each time a write is performed to some destination register in SM, its corresponding entry in *Rwrite* is decremented. If the value for a given register in *Rwrite* table entry becomes less than 0, a nonpredicted write has happened and violation occurs. Then, all subsequent threads must be squashed, while all physical registers not shared with the previous thread need to be released [33].

Trace introduces a selective reissuing model for handling misspeculation when misprediction of source register values happens. When computed values are seen on the global result buses, the live-in predictions are validated. If the predicted live-in values and computed values do not match,

Table 1.6 Misprediction Recovery Support

CMP	Misprediction Recovery Support
SM [16]	*Rwrite* table
Trace [15]	Selective reissuing mechanism
Atlas [35]	Fine-grained recovery model
Mitosis [19]	RVS for *p*-slice validation

the misspeculation occurs and instructions that used the predicted live-ins have to be reissued with the new values for their operands. The existing issue mechanism in Trace reissues only the instructions along the dependence chain [15].

Atlas exploits fine-grained recovery model in case of misprediction to reexecute only those instructions dependent on incorrect data. Consequently, the successor speculative threads will not be squashed, which will allow their correct completion even in the presence of a less speculative register value misprediction [22].

If a misspeculation occurs in Mitosis, the violating speculative thread and all its successors are squashed. Mitosis explicitly tracks the consumed live-ins with additional RVS structure per each core, which is used for validation of predicted register values. The incorrect live-in register values produced by *p*-slice, but not consumed by a speculative thread, will not cause a violation. Mitosis is relatively insensitive to squash overhead since prediction of live-ins in system is highly accurate [19].

Table 1.6 summarizes the different misprediction recovery support in speculative CMPs that use value prediction techniques to resolve interthread register dependencies.

4.4. Performance and Scalability

4.4.1 Performance Issues

Evaluations of the speculative CMPs that support interthread register-level communication were performed in dedicated simulation environments usually by different benchmarks. Although comparison of performance evaluation results of different architectures collected in such conditions seems to be quite difficult, it is still possible to comment on some performance indicators in these CMPs such as instructions per cycle (IPC), latencies and speedup against a single processor, or an ideal CMP configuration. Besides this, various illustrative performance results are presented for various CMPs related to hardware and/or software support for interthread register communication: a register file organization, a register bypass network, and the support for register synchronization.

4.4.2 Register File Organization

The evaluation on some signal, video, and image processing benchmarks has shown the efficiency of MAJC large unified register file that can hold any data. This in turn provides more registers for applications that involve dedicated data-type processing [17].

The hierarchical register file model exploited in Trace is evaluated against the nonhierarchical one with variations of either register communication bandwidth or register communication latency. It has been shown that the register hierarchical model significantly improves performance (IPC up to 6.8) since it off-loads much of register communication to local result buses [15].

The performance of IACOMA scoreboard (SS) is compared to an ideal environment with zero communication latency. The complexity of each register file is quite modest since only one read and one write port is added for each register file. Hence, only one value can be read from or written to SS bus in a given cycle, which in turn has a little impact on performance. Also, replicating the availability, last-copy control, and check–on–store logic for each register implies an extra overhead. However, it was shown that IACOMA requires slightly a larger area than a 12-issue superscalar processor [9].

Mitosis MRF structure design met the expected performance since an average latency of register access was equal to the latency experienced in a particular LRF, that is, 99% of the register accesses in evaluated benchmarks have been satisfied from LRF structure. This confirms the accuracy of p-slice concept since most of the register values needed during speculative thread execution are produced by corresponding p-slice [19].

4.4.3 Register Bypass Network

The performance of modest Multiscalar register file configurations with a low communication bandwidth between adjacent PUs of 1 register per cycle is quite comparable to the performance of ideal configuration with infinite communication bandwidth. It has been shown that less than a fourth of the available bandwidth is actually used during the execution, while the queues among the PUs contain no more than a single register most of the time. Also, the negligible increase in communication latency between adjacent PUs has insignificant impact on Multiscalar performance [14].

The efficiency of NEKO register communication support is evaluated for different datapath configurations with variable update latency, propagate latency, and update and propagation bandwidth. Also, for comparison reasons, the evaluation is performed for a datapath configuration that exploits more sophisticated scheduling where registers whose consumer is waiting in the reservation station have to be scheduled first. The variation in latency and bandwidth of update and propagate datapath has shown that the performance is more sensitive to latency and bandwidth of update than of propagate datapath since most of interthread register dependencies exist between two adjacent threads. However, the increase of update bandwidth in datapath configuration requires additional ports in register file and renames map indicating that the datapath configuration with a sophisticated scheduling applied might be a better design decision. The achieved performance in terms of IPC is degraded only by 6% in average compared to an ideal datapath configuration with zero latency and unlimited bandwidth [22].

The sensitivity of register file organization in Trace to global bus communication latency is measured while the global bus bandwidth was kept unconstrained in order to isolate the effect of latency. The results have shown that the nonhierarchical register file model decreased IPC by 20% to 35% since it penalized all values uniformly. On the other hand, the hierarchical register file model that penalized only the global values reduced this performance loss by more than half. Furthermore, the evaluation results have shown that Trace benefits on both control flow and data flow hierarchy to overcome complexity and architectural limitations of conventional superscalar processors [15].

The evaluation of IACOMA SS bus bandwidth requirements has shown that increase of bandwidth beyond one word per cycle has only a very modest effect on performance. The ideal environment with infinite bandwidth is less than 5% faster than SS bus with one register per cycle bandwidth. Moreover, even the highest experienced three-cycle SS bus latency between processors that are located far apart does not degrade the performance. This shows that the communication between producer and consumer threads occurs between adjacent processors of IACOMA in spite of the fact that the shared bus is used as register bypass network instead of the ring [9].

The lower sensitivity of performance to latency and bandwidth of propagate datapath indicates that either a ring interconnect or shared bus is sufficient for efficient handling of register communication in speculative CMPs.

4.4.4 Speculative CMP Versus Single Processor

It would be very interesting to compare the performance of speculative CMPs, but there is no available comparative evaluation even for two of them. Each system is separately evaluated in different evaluation environments and with different methodologies, making a comparison on a fair ground practically impossible. In addition, the results almost always express the combined effects of speculation on both memory and register level, and effects of register communication are hard to isolate. Nevertheless, with all these constraints in mind, Table 1.7 represents a cross compilation of results of various performance evaluation studies that focuses on one of the most expressive performance indicators in parallel systems—the speedup against single processor.

The results provide a clear evidence of a potential of speculative CMPs to extract parallelism from sequential applications and to run them faster. The speedup naturally depends on the type of application. It is typically higher for floating-point than for integer benchmarks since in integer benchmarks, most of the loops have lower iteration counts and much more frequent intrathread control instructions. The examples of Multiscalar and NEKO imply that higher core issue width is not beneficial for speedup. In prediction-based systems, the accuracy of prediction is crucial for performance (e.g., Trace).

4.4.5 Scalability Issues

The register-level synchronization and communication support are also analyzed from the scalability point of view. The relevant scalability issues are related to register file organization, register bypass network, and support for register synchronization.

4.4.5.1 Register File Organization

Although the GRF organization (e.g., in MP98 (Merlot) and MAJC) saves the bandwidth in extremely small multiprocessor designs like CMPs, it imposes complex wiring, increases in number of read and write ports, and affects the cycle time and latencies. Hence, most of speculative CMP designs exploit distributed register structures to alleviate aforementioned issues noticed in designs with a shared register file organization.

4.4.5.2 Support for Register Communication

The hardware support for register value communication in Multiscalar, Multiplex, and NEKO requires additional register storage banks and sets of bit masks per each core, which results in complex core designs. The

Table 1.7 Speculative CMPs Speedups versus Single Processor

CMP	PUs	Issue width	Instruction execution	Speedup (on avg.)	Remarks	Benchmarks
Multiscalar [14]	4	1 2	In-order	1.9 1.7	Sophisticated compiler support improves performance on register communication up to 67% (in-order PUs) and 59% (out-of-order PUs)	SPEC92 suite GNU diffutils2.6 GNU textutils1.9
	8	1 2	In-order	2.8 2.6		
	4	1 2	Out-of-order	2 1.6		
	8	1 2	Out-of-order	3 2.4		
Multiplex [8]	4	2	Out-of-order	2.63	Matches or outperforms implicit-only or explicit-only CMP for almost all benchmarks	SPECfp95 suite Perfect suite
SM [16]	4	4	In-order	1–3	Speedup is higher for floating-point applications	SPEC95 suite
MP98 (Merlot) [18]	4	2	In-order	3	Unnecessary processors are turned off when application load is lower	Speech recognition Inverse discrete cosine transform code
MAJC [17]	2	4	In-order	1.6	Parallelism at multiple levels (instruction, data, thread, and process) with fast communication mechanism	Video and image processing applications

Name					Description	Benchmark suite
Trace [15]	8	4	Out-of-order	1.1–1.25	No data prediction	SPECint95 suite
				1.08	Real data prediction diminishes performance gain	
				1.45	Perfect data prediction increase performance for almost all benchmarks	
IACOMA [9]	4	4	Out-of-order	1–2	For floating-point applications, speedup is almost twice higher on average	SPEC92 suite SPEC95 suite MediaBench suite
Atlas [35]	8	1	In-order	3.4	Accurate value and control prediction, a fast misprediction recovery mechanism, and efficient thread partitioning	SPECint95 suite
NEKO [22]	4/2	8/2	Out-of-order	1.22 1.28 1.24 1.32	Integration of narrower issue width cores increases throughput and keeps high performance in sequential applications during speculative execution	SPECint95 suite
Pinot [23]	4	4	Out-of-order	3.7	Exploiting coarse-grained parallelism is essential to improve performance	SPEC95 suite MiBench suite
Mitosis [19]	4	6	Out-of-order	2.2	Highly accurate dependence prediction and efficient data communication between threads	Olden suite

support for speculative execution and prediction in SM is completely based on hardware mechanisms, which in turn heavily increases the complexity of the overall design. Atlas uses on-chip value/control predictor that communicates with the other components through a shared bus, which impacts also area and power efficiency.

Since augmentation of the SS in IACOMA depends on the number of cores, it would not be scalable due to the increase of hardware complexity of LC, register availability, and check-on-store logic, placed per each core. Also, the increase of number of TUs in the Mitosis will cause an increase in size of the RVT structure since one of its dimensions is related to the number of TUs.

4.4.5.3 Register Bypass Network

The ring interconnect, as a natural choice for TLS technique, is exploited for register transfer between cores at Multiscalar, Multiplex, SM, Atlas, NEKO, and Pinot. Although its hardware cost and latency hop are small, it limits the ability to optimize data locality and to perform efficient multiprogramming. Also, the ring suffers from a fundamental scaling problem since it does not scale with the number of nodes. The scalability evaluation of different Atlas architecture layouts of 4, 8, and 16 nodes has shown that an efficient architecture for execution of sequential binaries can be attained. However, the increase in number of cores (over 16 cores) results in worse performance (control and data become less predictable), area, and power efficiency than in a uniprocessor [21].

Trace, IACOMA, and Mitosis employ either set of global buses or shared bus between processor cores for register-level communication. The overall performance depends not only on the amount of data transferred but also on the bus protocol, the bus design parameters (bus width, priorities, data block size, arbiter handshake overhead, etc.), clock frequency (which depends on complexity of the interface logic, routing of the wires, and placement of the various components), and the components' activity. The simple bus would be sufficient to handle a small number (4–8) of processor cores in a CMP, but more cores or even faster cores would require higher bandwidth, which in turn demands either more buses or hierarchy of buses. Since communication over a bus can be a costly solution, this is likely a limitation factor for PE complexity and overall scalability and performance for those processors.

Finally, the scalability issues in the aforementioned speculative CMP architectures that support register-level communication are summarized in Table 1.8.

Table 1.8 Scalability Isues

CMP	Scalability Issues
Multiscalar [14]	Complex support for register synchronization and communication per each core Ring interconnect for register transfer
Multiplex [8]	Complex support for register synchronization and communication per each core Ring interconnect for register transfer
SM [16]	Hardware mechanisms for speculation and prediction Ring interconnect for register transfer
MP98 (Merlot) [18]	Tightly coupled architecture Global register file, port requirements, long wires
MAJC [17]	Tightly coupled architecture Global register file, port requirements, long wires
Trace [15]	Global register file, port requirements, long wires Global and local result buses
IACOMA [9]	Register availability logic per each core Last-copy control logic per each core Check-on-store logic per each core Shared bus
Atlas [35]	Value control predictor Shared bus Ring interconnect for register transfer
NEKO [22]	Complex support for register synchronization and communication per each core Ring interconnect for register transfer
Pinot [23]	Ring interconnect for register transfer
Mitosis [19]	RVT structure Ring interconnect for register transfer

5. CASE STUDY: SIC AND ESIC PROTOCOLS

It is obvious from the previous discussion that the support for inter-thread register communication is rather complex. The rest of this chapter describes two variants of a protocol that supports the register communication in a speculative CMP. These protocols are intended to offer simplicity, scalability, and better cost-effectiveness compared to the similar approaches from literature (e.g., IACOMA and NEKO). The proposed protocols are envisaged for a generic speculative CMP architecture and hence employ only necessary support for speculative execution. The underlying CMP architecture consists of four processor cores with private L1 caches sharing an on-chip L2 cache. The interthread communication is achieved through both registers and shared memory. The register communication is complemented with memory-level communication protocol that integrates the speculation and cache coherence—SISC (speculation integrated with snoopy coherence) [49].

The speculation model assumes that the threads are identified as the loop iterations. One nonspeculative thread and up to three successor speculative threads can run in parallel. The threads keep their speculation states locally. The threads strictly commit in order to preserve the sequential semantics of the application program. A thread waits to reach the nonspeculative status before it can complete and a new thread can be started on the same processor. In case of incorrect speculation, the thread and its successors are squashed.

The register communication is intended to incur minimal additional hardware complexity while keeping the communication latency as low as possible. It avoids complex multiported shared register files, the additional banks of registers for saving the correct values, the prediction schemes, the demanding communication mechanisms, and additional bits for keeping track of the register status.

The technique includes both producer- and consumer-initiated communication of the register values. It not only is implemented in hardware but also relies on some off-line software support. The dedicated shared bus is used for propagation of the register values. Consequently, the speculation support is based on snoopy protocols [50]. There are two variants of the protocol: (a) basic version, the SIC protocol [51], and (b) enhanced version, the ESIC protocol [52].

5.1. SIC Protocol

The SIC[1] protocol is a conservative approach that propagates only the safe register values to the successor threads. Its software support, hardware infrastructure, and the protocol itself are described in this section.

---

[1] "*sic*"—Latin word meaning "thus," "so," "as such," or "in such a manner."

5.1.1 SIC Software Support

The speculation method and approach is similar to IACOMA. The software support in the form of binary annotator works on sequential binary code. The advantage of avoiding a need for source code and a need for source recompilation is significant. As in IACOMA, the annotator identifies threads, finds the register write instructions that produce the safe values for propagation to the successors, and annotates the binary code accordingly.

The identification of the speculative threads is relatively simple since they are restricted to loop iterations and, hence, the code of threads running in parallel is the same. Only entry and exit points have to be marked. The analysis of register writes is more demanding. First, the annotator recognizes which registers are live at the loop entry and exit points and may be written into within the loop (referred to as *loop-live registers*). The registers that can only be read within the loop are referred to as *non-loop-live registers*. Finally, the write instructions to the loop-live registers need to be annotated. Those writes can be regarded as *nonfinal* or *final* (see Fig. 1.19). The *nonfinal* writes (NFWs) produce the register values that might be overwritten during

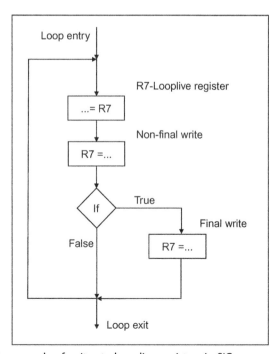

Figure 1.19 An example of writes to loop-live registers in SIC.

current loop iteration, while the *final* writes (FWs) produce the register values that cannot be overwritten in any case in the current loop iteration.

5.1.2 SIC Hardware Support

The hardware infrastructure imposed by the SIC protocol for each core consists of the logic for keeping thread speculation status, a register directory for keeping state of each register, the control logic for performing protocol state transitions, and a shared bus interface used for exchanging the register values between processors (see Fig. 1.20). A dedicated snoopy shared bus is used to transfer the register values between cores and local directories for keeping the status of registers in terms of their validity, availability for propagation, etc. A directory entry per each register is only several bits wide.

The speculation status of a thread currently running on a processor is kept in a special register. Since four threads can run in parallel, thread status appears as a 2-bit mask. The nonspeculative thread (mask 00) executes the current iteration of the loop, while the speculative successors execute the first (mask 01), second (mask 10), and third (mask 11) successive speculative iterations, respectively. After the nonspeculative thread is finished, its immediate successor thread becomes nonspeculative while the masks of the remaining running threads are decremented. A new thread is initiated on the freed processor and it obtains the most speculative status (mask 11).

The register directory has an entry per register for keeping its current state. A loop-live register can be in one of four states: *invalid* (INV),

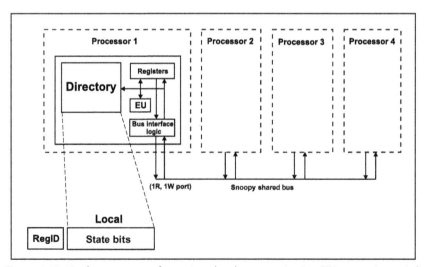

Figure 1.20 Hardware support for register-level communication (EU, execution units).

valid-unsafe (VU), *valid-safe* (VS), and *last-copy* (LC). Non-loop-live registers can be either in *invalid* (INV) or *valid-safe* (VS) state. Therefore, three bits per register are provided in local directory (Fig. 1.20), one for distinguishing between loop-live and non-loop-live registers and two for coding of four states.

The INV state indicates that a register value is not valid and cannot be used by a local thread or propagated to others. The VU state indicates that a register value is valid for current thread, but it is not a final value produced by this thread and cannot be safely forwarded to the successor threads. The VS state indicates that a register value is valid for current thread, and it is also final and safe to be forwarded to the successor threads. The LC state indicates that a valid register value is the only copy across all processor cores.

The register-level communication is carried on over a dedicated shared bus. It encompasses address lines for a register address, data lines for register values, and some control lines. The control part includes *BusR*, *BusW*, *Mask*, and *Shared* signals.

BusR signal denotes the bus read transaction caused by a processor read request for a register in the INV state. The read request is issued on the bus along with the mask code in order to get the requested register value.

BusW signal denotes the bus write transaction caused by a processor write request either when a speculative thread reaches the VS state for a given register or when a register value in the LC state is sent over the bus. The register value is sent over the bus, so the consumer thread can load it. In both cases, the register value is transferred on nondemand base (producer-initiated communication).

Mask signals are set on the bus during bus read transaction when a thread requests the register value from its nearest predecessor. Each predecessor thread, with the requested register value in the VS state, replies by posting its mask on the bus mask lines, which are realized as wired-OR lines. Consequently, the bus interface logic in each processor core can sense whether any other predecessor posted its mask on the bus. The mechanism of distributed arbitration chooses the nearest, most recent predecessor thread, which is allowed to provide the valid requested register value on the bus.

Shared signal, which is also sent over a wired-OR bus line, is raised by a consumer thread when it responds to a nondemand producer-initiated transaction for sending a register value, which is in the VS or LC state. When this line is raised by a consumer, the producer is informed that the register value sent on the bus is also loaded by some other processor and that it is not the last and only copy.

5.1.3 Description of SIC Protocol

As for an access to a register, a processor can issue two types of requests: read (R) or write. Writes can be the *final* or the *nonfinal* as annotated by the binary annotator. The SIC protocol includes both producer-initiated and consumer-initiated register-level communication. This protocol is based on previously defined states and transitions between them. The protocol handles the accesses to loop-live and non–loop-live registers differently. The processor-induced and bus-induced state transitions for loop-live registers are presented in Fig. 1.21.

The protocol mechanism for loop-live registers works as follows:
1. *Read hit.* If a speculative or nonspeculative thread issues a read request for a register in a valid state (VU, VS, or LC), the request is satisfied locally and that register remains in the same state.
2. *Read miss.* A read request for a register in the INV state causes the read miss and initiates *BusR* transaction. The read request for this register is issued on the bus along with the mask code of its speculative thread. Consequently, read miss incurs a consumer-initiated interthread communication. All possible suppliers, that is, predecessors (nonspeculative thread and/or earlier speculative threads) that have a requested register in either the VS or LC state, reply with posting their mask codes on the bus and a distributed arbitrator chooses the nearest predecessor. Then, the chosen predecessor thread supplies the requested register value over

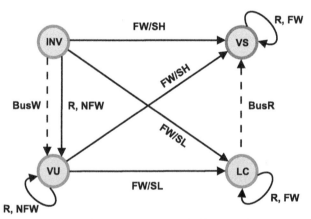

Figure 1.21 Processor-initiated state transitions (solid lines) and bus-induced state transitions (dashed lines) for loop-live registers in the SIC protocol. Processor reads are denoted with R. Notation A/B means that processor writes (*final* write, FW, or *nonfinal* write, NFW) are observed in relation to the *Shared* signal either high (SH) or low (SL). (For color version of this figure, the reader is referred to the online version of this chapter.)

the bus. The requested register is loaded in the VU state in the local directory of the speculative thread that issued a read request. If the requested register was in the LC state at the supplier's side, its state changes from the LC to the VS state. If there is no supplier available when a consumer thread issues the read request on the bus, the consumer thread is blocked and it waits until the safe value is produced elsewhere and sent by the producer.

3. *Write hit.* If a register value is in the VU state when a thread (either non-speculative or speculative) performs the NFW, the register is updated locally and remains in the VU state. However, if a register value is in the VU state when a processor performs the FW, the register is updated and state is changed from the VU to the VS. Also, the FW incurs the producer-initiated communication by sending the register value on the bus for the immediate successor thread. If the value is loaded into the register of its immediate successor thread, it changes the register state from the INV to VU and raises *Shared* line, informing the producer that the value is loaded. Also, if the successor was blocked waiting for this particular register value, it continues the execution. If the shared line remains inactive (low), the producer changes the state for this register from the VS to LC, indicating the only valid copy.

4. *Write miss.* A write, either *final* or *nonfinal*, to a register value in the INV state causes the write miss. The protocol actions for both FWs and NFWs are the same as in the previously described corresponding cases of write hit. The destination states of state transitions are also the same, while the source state is INV (instead of VU in the case of write hit).

Since non-loop-live registers can only be read within a thread, the protocol mechanism for them works as follows:

1. *Read hit.* If a register value is in the VS state when a thread, either speculative or nonspeculative, issues a read request, this hit is satisfied locally and the register remains in the VS state.

2. *Read miss.* This case can happen only when a processor runs a speculative thread for the first time following some sequential section of the application. A read request for a register in the INV state initiates *BusR* transaction. Then, nonspeculative or some other speculative thread supplies the requested register value, which is loaded in the VS state by the consumer thread. At the same time, the other successor threads that also have the same register in the INV state snoop the bus and, on this occasion, load the sent value in the VS state by means of the read snarfing technique [50].

5.1.4 Thread Initiation and Completion

When a processor initiates a new speculative thread (the most speculative one), it is necessary to invalidate all loop-live registers by setting their state to INV. However, the non-loop-live registers remain in their current state. When a thread is about to complete, a search for last copies (the LC state) in local directory is carried out. The thread is allowed to complete only if there are no such register values. Otherwise, each register value in the LC state must be saved by sending it over bus to its successor, as in processing of the FW in producer-initiated communication.

5.2. ESIC Protocol

In strive to improve the SIC protocol performance, blocking of a consumer thread while waiting for a register value from a producer was recognized as a main obstacle. The SIC protocol is fully speculation conservative since during both the producer- and consumer-initiated communication, only finally written, safe values are communicated. However, there are cases (especially when conditional execution is encountered) where the safe values cannot be unambiguously identified by the binary annotator. The register write, which immediately precedes the If-statement, can turn out to be not only *final* if the condition is false but also *nonfinal* if the condition is true, as illustrated in Fig. 1.22. The SIC annotator cannot resolve it in advance and it conservatively annotates this write as *nonfinal*. It can incur some unnecessary blocking of a successor speculative thread that requests this register if the condition in run time occurs to be true.

In order to exploit this potential for performance improvement, the ESIC protocol is proposed. Unlike SIC, it relies on speculative forwarding of the possibly safe register values. The following description concentrates on the ESIC enhancements to the SIC protocol.

5.2.1 ESIC Software Support

The ESIC protocol requires further modifications of the binary annotator. The classification of the writes is refined with recognition of *possibly final* writes (PFWs) (Fig. 1.22). As before, the NFW is one that is followed by at least one write to the same register, while the FW is the last one in a thread. The PFW is one that might be either *final* or *nonfinal* depending on the control flow. In case when a consumer thread requested the register value that has not been produced yet, the possibly final register value can be forwarded to the consumer thread to satisfy the request and to prevent the blocking. Subsequently, if producer thread reaches the FW for earlier

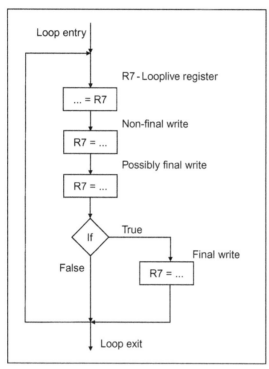

Figure 1.22 Examples of *nonfinal, possibly final,* and *final* writes found by the ESIC annotator.

forwarded possibly final register value, it sends the squash signal to the consumer thread that has already used it to undo the effects of misspeculation.

The performance benefit of such an aggressive speculation directly depends on the probability that a write labeled as PFW by annotator turns out to be *final* during run time and that speculation succeeds. Otherwise, wrong speculation introduces a certain overhead. This probability can be estimated by profiling the application. Therefore, in order to obtain the best performance, the preprocessing of an application also encompasses further steps:

- By profiling of an application for each write labeled as PWF by the annotator, the statistics is collected on how many times (*fcnt*) this write indeed occurred to be the *final* across all *n* iterations during run time.
- If the probability of speculation success (*fcnt/n*) is above the prespecified threshold for a specific PFW, the speculation can be beneficial and this write stays labeled as PFW. Otherwise, this write is relabeled to NFW, since too aggressive speculation can be even counterproductive.

The specific threshold value is application– and system–dependent and can be determined by means of simulation.

5.2.2 ESIC Hardware Support

Loop-live registers in ESIC protocol can be found in one of the following states: *invalid* (INV), *valid-unsafe* (VU), *valid-safe* (VS), *valid-possibly-safe* (VPS), *valid-possibly-safe-forwarded* (VPSF), and *last-copy* (LC). Non–loop-live registers can be in either *invalid-others* (INVO) or *valid-safe-others* (VSO) states.

The INV, VU, VS, LC, INVO, and VSO states are inherited from the SIC protocol, while the VPS and VPSF states are unique to the ESIC protocol. The VPS state denotes that a register value is valid for the current thread, and, as a possibly safe value, it can be speculatively forwarded to the successor threads on demand. The VPSF state indicates that a given register value is valid for the current thread and it has been speculatively forwarded to the successor threads on their request. This state makes it possible to track the possible misspeculation and to detect violation.

In addition to *BusR*, *BusW*, *Mask*, and *Shared* signals, the control part of shared bus also includes *Squash* (Sq) signal. This signal is issued on the bus as a consequence of a processor write to a given register found in the VPSF state. The successor consumer thread, which loaded a given register prematurely, is squashed when the squash signal for this register is detected on the bus.

5.2.3 Description of ESIC Protocol

The register communication between threads in ESIC can be producer-initiated and consumer-initiated as in SIC protocol. The processor-induced and bus-induced state transitions for loop-live registers in ESIC protocol are presented in Fig. 1.23.

The protocol for loop-live registers works as follows:

1. *Read hit.* As in the SIC, the read request for a register in a valid state (here also including VPS and VPSF) is satisfied locally without state change.
2. *Read miss.* A read request for a register in the INV state initiates *BusR* transaction, as in the SIC. The procedure is the same and only difference is that possible supplier can be also a predecessor thread with requested register in the VPS state. If the requested register was in the VPS state at the supplier's side, it goes from VPS to VPSF state to keep track of speculative forwarding. The requested register is loaded in the VU state at the consumer's side.

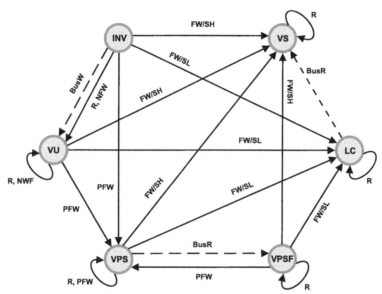

Figure 1.23 Processor-induced and bus-induced state transitions for loop-live registers in the ESIC protocol. Notation A/B means that processor writes (FW, PFW, and NFW) are observed in relation to Shared signal either high (SH) or low (SL). Processor reads are denoted with R. Dashed line indicates bus-induced transitions, while solid line indicates processor-induced transitions. (For color version of this figure, the reader is referred to the online version of this chapter.)

In the SIC protocol, a consumer thread is blocked if there is no supplier of a safe value available when the consumer's read request is issued on the bus. However, in the same situation, the ESIC protocol prevents blocking if there is a supplier of a possibly safe value. A consumer thread in the ESIC blocks only if there is no supplier of neither a safe nor a possibly safe value.

3. *Write hit.* The reaction in cases of the NFW request to a register value in the VU state and of the FW request to a register value in the VU or VPS state is the same as in the SIC. However, if a FW request finds a register value in the VPSF state, the thread first sends the *Squash* signal on the bus to the successor thread(s) that loaded a given register value earlier to undo the effects of incorrect speculation. After that, it repeats the same procedure as in the case of the FW request to the VPS state to provide a safe value to the successors.

In case of the PFW request to a register value in the VU state, the register is updated locally and its state is changed from the VU to VPS. If the PFW request finds a register value in the VPS state, the register is updated locally and it remains in the VPS state. Finally, when the PFW finds a register value in the VPSF state, the thread issues the *Squash* signal on the bus for successor thread(s) that loaded a given register value earlier. Then, the register is updated locally and goes from VPSF to VPS.

4. *Write miss.* A thread's NFW to a register value in the INV state only updates the register value avoiding the *BusW* transaction. The register state is modified from the INV to VU state. The same reaction occurs when a thread performs the PFW to a register value in the INV state but the destination state is the VPS. The FW request to a register in the INV state updates the register value and changes its state from the INV to VS state. Also, it incurs a producer-initiated interthread communication in form of a *BusW* transaction. The producer thread puts the register value on the bus and if the successor thread loaded the sent value, it raises *Shared* signal and sets the state to the VU. The destination state in the producer thread is either VS or LC depending on observed *Shared* signal.

The protocol for non-loop-alive registers works in the same way as in the SIC.

5.2.4 Thread Initiation, Completion, and Squashing

When a processor initiates a new speculative thread, it is necessary to invalidate all loop-live registers in the LC, VU, VPS, or VPSF state in a local directory by setting their states to INV. However, the other registers remain in their current states during the new thread initiation.

The thread is allowed to complete only if there are no registers in either the VPS or LC state in its local directory. Otherwise, each register value in either the VPS or LC state must be saved by sending it over bus to its successor, in the same way as in the handling of a FW in producer-initiated communication.

When a producer thread performs write for a register value in the VPSF state, the Squash signal is issued on the bus in order to squash a consumer thread that has already loaded a given register value. During the thread squash, the non-loop-live registers in a local directory remain in their current states, while loop-live registers, except those in the LC state, are invalidated.

5.3. SIC Versus ESIC

Comparison between two protocols (SIC and ESIC) from complexity and performance points of view is in order. Software support for the ESIC

protocol requires only slight modifications in the binary annotator for identification of PFWs. This is not a new issue since the tracing of writes to the
registers is one of the basic activities of the binary annotator. The ESIC protocol does not impose any directory overhead compared to SIC. While the
SIC uses 3 bits (2 bits for coding four states and 1 bit for denoting loop-live
and non-loop-live registers), the ESIC uses 3 bits for coding six states for
loop-live and two for non-loop-live registers. As for the bus structure, only
one additional control signal is needed (*Squash* signal). State machine in the
ESIC controller is more complex than in SIC, but the experience from similar designs tells that this extra logic is not significant.

Although the final conclusion on performance can be drawn only from
an evaluation study with real benchmarks, there is a potential performance
gain of the ESIC compared to SIC. This is a consequence of decreased
blocking of the consumer threads in idle waiting for safe final values from
the producer threads. On the other side, squashing can have adverse effects
on performance. In order to avoid the chance of performance degradation,
profiling information is used to apply speculation only when its success is
probable.

Precise comparison with some other register communication schemes is
difficult because of quite different architectures and approaches. Still, some
brief qualitative comparison to IACOMA [9] (as an existing solution of the
similar kind) can be made. While software support is practically the same, as
for the hardware support for register-level communication, the SIC and
ESIC protocols significantly reduce the directory overhead and an extra
logic for checking the register availability and last-copy status for each register. Besides that, mechanism of distributed arbitration allows to find the
closest predecessor in a faster, nonsequential way compared to IACOMA.
Finally, in the SIC and ESIC protocols, the bus read snarfing decreases
the number of invalidation misses to non-loop-live registers.

It can also be noticed that the SIC and ESIC protocols are better scalable
from the complexity point of view. While in IACOMA overhead in terms
of local directory size and the hardware logic increases for higher number of
processor cores, in these protocols, it stays nearly constant.

6. CONCLUSION

Some earlier studies have shown that the register-level communication brings a considerable performance benefit for speculative multithreading in the CMP architectures. Consequently, this low-latency

transfer mechanism has been employed in a number of CMPs com-
plementing the memory-level communication. The different approaches
and systems and relevant issues in speculative communication of the register
values between threads in existing solutions are surveyed and extensively
discussed in the first part of this chapter.

Most of the systems exploit local distributed register files in different PUs
interconnected by the ring and shared bus, while a few of them employ
shared GRF to some extent. The speculative threads of different granularities are identified with special hardware and/or software support. Register
interthread dependencies are resolved by speculative forwarding of register
values, aggressive value prediction techniques, or inheritance. The misspeculation and misprediction recovery usually results in nonselective or
selective squashing and reexecution.

The second part of the chapter describes a case study, which tries to propose a simple and scalable solution. The proposal includes two variants of the
snoopy-based protocol that exchanges the register values over a dedicated
bus and implies low overhead. It relies on an off-line analysis of register
writes and their proper annotation in binary code. The basic SIC variant
communicates only the safe register values, while the ESIC protocol applies
speculation more aggressively. Both variants enable the producer- and
consumer-initiated communication. The future research directions should
be oriented towards an evaluation of the proposed protocols by means of
simulation. An interesting issue is also to check the viability of run-time
hardware-supported determination of an optimal threshold for speculation
in ESIC protocol instead of using profiling information. Finally, an extension of the protocol functionality to allow the binary annotator tool to deal
with other kinds of speculations (e.g., on subprogram calls) would be very
desirable.

ACKNOWLEDGMENTS

The authors would like to give special thanks to Stefanos Kaxiras of University of Patras for
his vital encouragement and valuable advices. The authors are also very thankful to Sylvain
Girbal from Thales Research and Technologies for his help in implementation of application
profiling.

REFERENCES

[1] T. Knight, An architecture for mostly functional languages, in: ACM Lisp and Functional Programming Conference, 1986, pp. 500–519.
[2] J. Torrellas, Thread-Level Speculation, Encyclopedia of Parallel Computing, Springer
Science+Business Media LLC, New York, NY, 2011, 1894–1900.

[3] M. Tomašević, M.B. Radulović, Speculative chip multiprocessors, in: Proceedings of the Symposium on 25th Anniversary of Faculty of Natural Sciences and Mathematics, University of Montenegro, Podgorica, 2005, pp. 168–186.

[4] C.B. Colohan, A. Ailamaki, J.G. Steffan, T.C. Mowry, CMP support for large and dependent speculative threads, IEEE Trans. Parallel Distrib. Syst. 18 (8) (2007) 1041–1054.

[5] V. Packirisamy, Y. Luo, W.-L. Hung, A. Zhai, P.-C. Yew, T.-F. Ngai, Efficiency of thread-level speculation in SMT and CMP architectures—Performance, power and thermal perspective, in: 26th International Conference on Computer Design, 2008, pp. 286–293.

[6] C. Madriles, P. López, J.M. Codina, et al., Boosting single-thread performance in multicore systems through fine-grain multithreading, in: Proceedings of the 36th Annual International Symposium on Computer Architecture, 2009, pp. 474–483.

[7] K. Olukotun, L. Hammond, J. Laudon, Chip Multiprocessor Architecture: Techniques to Improve Throughput and Latency, Morgan & Claypool, San Rafael, California (USA), 2007, Synthesis Lectures on Computer Architecture #3.

[8] C.L. Ooi, S.W. Kim, I. Park, R. Eigenmann, B. Falsafi, T.N. Vijaykumar, Multiplex: Unifying conventional and speculative thread-level parallelism on a chip multiprocessor, in: ICS-15, 2001, pp. 368–380.

[9] V. Krishnan, J. Torrellas, A chip-multiprocessor architecture with speculative multithreading, IEEE Trans. Comput. 48 (9) (1999) 866–880.

[10] V. Packirisamy, A. Zhai, W.-C. Hsu, P.-C. Yew, T.-F. Ngai, Exploring Speculative Parallelism in SPEC2006, 2009, pp. 77-88.

[11] C.E. Oancea, A. Mycroft, Software thread-level speculation—An optimistic library implementation, in: Proceedings of the 1st International Workshop on Multicore Software Engineering, ACM, New York, NY, 2008, pp. 23–32.

[12] L. Ziarek, S. Jagannathan, M. Fluet, U.A. Acar, Speculative N-Way Barriers, ACM, New York, NY, 2009, 1–12.

[13] F. Warg, Techniques to Reduce Thread-Level Speculation Overhead, Department of Computer Science and Engineering, Chalmers University of Technology, 2006, Ph.D. thesis.

[14] G.S. Sohi, S. Breach, T.N. Vijaykumar, Multiscalar processors, in: Proceedings of the 22nd ISCA, 1995, pp. 414–425.

[15] E. Rotenberg, Q. Jacobson, Y. Sazeides, J. Smith, Trace processors, in: 30th International Symposium on Microarchitecture, 1997, pp. 138–148.

[16] P. Marcuello, A. Gonzalez, J. Tubella, Speculative multithreaded processors, in: Proc. 12th Int'l Conf. Supercomputing (ICS), 1998, pp. 77–84.

[17] M. Tremblay, et al., The MAJC architecture: A synthesis of parallelism and scalability, IEEE Micro 20 (6) (2000) 12–25.

[18] M. Edahiro, S. Matsushita, M. Yamashina, N. Nishi, A single-chip multiprocessor for smart terminals, IEEE Micro 20 (4) (2000) 12–30.

[19] C. Madriles, C. García-Quinones, J. Sanchez, P. Marcuello, A. Gonzalez, D.M. Tullsen, H. Wang, J.P. Shen, Mitosis: A speculative multithreaded processor based on precomputation slices, IEEE Trans. Parallel Distrib. Syst. 19 (7) (2008) 914–925.

[20] J. Gregory Steffan, Christopher B. Colohan, Antonia Zhai, Todd C. Mowry, The STAMPede approach to thread-level speculation, ACM Trans. Comput. Syst. 23 (3) (2005) 253–300.

[21] Peter G. Sassone, D. Scott Wills, Scaling up the atlas chip-multiprocessor, IEEE Trans. Comput. 54 (1) (2005) 82–87.

[22] N.D. Barli, et al., A register communication mechanism for speculative multithreading chip multiprocessors, in: Symposium on Advanced Computer Systems and Infrastructures, 2003, pp. 275–282.

[23] T. Ohsawa, M. Takagi, S. Kawahara, S. Matsushita, Pinot: Speculative multi-threading processor architecture exploiting parallelism over a wide range of granularities, in: Proc. 38th Int'l Symp. Microarchitecture (MICRO), 2005, pp. 81–92.

[24] J.G. Steffan, C.B. Colohan, A. Zhai, T.C. Mowry, A scalable approach to thread-level speculation, in: Proceedings of the 27th International Symposium on Computer Architecture, 2000, pp. 1–12.

[25] J.-Y. Tsai, J. Huang, C. Amlo, D.J. Lilja, P.-C. Yew, The Superthreaded Processor Architecture, IEEE Transactions on Computers, 1999, 881–902, Special Issue on Multithreaded Architectures and Systems, Washington, DC, USA.

[26] S. Keckler, et al., Exploiting fine-grain thread level parallelism on the MIT ALU processor, in: Proc. of the 25th ISCA, 1998, pp. 306–317.

[27] V. Krishnan, J. Torellas, Hardware and software support for speculative execution of binaries on a chip-multiprocessor, in: Proc. of 1998 Int. Conf. on Supercomputing, 1998, pp. 85–92.

[28] D.A. Patterson, J.L. Hennessy, Computer Organization and Design: The Hardware/Software Interface, Morgan Kaufman, San Francisco, CA, USA, 2007.

[29] I. Bell, N. Hasasneh, C. Jessope, Supporting microthread scheduling and synchronization in CMPs, Int. J. Parallel Prog. 34 (4) (2006) 343–381.

[30] Y. Tanaka, H. Ando, Reducing register file size through instruction preexecution enhanced by value prediction, in: IEEE International Conference on Computer Design, 2009, pp. 238–245.

[31] M. Alipour1, H. Taghdisi, Effect of thread-level parallelism on the performance of optimum architecture for embedded applications, IJESA 2 (2012) 15–24.

[32] S.E. Breach, T.N. Vijaykumar, G.S. Sohi, The anatomy of the register file in a multiscalar processor, in: 27th Annual International Symposium on Microarchitecture (MICRO-27), 1994, pp. 181–190.

[33] P. Marcuello, J. Tubella, A. Gonzalez, Value prediction for speculative multithreaded architectures, in: Proc. of the 32th. Int. Conf. on Microarchitecture, 1999, pp. 230–236.

[34] P. Marcuello, Speculative Multithreaded Processors, Universitat Politecnica de Catalunya, Barcelona, Spain, 2003, Ph.D. thesis.

[35] L. Codrescu, D. Scott Wills, Architecture of the atlas chip-multiprocessor: Dynamically parallelizing irregular applications, IEEE Trans. Comput. 50 (1) (2001) 67–82.

[36] L.D. Hung, H. Miura, C. Iwama, D. Tashiro, N.D. Barli, S. Sakai, H. Tanaka, A hardware/software approach for thread level control speculation, IPSJ SIG technical reports 2002-ARC-149, 15th Annual Workshop, Summer United Workshops on Parallel, Distributed, and Cooperative Processing (SWoPP), Yufuin, Japan, vol. 2002, No. 12, (2002) 67–72.

[37] N.D. Barli, Designing NEKO: A Speculative Multithreading Chip MultiProcessor, The University of Tokyo, 2004, Ph.D. thesis.

[38] V. Krishnan, J. Torrellas, Executing sequential binaries on a multithreaded architecture with speculation support, in: Workshop on Multi-Threaded Execution, Architecture and Compilation (MTEAC'98), 1998.

[39] V. Krishnan, J. Torrellas, The need for fast communication in hardware-based speculative chip multiprocessors, Int. J. Parallel Process. 29 (1) (2001) 3–33.

[40] S. Vajapeyam, T. Mitra, Improving superscalar instruction dispatch and issue by exploiting dynamic code sequences, in: 24th International Symposium on Computer Architecture, 1997, pp. 1–12.

[41] K. Sundararaman, M. Franklin, Multiscalar execution along a single flow of control, in: International Conference on Parallel Processing, 1997, pp. 106–113.

[42] E. Rotenberg, J. Smith, Control independence in trace processors, in: 32nd International Symposium on Microarchitecture, 1999, pp. 4–15.

[43] S. Matsushita, et al., Merlot: A single-chip tightly coupled four-way multi-thread processor, in: Proc. Cool Chips III Symp, 2000, pp. 63–74.

[44] MAJC Architecture Tutorial. Sun Microsystems, White Paper, 1999.

[45] S. Sudharsanan, MAJC-5200: A high performance microprocessor for multimedia computing, in: Proc. IPDPS Workshops, 2000, pp. 163–170.

[46] W. Blume, R. Doallo, R. Eigenmann, J. Grout, J. Hoeflinger, T. Lawrence, J. Lee, D. Padua, Y. Paek, B. Pottenger, L. Rauchwerger, P. Tu, Parallel programming with Polaris, IEEE Comput. 29 (1996) 78–82.

[47] L. Codrescu, S. Wills, On dynamic speculative thread partitioning and the MEM-slicing algorithm, in: Proc. Int'l Conf. Parallel Architectures and Compilation Techniques (PACT99), 1999, pp. 40–46.

[48] L. Codrescu, S. Wills, The AMA correlated value predictor, Pica group technical report 10-98, 1998).

[49] M.B. Radulović, M. Tomašević, Towards an improved integrated coherence and speculation protocol, in: IEEE EUROCON 2007, Warsaw, Poland, 2007, pp. 405–412.

[50] M. Tomašević, V. Milutinović, Cache Coherence Problem in Shared-Memory Multiprocessors: Hardware Solutions, IEEE Computer Society Press, Los Alamitos, CA, 1993.

[51] M.B. Radulović, M. Tomašević, A proposal for register-level communication in a speculative chip multiprocessor, in: XLIX ETRAN Conference, Budva, Serbia and Montenegro, 2005, pp. 88–91, Reprinted in ETF J. Electr. Eng. 15 (1) (2006) 91–98.

[52] M.B. Radulović, M. Tomašević, An aggressive register-level communication in a speculative chip multiprocessor, in: IEEE EUROCON2005 Conference, Belgrade, Serbia and Montenegro, 2005, pp. 689–692.

ABOUT THE AUTHORS

Milan B. Radulović was born in Nikšić, Montenegro. He received his B.Sc. in Electrical Engineering and M.Sc. in Robotics and Artificial Intelligence from the University of Montenegro, Montenegro, in 1992 and 1996, respectively. He is enrolled on Ph.D. studies at the Department of Computer Engineering, School of Electrical Engineering, University of Belgrade, Serbia. He is currently working with Crnogorski Telekom A.D., Montenegro. He was previously with the University of Montenegro, Montenegro, for over a decade where he was involved both in teaching process and many research and development projects (robotics and artificial intelligence, electronics, telecommunications, and real-time control systems). He was with the University Mediterranean, Montenegro, for 4 years as a part-time assistant. He was included in several research projects at the universities abroad: University of Warwick, University of Granada, and University of Siena. His current research interests are mainly in computer architecture (especially chip multiprocessor systems with thread-level speculation support), coherence and speculation protocols, transactional memory, compilers, parallel programming, and real-time systems. He is the member of HiPEAC group.

Milo Tomašević was born in Nikšić, Montenegro. He received his B.Sc. in Electrical engineering and M.Sc. and Ph.D. in Computer

Engineering from the University of Belgrade, Serbia, in 1980, 1984, and 1992, respectively. He is currently an Associate Professor and Head of Department of Computer Engineering, School of Electrical Engineering, University of Belgrade, Serbia. He was previously with the Pupin Institute, Belgrade, for over a decade where he was involved in many research and development projects. His current research interests are mainly in computer architecture (especially multiprocessor systems), parallel programming, cryptography, and algorithms and data structures. In these areas, he published almost 100 papers in international scientific journals, books, and proceedings of international and domestic conferences. He served as a reviewer for several journals and conferences and delivered tutorials at major conferences from the field of computer architecture and companies.

Veljko Milutinović received his Ph.D. in Electrical Engineering from University of Belgrade in 1982. During the 1980s, for about a decade, he was on the faculty of Purdue University, West Lafayette, Indiana, USA, where he coauthored the architecture and design of the world's first DARPA GaAs microprocessor. Since the 1990s, after returning to Serbia, he is on the faculty of the School of Electrical Engineering, University of Belgrade, where he is teaching courses related to computer engineering, sensor networks, and data mining. During the 1990s, he also took part in teaching at the University of Purdue, Stanford and MIT. After the year 2000, he participated in several FP6 and FP7 projects through collaboration with leading universities and industries in the EU/US, including Microsoft, Intel, IBM, Ericsson, especially Maxeler. He has lectured by invitation to over 100 European universities. He published about 50 papers in SCI journals and about 20 books with major publishers in the United States. Professor Milutinović is a Fellow of the IEEE and a Member of Academia Europaea.

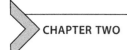

CHAPTER TWO

Survey on System I/O Hardware Transactions and Impact on Latency, Throughput, and Other Factors

Steen Larsen*,†, Ben Lee*
*School of Electrical and Engineering Computer Science, Oregon State University, Corvallis, Oregon, USA
†Intel Corporation, Hillsboro, Oregon, USA

Contents

Abstract

Computer system input/output (I/O) has evolved with processor and memory technologies in terms of reducing latency, increasing bandwidth, and other factors. As requirements increase for I/O, such as networking, storage, and video, descriptor-based direct memory access (DMA) transactions have become more important in high-performance systems to move data between I/O adapters and system memory buffers. DMA transactions are done with hardware engines below the software protocol abstraction layers in all systems other than rudimentary embedded controllers. Central processing unit (CPUs) can switch to other tasks by offloading hardware DMA transfers to the I/O adapters. Each I/O interface has one or more separately instantiated descriptor-based DMA engines optimized for a given I/O port. I/O transactions are optimized by accelerator functions to reduce latency, improve throughput, and reduce CPU overhead. This chapter surveys the current state of high-performance I/O architecture advances and explores benefits and limitations. With the proliferation of CPU multicores within a system, multi-GB/s ports, and on-die integration of system functions, changes beyond the techniques surveyed may be needed for optimal I/O architecture performance.

ABBREVIATIONS

ARM Acorn RISC Machine

BIOS basic input/output system—allows access by the operating system to low-level hardware

BW bandwidth supported by an interface, usually synonymous with throughput capability

CNI coherent network interface

CPU central processing unit—consisting of potentially multiple cores, each with one or more hardware threads of execution

CRC cyclic redundancy check

CQE completion queue entry—used in RDMA to track transaction completions

DCA direct cache access

DDR double data rate—allows a slower clock to transmit twice the data per cycle. Usually based on both the rising and falling edge of a clock signal

DDR3 3rd generation memory DDR interface

DLP data layer protocol in PCIe, which is similar to networking IP layer

DMA direct memory access—allows read or write transactions with system memory

DSP digital signal processing

FPGA field-programmable gate array

FSB front-side bus—a processor interface protocol that is replaced by Intel QPI and AMD HyperTransport

GbE gigabit Ethernet

GBps gigabytes per second

Gbps gigabits per second (GBps x8)

GHz gigahertz

GOQ global observation queue

GPU graphic processing unit

HPC high-performance computing—usually implies a high-speed interconnection of high-performance systems

HW hardware

ICH Intel I/O controller hub—interfaced to the IOH to support slower system protocols, such as USB and BIOS memory

I/O input/output

IOH Intel I/O hub—interfaces between QPI and PCIe interfaces

iWARP Internet wide area RDMA protocol—an RDMA protocol that supports lower level Ethernet protocol transactions

kB kilobyte, 1024 bytes. Sometimes reduced to "K" based on context

L1 cache level 1 cache

L2 cache level 2 cache

LCD liquid crystal display

LLC last-level cache—level 3 cache

LLI low latency interrupt

LLP link layer protocol—used PCIe

LRO large receive offloading

LSO large segment offload

MB megabytes

MESI(F) modified, exclusive, shared, invalid, and optionally forward—protocol to maintain memory coherency between different CPUs in a system

MFC memory flow controller—used to manage SPU DMA transactions

MMIO memory-mapped I/O

MPI message passing interface—a protocol to pass messages between systems often used in HPC

MSI message signaled interrupt—used in PCIe to interrupt a core

MTU maximum transmission unit

NIC network interface controller

NUMA nonuniform memory architecture—allows multiple pools of memory to be shared between CPUs with a coherency protocol

PCIe Peripheral Component Interconnect express—defined at www.pcisig.com. Multiple lanes (1–16) of serial I/O traffic reaching 16 Gbps per lane. Multiple generations of PCIe exist, represented by Gen1, Gen2, Gen3, and Gen4. PCIe protocol levels have similarities with networking ISO stack

PHY PHYsical interface defining the cable (fiber/copper) interfacing protocol

PIO programmed I/O—often synonymous with MMIO

QDR quad data rate—allows four times the data rate based on a slower clock frequency

QoS quality of service—a metric to define guaranteed minimums of service quality

QP queue pair—transmit queue and receive queue structure in RDMA to allow interfacing between two or more systems

QPI QuickPath Interconnect—Intel's proprietary CPU interface supporting MESI(F) memory coherence protocol

RAID redundant array of independent disks

RDMA remote direct memory access—used to access memory between two or more systems

RSS receive side scaling

RTOS real-time operating system

RX reception from a network to a system

SAS storage array system

SCC single-chip cloud

SCSI small computer system interface

SMT simultaneous multithreading

SPE synergistic processing element in the cell processor

SPU synergistic processing unit in cell SPE

SSD solid-stated disk

SW software

TCP/IP transmission control protocol and Internet protocol networking stack

TLP transaction layer protocol of PCIe stack

TOE TCP/IP offload engine

TX transmission from a system to a network
USB universal serial bus
WQE work queue entry—used in RDMA to track transaction parameters

1. INTRODUCTION

Input/output (I/O) is becoming a peer to processor core (or simply *core*) and memory in terms of latency, bandwidth, and power requirements. Historically, when a core was simpler and more directly I/O focused, it was acceptable to "bit-bang" I/O port operations using port I/O or memory-mapped I/O (MMIO) models [1]. However, with complex user interfaces and programs using multiple processes, the benefit of offloading data movement to an I/O adapter became more apparent. Since I/O devices are much slower than the core–memory bandwidth, it makes sense to move data at a pace governed by the external device.

Typically, I/O data transfer is initiated using a descriptor containing the physical address and size of the data to be moved. This descriptor is then posted (i.e., sent) to the I/O adapter, which then processes the direct memory access (DMA) read/write operations as fast as the core–memory bandwidth allows. The descriptor-based DMA approach makes sense when the I/O bandwidth requirements are much lower than the core–memory bandwidth. However, with the advent of multicore processors and simultaneous multithreading (SMTs), the I/O device capability can be scaled as the number of cores scale per central processing unit (CPU). A CPU can consist of multiple cores and other related functions but is unified on a single silicon die. Figure 2.1 shows how CPU scaling and the integration of the memory controller have exceeded I/O bandwidth gains during the period from 2004

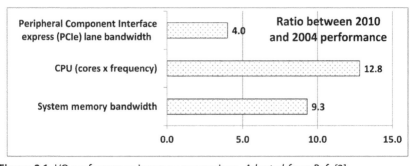

Figure 2.1 I/O performance increase comparison. *Adapted from Ref. [2].*

to 2010 [2]. As can be seen, I/O bandwidth has improved at a much lower rate than CPU and memory performance capabilities. I/O also needs quality of service (QoS) to provide low latency for network interfaces and graphics accelerators and high bandwidth support for storage interfaces.

The movement of data between CPUs and I/O devices is performed using variety methods, each often optimized based on the traffic type. For example, I/O devices such as storage disk drives typically move large blocks of data (>4 kB) for throughput efficiency but result in poor latency performance. In contrast, low latency is crucial in a scenario, such as a cluster of internetworked systems, where messages may be small (on the order of 64 bytes). Therefore, this chapter provides a survey on existing methods and advances in utilizing the I/O performance available in current systems. Based on our measurements and analysis, we also show how I/O is impacted by latency and throughput constraints. Finally, we suggest an option to consider based on these measurements to improve I/O performance.

The chapter is organized as follows: Section 2 provides a general background on I/O operation and how the DMA transactions typically occur between I/O adapters and higher-level software layers. This is followed by a detailed measurement and analysis of typical current high-performance I/O devices in Section 3. Section 4 provides a survey on how various current systems perform I/O transactions. Finally, Section 5 suggests areas for improvement and optimization opportunities.

2. BACKGROUND AND GENERAL DISCUSSION

Current I/O devices, such as network interface controllers (NICs), storage drives, and universal serial bus (USB), are orders of magnitude lower in bandwidth than the core–memory complex. For example, a modern 64-bit core running at 3.6 GHz compared to a 1.5 Mbps USB1.1 mouse has 153,600 times higher bandwidth. CPUs with multiple cores and SMT make this ratio even higher. Therefore, it makes sense to off-load the cores by allowing the I/O adapters some control over how I/O data are pushed/pulled to/from memory. This allows a core to switch to other tasks while the slower I/O adapters operate as efficiently as they are capable.

Figure 2.2 shows a diagram of the internal system components of a current high-performance system based on the Intel 5520 chipset [3]. The 8-core system contains two quad-core processors, each with 8 MB L3 cache, memory interface, and QuickPath Interconnect (QPI) coherent memory interface. The speed of each core (3.2 GHz) is not directly applicable to

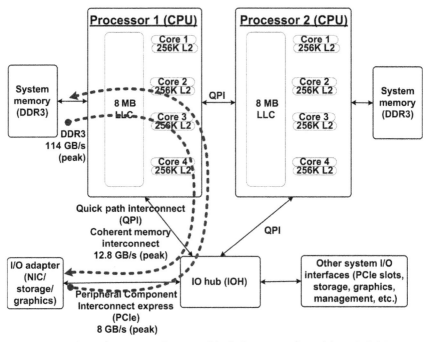

Figure 2.2 High-performance I/O system block diagram. *Adapted from Ref. [3].*

the discussion as we will see that I/O transaction efficiency is governed more directly by the I/O device controllers. The two dotted arrows between the I/O adapter and a CPU indicate the path and bandwidth available for the I/O adapter to read data to be transmitted from system memory and write received data to system memory.

The I/O hub (IOH) interfaces between the QPI interface and multiple Peripheral Component Interconnect express (PCIe) interfaces. This flexible design allows one to four CPUs to be configured using one to two IOHs for a variety of I/O expansion capabilities. In addition, each IOH has basic input/output system (BIOS) controlled registers to define the PCIe lane configuration, allowing the system to have either multiple low bandwidth PCIe interfaces or fewer high bandwidth PCIe interfaces, such as graphics engines. In previous generations of Intel and AMD systems, the IOH was termed "Northbridge" and included a memory controller allowing the processor silicon to be dedicated to core and cache functions. Advances in silicon die technology have allowed the memory controller to be integrated on the same silicon die with the cores and cache for improved memory performance. This performance improvement is mainly due to the removal of the old "Northbridge" and the related protocol overhead.

In 2012, Intel launched products that integrate the IOH onto the same CPU. This integration reduces system power and form factor size, but not other factors such as latency and throughput. Our measurements show that it is the PCIe interface capabilities that define the latency between the system components and not whether or not the IOH is integrated. For this reason, our measurement analysis discussed in Section 3 is based on the more recent platform shown in Fig. 2.2.

High-performance I/O adapters connect directly to the IOH, while more basic I/O adapters are interfaced with the I/O controller hub (ICH). The ICH, which was often termed "southbridge" in previous system generations, supports the interface hardware to BIOS boot flash memory, direct attached storage, USB, and system management modules that include temperature, voltage, and current sensors. Our focus is on I/O devices connected to the IOH interface and not ICH-connected devices.

An NIC is used as the baseline I/O device since it offers a wide variety of I/O performance factors to study. For storage, throughput is more important than latency, and several techniques can be incorporated into NICs to enhance storage over the network. For clusters and high-performance computing, latency is often a critical component; thus, different techniques can be applied. Table 2.1 lists the performance focus and reference section.

Note that although power minimization is always a concern, it is common practice to disable power-saving states to maintain a low (and predictable) I/O latency. This baseline NIC for I/O transactions can be extended to other high-performance devices, such as disk storage controllers and graphics adapters. These devices all share the descriptor-based DMA transactions that will be discussed in detail in the rest of this section.

Table 2.1 NIC Performance Accelerator Examples

Performance Focus	Techniques to Improve Performance	Chapter Reference
Throughput	CPU DMA	4.1.2
Throughput	Interrupt moderation	4.2.2
Throughput	RSS, LRO, LSO	4.3.1
Latency	LLI	4.2.2
Latency	Infiniband	4.4.3
Latency	User-based I/O	4.2.1

Figure 2.3 illustrates a typical I/O transmission for an Ethernet NIC (either wired or wireless). The following sequence of operations occurs to transmit an Ethernet packet between two connected systems (i.e., kernel sockets have been established and opened):

1. The kernel software constructs the outgoing packet in system memory. This is required to support the protocol stack, such as transmission control protocol and Internet protocol (TCP/IP), with proper headers, sequence numbers, and checksums.

2. A core sends a *doorbell request* on the platform interconnect (e.g., PCIe, but this also applies to any chip-to-chip interconnect within a platform) to the NIC indicating that there is a pending packet transmission. This is a write operation by a core to the memory space reserved for the I/O adapter, which is uncacheable with implications that other related tasks that are potentially executing out-of-order must be serialized until the uncacheable write completes. The core then assumes the packet will be transmitted, but will not release the memory buffers until confirmed by the NIC that the packet has been transmitted.

3. The doorbell request triggers the NIC to initiate a DMA request to read the descriptor containing the physical address of the transmit payload.

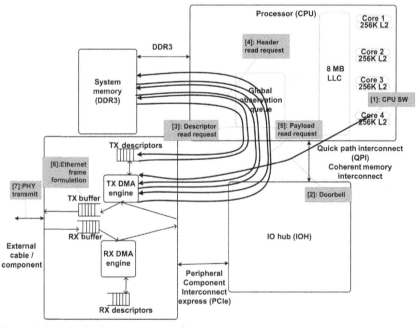

Figure 2.3 Typical Ethernet transmit flow.

The descriptor for the payload is not included in the doorbell request because there are two separate descriptors for header and payload in an Ethernet packet definition, and a larger network message will require more descriptors (e.g., maximum payload for Ethernet is 1460 bytes). A tracking mechanism called a global observation queue (GOQ) in the CPU controls memory transaction coherency such that on-die cores or other CPUs correctly snoops the (system) bus for memory requests. The GOQ also helps avoid memory contention between I/O devices and the cores within the system.

4. A memory read request for the descriptor(s) returns with the physical addresses of the header and payload. Then, the NIC initiates a request for the header information (e.g., IP addresses and the sequence number) of the packet.

5. After the header information becomes available, a request is made to read the transmit payload using the address of the payload in the descriptor with almost no additional latency other than the NIC state machine.

6. When the payload data return from the system memory, the NIC state machine constructs an Ethernet frame sequence with the correct ordering for the bitstream.

7. Finally, the bitstream is passed to a PHYsical (PHY) layer that properly conditions the signaling for transmission over the medium (copper, fiber, or radio).

The typical Ethernet receive flow is the reverse of the transmit flow and is shown in Fig. 2.4. After a core prepares a descriptor, the NIC performs a DMA operation to transfer the received packet into the system memory. After the transfer completes, the NIC interrupts the processor and updates the descriptor.

1. The NIC prefetches a descriptor associated with the established connection and matches an incoming packet with an available receive descriptor.

2. The received packet arrives asynchronously to the NIC adapter.

3. The NIC performs a DMA write to transfer the packet contents into the system memory space pointed to by the receive descriptor.

4. After the memory write transaction completes, the NIC interrupts the core indicating a new packet has been received for further processing.

5. As part of the interrupt processing routine, the core driver software issues a write to the NIC to synchronize the NIC adapter descriptor ring with the core descriptor ring. This also acts as a confirmation that the NIC

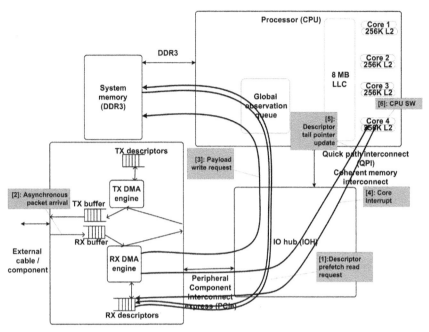

Figure 2.4 Typical Ethernet receive flow, which is similar to the transmit flow but in reverse.

packet has been successfully moved from the I/O adapter to system memory.

6. Finally, the kernel software processes the received packet in the system memory.

3. MEASUREMENTS AND QUANTIFICATIONS

In order to quantify various I/O design aspects of current servers and workstations and explore potential changes, a conventional NIC was placed in an IOH slot of a platform described in Section 2. A PCIe protocol analyzer was used to observe the PCIe transactions, which are summarized in Table 2.2. Using measurements on a real (and current) system offers validity in extrapolations and conclusions that are less certain in simulated environments.

The following subsections discuss the measurements and analysis in more detail. By observing the latency breakdown and bandwidth–per–pin utilization, we can explore requirements and inefficiencies in the current model.

Table 2.2 Quantified Metrics of Current Descriptor-Based DMA Transactions

	Latency	Bandwidth-Per-Pin
Description	Latency to transmit a TCP/IP message between two systems	Gbps per serial link
Measured value	8.6 μs	2.1 Gbps/link
Descriptor-related overhead	18%	17%
See Section	3.1	3.2

3.1. Latency

Latency is a critical aspect in network communication that is easily masked by the impact of distance. However, when interplatform flight time of messages is small, the impact of latency within a system is much more important. One such example is automated stock market transactions (arbitrage and speculation) as demonstrated by Xasax claiming 30 μs latency to the NASDAQ trading floor [4]. Another example is in high-performance computing (HPC) nodes where LINPACK Benchmark (used to define the Top500 supercomputers) shares partial calculations of linear algebra matrix results among nodes [5].

Figure 2.5 shows a typical 10 gigabit Ethernet (GbE) latency between a sender (TX) and a receiver (RX) in a data center environment where the

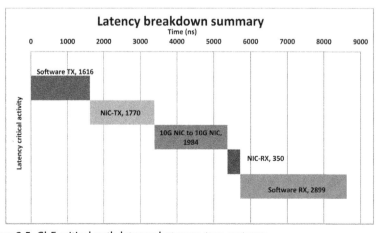

Figure 2.5 GbE critical path latency between two systems.

fiber length is on the order of 3 m. These results are based on PCIe traces of current 10 GbE Intel 82598 NICs (code named Oplin) on PCIe x8 Gen1 interfaces [6]. The latency benchmark NetPIPE is used to correlate application latencies to latencies measured on the PCIe interface for 64-byte messages. The 64-byte size was used since it is small enough to demonstrate the critical path latencies but also large enough to represent a minimal message size that can be cache line-aligned.

End-to-end latency consists of both hardware and software delays and depends on many aspects not directly addressed in this chapter, such as core and memory clock frequencies, bandwidth, and cache structure. The critical path latency of the software stack is around 1.61 and 2.9 μs for send and receive, respectively, and is not related to descriptor-based I/O communication since it is only associated with how a core handles I/O traffic data that is already in system memory. Software latency in terms of the core cycles required to formulate TCP/IP frames for transmit and processing received TCP/IP frames is described in more detail in Ref. [7]. On the other hand, hardware latency can be split into three portions. First, the TX NIC performs DMA reads (NIC TX) to pull the data from the system memory to the TX NIC buffer, which is around 1.77 μs. This is followed by a flight latency of 1.98 μs for the wire/fiber and the TX/RX NIC state machines (NIC to NIC). Finally, the RX NIC requires 0.35 μs to perform DMA writes (NIC-RX) to push the data from the RX NIC buffer into the system memory and interrupt a core for software processing. The total latency, $Latency_{Total}$, is 8.6 μs and can be expressed by the following equation:

$$Latency_{Total} = Tx_{SW} + Tx_{NIC} + fiber + Rx_{NIC} + Rx_{SW}$$

The latency for the Tx_{NIC} portion can be further broken down using PCIe traces as shown in Fig. 2.6. A passive PCIe interposer was placed between the platform PCIe slot and the Intel 82598 NIC. PCIe traces were taken from an idle platform and network environment. These latencies are averaged over multiple samples and show some variance, but it is under 3%. The variance is due to a variety of factors, such as software timers and PCIe transaction management. Based on a current 5500 Intel processor platform with 1066 MB/s double data rate (DDR3) memory, the doorbell write takes 230 ns, the NIC descriptor fetch takes 759 ns, and the 64 B payload DMA read takes 781 ns. The core frequency is not relevant since the PCIe NIC adapter controls the DMA transactions. Note that 43% and 44% of the transmit HW latency (Tx_{NIC}) are used by the descriptor fetch (and decode) and

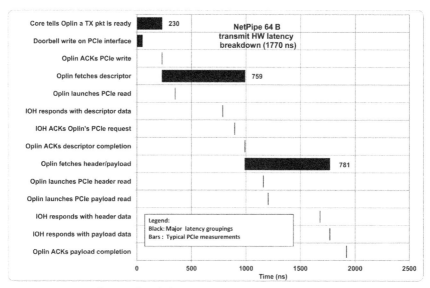

Figure 2.6 NIC TX latency breakdown.

payload read, respectively. This is important in the scope of getting a packet from memory to the wire, and assuming the core could write the payload directly to the NIC, 1770 ns could be nearly reduced to 230 ns. This results in about 18% reduction in total end-to-end latency as shown in Table 2.2.

3.2. Throughput and Bandwidth Efficiency

The Iperf bandwidth benchmark was used on a dual 10 GbE Intel 82599 Ethernet adapter (code name Niantic) [8] on an Intel 5500 server. The primary difference between the 82,598 and the 82,599 Intel NIC is the increase in PCIe bandwidth. This does not impact the validity of the previous latency discussion, but allows throughput tests up to the theoretical 2×10 GbE maximum. PCIe captures consisted of more than 300,000 PCIe x8 Gen2 packets, or 10 ms of real-time trace, which gives a statistically stable data for analysis.

Figure 2.7 shows a breakdown of transaction utilization in receiving and transmitting data on a PCIe interface for a dual 10 GbE NIC. The four stacked bars show extreme cases of TCP/IP receive (RX_) and transmit (TX_) traffic for small (_64B_) and large (_64KB_) I/O message sizes. Since throughput is lower than the link rate for small message sizes, we also show the aggregate throughput (1 Gbps, 18 Gbps, 400 Mbps, and 19 Gbps) across both 10 GbE ports when using the Iperf benchmark. The traffic is normalized to 100% to illustrate the proportion of nonpayload-related traffic across the PCIe interface.

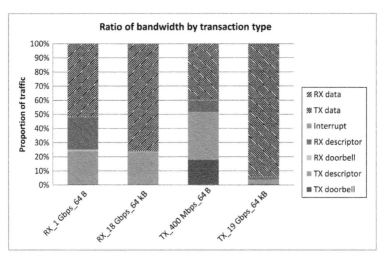

Figure 2.7 Proportions of PCIe transaction bandwidths.

Receive traffic performance is important for applications such as backup and routing traffic, while transmit traffic performance is important in serving files and streaming video. I/O operation on small messages is representative of latency sensitive transactions, while large I/O is representative of storage types of transactions. Figure 2.8 highlights the impact of nonpayload-related PCIe bandwidth when the PCIe frame overhead is factored in to account for the actual bandwidth required for each frame. This figure shows that descriptors and doorbell transactions for small messages represent a significant portion of the total PCIe bandwidth utilized in this measurement. This includes PCIe packet header and cyclic redundancy check (CRC) data along with PCIe packet fragmentation. If descriptor and doorbell overhead were to be removed, the bandwidth could be improved by up to 43% as indicated by the TX_400Mbps_64 case. In the case of I/O receive for small payload sizes, the inefficiency due to descriptors and doorbells is only 16% since 16-byte descriptors can be prefetched in a 64-byte cache-line read request. For large I/O message sizes, the available PCIe bandwidth is efficiently utilized with less than 5% of the bandwidth used for descriptors and doorbells.

4. SURVEY OF EXISTING METHODS AND TECHNIQUES

Computer systems utilize a broad range of I/O methods depending on the external usage requirements and the internal system requirements. Since the scope of this chapter is on the hardware I/O transactions that are

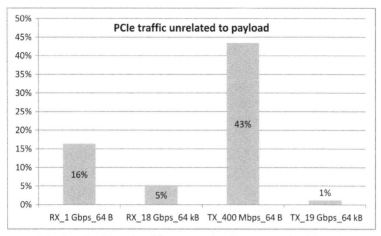

Figure 2.8 PCIe bandwidth utilized for nonpayload versus payload bandwidth.

essentially common regardless of application, the survey is structured based on system complexity for the following four categories: (1) simple systems, (2) workstations and servers, (3) data centers and HPC clusters, and (4) system interconnects and networks. Note that an alternative I/O survey organization could be based on different I/O usages (such as networking, storage, and video applications). However, this would add an orthogonal dimension to the survey, and thus is not considered.

4.1. Simple Systems: Direct I/O Access and Basic DMA Operations

This subsection discusses I/O for systems that access I/O directly by the CPU without DMA, sometimes termed programmed I/O (PIO), as well as systems that have DMA engines directly associated with CPUs. These include embedded systems, systems with digital signal processing (DSP), and graphics subsystems. These systems may either access I/O directly using the CPU instruction set or set up a DMA operation that is associated directly with a CPU. Real-time operating systems (RTOS) are part of this classification since the I/O performance characterization is a critical part of system performance.

4.1.1 Embedded Systems

The simplest method of system I/O, which is usually found in slower systems with a single dedicated function, is found in embedded controllers with dedicated memory locations for I/O data. An example would be a clock radio where outputs are LCD segment signals and inputs are buttons with dedicated signals that can be polled or interrupt a basic software routine. Example controllers used for such functions include device families around the Intel 8051, Atmel AVR, ARM, and Microchip PIC, where no operating system is used to virtualize hardware.

This direct access of I/O by a microcontroller can support I/O protocols at very low bandwidths such as "bit-banging" mentioned in Section 1 as implemented with Softmodem [1].

4.1.2 CPU DMA and DSP Systems

An extension of the direct I/O control is to have a DMA engine configured and controlled by the CPU. This is common in DSP systems where large amounts of data need to be moved between I/O, signal processing function blocks, and memory. The basic operations consist of the following:

1. CPU determines via interrupt or other control a need to move N bytes from location X to location Y, often in a global memory-mapped address space.
2. CPU configures the DMA engine to perform the data transfer.
3. CPU either polls or waits for DMA interrupt for completion.

An example of such a system is the IBM/TI cell processor shown in Fig. 2.9, which consists of power processing element (PPE) and eight synergistic processing elements (SPEs) or cores [9,10]. Each SPE has a synergistic processing unit (SPU) and a memory flow controller (MFC), which is used to handle the SPE DMA transactions.

Each SPE has 256 kB of local on-die memory. If an SPE requires non-local memory access, it can either request the PPE for a kernel/OS service or configure DMA to perform I/O transaction from the system memory to and from the SPE. To reduce the SPE DMA programming overhead, Ionkov et al. [9] proposed using coroutines to manage I/O transactions between

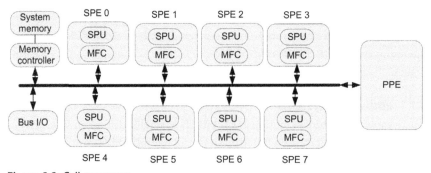

Figure 2.9 Cell processor.

SPEs and system memory. This removes the requirement to program each SPE DMA transaction but adds a software layer that requires tracking coroutine state that impacts the number of coroutines that can be supported and the switch time between coroutines. There is no memory coherency structure, as found in x86 CPUs, reducing intercore communication requirements. The cell processor architecture shows how data movement via core-controlled DMAs is effective for graphics processing in current workloads.

Further examples of core-based DMA control are presented in Refs. [11,12] covering typical embedded DMA processing. Katz and Gentile [13] provide a similar description of DMA on a Texas Instruments Blackfin digital signal processor. These systems use DMA descriptors to define physical payload status and memory locations similar to legacy Ethernet I/O processing described in Section 2.

4.1.3 General CPU Controlled DMA Engines

An alternative to the simple embedded controller system cases discussed thus far is Intel's DMA offload engine in server CPUs called QuickData Technology, which is a method to improve I/O performance for storage and redundant array of independent disks (RAID) [14]. Certain RAID configurations will use XOR bit-level calculations to regenerate data on failed disk drives [15]. Often, an expensive RAID storage controller will execute the XOR functions, but the Intel QuickData Technology allows standard disks to be attached in a RAID configuration and support in-flight XOR calculations. Currently, it is implemented in the IOH shown in Fig. 2.2 and with a large and cumbersome 64-byte descriptor. Obviously, there is inefficiency in handling asynchronous variable-sized data common in networking that needs to be set up before any DMA copies can be made between I/O adapter and memory. As a result, the DMA engine is often used for memory-to-memory copies, such as between kernel space and user space. In networking, this shows little if any benefit to CPU utilization [16], in part because memory accesses can be pipelined and thus hide a software core-controlled memory-to-memory copy.

4.1.4 PCIe Bandwidth Optimization

Yu et al. [17] described how existing DMA transfer speed can be improved by increasing buffer efficiencies for large block DMA transfers on a particular PCIe implementation (PEX8311). The speedup is achieved primarily by expanding the PCIe packet frame size. An analogy could be made to the use of jumbo frames on Ethernet that exceed the default 1500-byte maximum transmission unit (MTU). PCIe transactions normally have a maximum frame payload of 256 bytes because larger maximum frame payloads would require more silicon on both ends of the PCIe interface. The selection of 256 bytes is an industry norm since often each end of the PCIe interface can be populated by silicon from various companies. The PCIe protocol specifies three headers for each transaction [18]: transaction layer protocol (TLP), data layer protocol (DLP), and link layer protocol (LLP), which combined add 24 bytes to each PCIe transaction reducing the effective bandwidth.

Tumeo *et al.* [19] provide details on optimizing for *double buffering* and how this technique can be used to optimize latency in a multicore field-programmable gate array (FPGA) with each core having a DMA engine to move data between system memory and core memory. The basic idea is to pipeline multiple DMA transactions such that the PCIe interface is optimally utilized. While this allows DMA transactions to be set up, executed, and terminated in parallel, it can be detrimental to latency and predictability of latency as discussed in Section 4.1.5.

4.1.5 Predictability and RTOS

In RTOS, *I/O latency prediction* is an important factor to guarantee predictable operations. If an I/O transaction cannot be predicted to occur within a certain time interval, the degree of deterministic behavior by the operating system cannot be defined. The smaller variability in latency prediction of an I/O transaction results in better overall RTOS performance. Several papers present models on how to accurately predict and bound the DMA latency when controlled by the I/O adapter [20–24]. Worst-case execution time (WCET) is the most critical parameter to consider. Current I/O transactions use multiple DMA engines in different clock domains throughout the system and each engine may have different I/O transaction queuing and QoS characteristics. Based on this, the predictability of I/O transactions is generally inversely proportional to system complexity.

A more predicable I/O transaction can involve the core directly accessing the I/O device using PIO. However, I/O adapter DMA engines remain common in systems with RTOS since standard "bit-banging" by the core results in poor I/O performance. For example, Salah and El-Badawi compared PIO to DMA, where PIO resulted in only 10% throughput compared to DMA throughput measurements [20].

4.1.6 Other DMA-Related Proposals

The *dynamic compression of data* for memory accesses discussed in Ref. [25] is an option to reduce I/O latency and reduce the chip-to-chip bandwidth. However, there is added logic complexity required to compress and decompress payload data. In addition, the I/O device is often clocked at a much slower rate than the memory interface, such as the Intel 82599 NIC internal frequency of 155 MHz [8].

One method to overcome the problem with a common clock DMA engine to transfer data between memory devices is to use *asynchronous DMA*. With asynchronous DMA, the transfer occurs as soon as the producer has the data to transfer and requires the consumer to be available without a defined clock boundary. The challenges of asynchronous DMA are discussed in Refs. [26,27], where it can yield lower latencies across a DMA interface, which typically requires scheduling by a DMA controller. Their results show that asynchronous DMA is more appropriately targeted for a heterogeneous clock domain, which would reduce latency by a few clock cycles in the system shown in Fig. 2.2.

Table 2.3 summarizes how simple systems implement I/O transactions, their primary benefits and costs, and example implementations.

4.2. Generic Workstations and Servers

Systems that run standard multiuser and multiprocessing operating systems, such as Unix and Windows, use more complex I/O structures. Since application software is usually an abstraction of hardware capability to virtualize the I/O ports, the CPU can be utilized very effectively during I/O transactions on other tasks. This has led to the distributed I/O model where each I/O port may have a DMA engine to move incoming/outgoing data to/from system memory. Offloading I/O transactions to a DMA engine is very effective since the I/O device is typically a 100 MHz state machine, while the CPU operates in multi-GHz range allowing the I/O to proceed as fast as it can transfer data (network, storage, or video).

Since CPU and memory performance capabilities have increased faster than I/O performance, the descriptor-based DMA mechanism described in Section 2 is used for a variety of devices in the system. These include not just add-in cards but also the on-board NIC, USB, and storage controllers on current desktop and workstation systems. This section discusses the I/O issues of such systems and how they are addressed.

Table 2.3 Simple System I/O Transactions

Simple Systems	Key Benefits	Key Costs	Example Implementation
Embedded systems	No DMA—allows direct interaction between controller and I/O interface	Core overhead to read and write directly to I/O interface	Clock radio
CPU DMA and DSP	Each core has a dedicated DMA engine close to core to service data movement saving core cycles and power	Per core silicon area and power	Cell processor and 1980s personal computers
General CPU DMA engine	Shared DMA engine between cores and CPUs saves silicon area and power	DMA transaction complexity and increased latency	Intel QuickData technology
PCIe bandwidth optimization	Reducing PCIe protocol overhead allows lower I/O latency	Requires larger PCIe buffers that consume more silicon area and power	Research proposals [17,19]
Predictability and RTOS	More predictable latency bounds and throughput minimums by removing DMA variability	Overall lower system throughput	RTOS research to optimize worst-case execution time (WCET)
Other DMA proposals	I/O data compression and asynchronous DMA may allow lower latencies	Silicon complexity and power	Research proposals [25–27]

4.2.1 Operating System Virtualization Protection

The mechanism to place a kernel barrier between a user application program and hardware makes sense when there are multiple potential processes requesting I/O services; however, there is a penalty in performance. Latency increases because the application software needs to first request kernel services to perform I/O transactions. Throughput may also decrease since buffers need to be prepared and managed using system calls, which often include CPU context switches.

An alternative to always having kernel interaction with system I/O is carefully controlling *user-mode DMA I/O*. The two proposals discussed in Refs. [28,29] describe how to bring kernel-based system calls for moving data into user space so that it can be accessed by user applications. Significant performance improvement can be obtained for small I/O messages by having a user application directly control data movement rather than using system calls. However, there are serious security risks in that any user application can access physical memory. The risk grows when systems are interconnected, potentially allowing physical memory access not just from other processes within a system but also from processes on other systems.

4.2.2 Interrupts and Moderation

Interrupt methods have advanced over the past several years. Traditionally, an interrupt signal or connection was asserted upon requiring CPU software services. This requires a core context switch and parsing through the available interrupt sources within a system. Since other interrupt sources could be I/O devices on slow interfaces, polling for interrupt would require many core cycles. In current systems, message signaled interrupts (MSIs) use a message on the PCIe interface rather than a separate signal for a device interrupt, which saves circuit board resource and allows up to 32 interrupt sources to be defined in the message [18]. MSI was extended to MSI-X that allows up to 2048 sources since there can often be more than 32 interrupt sources in a system. As a result, a core being interrupted can directly proceed to the needed interrupt vector software.

Interrupt moderation, which is also referred to as interrupt coalescing or interrupt aggregation, allows multiple incoming data (e.g., Ethernet packets) to be processed with a single interrupt. This results in relatively low latency and reduces the number of context switches required for received network traffic. Common methods are discussed in Ref. [7] where two timers can be used as follows: one absolute timer with a default, yet configurable, interval of 125 µs to interrupt after any received data arrival and another per packet timer that can expire based on each received packet arrival.

Since network traffic can be both latency and throughput sensitive, adaptive interrupt moderation has been an ongoing area of research and implementations. For example, Intel's 82599 NIC allows interrupt filtering control based on frame size, protocol, IP address, and other parameters [8]. This low latency interrupt (LLI) moderation uses credits based on received packet event control rather than on timer control.

Table 2.4 Generic Workstation and Server I/O Transactions

Generic Workstations and Servers	Key Benefits	Key Costs	Example Implementation
Operating system virtualization protection	Protection from I/O generated access to system resources	Latency and CPU overhead to authorize user access to operating system-controlled transactions	Linux and Windows OS protection layers
Interrupts and moderation	Reduced CPU overhead to manage I/O transactions	Added latency per I/O transaction	10 GbE network interface controllers

Table 2.4 summarizes how generic workstations and servers implement I/O transactions, their primary benefits and costs, and example implementations.

4.3. Data Centers and HPC Cluster Systems

Systems that are used in data centers and HPC clusters have requirements beyond general stand-alone workstations and servers. Often, these systems are composed of high-end servers using multiple 10 GbE interconnects, 15,000 RPM disks, multiple graphic processing units (GPUs), and solid-state drive (SSD) clusters. This drives the internal system requirements to use high-performance scalable protocols, such as Serial Attached SCSI (SAS) for storage and low latency Ethernet or InfiniBand [30] for internode communications. Some HPCs will have front-end CPUs to prepare the I/O in memory for high-speed processing. An example would be an environmental simulation that loads the working set into memory and after simulation outputs a completed working set.

Since Ethernet is ubiquitous and flexible as a network and storage interface, this subsection considers some of the high-end capabilities found in data centers as link speeds increase to 10 GbE and beyond. We first review I/O receive optimizations followed by I/O transmit optimizations, ending with more complex bidirectional improvements.

4.3.1 Device I/O Optimizations

Receive side scaling (RSS) is the ability to demultiplex Ethernet traffic and effectively spread the traffic flow across multiple available cores within a system [31]. An example would be a web server supporting thousands of simultaneous TCP sessions. Each session is hashed using a Toeplitz hash table to properly direct the receive interrupt and traffic to a core that presumably maintains context for the related TCP session. An additional benefit of RSS is that a given TCP session will often be serviced by a persistent core that may well have the connection context in cache.

Large receive offloading (LRO), also called receive side coalescing by Intel [8], is a receive mechanism to clump sequenced frames together, presenting them to the operating system as a single receive frame [32]. This effectively allows creation of a jumbo frame avoiding the higher-level software layer to patch the discrete smaller Ethernet frames (typically 1500 bytes) together.

Large segment offload (LSO), also called TCP segmentation offload or generic segmentation offload, allows an I/O device to be given a pointer to a segment of data much larger than a single frame (e.g., 64 kB) and stream the data for transmits [33]. With 64 kB sized messages, LSO can improve performance by up to 50%.

4.3.2 Descriptor Packing

Descriptor coalescing can be used to reduce the overall receive latency. For example, an Ethernet descriptor size is typically 16 bytes, and thus, multiple descriptors can be read from a single doorbell [34] (e.g., four descriptors would be read at once for a cache-line size of 64 bytes). This works well when the NIC is prefetching descriptors to DMA packets that will be received in the future.

However, a server supporting web or database transactions for thousands of sessions over multiple descriptor queues may not allow for transmit descriptor bundling. This is because organizing the transmit descriptors for packing over thousands of sessions may not be productive since transmit messages need to be formulated in system memory before the descriptor can be defined. In contrast, transmit descriptor coalescing may be beneficial when large multiframed messages are being processed. For example, a data center where multiple systems are physically colocated may simply choose to enable jumbo frames, which again may cause the transmit descriptor serialization described earlier, leading to longer latencies.

4.3.3 TCP/IP Offload Engine and Other Offload Engines

Offloading the entire TCP/IP stack onto an I/O adapter can reduce the stack protocol overhead on the CPU [35]. Figure 2.10 shows an example of TCP/IP offload engine (TOE).

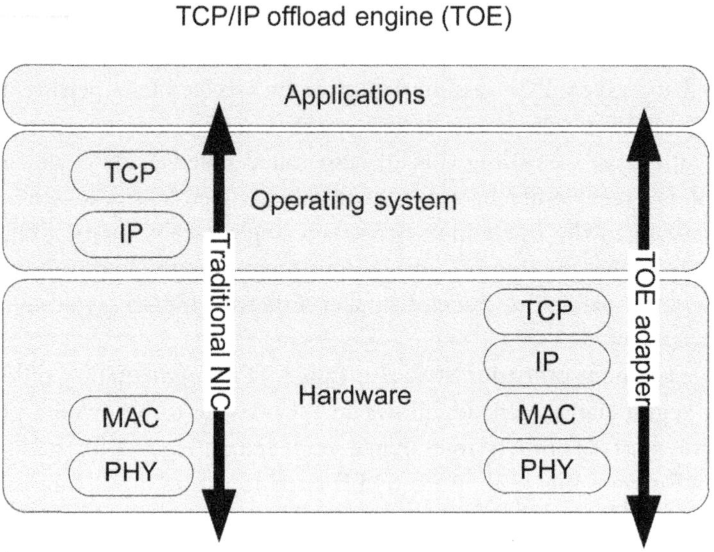

TCP/IP offload engine (TOE)

Figure 2.10 Basic TOE comparison to software-based implementation.

This approach is beneficial for large blocks of I/O, such as storage with average block size greater than 4 kB. The downside of this approach is that HPC and data center servers have to also process small messages. For example, virtualizing multiple operating systems within a single system is common due to increased capabilities of CPUs and memory. This leads to a single I/O adapter processing small packets over thousands of TCP connections. The TOE also processes frames at slower frequencies (typically in the order of 100 MHz) than a modern CPU with multi-GHz frequencies. This adds significant amount logic complexity and connection context memory requirements to the less flexible TOE I/O adapter [35].

In general, any higher-level software I/O protocol may be implemented in an I/O adapter. For instance, the Intel 82599 does not off-load the TCP stack, but does off-load IPsec and Fibre Channel over Ethernet protocols [8]. Myrinet is another type of TOE engine that provides a commonly used HPC interconnect using low-cost Ethernet over a non-TCP/IP proprietary fabric [36]. Since a proprietary protocol is used, Myrinet-specific routing devices between nodes are required.

4.3.4 Coherent Network Interface

Mukherjee *et al.* proposed a coherent NIC interface (CNI) [37], which was followed by an implementation on the front-side bus (FSB) architecture by

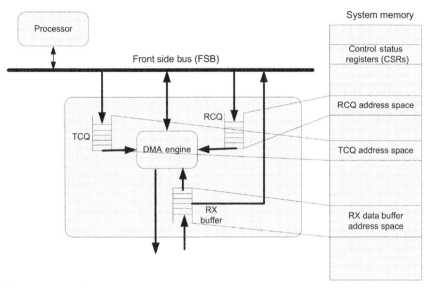

Figure 2.11 NIC system memory apertures.

Schlansker *et al.* [38]. A block diagram of the coherent memory implementation is shown in Fig. 2.11, which consists of transmit command queue (TCQ), receive command queue (RCQ), and Rx data buffer that are all memory-mapped to coherent memory address space. This approach makes the NIC a peer to core memory communication by exposing some of the NIC buffers as coherent system memory. The implementation in coherent memory removes the need for DMA transactions since the core directly reads or writes to the NIC pointers and buffers. They implemented a prototype design and tested on a CPU socket using an FPGA.

The TCQ maintains the transmit descriptor information such that as soon as the CPU software writes the location of the transmit packet in system memory, the DMA engine fetches the packet for transmission. This removes the requirement to fetch a descriptor for transmitting a network packet.

The RCQ is updated as soon as a received packet is placed in the Rx data buffer. Both regions are in coherent memory allowing the CPU software to access the CNI received packets without the traditional DMA operation into system memory. When the CPU, either through polling or interrupt, is signaled with a receive operation, the Rx data buffer points to the appropriate memory location for the received packet.

The key detriment to this implementation is the additional coherency traffic since CNI has to perform snoops and write-back operations between cores and NIC buffers. This additional traffic conflicts with CPU-related traffic between cores on the FSB [39].

4.3.5 CPU Caching Optimizations

One optimization to I/O DMA is direct cache access (DCA), where an I/O device can write to a processor's last-level cache (LLC) by either directly placing data in a cache or hinting to a prefetcher to pull the data from the system memory to a cache [40]. However, this method still requires a descriptor fetch for the I/O device to determine where to place the data in physical memory.

Work by Dan et al. explores the idea of having a separate I/O DMA cache structure, allowing DMA traffic to be cached separately from non-I/O-related data [41]. Similar to DCA, this allows a CPU to have access to receive traffic with an on-die cache and to transmit without requiring the system memory transactions. A criticism of DCA is the risk of cache pollution where the cache becomes a dumping site for I/O evicting more critical data. This risk of pollution can be lowered by having a dedicated I/O cache or partitioning the cache structure into I/O cache and general cache. Nevertheless, a dedicated I/O DMA cache would require more CPU silicon resources and benefits would be small for systems with small I/O.

4.3.6 CPU Network Interface Integration

One approach that is assumed to improve performance is the integration of I/O adapters closer to the CPU. By integrating I/O adapters on the same silicon as the CPU, there are no chip-to-chip requirements such as the PCIe frame protocol that can impact latency and throughput. The design of Sun's Niagara2 processor with integrated 10 GbE showed that the internal architecture needs to be carefully considered to match the desired network performance [42]. In both transmit and receive directions, the integrated NIC shows marginal, if any, improvement over the discrete NIC in terms of bandwidth and CPU utilization.

As a result, simply gluing I/O adapters to processors can often be a waste of die area, power, and development time with little performance improvement.

Table 2.5 summarizes how data center and HPC cluster systems implement I/O transactions, their primary benefits and costs, and example implementations.

Table 2.5 Data Center and HPC Cluster I/O Transactions

Data Centers and HPC Clusters	Key Benefits	Key Costs	Example Implementation
Device I/O optimizations	Higher I/O throughput by adding offload accelerators	I/O device silicon area and power for large I/O transactions	RSS, LRO, LSO on Intel and other NIC devices
Descriptor packing	Increased throughput based on lower PCIe interface overhead	Increased latency	Receive descriptor prefetching on Intel 10 GbE NIC devices
TOE and other offloads	Offload stack protocol processing to I/O device saving CPU cycles	Increased latency, silicon area, and power	Broadcom and Chelsio 10 GbE
Coherent network interfaces	Reduced latency and higher throughput	Increased silicon area and power with nonstandard I/O interfaces	Research proposals [37,38]
CPU caching optimizations	Lower latency and higher throughput	Probable cache inefficiencies and more coherency transactions	Intel direct cache access
CPU network interface integration	Lower latency and higher throughput	Architectural risk of fixing a CPU with a lower volume I/O device	Oracle/Sun Niagara2

4.4. System Interconnects and Networks

Since we are examining how data can be moved optimally within a system, this section considers the important role interconnect architectures play in moving data within a larger, more monolithic system (as opposed to a cluster of systems) and between systems. A particular emphasis is given to HPC environment since this area bears more importance on latency and bandwidth performance characteristics. HPCs prioritize CPU-to-CPU communications rather than moving data into and out of a system, so we discuss the system I/O-oriented communication aspects.

4.4.1 CPU Socket Interconnect

AMD HyperTransport [43] and Intel QPI [14] CPU interconnects are two widely accepted and competitive implementations of data movement between multiple CPUs. These interconnects enable the increasing number of cores in a system to interface with each other, memory, and I/O. Not only are there multiple cores, but also memory is distributed using nonuniform memory access (NUMA) architectures. For example, Fig. 2.2 shows only two NUMA nodes (current platforms can have many more) for a total of 8 cores (where each can operate as two logical cores to the operating system with SMT). Communication between cores is usually done using the memory coherency specified by the MESI(F) protocol [44]. Both HyperTransport and QPI use snoops and coherence directories to determine common states of all memory locations. While they both address similar architecture concerns, there are differences that make them incompatible.

While these interconnects could be used for system I/O transactions, there has not been any widespread demand for using them as I/O interface. Presumably, part of the reason is that a coherent I/O interface would need to address the coherency overhead discussed in Section 4.3.4.

4.4.2 Messaging Between Cores

Intel has explored *I/O messaging* with the single-chip cloud computer (SCC) [45]. This defines a new noncoherent memory type for I/O where software controls what is written and read from a message passing buffer shown in Fig. 2.12. This allows for efficient movement of data between cores while avoiding cache coherency overhead in the form of snoops and data write backs. By using the message memory type, the coherency issues with write-back and write-through memory are avoided, and the core interfaces are not impacted with irrelevant intercore traffic. In SCC, this is accomplished by reserving space in the level 1 cache (L1 cache) as noncoherent memory. For core A to pass a message to core B, the L1 cache line has to be first moved to a noncoherent space, after which the message can be moved to a message passing buffer to be moved into core B's noncoherent L1 cache space. This becomes particularly important as the core count increases to 48, as is the case for SCC, and beyond. While this is similar in architecture to the well-established message passing interface (MPI) standard [46], MPI defines only the higher software layer that uses TCP/IP or other interconnect fabrics and does not define any of the hardware details.

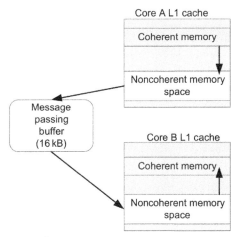

Figure 2.12 SCC message data types.

4.4.3 Remote Direct Memory Access: InfiniBand and iWARP

Remote direct memory access (RDMA) is a method to allow remote access directly into a system memory without involving OS overhead. This reduces latency and increases throughput that is important particularly in data centers and HPC clusters. In the two systems shown in Fig. 2.13, once a connection has been established with proper authentications, a user application can access the remote system's user application space with no requirement for system calls to the OS on either system. This is basically an offload engine where the I/O adapter grants physical access to system memory. Protection is ensured by the hardware interfaces and the software protocol.

InfiniBand and Internet wide area RDMA protocol (iWARP) are both implementations of RDMA. iWARP implements RDMA over the standard Ethernet protocol, which allows iWARP clusters to utilize standard Ethernet routers and interconnect frameworks. In contrast, InfiniBand uses a redesigned network that is not compatible with Ethernet.

InfiniBand is considered a premier high bandwidth and low latency system interconnect [8]. The non-Ethernet protocol allows latencies as low as 1 μs for Mellanox ConnectX, which is the 1999 merger of two competing specifications from future I/O and next-gen I/O [47]. It shares many similarities with TOE/Myrinet/I2O in that transmit and receive queues are processed without the OS involvement in that the session connection is off-loaded to the I/O device adapter. Figure 2.13 shows how two I/O devices communicate across an RDMA fabric with each adapter having a work queue entry (WQE) for each communication session. To provide

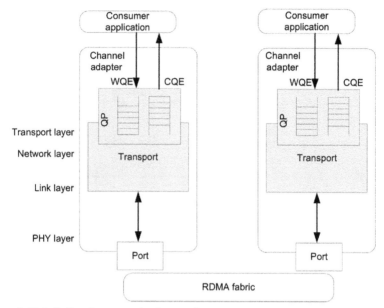

Figure 2.13 InfiniBand communication stack.

session reliability, the completion queue entry (CQE) supports transaction acknowledgments. Thus, each RDMA session is basically represented by two queues where the WQE queue generates the outgoing work requests and the CQE queue tracks completion of outstanding WQE transactions. These two queues are usually termed a queue pair (QP) and are repeated for the sessions used by the higher-level application software.

InfiniBand is a performance reference not only in latency but also in throughput. In a comparison of InfiniBand DDR (at 8 Gbps) and quad data rate (QDR at 16 Gbps) I/O adapters on Intel platforms [48], the internode bandwidth requirements start to exceed the available intranode bandwidth. In particular, DDR intersystem bandwidth exceeded the PCIe Gen1 host interface of 16 Gbps for traffic of small (less than 1 kB) messages.

InfiniBand adds hardware complexity to the I/O adapter to track the connection context and lacks broad popularity due to the high porting cost in both hardware and software when compared to the ubiquitous Ethernet protocol. This can be seen in the Top500 supercomputer interconnect listings where 44% are Ethernet-based and only 42% are InfiniBand-based[5].

Table 2.6 System Interconnect and Network I/O Transactions

System Interconnects and Networks	Key Benefits	Key Costs	Example Implementation
CPU socket interconnect	Higher I/O throughput	I/O device complexity and memory coherency transaction overhead	Intel QPI and AMD HyperTransport
Messaging between cores	Higher I/O throughput and lower latency	Dedicated core silicon area and power	Intel SCC
RDMA InfiniBand and iWARP	Lower latency and reduced CPU overhead	Increased I/O device silicon area and power	Mellanox Infiniband I/O adapters
SiCortex fabric	Network optimized communication between nodes	Customized I/O interfaces with low volume	SiCortex clusters

4.4.4 SiCortex and Other Fabrics

SiCortex uses a custom fabric using a Kautz graph to connect 5832 cores on 972 nodes of 6 cores each [49]. An important point of this architecture is that relatively low-performance cores were used and the network hops between cores were optimized. Based on their HPC benchmark results, bimodal message size patterns of 128 bytes and 100 kB were found. In this case, PIO would be better for small messages with a CPU I/O engine support for large messages.

A popular fabric is the 3-dimension torus in the IBM Blue Gene/P to interconnect 36,864 nodes, each with 4 cores [50]. Each node has a DMA engine to communicate with other nodes, which is similar to the engine discussed in Section 4.1.3. The Blue Gene/P DMA engine services the core-to-core communications instead of serving general purpose I/O.

Table 2.6 summarizes how system interconnects and network I/O transactions can impact I/O transactions.

5. POTENTIAL AREA OF PERFORMANCE IMPROVEMENT

The prior sections have shown that most I/O implementations rely on DMA engines on the I/O adapters to move network, storage, and video data within a system. As CPU and memory performance increases faster than I/O requirements, it is important to reconsider the premise that I/O tasks should always be off-loaded to I/O devices as in the descriptor-based DMA method. As shown in Section 3, the primary advantage of not relying on an I/O adapter's DMA engine and removing descriptor handling is that latency can be reduced. If the DMA engine of the I/O device can be integrated on the CPU, it is possible to reduce end-to-end latency by 18% and also reduce the size of the I/O device memory buffer.

Typical network traffic exhibits a bimodal packet size with concentrations of small and large Ethernet frames [51]. Based on this assumption and projecting that small and large impacts can be averaged, our measurements summarized in Fig. 2.7 show the potential benefits of removing descriptor-related PCIe traffic. The 17% bandwidth reduction due to removal of descriptor, doorbell, and interrupt from the PCIe interface would allow for more payload transfers across the interface. Therefore, this section suggests a CPU-based *integrated DMA* (iDMA) engine and presents several benefits of this design.

The iDMA can be implemented as a simple microcontroller or enhanced state machine that manages the data flow between an arbitrary I/O device and system memory and would basically act as a heterogeneous or SoC core to the larger application generic cores. Figure 2.14 shows the placement of iDMA within a CPU. The arrow from the I/O adapter shows the iDMA pulling receive traffic from an I/O adapter into system memory. The arrows from

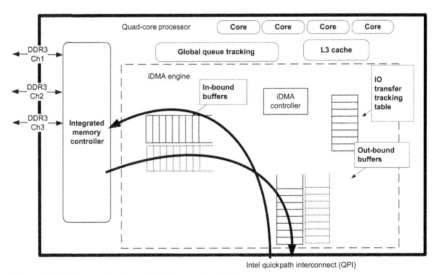

Figure 2.14 An option for CPU integrated DMA.

system memory show the iDMA reading memory and pushing transmit traffic to the I/O adapter, and vice versa. Since I/O messages and cache-line memory accesses occur at different times and with different sizes, basic buffers are needed to support arbitration and fragmentation of off-chip interfaces.

Other less quantifiable improvements of removing descriptor-based DMA transactions include the following and are discussed in more detail by Larsen and Lee [52]. Potential performance improvements are tabulated in Table 2.7.

Table 2.7 Potential Benefits for Nondescriptor DMA

Factor	Description	Measured Value	Descriptor-Related Overhead	Comments/ Justification
Latency	Latency to transmit a TCP/IP message between two systems	8.6 μs	18%	Descriptors are no longer latency critical
BW-per-pin	Gbps per serial link	2.1 Gbps/link	17%	Descriptors no longer consume chip-to-chip bandwidth
BW-right-sizing	Not quantifiable	N/A	N/A	Reduced platform silicon area and power
Power efficiency	Normalized core power relative to maximum power	100%	71%	Power reduction due to more efficient core allocation for I/O
Quality of service	Time required to control connection priority from software perspective	600 ns	92%	Round-trip latency to queuing control reduced between PCIe and system memory
Multiple I/O complexity	Die cost reduction	100%	>50%	Silicon, power regulation, and cooling cost reduction of multiple I/O controllers into a single iDMA instance
Security	Not quantifiable	N/A	N/A	Not quantifiable

1. *Matched I/O and core–memory bandwidths*: In current systems, I/O bandwidth and core and memory bandwidths are not matched, and often, systems can be found with too little I/O capability or inflexible in expanding I/O bandwidth and latency capabilities. Although there are a variety of reasons for the I/O mismatch to core and memory service capabilities, this problem is exacerbated by having multiple CPUs with possibly integrated IOHs. With iDMA, a dual-core processor could be matched with a lower bandwidth iDMA engine than a 4- or 8-core processor. Similarly, a platform that may need higher processor performance relative to I/O performance may need many cores with a lower-capacity iDMA engine.

2. *Power management efficiency*: Mechanisms like RSS can spread I/O traffic across all available cores, thereby wasting system power that could be localized to a subset of cores when I/O traffic is low.

3. *System-level quality-of-service guarantees*: As I/O increases in bandwidth and complexity, having independent DMA engines contending for memory bandwidth reduces quality control. By having a central observation and control point for I/O transactions, the system can prioritize and deliver transactions more appropriately.

4. *Silicon cost and complexity*: Not having independent DMA engines servicing I/O transactions can reduce silicon cost and complexity.

5. *Security*: Security can be improved since iDMA would provide more control over which I/O device reads/writes from/to physical memory.

6. CONCLUSIONS

This survey of I/O methods and existing optimizations illustrates the historical development of I/O transactions for variety of computing systems. In simple systems, I/O is directly addressed by the processor using either PIO or DMA engines associated with the cores, which eliminates the need to set up descriptors to post DMA requests. However, to reduce the CPU management overhead, I/O transaction distribution using DMA engines on the I/O devices became the optimal system design. This DMA offloading approach has continued as I/O transfer optimizations techniques surveyed continue to drive for I/O performance improvements. Based on our measurements and analysis of latency and throughput efficiency, there is an argument to revisit processor-based I/O transactions suggesting quantifiable latency and bandwidth-per-pin advantages and potential benefits in power, QoS, silicon area, and security for future data center server architecture.

ACKNOWLEDGMENTS

This work was supported in part by Ministry of Education Science and Technology (MEST) and the Korean Federation of Science and Technology Societies (KOFST).

REFERENCES

[1] Softmodem description, 2013. Available from: http://en.wikipedia.org/wiki/Softmodem.
[2] H. Newman, I/O Bottlenecks: Biggest Threat to Data Storage, 2009. Available from: http://www.enterprisestorageforum.com/technology/features/article.php/3856121.
[3] Intel 5520 Chip-Set Datasheet, 2010. Available from: http://www.intel.com/assets/pdf/datasheet/321328.pdf.
[4] D. Harris, Banks and Outsourcing: Just Say 'Latency', 2008. Available from: http://www.hpcwire.com/features/Banks_and_Outsourcing_Just_Say_Latency_HPCwire.html.
[5] Top500, 2012. Available from: http://i.top500.org/stats.
[6] Intel 82598 10GbE NIC, 2012. Available from: http://www.intel.com/assets/pdf/prodbrief/317796.pdf.
[7] S. Larsen, et al., Architectural breakdown of end-to-end latency in a TCP/IP network, Int. J. Parallel Program. 37 (6) (2009) 556–571.
[8] Intel 82599 10GbE NIC, 2012. Available from: http://download.intel.com/design/network/prodbrf/321731.pdf.
[9] L. Ionkov, A. Nyrhinen, A. Mirtchovski, CellFS: taking the "DMA" out of cell programming, in: Proceedings of the 2009 IEEE International Symposium on Parallel and Distributed Processing, IEEE Computer Society, Rome, Italy, 2009, pp. 1–8.
[10] F. Khunjush, N. Dimopoulos, Extended characterization of DMA transfers on the Cell BE processor, in: IEEE International Symposium on Parallel and Distributed Processing (IPDPS), 2008.
[11] Z.D. Dittia, G.M. Parulkar, J.R. Cox Jr., The APIC approach to high performance network interface design: protected DMA and other techniques, in: INFOCOM '97. Sixteenth Annual Joint Conference of the IEEE Computer and Communications Societies, Proceedings IEEE, 1997.
[12] L. Yuan, H. Li, C. Duan, The design and implementation of MPI based on link DMA, in: Fifth IEEE International Symposium on Embedded Computing, SEC '08, 2008.
[13] Using DMA effectively, 2012. Available from: http://www.embedded.com/columns/technicalinsights/196802092fire-questid=228429.
[14] Intel QuickPath Interconnect, 2012. Available from: http://en.wikipedia.org/wiki/Intel_QuickPath_Interconnect.
[15] Wikipedia. RAID, 2013. Available from: http://en.wikipedia.org/wiki/RAID.
[16] IOAT Performance, 2012. Available from: http://www.linuxfoundation.org/collaborate/workgroups/networking/i/oat.
[17] P. Yu, et al., A high speed DMA transaction method for PCI express devices testing and diagnosis, in: IEEE Circuits and Systems International Conference on ICTD, 2009.
[18] PCIe Base 3.0 Specification, 2012. Available from: http://www.pcisig.com/specifications/pciexpress/base3/.
[19] A. Tumeo, et al., Lightweight DMA management mechanisms for multiprocessors on FPGA, in: International Conference on Application-Specific Systems, Architectures and Processors, ASAP 2008, 2008.

[20] K. Salah, K. El-Badawi, Throughput-delay analysis of interrupt driven kernels with DMA enabled and disabled in high-speed networks, J. High Speed Netw. 15 (2006) 157–172.

[21] J. Hahn, et al., Analysis of worst case DMA response time in a fixed-priority bus arbitration protocol, Real-Time Syst. 23 (3) (2002) 209–238.

[22] T.-Y. Huang, C.-C. Chou, P.-Y. Chen, Bounding the execution times of DMA I/O tasks on hard-real-time embedded systems, in: J. Chen, S. Hong (Eds.), Real-Time and Embedded Computing Systems and Applications, Springer Berlin, Heidelberg, 2004, pp. 499–512.

[23] T.-Y. Huang, J.W.-S. Liu, D. Hull, A method for bounding the effect of DMA I/O interference on program execution time, in: Proceedings of the 17th IEEE Real-Time Systems Symposium, IEEE Computer Society, Rome, Italy, 1996, p. 275.

[24] C. Pitter, M. Schoeberl, Time predictable CPU and DMA shared memory access, in: International Conference on Field Programmable Logic and Applications, FPL 2007, 2007.

[25] B. Rogers, et al., Scaling the bandwidth wall: challenges in and avenues for CMP scaling, in: ISCA '09: Proceedings of the 36th Annual International Symposium on Computer Architecture, 2009.

[26] A. Bardsley, D. Edwards, Synthesising an asynchronous DMA controller with balsa, J. Syst. Architect. 46 (14) (2000) 1309–1319.

[27] F. Aghdasi, A. Bhasin, DMA controller design using self-clocked methodology, in: AFRICON, 2004. 7th AFRICON Conference in Africa, 2004.

[28] E. Markatos, M. Katevenis, User-level DMA without operating system kernel modification, in: Third International Symposium on High-Performance Computer Architecture, 1997.

[29] M.A. Blumrich, et al., Protected, user-level DMA for the SHRIMP network interface, in: Second International Symposium on High-Performance Computer Architecture Proceedings, 1996.

[30] Infiniband Architecture Specification Version 1.2.1, 2008, 2010. Available from: http://members.infinibandta.org/kws/spec/.

[31] M. Corporation, Introduction to Receive Side Scaling, 2012. Available from: http://msdn.microsoft.com/en-us/library/ff556942.aspx (cited June 2012).

[32] T. Hatori, H. Oi, Implementation and analysis of large receive offload in a virtualized system, in: Proceedings of the Virtualization Performance: Analysis, Characterization, and Tools (VPACT'08), 2008.

[33] G. Regnier, et al., TCP onloading for data center servers, Computer 37 (11) (2004) 48–58.

[34] M. Ross, A. Bechtolsheim, M.T. Le, J. O'Sullivan, FX1000: a high performance single chip Gigabit Ethernet NIC, in: Compcon '97. Proceedings, IEEE, vol., no., 1997, pp. 218, 223, 23–26 Feb, http://dx.doi.org/10.1109/CMPCON.1997.584711.

[35] TCP Offload Engine, 2012. Available from: http://en.wikipedia.org/wiki/TCP_Offload_Engine.

[36] R.A.F. Bhoedjang, T. Ruhl, H.E. Bal, User-level network interface protocols, Computer 31 (11) (1998) 53–60.

[37] M.D. Hill, B. Falsafi, D.A. Wood, S.S. Mukherjee, Coherent network interfaces for fine-grain communication. in: Computer Architecture, 1996, 23rd Annual International Symposium on , vol., no., 1996, pp. 247, 22–24 May, http://dx.doi.org/10.1109/ISCA.1996.10009.

[38] M. Schlansker, et al., High-performance Ethernet-based communications for future multi-core processors, in: Proceedings of the 2007 ACM/IEEE Conference on Supercomputing, SC '07, 2007.

[39] N. Chitlur, S. Larsen (Eds.), 2011. Private conversation with Intel architect N. Chitlur.

[40] IOAT Description, 2012. Available from: http://www.intel.com/network/connectiv ity/vtc_ioat.htm.
[41] T. Dan, et al., DMA cache: using on-chip storage to architecturally separate I/O data from CPU data for improving I/O performance, in: 2010 IEEE 16th International Symposium on High Performance Computer Architecture (HPCA), 2010.
[42] L. Guangdeng, L. Bhuyan, Performance measurement of an integrated NIC architecture with 10 GbE, in: 17th IEEE Symposium on High Performance Interconnects, HOTI 2009, 2009.
[43] HyperTransport IO Link Specification Rev3.10, 2008. Available from: http://www.hypertransport.org/docs/twgdocs/HTC20051222-00046-0028.pdf.
[44] MESI Protocol, 2012. Available from: http://en.wikipedia.org/wiki/MESI_protocol.
[45] J. Mellor-Crummey, Intel Single Chip Cloud Computer, 2010. Available from: http://www.cs.rice.edu/johnmc/comp522/lecture-notes/COMP522-2010-Lecture5-SCC.pdf.
[46] Message Passing Interface. Available from: http://en.wikipedia.org/wiki/Message_Passing_Interface (cited July 29, 2012).
[47] Infiniband Overview, 2012. Available from: http://en.wikipedia.org/wiki/InfiniBand.
[48] H. Subramoni, M. Koop, D.K. Panda, Designing next generation clusters: evaluation of InfiniBand DDR/QDR on Intel computing platforms, in: 17th IEEE Symposium on High Performance Interconnects, HOTI 2009, 2009.
[49] N. Godiwala, J. Leonard, M. Reilly, A network fabric for scalable multiprocessor systems, in: 16th IEEE Symposium on High Performance Interconnects, HOTI '08, 2008.
[50] B. Barney, Using the Dawn BP/P System, 2012. Available from: https://computing.llnl.gov/tutorials/bgp/.
[51] P. Hurtig, W. John, A. Brunstrom, Recent trends in TCP packet-level characteristics, in: ICNS 2011, 2011.
[52] S. Larsen, B. Lee, Platform IO DMA transaction acceleration, in: International Conference on Supercomputing (ICS) Workshop on Characterizing Applications for Heterogeneous Exascale Systems (CACHES), 2011.

ABOUT THE AUTHORS

Steen Larsen, Ph.D. student, received his BS and MS EE at OSU in 1999 and MST at OHSU/OGI 2003 before going back to architectural aspects of I/O communication in a Ph.D. program to optimize platform I/O interconnect over PCIe and other fabrics. This involves applying theories in FPGA designs and low-level operating system device driver control and optimizations. Steen's interest spans latency reduction, CPU overhead reduction, energy savings, and I/O transaction simplification. During much of the day, Steen works at Intel doing applied research in communications and emulating next-generation CPUs.

Ben Lee received his B.E. degree in Electrical Engineering in 1984 from the Department of Electrical Engineering at State University of New York (SUNY) at Stony Brook, and his Ph.D. degree in Computer Engineering in 1991 from the Department of Electrical and Computer Engineering at the Pennsylvania State University. He is currently a Professor of School of

Electrical Engineering and Computer Science at Oregon State University. He has published over 100 conference proceedings, book chapters, and journal articles in the areas of embedded systems, computer architecture, multithreading and thread-level speculation, parallel and distributed systems, and wireless networks. He received the Loyd Carter Award for Outstanding and Inspirational Teaching and the Alumni Professor Award for Outstanding Contribution to the College and the University from the OSU College of Engineering in 1994 and 2005, respectively. He also received the HKN Innovative Teaching Award from Eta Kappa Nu, School of Electrical Engineering and Computer Science, 2008. He has been on the program and organizing committees for numerous international conferences, including 2003 International Conference on Parallel and Distributed Computing Systems (PDCS), 2005–2011 IEEE Workshop on Pervasive Wireless Networking (PWN), and 2009 IEEE International Conference on Pervasive Computing and Communications. He is also a Keynote speaker at the 2014 International Conference on Ubiquitous Information Management and Communication. His research interests include wireless networks, embedded systems, computer architecture, multithreading and thread-level speculation, and parallel and distributed systems.

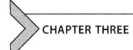

CHAPTER THREE

Hardware and Application Profiling Tools

Tomislav Janjusic*, Krishna Kavi†
*Oak Ridge National Laboratory, Oak Ridge, Tennessee
†University of North Texas, Denton, Texas

Contents

Abstract

This chapter describes hardware and application profiling tools used by researchers and application developers. With over 30 years of research, there have been numerous tools developed and used, and it will be too difficult to include all of them here. Therefore, in this chapter, we describe various areas with a selection of widely accepted and recent tools. This chapter is intended for the beginning reader interested in exploring more

Advances in Computers, Volume 92
ISSN 0065-2458
http://dx.doi.org/10.1016/B978-0-12-420232-0.00003-9

about these topics. Numerous references are provided to help jump-start the interested reader into the area of hardware simulation and application profiling.

We make an effort to clarify and correctly classify application profiling tools based on their scope, interdependence, and operation mechanisms. To visualize these features, we provide diagrams that explain various development relationships between interdependent tools. Hardware simulation tools are described into categories that elaborate on their scope. Therefore, we have covered areas of single to full-system simulation, power modeling, and network processors.

ABBREVIATIONS
ALU arithmetic logic unit
AP application profiling
API application programming interface
CMOS complementary metal-oxide semiconductor
CPU central processing unit
DMA direct memory access
DRAM dynamic random access memory
DSL domain-specific language
FS full system
GPU graphics processing unit
GUI graphical user interface
HP hardware profiling
HPC high-performance computing
I/O input/output
IBS instruction-based sampling
IR intermediate representation
ISA instruction set architecture
ME microengine
MIPS microprocessor without interlocked pipeline stages
MPI message passing interface
NoC network on chip
OS operating system
PAPI performance application programming interface
PCI peripheral component interconnect
POSIX portable operating system interface
RAM random access memory
RTL register transfer level
SB superblock
SCSI small computer system interface
SIMD single instruction, multiple data
SMT simultaneous multithreading
TLB translation lookaside buffer
VC virtual channel
VCA virtual channel allocation
VLSI very large-scale integration
VM virtual machine

1. INTRODUCTION

Researchers and application developers rely on software tools to help them understand, explore, and tune new architectural components and optimize, debug, or otherwise improve the performance of software applications. Computer architecture research is generally supplemented through architectural simulators and component performance and power efficiency analyzers. These are architecture-specific software tools, which simulate or analyze the behavior of various architectural devices. They should not be confused with emulators, which replicate the inner workings of a device. We will refer to the collective of these tools simply as hardware profilers. To analyze, optimize, or otherwise improve an application's performance and reliability, users utilize various application profilers. In the following subsections, we will distinguish between various aspects of application and hardware analysis, correctness, and performance tuning tools. In Section 2, we will discuss application profiling (AP) tools. In Section 3, we will discuss hardware profiling (HP) tools. Sections 2 and 3 follow the diagrams in Fig. 3.1. Finally, we will conclude the chapter in Section 4.

1.1. Taxonomy

Many tools overlap in their scope and capabilities; therefore, some tools covered in this chapter are not mutually exclusive within the established categories. For example, both instrumentation tools and profiling libraries can

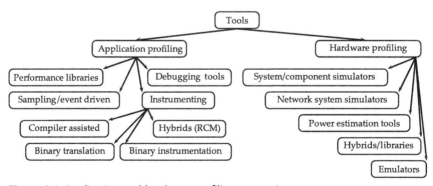

Figure 3.1 Application and hardware profiling categories.

analyze an application's memory behavior, albeit from different perspectives. We must also note that several other tools are built on top of libraries; however, they are classified into different groups based on their scope of application. Likewise, hardware profilers can profile memory subcomponent behavior for a given application. Assuming the simulation environment resembles the native system's hardware, one can expect the profiled behavior to be similar to an actual execution behavior. In this chapter, we classify the tools based on their scope of application.

Our categorization starts by distinguishing between AP and HP. Hardware profiling tools are divided into system and component simulators, power estimation tools, network-system simulators, and architectural emulators. We must note that the terms emulation and simulation are sometimes used interchangeably, but the difference is often seen in completeness. Emulators are faithful imitations of a device, whereas simulators may simulate only certain behaviors of a device. The usefulness of emulators is primarily in their ability to run software, which is incompatible with host hardware (e.g., running codes designed for microprocessor without interlocked pipeline stages (MIPS) processors on Intel x86 processors). Researchers and developers use simulators when interested in a subset of behaviors of a system without worrying about other behaviors; the goal is to simulate faithfully the behaviors of interest. For example, cycle-accurate simulators can be used to observe how instructions flow through a processor execution cycles but may ignore issues related to peripheral devices. This subcategory will be annotated with an s or e in our table representation.

Technically speaking, network-system simulators and power estimation tools should be considered as simulators. We felt that a separate category describing these tools is appropriate because most tools in this category are very specific in their modeling that they distinguish themselves from other generic instruction set simulators.

Some tools are closely related to tool suites and thus cannot be pigeonholed into a specific group. We will list these tools in the category of hybrids/libraries. The category of hybrids includes a range of application and hardware profilers. For example, the Wisconsin Architectural Research Tool Set [1] offers profilers and cache simulators and an overall framework for architectural simulations. Libraries are not tools in the sense that they are readily capable of executing or simulating software or hardware, but they are designed for the purpose of building other simulators or profilers. Table 3.1 lists a number of HP tools listed in Section 6.

We will cover detailed tool capabilities in the subsequent sections. Figure 3.1 is a graphic representation of our tool categories. The tools, which are described in this chapter, are placed in one of the earlier mentioned categories. For example, emulators and simulators are more closely

Table 3.1 Hardware Profilers
Hardware Profilers

System/component simulators	Network–system simulators
DRAMSim [2]	NepSim [3]
DineroIV [4]	Orion [5]
EasyCPU [6]	Garnet [7]
SimpleScalar [8]	Topaz [9]
ML_RSIM [10]	MSNS [11]
M-Sim [12]	Hornet [13]
ABSS [14]	**Power estimation tools**
AugMINT [15]	CACTI [16]
HASE [17]	WATTCH [18]
Simics [19]	DSSWATCH [20]
SimFlex [21]	SimplePower [22]
Flexus [23]	AccuPower [24]
SMARTS [25]	**Frameworks**
Gem5 [26]	CGEN [27]
SimOS [28]	LSE [29]
Parallel SimOS [30]	SID [31]
PTLsim [32]	
MPTLsim [33]	
FeS$_2$ [34]	
TurboSMARTS [35]	

related to each other than to AP tool; thus, they are listed under hardware profilers. The list of all tools mentioned in this chapter is summarized in Sections 5 and 6. The tables categorize the tools based on Fig. 3.1.

Software profilers and libraries used to build profiler tools are categorized based on their functionality. We felt that application profilers are better distinguished based on their profiling methodology because some plug-in and tools built on top of other platforms have some common functionalities. Consider tools, which may fall under the category of instrumenting tools; these tools could provide the same information as library-based tools that use underlying hardware performance counters. The difference is in how the profiler obtains the information. Most hardware performance counter libraries such as performance application programming interface (PAPI) [36] can provide a sampled measurement of an application's memory behavior. Binary instrumentation tool plug-ins such as Valgrind's Cachegrind or Callgrind can give the user the same information but may incur overheads. Some recent performance tools utilize both performance libraries and instrumentation frameworks to deliver performance metrics. Therefore, a user attempting to use these tools must choose the appropriate tool depending on the required profiling detail, overhead, completeness, and accuracy.

Table 3.2 outlines the tools from Section 5 categorized as instrumenting tools and sampling/event-driven tools and performance libraries and interfaces.

1.2. Hardware Profilers

The complexity of hardware simulators and profiling tools varies with the level of detail that they simulate. Hardware simulators can be classified based on their complexity and purpose: simple-, medium-, and high-complexity system simulators, power management and power-performance simulators, and network infrastructure system simulators.

Simulators that simulate a system's single subcomponent such as the central processing unit's (CPU) cache are considered to be simple simulators (e.g., DineroIV [4], a trace-driven CPU cache simulator). In this category, we often find academic simulators designed to be reusable and easily modifiable.

Medium-complexity simulators aim to simulate a combination of architectural subcomponents such as the CPU pipelines, levels of memory hierarchies, and speculative executions. These are more complex than single-component

Table 3.2 Application Profilers
Application Profilers

Instrumenting	Sampling/event-driven	Performance libraries/kernel interfaces
gprof [37]	OProfile [38]	PAPI [36]
Parasight [39]	AMD CodeAnalyst [40]	perfmon [41]
Quartz [42]	Intel VTune [43]	perfctr
ATOM [44]	HPCToolkit [45]	Debuggers
Pin [46]	TAU [47]	gdb [48]
DynInst [49]	Open SpeedShop [50]	DDT [51]
Etch [52]	VAMPIR [53]	
EEL [54]		
Valgrind [55]		
DynamoRIO [56]		
Dynamite [57]		
UQBT [58]		

simulators but not complex enough to run full-system (FS) workloads. An example of such a tool is the widely known and widely used SimpleScalar tool suite [8]. These types of tools can simulate the hardware running a single application and they can provide useful information pertaining to various CPU metrics (e.g., CPU cycles, CPU cache hit and miss rates, instruction frequency, and others). Such tools often rely on very specific instruction sets requiring applications to be cross compiled for that specific architecture.

To fully understand a system's performance under reasonable-sized workload, users can rely on FS simulators. FS simulators are arguably the most complex simulation systems. Their complexity stems from the simulation of all the critical system's components, as well as the full software systems including the operating system (OS). The benefit of using FS simulators is that they provide more accurate estimation of the behaviors and component interactions for realistic workloads. In this category, we find the widely used Simics [19], Gem5 [26], SimOS [28], and others. These simulators are capable of full-scale system simulations with varying levels of detail. Naturally, their accuracy comes at the cost of simulation times; some simulations may take several hundred times or even several thousand times longer than the time it takes to run the workload on a real hardware system [25]. Their features and performances vary and will be discussed in the subsequent sections.

Energy consumed by applications is becoming very important for not only embedded devices but also general-purpose systems with several processing cores. In order to evaluate issues related to power requirements of hardware subsystems, researchers rely on power estimation and power management tools. It must be noted that some hardware simulators provide power estimation models; however, we will place power modeling tools into a different category.

In the realm of hardware simulators, we must touch on another category of tools specifically designed to simulate accurately network processors and network subsystems. In this category, we will discuss network processor simulators such as NePSim [3]. For large computer systems, such as high performance computers, application performance is limited by the ability to deliver critical data to compute nodes. In addition, networks needed to interconnect processors consume energy, and it becomes necessary to understand these issues as we build larger and larger systems. Network simulation tools may be used for those studies.

Lastly, when available simulators and profiling tools are not adequate, users can use architectural tool-building frameworks and architectural tool-building libraries. These packages consist of a set of libraries specifically designed for building new simulators and subcomponent analyzers. In this category, we find the liberty simulation environment (LSE) [29], Red Hat's SID environment [31], SystemC, and others.

1.3. Application Profilers

Simulators are powerful tools that give insight into a device behavior under varying runtime circumstances. However, if a user is trying to understand an application's runtime behavior, which is a crucial step when trying to optimize the code, the user needs to rely on different class of tools. AP refers to the ability to measure an application's performance, diagnose potential problems, or otherwise log an application's runtime information. For example, a user may want to reduce an application's memory consumption, which is a common optimization required in embedded applications, and improve an application execution speed, which is a requirement for high-performance scientific applications, or the user simply needs to improve an application's reliability and correctness by tracking active and potential program errors.

For such tasks, application developers rely on debugging tools, profiling tools, and other performance libraries capable of delivering the needed information. These tools vary in their accuracy, profiling speed, and capabilities. Profiling generally involves a software tool called a profiler that analyzes the application. This is achieved either through analyzing the source code statically or at runtime using a method known as dynamic program translation.

Profiling tools can be further categorized into event-driven profiling, sampling profiling, and instrumented profiling. Event-driven profiling collects information about user-defined events, which may require hooks into the OS. When a desired event is triggered, the tool will collect program characteristic related to that event. Event-driven profiling tools have a tendency to rely on the OS to collect necessary information. Sampled profiling aims at collecting information at specified intervals or frequency. The goal is to collect enough samples to acquire a statistically accurate picture of the application. Note that some profiling libraries may be classified as sampling profilers although we must not confuse the libraries and tools that rely on the libraries for functionality. There are various commercial sampling profilers such as AMD CodeAnalyst [40], Intel VTune [43], and others.

Lastly, instrumentation profiling encompasses several subcategories that involve insertion or transformation of source code at strategic sections, usually driven and limited by the instrumenting tool. Instrumenting tools can be further categorized into compiler-assisted instrumentation (e.g., gprof [37]), binary translation, binary instrumentation (e.g., Pin [46], DynInst [49], ATOM [44]), and hybrids (e.g., Valgrind [55] and DynamoRIO [56]). We will discuss the details of each of these categories in the subsequent sections. It should be noted that many tools fit multiple categories; sometimes, this is due to evolution of tools based on need, and sometimes, this is due to the very nature of the profiling. However, we categorized the tools based on their primary functionality or capabilities.

1.4. Performance Libraries

Understanding application's runtime behavior is generally supplemented through AP tools. AP tools come in various forms such as debuggers, profilers, or libraries. From a user's perspective, a profiling tool is software that manipulates an application by injecting foreign code fragments at strategic locations of an application's source code or executable code. The injected code executes at the desired section and collects information on a number of application-triggered events or other application-specific timing information. Similarly, profiling libraries refer to a subset of AP tools that offer specific application programming interfaces (APIs), which can be called from the client application. In a general sense, profiling libraries are a bridge between profiling tools and specialized hardware units called hardware performance counters, or simply hardware counters, used for hardware performance measurement. We will not list profiling libraries as part of hardware profilers because performance counters are, more often than not, used for software tuning. Implicitly, they provide information about the host hardware during an application execution, but their intent is not driven by hardware research. Another reason why profiling libraries are listed as application profilers is because they cannot distinguish, unless user corrections are applied, between application-triggered metrics and system noise during the application's execution.

2. APPLICATION PROFILING

2.1. Introduction

To our knowledge, the first paper on profiling was published in the early 1980s, gprof: a call graph execution profiler [37]. The need for gprof arose out of the necessity to adequately trace the time spent on specific procedures or subroutines. At that time, profilers were fairly simple and the tools only reported very limited information such as how many times a procedure was invoked. Gprof extended this functionality by collecting program timing information. At compile time, gprof inserts timers or counters, and during execution, the time spent within functions is aggregated. The end results, a collection of time spent within each function, may be analyzed off-line. The information provided by gprof is timing and function call counts with respect to subroutines as a percentage of an application's total executed time. Gprof was unique for its time (and still useful today) because it allowed the programmer to see where the majority of the execution time is spent. The idea of gprof is to allow programmers to tune individual program routines. Gprof is an example of a compiler-assisted profiling tool. Note that modern compilers ship with gprof and other analysis tools. Compiler-assisted profiling inserts profiling calls into the application during compilation process. The inserted profiling routines are invoked when the application executes. This means that the application will incur extra overhead. Gprof's development launched the research area of program profiling. Similar tools were developed soon after (e.g., Parasight [39] and Quartz [42]). They are similar to gprof, but these tools targeted tuning of parallel applications.

Binary instrumentation tool research accelerated after the development of the ATOM tool [44]. Binary translation tools translate a binary code into a machine code. Their functionality is similar to a compiler. The difference is that unlike compilers their input is a precompiled binary image. As the name suggests, binary translators operate on a binary file, unlike compilers that operate on the source code. Another difference is that the translation tries to gather other information about the code during the translation processes using an interpreter. If a binary translation tool inserts, removes, or otherwise modifies code from the original binary image, then we can call that tool as a code manipulation tool. Binary translation comes in two forms: static binary translation and dynamic binary translation. Binary translators are usually used as optimization frameworks, for example, DIXIE [59] and UQBT [58], because of their ability to translate and modify compiled code. The limitation of static binary translation is the inability to accurately account for all the code because some code paths cannot be predicted statically. When higher accuracy is needed, we should utilize dynamic binary translation. Dynamic translation is slower than static, but dynamic translation is superior to static translation in terms of code coverage. We must note that dynamic translation is not always 100% accurate because it is possible that code paths may be dependent on a specific set of input parameters. While dynamic translators are better at coverage, or predicting taken code paths, they suffer in terms of performance. This is because they must translate blocks of source code on the fly and then execute the translated segments. The reason behind the performance degradation is that in dynamic translation, the translation is performed at runtime and program registers and its state needs to be preserved. Copying and preserving the program registers adds to the total cost of the application's wall-clock time. Since the dynamic translation needs to be fast, complex optimizations are not performed; thus, the translated code may be less efficient. However, the benefits of dynamic translation often outweigh these drawbacks: dynamic translators are more accurate than static because they have runtime knowledge of the taken code paths and this results in better optimizations or analysis for tools that utilize binary translators. Some speedup can be achieved by caching translated code and thus eliminate repeated translations of code segments. This is similar to the idea of CPU caches. Utilizing a code cache reuses frequently used translated blocks. Only portions of the code need to be kept in memory at any one time, thereby improving performance at the expense of memory requirements.

Binary instrumentation tools are different from other profiling tools because their main approach lies in injecting program executable with additional code. The inserted code is then passed on to various plug-in tools for additional analysis. Binary instrumentation similar to binary translation comes in two forms: static binary instrumentation and dynamic binary instrumentation. The trade-offs between the two mechanisms are also in terms of performance and accuracy. Static binary instrumentation is faster but less accurate, and dynamic binary instrumentation is slower but more accurate. It is important to note that ATOM and most other instrumenting tools are considered a tool-building system. This means that the underlying functionality of binary instrumentation tools allows for other plug-in tools to run on top of the framework. Development of ATOM has inspired other developers to build other more capable tools. We can consider these five instrumentation technique categories: manual, compiler-assisted, binary translations, runtime instrumentation, and hybrids.

In addition, programmers can manually instrument their code. Functions that will collect some type of runtime information are manually inserted into the application's source code. These vary from simple print statements to complex analysis routines specifically developed for debugging and profiling purposes.

For clarity purposes, however, we can group binary translation, binary instrumentation, and hybrids of these tools simply into runtime instrumentation tools. Runtime instrumentation is the predominant technique among modern profiling tools. It involves an external tool that supervises the application being instrumented. The instrumented code may be annotated or otherwise transformed into an intermediary representation. The plug-in tools that perform various types of analyses use annotated code or the intermediate representation. This also implies that the extent, accuracy, and efficiency of the plug-in tools are limited by the capabilities provided by the framework. The benefit of runtime instrumentation, particularly binary instrumentation, is the level of binary code detail that plug-in tools can take advantage of. Example frameworks in this area are Pin [46], Valgrind [55], DynamoRIO [56], DynInst [49], and others.

2.2. Instrumenting Tools

Instrumentation is a technique that injects analysis routines into the application code to either analyze or deliver the necessary metadata to other analysis tools. Instrumentation can be applied during various application development cycles. During the early development cycles, instrumentation comes in the form of various print statements; this is known as manual instrumentation. For tuning and optimization purposes, manual instrumentation may invoke underlying hardware performance counters or OS events.

Compiler-assisted instrumented utilizes the compiler infrastructure to insert analysis routines, for example, instrumentation of function boundaries, to instrument the application's function call behavior.

Binary translation tools are a set of tools that reverse compile an application's binary into intermediate representation (IR) suitable for program analysis. The binary code is translated, usually at basic-block granularity, interpreted, and executed. The translated code may simply be augmented with code that measures desired properties and resynthesized (or recompiled) for execution. Notice that binary translation does not necessarily include any instrumentation to collect program statistics. The instrumentation in this sense refers to the necessity to control the client application by redirecting code back to the translator (i.e., every basic block of client application must be brought back under the translator's control).

Instrumentation at the lowest levels is applied on the application's executable binaries. Application's binary file is dissected block by block or instruction by instruction. The instruction stream is analyzed and passed to plug-in tools or interpreters for additional analysis.

Hybrids are tools that are also known as runtime code manipulation tools. We opted to list hybrid tools as a special category because some tools in this group are difficult to categorize. Hybrid tools apply binary translation and binary instrumentation. The translation happens in the framework's core and the instrumentation is left to the plug-in tools (e.g., Valgrind [55]) (Table 3.3).

2.2.1 Valgrind

Valgrind is a dynamic binary instrumentation framework that was initially designed for identifying memory leaks. Valgrind and other tools in this realm are also known as shadow value tools. That means that they shadow every register with another descriptive value. Valgrind belongs to a complex or heavyweight analysis tools in terms of both its capabilities and the complexities. In our taxonomy, Valgrind is an instrumenting profiler that utilizes a combination of binary translation and binary instrumentation. Referring to the chart in Fig. 3.1, Valgrind falls into the hybrid category. The basic Valgrind structure consists of a core tool and plug-in tools. The core tool is responsible for disassembling the client application's binary file into an

Table 3.3 Application Profiling Instrumenting Tools
Instrumenting Tools

Compiler-Assisted	Binary Translation	Binary Instrumentation	Hybrids/Runtime Code Manipulation
gprof [37]	Dynamite [60]	DynInst [49]	DynamoRIO [57]
Parasight [39]	UQBT [58]	Pin [46]	Valgrind [55]
Quartz [42]		ATOM [44]	
		Etch [52]	
		EEL [54]	

IR specific to Valgrind. The client code is partitioned into superblocks (SBs). An SB, consisting of one or more basic blocks, is a stream of approximately 50 instructions. The block is translated into an IR and passed on to the instrumentation tool. The instrumentation tool then analyzes every SB statement and inserts appropriate instrumented calls. When the tool is finished operating on the SB, it will return the instrumented SB back to the core tool. The core tool recompiles the instrumented SB into machine code and executes the SB on a synthetic CPU. This means that the client application never directly runs on the host processor. Because of this design, Valgrind is bound to a specific CPU and OS. Valgrind supports several combinations of CPUs and OS systems including AMD64, x86, ARM, and PowerPC 32/64 running predominately Linux/Unix systems.

Several widely used instrumentation tools come with Valgrind, while others are designed by researchers and users of Valgrind:

- Memcheck: Valgrind's default tool Memcheck enables the user to detect memory leaks during execution. Memcheck detects several common C and C++ errors. For example, it can detect accesses to restricted memory such as areas of heap that were deallocated, using undefined values, incorrectly freed memory blocks, or a mismatched number of allocation and free calls.

- Cachegrind: Cachegrind is Valgrind's default cache simulator. It can simulate a two-level cache hierarchy and an optional branch predictor. If the host machine has a three-level cache hierarchy, Cachegrind will simulate the first and third cache level. The Cachegrind tool comes with a third-party annotation tool that will annotate cache hit/miss statistics per source code line. It is a good tool for users who want to find potential memory performance bottlenecks in their programs.

- Callgrind: Callgrind is a profiling tool that records an application's function call history. It collects data relevant to the number of executed instructions and their relation to the called functions. Optionally, Callgrind can also simulate the cache behavior and branch prediction and relate that information to function call profile. Callgrind also comes with a third-party graphic visualization tool that helps visualize Callgrind's output.
- Helgrind: Helgrind is a thread error detection tool for applications written in C, C++, and Fortran.

  It supports portable operating system interface (POSIX) pthread primitives. Helgrind is capable of detecting several classes of error that are typically encountered in multithreaded programs. It can detect errors relating to the misuse of the POSIX API that can potentially lead to various undefined program behavior such as unlocking invalid mutexes, unlocking a unlocked mutex, thread exits still holding a lock, and destructions of uninitialized or still waited upon barriers. It can also detect error pertaining to an inconsistent lock ordering. This allows it to detect any potential deadlocks.
- Massif: Massif is a heap profiler tool that measures an application's heap memory usage. Profiling an application's heap may help reduce its dynamic memory footprint. As a result, reducing an application's memory footprint may help avoid exhausting a machine's swap space.
- DHAT: DHAT is a dynamic heap analysis tool similar to Massif. It helps identify memory leaks and analyze application allocation routines that allocate large amounts of memory but are not active for very long, allocation routines that allocate only short lived blocks or allocations that are not used or used incompletely.
- Lackey: Lackey is a Valgrind tool that performs various kinds of basic program measurements. Lackey can also produce very rudimentary traces that identify the instruction and memory load/store operations. These traces can then be used in a cache simulator (e.g., Cachegrind operates on a similar principle).
- Gleipnir: Gleipnir is a program profiling and tracing tool built as a third-party plug-in tool [61]. It combines several native Valgrind tools into a tracing–simulating environment. By taking advantage of Valgrind's internal debug symbol table parser, Gleipnir can trace memory accesses and relate each access to a specific program internal structure such as thread; program segment; function, local, global, and dynamic data structure; and scalar variables. Gleipnir's ability to collect fine-grained

memory traces and associate each access to source level data structures and elements of these structures makes it a good candidate tool for advanced cache memory simulation and analysis. The data provided by Gleipnir may be used by cache simulators to analyze accesses to data structure elements or by programmers to understand the relation between dynamic and static memory behavior. The goal of Gleipnir is to provide traces with rich information, which can aid in advanced analysis of memory behaviors. Gleipnir aims to bridge the gap between a program's dynamic and static memory behavior and its impact on application performance.

2.2.2 DynamoRIO

DynamoRIO [56] is a dynamic optimization and modification framework built as a revised version of Dynamo. It operates on a basic-block granularity and is suitable for various research areas: code modification, intrusion detection, profiling, statistical gathering, sandboxing, etc. It was originally developed for Windows OS but has been ported to a variety of Linux platforms. The key advantage of DynamoRIO is that it is fast and it is designed for runtime code manipulation and instrumentation. Similar to Valgrind, DynamoRIO is classified as a code manipulation framework and thus falls in the hybrid category in Fig. 3.1. Unlike other instrumentation tools, Dynamo does not emulate the incoming instruction stream of a client application but rather caches the instructions and executes them on the native target. DynamoRIO intercepts control transfers after every basic block because it operates on basic-block granularity. Performance is gained through various code block stitching techniques, for example, basic blocks that are accessed through a direct branch are stitched together so that no context switch, or other control transfer, needs to occur. Multiple code blocks are cached into a trace for faster execution. The framework employs an API for building DynamoRIO plug-in tools. Because DynamoRIO is a code optimization framework, it allows the client to access the cached code and perform client-driven optimizations.

In dynamic optimization frameworks, instruction representation is key to achieving fast execution performance. DynamoRIO represents instructions at several levels of granularity. At the lowest level, the instruction holds the instruction bytes, and at the highest level, the instruction is fully decoded at machine representation level. The level of detail is determined by the routine's API used by the plug-in tool. The levels of details can be automatically and dynamically adjusted depending on later instrumentation and optimization needs.

The client tools operate through hooks that offer the ability to manipulate either basic blocks or traces. In DynamoRIO's terminology, a trace is a collection of basic blocks. Most plug-in tools operate on repeated executions of basic blocks also known as hot code. This makes sense because the potential optimization savings are likely to improve those regions of code. In addition, DynamoRIO supports adaptive optimization techniques. This means that the plug-in tools are able to reoptimize code instructions that were placed in the code cache and ready for execution.

Dynamic optimization frameworks such as DynamoRIO are designed to improve and optimize applications. As was demonstrated in Ref. [56], the framework improves on existing high-level compiler optimizations.

The following tools are built on top of the DynamoRIO framework:

- TaintTrace: TaintTrace [62] is a flow tracing tool for detecting security exploits.
- Dr. Memory: Dr. Memory [63] is a memory profiling tool similar to Valgrind's Memcheck. It can detect memory-related errors such as accesses to uninitialized memory, accesses to freed memory, improper allocation, and free ordering. Dr. Memory is available for both Windows and Linux OSs.
- Adept: Adept [64] is a dynamic execution profiling tool built on top of the DynamoRIO platform.

It profiles user-level code paths and records them. The goal is to capture the complete dynamic control flow, data dependencies, and memory references of the entire running program.

2.2.3 Pin

Pin [46] is a framework for dynamic binary program instrumentation that follows the model of the popular ATOM tool (which was designed for DEC Alpha-based systems, running DEC Unix), allowing the programmer to analyze programs at instruction level. Pin's model allows code injection into client's executable code. The difference between ATOM and Pin is that Pin dynamically inserts the code while the application is running, whereas ATOM required the application and the instrumentation code to be statically linked. This key feature of Pin allows it to attach itself to already running process, hence the name Pin. In terms of taxonomy, Pin is an instrumenting profiler that utilizes dynamic binary instrumentation. It is in many ways similar to Valgrind and other dynamic binary instrumentation tools; however, Pin does not use an intermediate form to represent the instrumented instructions. The primary motivation of Pin is to have an easy to use, transparent, and efficient tool-building system.

Unlike Valgrind, Pin uses a copy and annotates IR, implying that every instruction is copied and annotated with metadata. This offers several benefits as well as drawbacks. The key components of a Pin system are the Pin virtual machine (VM) with just-in-time (JIT) compiler, the Pintools, and the code cache. Similar to other frameworks, a Pintool shares a client's address space, resulting in some skewing of address space; application addresses may be different when running with Pin compared to running without Pin. The code cache stores compiled code waiting to be launched by the dispatcher. Pin uses several code optimizations to make it more efficient.

For a set of plug-in tools, an almost necessary feature is its access to the compiler-generated client's symbol table (i.e., its debug information). Unlike Valgrind, Pin's debug granularity ends at the function level. This means that tracing plug-in tools such as Gleipnir can map instructions only to the function level. To obtain data-level symbols, a user must rely on debug parsers built into the plug-in tool.

Pin uses several instrumentation optimization techniques that improve the instrumentation speed. It is reported in Refs. [46,55] that Pin outperforms other similar tools for basic instrumentation. Pin's rich API is well documented and thus attractive to users interested in building Pin-based dynamic instrumentation. Pin comes with many examples; Pintools can provide data on basic blocks, instruction and memory traces, and cache statistics.

2.2.4 DynInst

DynInst [65] is a runtime instrumentation tool designed for code patching and program performance measurement. It expands on the design of ATOM, EEL, and Etch by allowing the instrumentation code to be inserted at runtime. This contrasts with the earlier static instrumentation tools that inserted the code statically at postcompile time. DynInst provides a machine-independent API designed as part of the Paradyn Parallel Performance Tools project. The benefit of DynInst is that instrumentation can be performed at arbitrary points without the need to predefine these points or to predefine the analysis code at these points.

The ability to defer instrumentation until runtime and the ability to insert arbitrary analysis routines make DynInst good for instrumenting large-scale scientific programs. The dynamic instrumentation interface is designed to be primarily used by higher-level visualization tools.

The DynInst approach consists of two manager classes that control instrumentation points and the collection of program performance data. DynInst uses a combination of tracing and sampling techniques. An internal agent, the metric manager, controls the collection of relevant performance metrics. The structures are periodically sampled and reported to higher-level tools. It also provides a template for a potential instrumentation perturbation cost. All instrumented applications incur performance perturbation because of the added code or intervention by the instrumentation tool. This means that performance gathering tools need to account for their overhead and adjust performance data accordingly.

The second agent, an instrumentation manager, identifies relevant points in the application to be instrumented. The instrumentation manager is responsible for the inserted analysis routines. The code fragments that are inserted are called trampolines. There are two kinds of trampolines: base and mini trampolines. A base trampoline facilitates the calling of mini trampolines, and there is one base trampoline active per instrumentation point. Trampolines are instruction sequences that are inserted at instrumentation points (e.g., beginning and end of function calls) that save and restore registers after the analysis codes complete data collection. DynInst comes with an API that enables tool developers to build other analysis routines or new performance measurement tools built on top of the DynInst platform.

There are several tools built around, on top of, or utilizing parts of the DynInst instrumentation framework:

- TAU: TAU [47] is a comprehensive profiling and tracing tool for analyzing parallel programs. By utilizing a combination of instrumentation and profiling techniques, TAU can report fine-grained application performance data. Applications can be profiled using various techniques using TAU's API. For example, users can use timing, event, and hardware counters in combination with application dynamic instrumentation. TAU comes with visualization tools for understanding and interpreting large amounts of data collected.
- Open SpeedShop: Open SpeedShop [50] is a Linux-based performance tool for evaluating performance of applications running on single-node and large-scale multinode systems. Open SpeedShop incorporates several performance gathering methodologies including sampling,

call-stack analysis, hardware performance counters, profiling message passing interface (MPI) libraries and input/output (I/O) libraries, and floating-point exception analysis. The tool is supplemented by a graphical user interface (GUI) for visual data inspection.

- Cobi: Cobi is a DynInst-based tool for static binary instrumentation. It leverages several static analysis techniques to reduce instrumentation overheads and metric dilation at the expense of instrumentation detail for parallel performance analysis.

2.3. Event-Driven and Sampling Tools

Sampling-based tools gather performance or other program metrics by collecting data at specified intervals. One can be fairly conservative with our categories of sampling-based tools as most of them rely on other types of libraries or instrumentation frameworks to operate. Sampling-based approaches generally involve interrupting running programs periodically and examining the program's state, retrieving hardware performance counter data, or executing instrumented analysis routines. The goal of sampling-based tools is to capture enough performance data at reasonable number of statistically meaningful intervals so that the resulting performance data distribution will resemble the client's full execution. Sampling-based approaches are sometimes known as statistical methods when referring to the data collected. Sampling-based tools acquire their performance data based on three sampling approaches: timer-based, event-based, and instruction-based. Diagram in Fig. 3.2 shows the relationships of sampling-based tools.

- Timer-based performance measurements: Timer-based and timing-based approaches are generally the basic forms of AP, where the sampling is based on built-in timers. Tools that use timers are able to obtain a general picture of execution times spent within an application. The amount of time spent by the application in each function may be derived from the sampled data. This allows the user to drill down into the specific program's function and eliminate possible bottlenecks.
- Event-based performance measurements: Event-based measurements sample information when predetermined events occur. Events can be either software or hardware events, for example, a user may be interested in the number of page faults encountered or the number of specific system calls. These events are trapped and counted by the underlying OS library primitives, thereby providing useful 16 information back to the tool and ultimately the user. Mechanisms that enable

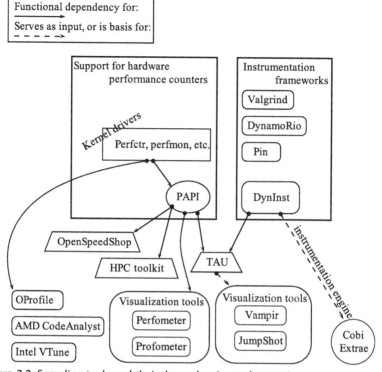

Figure 3.2 Sampling tools and their dependencies and extensions.

event-based profiling are generally the building blocks of many sampling-based tools.

- Instruction-based performance measurement: Arguably, the most accurate profiling representations are tools that use instruction-based sampling (IBS) approach. For example, AMD CodeAnalyst [40] uses the IBS method to interrupt a running program after a specified number of instructions and examine the state of hardware counters. The values obtained from the hardware counters can be used to reason about the program performance. The accuracy of instruction sampling depends on the sampling rate.

The basic components of sampling tools include the host architecture, software/hardware interfaces, and visualization tools. Most sampling tools use hardware performance counters and OS interfaces. We describe several sampling tools here.

2.3.1 OProfile

OProfile [38] is an open-source system-wide profiler for Linux systems. System-wide profilers are tools that operate in kernel space and are capable of profiling application and system-related events. OProfile uses a kernel driver and a daemon to sample events. Data collected on the events are aggregated into a file for postprocessing. The method by which OProfile collects information is through either hardware events or timing. In case the hardware performance counters are not available, OProfile resorts to using timers. The information is enough to account for time spent in individual functions; however, it is not sufficient to reason about application bottlenecks.

OProfile includes architecture-specific components, OProfile file system, a generic kernel driver, OProfile daemon, and postprocessing tools. Architecture-specific components are needed to use available hardware counters. The OProfile file system, oprofilefs, is used to aggregate information. The generic kernel driver is the data delivery management technique from the kernel to the user. The OProfile daemon is a user-space program that writes kernel data back to the disk. Graphic postprocessing tools provide user interfaces (GUIs) to correlate aggregated data to the source code.

It is important to note that to some extent, most open-source and commercial tools consist of these basic components, and virtually, all share the basic requirement of hardware performance counters or OS events, unless they rely on binary instrumentation.

2.3.2 Intel VTune

Intel VTune is a commercial system-wide profiler for Windows and Linux systems. Similar to OProfile, it uses timer and hardware event sampling technique to collect performance data that can be used by other analysis tools. The basic analysis techniques are timer analyses, which report the amount of time spent in individual functions, or specific code segments. Functions containing inefficiently written loops may be identified and optimized; however, the tool itself does not offer optimizations and it is left up to the user to find techniques for improving the code. Because modern architectures offer multiple cores, it is becoming increasingly important to fine-tune threaded applications. Intel VTune offers timing and CPU utilization information on application's threads. These data give programmers insights into how well their multithreaded designs are running. The information provided gives timing information for individual threads, time spent waiting for locks, and scheduling information. The more advanced analysis techniques are enabled with hardware event sampling. Intel VTune can use the host architecture performance counters to record statistics. For example, using hardware counters, a user can sample the processor's cache behavior, usually last-level caches, and relate poor cache performance back to the source code statements. We must stress that to take advantage of these reports, a programmer must be knowledgeable of host hardware capabilities and have a good understanding of compiler and hardware interactions. As the name implies, Intel VTune is specifically designed for the Intel processors and the tool is tuned for Intel-specific compilers and libraries.

2.3.3 AMD CodeAnalyst

AMD CodeAnalyst is very similar to Intel VTune except that it targets AMD processors. Like other tools in this group, AMD CodeAnalyst requires underlying hardware counters to collect information about an application's behavior. The basic analysis is the timing-based approach where application's functions are broken down by the amount of time spent in individual functions. Users can drill down to individual code segments to find potential bottlenecks in the code and tune code to improve performance. For multithreaded programs, users can profile individual threads, including core utilization and affinity. Identifying poor memory localities is a useful feature for nonuniform memory access (NUMA) platforms. The analyses are not restricted to homogeneous systems (e.g., general-purpose processors only). With the increasing use of graphics processing units (GPUs) for scientific computing, it is becoming increasingly important to analyze the behavior of GPUs. AMD CodeAnalyst can display utilization of heterogeneous systems and relate the information back to the application. Performance bottlenecks in most applications are memory-related; thus, recent updates to analysis tools address data-centric visualization. For example, newer tools report on a CPU's cache line utilizations in an effort to measure the efficiency of data transfers from main memory to cache. AMD CodeAnalyst can be used to collect many useful data including instructions per cycle (IPC), memory access behavior, instruction and data cache utilization, translation lookaside buffer (TLB) misses, and control transfers. Most, and perhaps all, of these metrics are achieved through hardware performance counters. Interestingly for Linux-based systems, CodeAnalyst is integrated into OProfile (a system-wide event-based profiler for Linux described earlier).

2.3.4 HPCToolkit

HPCToolkit [45] is a set of performance measuring tools aimed at parallel programs. HPCToolkit relies on hardware counters to gather performance data and relates the collected data back to the calling context of the application's source code. HPCToolkit consists of several components that work together to stitch and analyze the collected data:

- hpcrun: hpcrun is the primary sampling profiler that executes an optimized binary. Hpcrun uses statistical sampling to collect performance metrics.
- hpcstruct: hpcstruct operates on the application's binary to recover any debug-relevant information later to be stitched with the collected metrics.
- hpcprof: hpcprof is the final analysis tool that correlates the information from hpcrun and hpcprof.
- hpcviewer: hpcviewer is the toolkit's GUI that helps visualize hpcprof's data.

HPCToolkit is a good example of a purely sampling-based tool. It uses sampling to be as minimally intrusive as possible and minimal execution overhead for profiling applications.

2.4. Performance Libraries

Performance libraries rely on hardware performance counters to collect performance data. Due to their scope, we have listed performance libraries as application profilers rather than hardware profilers. As we will explain at the end of this subsection, performance libraries have been used by several performance measuring tools to access hardware counters.

Despite their claims of nonintrusiveness, it was reported in Ref. [66] that performance counters still introduce some data perturbations since the counters may still count events that are caused by the instrumentation code. And the perturbation is proportional to the sampling rate. Users interested in using performance libraries should ensure that the measured application (i.e., the original code plus inserted measurement routines) resembles the native application (i.e., unmodified application code) as closely as possible.

The benefit of using performance counters is that these tools are the least intrusive and arguably the fastest for AP. Code manipulative tools, such as instrumenting tools, tend to skew the native application's memory image by cloning or interleaving the application's address space or adding and removing a substantial amount of instructions as part of their instrumentation framework.

Generally, libraries and tools that use hardware counters to measure performance require the use of kernel interfaces. Therefore, most tools are tied to specific OS kernels and available interfaces. The approach is to use a kernel interface to access hardware performance counters and use system libraries to facilitate the calling convention to those units. And third-party tools are used to visualize the collected information. Among commonly used open-source interfaces are perfmon and perfctr. Tools such as PAPI [36] utilize the perfctr kernel interface to access hardware units. Other tools such as TAU [47], HPCToolkit [45], and Open SpeedShop [50] all utilize the PAPI performance libraries.

- PAPI: PAPI [36] is a portable API, often referred to as an interface to performance counters. Since its development, PAPI has gained widespread acceptance and is maintained by an active community of open-source developers.

  PAPI's portable design offers high-level and low-level interfaces designed for machine independence and portability. The perfctr kernel module handles the Linux kernel hardware interface. The high- and low-level PAPI interfaces are tailored for both novice users and application engineers that require a quick turnaround time for sampling and benchmarking.

  PAPI offers several abstractions. Event sets are PAPI abstractions to count, add, or subtract sets of hardware counters without incurring additional system overhead. PAPI event sets offer users the ability to correlate different hardware sets back to the application source. This is useful to understand application-specific performance metrics.

  Overflow events are PAPI features aimed at tool writers. Threshold overflow allows the user to trigger specific signals an event when a specific counter exceeded a predefined amount. This allows the user to hash instructions that overflowed a specific event and relate it back to application symbol information.

  The number of hardware counters is limited and the data collection must wait until the application completes execution. PAPI offers multiplexing to alleviate that problem by subdividing counter usage over time. This could have adverse affects on the accuracy of reported performance data.

2.5. Debugging Tools

While most of the focus of this chapter is on profiling tools and performance libraries, it is important to keep in mind another category of tools that help with program correctness. Virtually, everyone in the programming community is familiar with debugging tools. Programmers are usually confronted with either a compiler error or a logical error. Compiler errors tend to be syntactical in nature, that is, the programmer used a compiler unfriendly syntax. Logical errors are harder to find and they occur when a correctly compiled program errs during runtime. Debugging tools are used to identify logical errors in programs. Users can examine each code statement and logically traverse the program flow. There are a number of debuggers in use, and most integrated development environments (IDE) come with their own versions of program debuggers. For the common Unix/Linux user, gdb [48] will suffice.

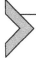

3. HARDWARE PROFILING

3.1. Introduction

Simulation of hardware (or processor architecture) is a common way of evaluating new designs. This in turn accelerates hardware development because software models can be built from scratch within months rather than years that it takes to build physical hardware. Simulations allow the designers to explore a large number of variables and trade-offs. The main drawback of simulators is the level of detail that is examined. To obtain accurate results, simulators will have to be very detailed, and such simulators will be very complex in terms of both their design and the amount of time needed to complete a simulation. As modern systems are getting more complex with large number of processing cores, network-on-chip (NoC), large multilevel caches, faithfully simulating such systems is becoming prohibitive. Many researchers limit their studies to a subsystem, such as cache memories. In such cases, one needs only to simulate the interested subsystem in detail while abstracting other components.

Many architectural simulators are available for academic and commercial purposes. As stated previously, the accuracy of the data generated by the simulators depends on the level of detail simulated, the complexity of the simulation process, and the nature of benchmarks that can be simulated. Simulators may simulate single components, multiple components, or entire computer system capable of running FS including OSs. A paper describing architectural simulators for academic and classroom purposes is described in Ref. [67].

In this section, we expose the reader to a variety of simulation and modeling tools, but we will constrain our review to architectural simulator based on their complexity and scope. We will introduce several simulators capable of simulating single component or FS. We will also treat simulation tools for modeling networks as well as modeling power consumption separately from architectural simulators. Figure 3.3 is a diagram that shows the various relationships between current and past tools. It also shows how various power modeling tools are used as interfaces with architectural simulators:

- Single-component simulators: Any simulator that simulates a single subsystem, regardless of accuracy or code complexity, is least complex among hardware simulators. In this category, we can find trace-driven tools such as the DineroIV cache simulator [4] or DRAMSim [2].
- Multiple-component simulators: Simulator tools that have the capability to simulate more than one subsystem are more complex than single-component simulators. An example of a simulator that can simulate

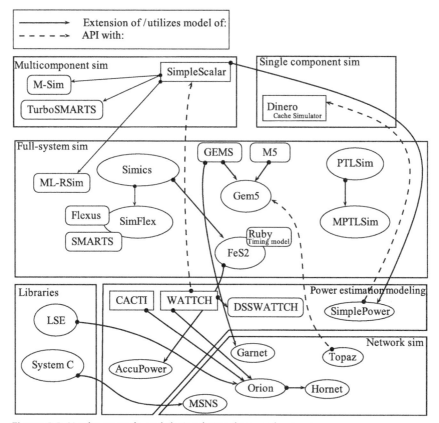

Figure 3.3 Hardware tools and their relationships and extensions.

multiple components is the widely used SimpleScalar [8] tool set that simulates a single CPU and several levels of memory systems.

- FS simulators: These are the most complex among architectural simulator as they simulate all subsystems, including multiple processing cores, interconnection buses, and multiple levels of memory hierarchy, and they permit simulation of realistic workloads under realistic execution environments. Note that the definition of an FS changes with time, since computing systems complexities in terms of the number of cores, complexity of each core, programming models for homogeneous and heterogeneous cores, memory subsystem, and interconnection subsystem are changing with time. Thus, today's FS simulators may not be able to simulate next-generation systems fully. In general, however, FS simulators simulate both hardware and software systems (including OSs and runtime systems).

- Network simulators: At the core of virtually every network router lies a network processor. They are designed to exploit packet-level parallelism by utilizing multiple fast execution cores. To study and research network processor complexity, power dissipation, and architectural alternatives, researchers rely on network simulators. Network simulators share many of the same features of other FS architectures, but their scope and design goals are specifically target network subsystem.

- Power estimation and modeling tools: Designing energy-efficient processors is a critical design pursued by current processor architects. With the increasing density of transistors integrated on a chip, the need to reduce power consumed by each component of the system becomes even more critical. To estimate the trade-offs between architectural alternatives in the power versus performance design space, researchers rely on power modeling and power estimation tools. They are similar to other simulators that focus on performance estimation, but power tools focus on estimating power consumed by each device when executing an application.

3.2. Single-Component Simulators

Although we categorize simulators that simulate a single component of a system as low-complexity simulators, they may require simulation of all the complexities of the component. Generally, these simulators are trace-driven: They receive input in a single file (e.g., a trace of instructions) and they simulate the component behavior for the provided input (e.g., if a given memory address causes a cache hit or miss or if an instruction requires a specific functional unit). The most common example of such simulators is memory system simulators including those that simulate main memory systems (e.g., Ref. [2] used to study RAM (random access memory) behavior) or caches (e.g., DineroIV [4]). Other simple simulators are used for educational purposes such as the EasyCPU [6].

3.2.1 DineroIV

DineroIV is a trace-based uniprocessor cache simulator [4]. The availability of the source code makes it easy to modify and customize the simulator to model different cache configurations, albeit for a uniprocessor environment. DineroIV accepts address traces representing the addresses of instructions and data accessed when a program is executed and models if the referenced addresses can be found in (multilevel) cache or cause a miss. DineroIV permits experimentation with different cache organizations including different block size, associativity, and replacement policy. Trace-driven simulation is an attractive method to test architectural subcomponents because experiments for different configurations of the component can be evaluated without having to reexecute the application through an FS simulator. Variations to DineroIV are available that extend the simulator to model multicore systems; however, many of these variations are either unmaintained or difficult to use.

3.3. Multiple-Component Simulators

Medium-complexity simulators model multiple components and the interactions among the components, including a complete CPU with in-order or out-of-order execution pipelines, branch prediction and speculation, and memory subsystem. A prime example of such a system is the widely used SimpleScalar tool set [8]. It is aimed at architecture research although some academics deem SimpleScalar to be invaluable for teaching computer architecture courses. An extension known as ML-RSIM [10] is an execution-driven computer system simulating several subcomponents including an OS kernel. Other extension includes M-Sim [12], which extends SimpleScalar to model multithreaded architectures based on simultaneous multithreading (SMT).

3.3.1 SimpleScalar

SimpleScalar is a set of tools for computer architecture research and education. Developed in 1995 as part of the Wisconsin Multiscalar project, it has since sparked many extensions and variants of the original tool. It runs precompiled binaries for the SimpleScalar architecture. This also implies that SimpleScalar is not an FS simulator but rather user-space single application simulator. SimpleScalar is capable of emulating Alpha, portable instruction set architecture (PISA) (MIPS like instructions), ARM, and x85 instruction sets. The simulator interface consists of the SimpleScalar ISA and POSIX system call emulations.

The available tools that come with SimpleScalar include sim-fast, sim-safe, sim-profile, sim-cache, sim-bpred, and sim-outorder:

- sim-fast is a fast functional simulator that ignores any microarchitectural pipelines.
- sim-safe is an instruction interpreter that checks for memory alignments; this is a good way to check for application bugs.
- sim-profile is an instruction interpreter and profiler. It can be used to measure application dynamic instruction counts and profiles of code and data segments.
- sim-cache is a memory simulator. This tool can simulate multiple levels of cache hierarchies.
- sim-bpred is a branch predictor simulator. It is intended to simulate different branch prediction schemes and measures miss prediction rates.
- sim-outorder is a detailed architectural simulator. It models a superscalar pipelined architecture with out-of-order execution of instructions, branch prediction, and speculative execution of instructions.

3.3.2 M-Sim

M-Sim is a multithreaded extension to SimpleScalar that models detailed individual key pipeline stages. M-Sim runs precompiled Alpha binaries and works on most systems that also run SimpleScalar. It extends SimpleScalar by providing a cycle-accurate model for thread context pipeline stages (reorder buffer, separate issue queue, and separate arithmetic and floating-point registers). M-Sim models a single SMT capable core (and not multicore systems), which means that some processor structures are shared while others remain private to each thread; details can be found in Ref. [12].

The look and feel of M-Sim is similar to SimpleScalar. The user runs the simulator as a stand-alone simulation that takes precompiled binaries compatible with M-Sim, which currently supports only Alpha APX ISA.

3.3.3 ML-RSIM

This is an execution-driven computer system simulator that combines detailed models of modern computer hardware, including I/O subsystems, with a fully functional OS kernel. ML-RSIM's environment is based on RSIM, an execution-driven simulator for instruction-level parallelism (ILP) in shared memory multiprocessors and uniprocessor systems. It extends RSIM with additional features including I/O subsystem support and an OS. The goal behind ML-RSIM is to provide detailed hardware timing models so that users are able to explore OS and application interactions. ML-RSIM is capable of simulating OS code and memory-mapped access to I/O devices; thus, it is a suitable simulator for I/O-intensive interactions.

ML-RSIM implements the SPARC V8 instruction set. It includes cache and TLB models, and exception handling capabilities. The cache hierarchy is modeled as a two-level structure with support for cache coherency protocols. Load and store instructions to I/O subsystem are handled through an uncached buffer with support for store instruction combining. The memory controller supports MESI (modify, exclusive, shared, invalidate) snooping protocol with accurate modeling of queuing delays, bank contention, and dynamic random access memory (DRAM) timing. The I/O subsystem consists of a peripheral component interconnect (PCI) bridge, a real-time clock, and a number of small computer system interface (SCSI) adapters with hard disks. Unlike other FS simulators, ML-RSIM includes a detailed timing-accurate representation of various hardware components. ML-RSIM does not model any particular system or device, rather it implements detailed general device prototypes that can be used to assemble a range of real machines.

ML-RSIM uses a detailed representation of an OS kernel, Lamix kernel. The kernel is Unix-compatible, specifically designed to run on ML-RSIM and implements core kernel functionalities, primarily derived from Net-BSD. Application linked for Lamix can (in most cases) run on Solaris. With a few exceptions, Lamix supports most of the major kernel functionalities such as signal handling, dynamic process termination, and virtual memory management.

3.3.4 ABSS

An augmentation-based SPARC simulator, or ABSS for short, is a multiprocessor simulator based on AugMINT, an augmented Mips interpreter. ABSS simulator can be either trace-driven or program-driven. We have described examples of trace-driven simulators, including the DineroIV, where only some abstracted features of an application (i.e., instruction or data address traces) are simulation. Program-driven simulators, on the other hand, simulate the execution of an actual application (e.g., a benchmark).

Program-driven simulations can be either interpretive simulations or execution-driven simulations. In interpretive simulations, the instructions are interpreted by the simulator one at a time, while in execution-driven simulations, the instructions are actually run on real hardware. ABSS is an execution-driven simulator that executes SPARC ISA.

ABSS consists of several components: a thread module, an augmenter, cycle-accurate libraries, memory system simulators, and the benchmark. Upon execution, the augmenter instruments the application and the cycle-accurate libraries. The thread module, libraries, the memory system simulator, and the benchmark are linked into a single executable. The augmenter then models each processor as a separate thread and in the event of a break (context switch) that the memory system must handle, the execution pauses, and the thread module handles the request, usually saving registers and reloading new ones. The goal behind ABSS is to allow the user to simulate timing-accurate SPARC multiprocessors.

3.3.5 HASE

HASE, hierarchical architecture design and simulation environment, and SimJava are educational tools used to design, test, and explore computer architecture components. Through abstraction, they facilitate the study of hardware and software designs on multiple levels. HASE offers a GUI for students trying to understand complex system interactions. The motivation for developing HASE was to develop a tool for rapid and flexible developing of new architectural ideas.

HASE is based in SIM++, a discrete-event simulation language. SIM++ describes the basic components and the user can link the components. HASE will then produce the initial code ready that forms the bases of the desired simulator. Since HASE is hierarchical, new components can be built as interconnected modules to core entities.

HASE offers a variety of simulations models intended for use for teaching and educational laboratory experiments. Each model must be used with HASE, a Java-based simulation environment. The simulator then produces a trace file that is later used as input into the graphic environment to represent interior workings of an architectural component. The following are few of the models available through HASE:

- Simple pipelined processor based on MIPS
- Processor with scoreboards (used for instruction scheduling)
- Processor with prediction
- Single instruction, multiple data (SIMD) array processors

- A two-level cache model
- Cache coherency protocols (snooping and directory)

3.4. FS Simulators

While lower-complexity systems described thus far are good at exploring and studying single components and component behavior under a smaller application load, for large-scale studies, we must employ FS simulators. In order to build large-scale system, a simulator must observe the scope and level of abstraction. The scope defines what the simulator is modeling, and the level defines the level of detail that is modeled. We can further refine the abstraction level by functionality and timing behavior. If we are trying to model a realistic workload, we must enlarge the scope to include an FS, including hardware and software systems. Each layer must be simulated in sufficient detail to run commercial systems and allow the researcher to tweak the hardware. Obviously, such systems are very complex and yet it is desirable that such systems complete simulations of realistic workloads in reasonable amount of time. For this reason, some FS simulators do not provide cycle-accurate simulations of the processor architecture. Some simulators permit the user to select between very detailed simulations of lower-level architectural components and abstractions of the architecture. The modular nature of some FS simulators allows users to include different ISAs, different microarchitectural designs, different memory system, or different OS kernels. Examples of FS simulator are the Simics simulator [19], Gem5 simulator [26], and SimOS [28].

3.4.1 Simics

'Simics is a widely used FS simulator. It simulates processors at the instruction level, and it is detailed enough to allow the booting of a variety of real OSs. Despite all of its complexity, it still offers performance levels to run realistic workloads. Simics supports a variety of processor architectures including Ultra-SPARC, Alpha, x86, x86-64, PowerPC, IPF Itanium, MIPS, and ARM. It can support Linux running on x86, PowerPC, and Alpha; Solaris on UltraSPARC; Tru64 on Alpha; and Windows 2000 on x86. Simics can be configured using command-level input. Since Simics simulates an FS, it includes device models capable of running real firmware and device drivers. For instance, Simics modeling the x86 architecture will correctly install and boot Windows XP OS.

Simics is unique in that it can connect several instances (viewed as nodes) and run distributed systems. A single Simics instance can simulate several nodes of a given instruction set architecture (ISA); but using multiple instances of Simics, communicating through Simics Central, can simulate heterogeneous systems.

At the core of each Simics' simulation is Simics Central, which synchronizes the virtual time between different Simics' simulators and nodes. Simics is configured through an object-oriented paradigm where each object instance is an instance of a processor or device. Any new object is derived using Simics API, which is defined in the configuration. It also supports a runtime Python interpreter for executing Python scripts, which can then be triggered at interesting breakpoints. Devices are a key component of any Simics' simulation; therefore, Simics supports devices that enable OS and firmware to boot and run, respectively. A few of the devices supported by Simics are timers, floppy controllers, keyboard/mouse controllers, direct memory access (DMA) controllers, interrupt controllers, RAM controller, and various other crucial devices needed for FS simulation.

A crucial feature of Simics is its ability to interface with other simulators. Because Simics does not natively support cycle-accurate simulations, it allows interfaces to clock cycle-accurate models written in hardware description languages (such as Verilog).

Another notable feature of Simics is its hindsight feature. A system simulation can progress in two ways, and this opens a new range of testing capabilities. Simics is capable of taking simulation snapshots, and any future simulations can be fast-forwarded to the snapshot and continue execution beyond the snapshot. This is practical for running large simulations at interesting sections multiple times from the saved snapshot.

Applications of Simics are manifold since it is useful for a variety of tasks such as microprocessor design, memory studies, device development, OS emulation and development, and more. Originally, Simics was used primarily for processor designs. Previous trace-based simulators have some known limitations, which Simics tries to resolve. The notable limitations are the inability to simulate multiprocessor systems and its interaction with other devices such as memory and OS memory management and scheduling.

Due to its complexity, Simics requires time to learn all of its features. Moreover, the acquisition of Virtutech by Wind River System and academic licenses do not provide source code, and in many cases, only older OS and processor models are provided to the academic institutions. Yet, Simics is a valuable simulator for conducting research on computer systems architecture.

3.4.2 SimFlex

SimFlex is a simulation framework to support the simulation of uni-processors, chip multiprocessors, and distributed shared memory systems; the project targets fast and flexible simulations of large-scale systems [21]. The core components of SimFlex are Flexus and SMARTS:

- Flexus: Flexus is the simulator framework, which relies on a set of well-defined components.
- SMARTS: SMARTS is a sampling method whose goal is to reduce the overall simulation time.

SimFlex is built around Simics and thus capable to running FS simulations. Unlike other modular component approaches to system design, SimFlex takes a compile-time component interconnect approach. This means that component interconnects can be optimized at compile time, reducing some runtime overheads. To further reduce simulation times, SimFlex applies SMARTS sampling methodology [25] instead of simulating every cycle.

The timing model around SimFlex is better than that provided natively in Simics. SimFlex operates on a stream of fetched instructions from Simics, allowing more accurate timing models for each instruction. Timing models for x86 and SPARC architectures, for both uniprocessor and multiprocessor configurations, are available with SimFlex.

SimFlex unique features are the notion of abstracting components through a layered approach while improving runtime performance. This is achieved through C++ template tricks around which the components are built, allowing compiler to optimize the overall system. Normally, simulation times of complex systems are reduced either by limiting the number of instructions simulated or by simulating a regularly sampled set of instructions. SimFlex takes the SMARTS [25] approach. SMARTS is a methodology to apply statistical sampling (similar to AP through hardware performance counters). SMARTS uses a coefficient of variation measure to obtain an instruction stream sample while maintaining accuracy of performance estimates. The system uses sampling to warm up components that are prone to have unpredictable state—this usually happens when simulation modes switch from highly accurate to simple models.

SimFlex is a good tool for modeling hardware where timing accuracy is critical.

3.4.3 Gem5 Simulator System

Gem5 simulator system is a combined effort of the previous work of GEMS (general execution-driven multiprocessor simulator) and M5 (a discrete event-driven simulator). It is written primarily in C++ and to a lesser extent Python. It is open source licensed under a BSD-style license.

Gem5 is primarily built for research environments and provides an abundance of components that work out of box (or without modifications). The Gem5 is modular enough to permit the study of new architectures. Gem5 is designed using object-oriented methodology. Nearly all major components (CPUs, buses, caches, etc.) are designed as objects, internally known as SimObjects. They share similar configurations, initialization, statistics collection, and checkpointing behavior. Internally, the nature of C++ provides for a complex but flexible system description of CPU interconnects, cache hierarchies, multiprocessor networks, and other subsystem. The Gem5 environment relies on domain-specific languages (DSLs) for specialized tasks. For defining ISA's, it inherited an ISA DSL from M5, and for specifying cache coherency, it inherited a cache coherency DSL from GEMS. These languages allow users to represent design issues compactly.

The ISA DSL allows users to design new ISAs through a series of class templates covering a broad range of instructions and arithmetic operations. Cache coherency DSL represents protocols through a set of states, events, and transitions. These features allow Gem5 to implement different coherency protocols through the same underlying state transitions, thus reducing the programmer effort. Gem5 operates on several interchangeable CPU models; a simple CPU model supports a basic 4-stage pipeline, a functional model, an in-order CPU model, while a more advanced out-of-order CPU model with SMT support is also available. It features a flexible event-driven memory system to model complex multilevel cache hierarchies.

Gem5 supports two modes of simulation (or modes of execution): an FS mode that simulates a complete system with devices and an OS and a user-space mode where user programs are serviced with system call emulation (SE). The two modes vary in their support for Alpha, ARM, MIPS, PowerPC, SPARC, and x86-64 targets.

3.4.4 SimOS (Parallel SimOS)

Developed in the late 1990s at Stanford University, SimOS is an FS simulator with features to simulate the OS at different abstraction levels. The development goals were to design a simulator to study FS workloads. Initial version of SimOS was capable of booting and running IRIX (an SGI SVR4 Unix implementation). Later versions permitted modeling of DEC Alpha machines with enough detail to boot DEC Unix systems. Other version of SimOS allowed x86 extensions. SimOS interfaces allow one to include different number of components. SimOS introduced the concept of dynamically adjustable simulation speed [28]. The simulation speed adjustment balances speed of execution with simulation detail. SimOS implements this through three different execution modes, defining different levels of detail. The three modes are the positioning mode (fastest mode) that offers enough functionality of boot operations and executes the basic OS operations; the rough characterization mode that offers a middle ground with more details but slightly slower than its predecessor; and the accurate mode that is the slowest but most detailed simulation mode. There are two different CPU models provided by SimOS: a basic single-issue pipeline model that provides the basic functionality and a more advanced superscalar dynamically scheduled processor model that supports privileged instructions, memory management unit executions, and exception handling.

The drawbacks of SimOS were addressed by its successor, Parallel SimOS. Parallel SimOS addresses SimOS' scalability issues. Thus, in many ways, Parallel SimOS is similar to the original SimOS, and it takes uses of multithreaded and shared memory capabilities of modern host processors to speedup simulations.

3.4.5 PTLsim

PTLsim is an x86-64 out-of-order superscalar microprocessor simulator [32]. One can think of PTLsim as a simulator and VM in one. It is capable of modeling a processor core at RTL (register transfer level) detail. It models the complete cache hierarchy and memory subsystems including any supportive devices with full-cycle accuracy. The instructions supported are x86- and x86-64-compatible including any modern streaming SIMD extension (SSE) instructions. PTLsim must run on the same host and target platform. Similar to SimOS, PTLsim supports multiple simulating modes.

PTLsim comes as a bare hardware simulator that runs in user space and a more advance version PTLsim/X, which integrates with the Xen hypervisor for full x86-64 simulations. PTLsim/X comes with full multithreading support, checkpointing, cycle-accurate virtual device timing models, and deterministic time dilation without the inherent simulation speed sacrifice. It is capable of booting various Linux distributions and industry standard heavy workloads.

C++ templated classes and libraries give PTLsim the flexibility to tweak and tune significant portions of the simulator for research purposes. It is licensed under a GNU free software license and thus is readily available for public use.

PTLsim employs a technique known as cosimulation, which means that the simulator runs directly on a host machine that supports the simulated instructions. This means that context switched between full-speed (native) simulation and simulated mode is transparent. Likewise, this provides an easy way for code verification. The drawback is that this limits the simulation to x86-based ISAs.

Cosimulation makes PTLsim extremely fast compared to other similar simulators, but other techniques to improve speed are also employed, particularly instruction vectorization. It comes with features to turn on or off various statistics to improve the simulation speed. Since PTLsim is a fast simulator, skipping streams of instructions used in sampling techniques is not necessary. The speed advantage that PTLsim makes is a very good candidate for HP under complex workloads, but because it requires the target platforms be compatible with simulated processors, PTLsim is not as flexible as other FS simulators described here.

Most simulators that were developed in the mid-2000s were designed to support the emergence of multicore architectures and SMT. MPTLsim [33] is an extension of PTLsim to permit SMT like threads.

3.4.6 FeS2

FeS2 is described as a timing-first, multiprocessor, x86 simulator built around Simics though many of its key features were also borrowed from other simulators (e.g., GEMS and PTLsim). It comes with all the standard features available with Simics, but it expands Simics' functionality with more accurate execution-driven timing model. The model includes cache hierarchy, branch predictors, and a superscalar out-of-order core. While the functionality is provided by Simics, the timing model is provided through Ruby, which was developed as part of the GEMS (now a part of Gem5) simulator.

The core is based on a microoperation (μop) model that decodes x86 instructions into a stream of RISC like μops.

FeS2 can be thought of as a separate simulator (technically a library) that wraps around Simics' functionality. The timing component is not FS-capable since it does not implement all the necessary devices required for FS simulation, such as SCSI controllers and disks, PCI and parallel bus interfaces, interrupt and DMA controllers, and temperature sensors (all of which are implemented by Simics).

3.4.7 TurboSMARTS

TurboSMARTS is a microarchitectural simulator that utilizes checkpointing to speed up overall simulation times [35]. In order to speedup simulation time, simulators often use sampling methods. Sampling involves collecting a large number of brief simulation windows to represent an accurate image of the application's runtime behavior. The problem arises when the collection of snapshots drifts from the native execution. This normally occurs because of instruction data-flow dependencies; normally a branch depends on precomputed values. However, if the values are not present during a sampled event, then the branch might execute a different path than it would if the correct data were present. Therefore, it becomes important to warm the system so that branches execute as if the program flow never halted.

TurboSMARTS provides accurate warmed up states that are stored as checkpoints in order to speedup simulation. It is based on observations that only a small amount of microarchitectural states is accessed during sampling and that checkpointing is a fast and more accurate method than other statistical sampling alternatives.

TurboSMARTS is derived from SimpleScalar's sim–outorder simulator (a superscalar out-of-order detailed simulator). Because of sampling, the simulations times are only a fraction of those using full out-of-order (OoO) simulators, yet the error rates (in terms of CPI) are in the range of $\pm 3\%$.

3.5. Network Simulators

3.5.1 NePSim

NePSim is a network processor simulator with a power evaluation framework [3]. Network processors are a special type of processors specifically used as network routers. A network processor consists of a few simple cores that exploit the inherent data-level parallelism associated with networking codes. With the increasing clock frequency of these chips, power dissipation becomes an issue that must be considered. NePSim offers a simulation environment to explore the design space of speed and power.

NepSim includes cycle-accurate simulations, a formal verification engine, and a power estimator for network processor clusters that may consist of several components (memory controllers, I/O ports, packet buffers, and buses). It implements the Intel IXP1200 system consisting of a StrongARM processor, six microengines (MEs), standards memory interfaces, and high-speed buses.

The input to NepSim is a stream of network packets generated through a traffic generator module. The core processor is not crucial in controlling critical data paths; thus, it is not simulated. The core simulation is the ME core. NepSim simulates the instruction lookup, instruction decoding and source register address formation, reading operands from the source register, arithmetic logic unit (ALU) operations, and writing results to destination registers. Memory timing information tries to resemble that of the Intel IXP1200s.

3.5.2 Orion

Orion is a power-performance simulator based on the LSE, a modularized microarchitectural simulator [29]. Guided by hierarchical modeling methodology described in Ref. [5], Orion abstracts a network model with building blocks (modules), which describe an interconnection between various parts of a network on chip system. Orion consists of two basic component classes: message transporting class and message processing class. Message-transporting classes consist of message sources and message sinks. Message processing classes consist of router buffers, crossbars, arbiters, and links.

Every module can be parameterized to represent various configurations at the design stage. The goal of Orion is to allow for an extensive range of architectural choices with relatively few reusable modules.

Power modeling in Orion is analytical based on components, which occupy the largest area (about 90%) such as first-in-first-out (FIFO) buffers, crossbars, and arbiters. The power model is based on a set of equations derived from a combination of cache access and cycle timing model tool (CACTI) [16] and WATTCH [18]. The goal is to provide reasonable power estimates through parameterized architectural-level power models. An updated version Orion 2.0 comes with some new features and an updated transistor technology database.

The hierarchical and modular composition of Orion allows us to explore different architectural compositions and workloads.

3.5.3 Garnet

Garnet is described as a cycle-accurate on-chip network model for an FS simulator [7]. The model utilizes the FS capabilities of the GEMS framework [68] modeling a five-stage pipelined router with a virtual channel (VC) flow control. Garnet enables researchers to evaluate system-level optimizations, new network processors simulated on an FS workload.

Garnet models a configurable classic five-stage VC router. The major components are the input buffers, route computation logic, virtual channel allocation (VCA), switch allocator, and a crossbar switch. Router's microarchitectural components consist of single-ported buffers and a single shared port into the crossbar from each input. Garnet's interaction between various memory systems (e.g., cache controllers) is handled by an interconnection network interface. This means that CPU cache misses are broken into lower-level units and passed onto the interconnect interface. To model a variety of coherency protocols, Garnet implements a system-level point-to-point ordering mechanism, meaning that a message sent from two nodes to a single destination is received in the same order as they were sent. Network power model is implemented from Orion [5]. Garnet records per component events and records them using power counters; these are then used to compute the final energy usage of various router components. There are several input parameters that can be adjusted to fit any desired interconnect such as network type, model detail, simulation type (network only vs. FS), number of router pipeline stages, VC buffer size, and number of bytes per flit (flit is the smallest measurable unit). The models are validated against results in previously published papers.

3.5.4 Topaz

Topaz is an open-source interconnection network simulator for chip multiprocessors and supercomputers [9]. To accommodate the growing need to efficiently simulate large chip interconnects, Topaz offers an open-source multithreaded cycle-accurate network simulator. The ability to interface with GEMS [68] and Gem5 [26] FS simulation frameworks allows Topaz to simulate network interconnects within an FS environment. Topaz was designed for use for studying supercomputers (off-chip network) systems, system-on-chip, to chip-multiprocessor systems.

Topaz is based on a previous simulator (SICOSYS [69]), but for reusability and modularity, the tool is designed using object-oriented methodology and is implemented in C++. The simulation phase consists of several phases. In the build phase, the system will hierarchically outline the network topology according to a set of parameters. During the execution phase, every component is visited and simulated every cycle. Lastly, the print phase will output the collected records of the simulation. The results can be configured to measure various network parameters.

The general simulator breakdown can be described in terms of object constructors, components and flows, traffic patterns, and simulator. Object constructs interpret the input parameters and are responsible for building the required objects for simulation. Components and flows represent hardware to be simulated (functional network units). Traffic patterns are responsible for injecting packets into the network for stand-alone simulation use. The simulator is the main driver and it is responsible for initialization and configuration interpretation.

To build a simulation environment, the user can specify the following parameters:

- Simulation parameters: the general simulation definition that defines traffic pattern and distribution, applied load, message length, etc.
- Network interconnect: this defines the network type through network topology, dimensions, and interconnection delays.
- Router microarchitecture: this describes the router elements such as memories, switches, and multiplexers. Topaz also comes with a few out-of-the-box models that the user can choose and build. To improve its scalability and optimize its performance, Topaz is designed as multi-threaded application. Synchronization between individual threads is done using barriers. For GEMS and Gem5 integration, Topaz provides an API allowing the user to integrate new designs effortlessly.

3.5.5 MSNS: A Top-Down MPI-Style Hierarchical Simulation Framework for Network on Chip

MSNS is an MPI-style network simulator, which aims at accurately simulating packet delays for NoC systems. Based on SystemC, MSNS implements simulation at various granularities from high-level abstraction to low RTL [11]. MSNS uses top-down approach of all network layers and utilizes wait() functions to guarantee cycle accuracy of individual layers. This leads to the following benefits of MSNS: It can simulate traffic of practical systems more precisely by ensuring an accurate abstraction of application's data transmission rates, it can accurately estimate dynamic power consumption, and it can provide methods to evaluate performances of parallel algorithms and high-performance applications on network infrastructure.

MSNS employs several interface levels. RTL modeling is performed at the link layer and network layer. The interface layer is composed of the MPI library, RTL description, and high-level abstraction descriptions. The simulator consists of two components: MSNS generator and MSNS simulator. By utilizing user supplied input files, the MSNS generator generates the network and application properties and stores them as a configuration file. To ensure highest possible accuracy, MSNS generator calculates wire latencies and bit-error probabilities through its built-in wire models. These delays are enforced by a wait function. When the libraries (SystemC, MPI, and design modules) are loaded into the MSNS simulator, they are combined with the previously generated configuration files and the simulation initiates. To calculate power at each individual layer MSNS provides a power estimation for the whole network infrastructure at the architectural level.

3.5.6 Hornet

Hornet is a parallel, highly configurable, cycle-level multicore simulator [13] intended to simulate many-core NoC systems.

Hornet supports a variety of memory hierarchies interconnected through routing and VC allocation algorithms. It also has the ability to model a system's power and thermal aspect.

Hornet is capable of running in two modes: a network-only mode and a full-multicore mode running a built-in MIPS core simulator. The goal of Hornet is the capability to simulate 1000 core systems.

Hornet's basic router is modeled using ingress and egress buffers. Packets arrive in flits and compete for the crossbar. When a port has been assigned, they pass and exit using the egress buffer. Interconnect geometry can be configured with pairwise connections to form rings, multilayer meshes, and tori. Hornet supports oblivious, static, and adaptive routing. Oblivious and adaptive routing are configurable using routing tables. Similarly VCA is handled using tables. Hornet also allows for internode bidirectional linking. Links can be changed at every cycle depending on dynamic traffic needs.

To accurately represent power dissipation and thermal properties, Hornet uses dynamic power models based on Orion [5], combined with a leakage power model, and a thermal model using HotSpot [70].

To speedup simulation, Hornet implements a multithreaded strategy to offload simulation work to other cores. This is achieved by tiling each simulated processor core to a single thread. Cycle accuracy is globally visible for simulation correctness.

Hornet simulates tiles where each tile is an NoC router connected to other tiles via point-to-point links.

The traffic generators are either trace-driven injectors or cycle-level MIPS simulators.

A simple trace injector reads a trace file that contains traces annotated with timestamps, packet sizes, and other packet information describing each packet. The MIPS simulator can accept cross compiled MIPS binaries. The MIPS core can be configured with varying memory levels backed by a coherency protocol.

3.6. Power and Power Management Tools

Computer architecture research revolves around estimating trade-offs between alternative architectural modifications. The trade-offs typically involve performance, hardware complexity, and power budgets. In order to estimate the power requirements of various design choices, researchers rely on power modeling and power management tools that offer validated models for power estimation.

3.6.1 CACTI

Perhaps the most widely used tool in this realm is the CACTI [16]. CACTI is an analytical model for a variety of cache components that contribute to the overall CPU memory subsystem. The earlier versions of CACTI modeled access and cycle times of on-chip caches. It supports both direct mapped and associative caches. CACTI is an extension to previous models that includes a tag array model, nonstep stage input slopes, rectangular stacking of memory subarrays, a transistor-level decoder model, column-multiplexed bitlines, cycle times and access times, and others. The analytical model in CACTI is validated through the HSPICE [71]. CACTI's access and cycle times are derived by estimating the delays in the following parameters: decoder, wordlines, bitlines, sense amplifiers, comparators, multiplexor drivers, and output drivers (data and valid signal output). Each delay is estimated separately, and the results are combined to estimate the final access and cycle times. Typically, the user describes cache parameters such as cache size, block size, and associativity, as well as process parameters. Describing the models of individual components is beyond the scope of this chapter; thus, the interested reader is referred to Ref. [16].

The tool evolved significantly over the past decade with enhancements to include an integrated approach: modeling access times, cycle times, area, aspect ratio, and power. As the fabrication technologies have changed over time, so have the models present within CACTI. CACTI's models have changed to reflect changes in feature sizes and technologies. CACTI now supports memories built using either SRAM or DRAM and even 3D packaging of DRAMs.

The latest CACTI tool focuses on the interconnect delays between cache subcomponents. The major extensions include the ability to model non-uniform cache access and the ability to model different types of wires. There is also a web-based GUI to facilitate a broader audience.

3.6.2 WATTCH

WATTCH is a framework for architectural-level power analysis and optimization [18]. The framework aims at facilitating power analysis and optimization early in the architectural design phase. Other tools offer highly accurate power estimates only after the initial layout or floor planning. In contrast, WATTCH offers power estimates early in the design phase.

The power models in WATTCH are interfaced with SimpleScalar. WATTCH uses a modified version of sim-outorder (a superscalar out-of-order processor simulator) to collect their results. SimpleScalar provides simulation environment that keeps track of units that are involved in each cycle. WATTCH records the total energy consumed by each unit on each instruction and accumulates the total energy consumed by an application. WATTCH power model includes four subcategories:

- Array structures: Data and instruction caches, cache tag arrays, register files, alias tables, branch predictors, and portions of instruction window and load/store queues
- Fully associative content-addressable memories: Instruction window/ reorder buffer wake-up logic, load/store order checks, and TLBs
- Combinational logic and wires: Functional units, instruction window selection logic, dependency check logic, and result buses
- Clocking: Clock buffers, clock wires, and capacitive loads

The models are similar to the early versions of CACTI tool with two key differences: WATTCH disregards the overall critical path but uses an expected critical path to determine a delay within a unit, and it only measures the capacitance of an entire unit to model power consumption rather than individual stages of a unit. WATTCH also offers models to measure varying conditional clocking styles. This means that WATTCH tracks the number of used ports and depending on the enabled option tracks full, low, or dynamic power consumptions.

Additional power estimation means adding additional overhead to sim-outorder; therefore, WATTCH performs at a 30% overhead well within a tolerable amount.

3.6.3 DSSWattch

DSSWattch [20] is a modification of WATTCH [18] framework. DSSWattch stands for Dynamic SimpleScalar; thus, DSSWattch is a tool for power estimation in dynamic SimpleScalar. The tool is simulates the PowerPC architecture. The tool operates on a new version of SimpleScalar that supports dynamic features for programs such as Jikes RVM Java VM. The additional features support actions such as dynamic compilation and dynamic memory mapping or programs that require dynamic linking.

The new features in DSSWattch are extended functionality of WATTCH through better register file modeling, floating-point capabilities, and support for the 32-bit mixed data-width PowerPC architecture.

Major differences between WATTCH and DSSWattch are the following:

- Operand harvesting to better serve the PowerPC architecture operand harvesting has been updated with new structures to accommodate the PowerPC instruction's ability to update special purpose registers as well as required additional operands.
- Handling of floating-point operands and population counting original WATTCH was unable to differentiate between floating point and integer registers. In order to estimate dynamic bus power usage, DSSWattch extends this functionality through the new operand harvesting data.
- Register file modeling: The original WATTCH tool only handled single integer register file of uniform word length. The PPC ISA requires both 32-bit integer and 64-bit floating-point register files. Therefore, DSSWattch extends this functionality by including multiple register files. Power consumed by these register files is computed separately and accumulated for overall power consumption.
- Differentiation of integer, floating-point, and address data widths: Along with the use of different register files, DSSWattch models different data widths for floating point and integer operations.

Since DSSWattch is an extension of the original WATTCH tool, the power models are based on WATTCH. The rename logic, instruction window, and the unified RUU (register update unit) reflect the microarchitectural state of the simulated out-of-order simulator.

3.6.4 SimplePower

SimplePower is a framework that utilizes several outstanding component-based simulators and combines them with power estimation models. It is an execution-driven, cycle-accurate, RTL-level power estimation tool.

SimplePower is based on a five-stage pipelined simulator with an integer ISA similar to SimpleScalar. The components of SimplePower are Simple-Power core, RTL power estimation interface, technology-dependent switch capacitance tables, cache/bus simulator, and loader. At each cycle, the core simulates the instructions and calls corresponding power units. The power estimation modules are C routines for each unit. With new technologies, only the technology-dependent capacitance tables need be changed, while the core remains intact. The cache simulation is interfaced with

DineroIII [4] cache simulator and integrated with a memory energy model. The bus simulator snoops appropriate lines and utilizes an interconnect power model to compute switch capacitance of the on-chip buses. The capacitance tables are based on the design of the functional units. The units can be bit-dependent or bit-independent. Bit-independent functional units are units where operations of one bit do not depend on the value of other bits. Examples of bit-independent units are pipeline registers, logic unit in the ALU, latches, and buses. Bit-dependent functional units are units where the value of one bit depends on the value of other bits in the vector. The transitional matrix to compute capacitance values for bit-dependent functional units becomes very large to efficiently estimate the consumed power. SimplePower uses a combination of an analytical model and functional unit partitioning to estimate the power for such units. For example, the memory module is modeled analytically, while adders, subtracters, multipliers, register files, decoders, and multiplexers are broken into subcomponents whose power is computed as the sum of the individual subcomponents using lookup tables.

3.6.5 AccuPower

Similar to WATTCH and SimplePower, AccuPower [24] is a tool to estimate power consumption for a superscalar microprocessor. AccuPower describes itself as a true hardware-level and cycle-level microarchitectural simulator with the ability to estimate power dissipation of actual complementary metal-oxide semiconductor (CMOS) layouts of critical data path. The ability to obtain transition counts from higher-level blocks such as caches, issue queues, reorder buffers, and functional units at RTL allows AccuPower to accurately estimate switching activity.

The benefit of AccuPower over its predecessors is that AccuPower does not rely on the original SimpleScalar simulator, which combines several critical data paths into a single unit. The problem with other tools is that in many cases, these critical components contribute to more than half of overall power dissipation.

Several AccuPower features include the following:

- It uses a cycle-level simulation of all major data path and interconnection components (issue queue, register files, reorder buffers, load–store queue, and forward mechanisms).
- It provides detailed and accurate on-chip cache hierarchy simulations.
- AccuPower models CPU-internal interconnections in great detail, for example, explicit data transfers and forwarding and clock distribution network.

- It supports three major built-in models of widely used superscalar data paths.
- It includes facilities to collect power and performance estimates at both individual subcomponent level per bit and byte and the entire processor.
- AccuPower uses subcomponent power coefficient estimates using SPICE.

The major components of AccuPower are a microarchitectural simulator, the very large-scale integration (VLSI) layouts for major data paths and caches, and power estimation modules that use energy coefficients obtained from SPICE.

- The microarchitectural simulator is really a greatly enhanced version of the SimpleScalar simulator.[1] The enhancements include implementations for the issue queue, reorder buffer, rename tables, physical register files, and architectural register files. The microarchitectural simulator is modified to fit three widely used versions of superscalar processors. The out-of-order simulator now supports a true cycle-by-cycle instruction execution. The CPU cache structure now supports a true cycle aware cache pipeline. Caches are also bus aware due to the possibility that instruction and data caches can access L2 at the same time. The ultimate goal is to design a simulator that closely resembles the real-world cycle-by-cycle-accurate superscalar processor.
- In order to get accurate energy and power coefficients, the power models rely on models derived from VLSI layouts using SPICE. To obtain accurate energy dissipation, CMOS layouts for on-chip caches, issue queues, physical register files, architecture register files, and reorder buffers are used to obtain real power coefficients.
- The tool's execution is sped up using multithreading. Analysis routines are handled in a separate thread.

AccuPower can be used to obtain

1. raw data collection pertaining to (a) bit-level data-path activity and (b) occupancy of individual data-path resources as measured by the number of valid entries,
2. record accurate data-path component-level power estimation,
3. exploration of power reduction techniques,
4. exploration of alternative circuit-level techniques,
5. exploration of alternative data-path architectures.

---

[1] According to authors, only 10% of the original code is untouched.

AccuPower remains a great tool to estimate power dissipation for various superscalar data paths as well as explore new microarchitectural innovations.

4. CONCLUSIONS

The topic of application tuning, optimization, and profiling and hardware simulation is vast, and with over 30 years of research, there is an abundance of literature covering this area. Our aim was to expose relevant information and popular tools to the reader. In this chapter, we have covered a variety of popular tools pertaining to hardware and AP.

In the chapter's introduction, we introduced a tool taxonomy and outlined their differences in scope and functionality. Furthermore, we have categorized the AP tools based on their data gathering methodology and categorized HP tools based on their scope. In the chapter's subsections, we provided diagrams that show various tool interdependencies and their categories related to our taxonomy. We have discussed several AP methods for performance tuning such as utilizing hardware performance counters and binary instrumentation and translation. To introduce and elaborate each method and category, we collected tools ranging from hardware performance libraries to binary instrumentation, translation, and code manipulation frameworks.

In the area of hardware simulation, we have covered widely known tools used for simulation and architectural research (e.g., SimpleScalar and Simics). To expose the reader to the chronological picture, we have covered several historical tools that are still used as the basis of many newer tools (e.g., SimpleScalar and SimOS). Because the area of hardware simulation is still growing, our aim was to correlate hardware profiler components and scope in a manner that will allow the reader to explore further in each area. For example, we categorized hardware profilers based on their complexity related to the number of hardware components simulated. Due to the various, often distinct, areas of hardware simulation, we also covered tools used for network interconnection simulations and power consumption. Network and power consumption research is increasingly important due to the advent of multicore and multiprocess machines. Accurate network simulators are becoming a vital part for system simulation and research in high-performance computing and network research areas. Therefore, we have covered several tools in that area.

Finally, as the density of transistors per processor die increases and the CMOS manufacturing technology shrinks, power estimation is becoming a critical part of future processor designs. Therefore, we have included some currently available tools for power estimation and modeling research. All tools that were picked in this chapter are summarized in Sections 5 and 6.

5. APPLICATION PROFILERS SUMMARY

Tool	Description
gprof	Compiler-assisted application profiler
Parasight	Parallel application profiler-based gprof
Quartz	A tool for tuning parallel program performance
ATOM	A tool for building static instrumentation analysis tools
Pin	A dynamic binary instrumentation tool for building analysis tools
DynInst	A dynamic binary instrumentation framework designed for code patching
Etch	A binary rewrite system for Windows32-based x86 executables
EEL	Machine- and system-independent executable editing library for building analysis tools
Valgrind	A dynamic binary instrumentation framework for code manipulation and error detection
DynamoRIO	Runtime code manipulation system for optimizations and error detection
Dynamite	A binary translation tool
UQBT	Static binary translation tool for RISC-, CISC-, and stack-based machines
OProfile	System-wide profiler for Linux (uses HW counters)
AMD CodeAnalyst	AMD chip-based performance analyzer
Intel VTune	Intel-based performance analysis tool
HPCToolkit	A parallel performance suite for measuring HPC applications
TAU	A portable profiling and tracing tool for parallel programs
Open SpeedShop	A open-source community-based multiplatform Linux-based performance analysis tool
VAMPIR	Visualization and Analysis tool for MPI Resources

PAPI	Portable application performance interface for hardware performance counters
perfmon	Kernel interface for hardware performance counters for performance analysis tools
perfctr	Linux-based hardware performance counter interface driver
gdb	The GNU debugger
DDT	An application debugger for large-scale parallel high-performance applications

 # 6. HARDWARE PROFILERS SUMMARY

Tool	Tool Description
DineroIV	Trace-driven single-process cache simulator
DRAMSim	Open-source DDR memory system simulator
EasyCPU	Educational tool for teaching computer organization
SimpleScalar	A superscalar simulator
SimpleScalar–Alpha	The SimpleScalar simulator ported to Alpha/Linux
SimplePower	Execution-driven data-path energy estimation tool based on SimpleScalar
ML_RSIM	Detailed execution-driven simulator running a Unix-compatible operating system
M-Sim	A multithreaded extension to SimpleScalar
ABSS	An augmentation-based SPARC simulator
AugMINT	An augmented MIPS interpreter
HASE	Hierarchical architecture design and simulation environment
Simics	An FS simulator
SimFlex	A system simulator that targets fast, accurate, and flexible simulation of large-scale systems
Flexus	The SimFlex framework component for FS simulation
Gem5	A collaborative simulation infrastructure targeting FS simulation

SimOS	A machine simulation environment designed for uni- and multiprocess machines
PTLsim	Open-source, FS, timing simulator. With SMP support, OoO core and AMD64 architecture
MPTLsim	Multithreaded version of PTLsim
FeS2	Timing-first, multiprocessor, x86 simulator, implemented as a module for Simics, uses PTLsim for decoding of μops
TurboSMARTS sim	A fast and accurate timing simulator
NepSim	A network processor simulator with power evaluation framework
Orion	Power-performance simulator based on LSE for NoC systems
Garnet	Network model within an FS simulator
Topaz	Open-source network interconnect simulator within an FS environment
MSNS	MPI-style network simulator targeting accurate packet delay measurement of NoC systems
Hornet	A parallel, highly configurable, cycle-level multicore simulator for many-core simulations
CACTI	Cache access and cycle time power estimation
WATTCH	A framework for architectural-level power analysis and optimization
DSSWATCH	Dynamic power analysis framework based on WATTCH
SimplePower	Execution-driven data-path energy estimation tool based on SimpleScalar
AccuPower	A hardware-level power estimation simulator
CGEN	Red Hat's CPU tools generator
LSE	Liberty simulation environment, framework for architectural component design

REFERENCES

[1] M.D. Hill, J.R. Larus, A.R. Lebeck, M. Talluri, D.A. Wood, Wisconsin architectural research tool set, SIGARCH Comput. Archit. News 21 (1993) 8–10.
[2] D. Wang, B. Ganesh, N. Tuaycharoen, K. Baynes, A. Jaleel, B. Jacob, DRAMsim: a memory system simulator, SIGARCH Comput. Archit. News 33 (4) (2005) 100–107.

[3] Y. Luo, J. Yang, L.N. Bhuyan, L. Zhao, NePSim: a network processor simulator with a power evaluation framework, IEEE Micro 24 (5) (2004) 34–44.

[4] M.D. Hill, J. Edler, DineroIV Trace-Driven Uniprocessor Cache Simulator. http://www.cs.wisc.edu/~markhill/DineroIV, 1997.

[5] X. Zhu, S. Malik, A hierarchical modeling framework for on-chip communication architectures [soc], in: IEEE/ACM International Conference on Computer Aided Design, 2002, ICCAD 2002, November, 2002, pp. 663–670.

[6] Holon Inst. Technology, Easy CPU H.I.T. http://www.hit.ac.il/EasyCPU/, 2008.

[7] N. Agarwal, T. Krishna, L.-S. Peh, N.K. Jha, Garnet: a detailed on-chip network model inside a full-system simulator, in: IEEE International Symposium on Performance Analysis of Systems and Software, 2009, ISPASS 2009, April, 2009, pp. 33–42.

[8] T. Austin, E. Larson, D. Ernst, SimpleScalar: an infrastructure for computer system modeling, Computer 35 (2002) 59–67.

[9] P. Abad, P. Prieto, L.G. Menezo, A. Colaso, V. Puente, J.-A. Gregorio, Topaz: an open-source interconnection network simulator for chip multiprocessors and supercomputers, in: 2012 Sixth IEEE/ACM International Symposium on Networks on Chip (NoCS), May, 2012, pp. 99–106.

[10] L. Schaelicke, M. Parker, ML-Rsim. http://www.cs.utah.edu/lambert/mlrsim/index.php, 2005.

[11] Z. Li, X. Ling, J. Hu, Msns: A top-down mpi-style hierarchical simulation framework for network-on-chip, in: WRI International Conference on Communications and Mobile Computing, 2009, CMC '09, vol. 2, January, 2009, pp. 609–614.

[12] J.J. Sharkey, D. Ponomarev, K. Ghose, Abstract M-SIM: a flexible, multi-threaded architectural simulation environment. http://www.cs.binghamton.edu/jsharke/m-sim/documentation/msim_tr.pdf, 2006.

[13] P. Ren, M. Lis, M.H. Cho, K.S. Shim, C.W. Fletcher, O. Khan, N. Zheng, S. Devadas, Hornet: a cycle-level multicore simulator, IEEE Trans. Comput. Aided Des. Integr. Circuits Syst. 31 (6) (2012) 890–903.

[14] M. Flynn, D. Sunada, D. Glasco, ABSS v2.0: a SPARC simulator, Technical Report, 1998.

[15] A.-T. Nguyen, M. Michael, A. Sharma, J. Torrella, The Augmint multiprocessor simulation toolkit for Intel x86 architectures, in: Proceedings of the 1996 International Conference on Computer Design, VLSI in Computers and Processors, ICCD '96, IEEE Computer Society, Washington, DC, 1996, p. 486.

[16] S.J.E. Wilton, N.P. Jouppi, CACTI: an enhanced cache access and cycle time model, IEEE J. Solid-State Circuits 31 (1996) 677–688.

[17] P.S. Coe, F.W. Howell, R.N. Ibbett, L.M. Williams, A hierarchical computer architecture design and simulation environment, ACM Trans. Model. Comput. Simul. 8 (1998) 431–446.

[18] V.T. Brooks, M. Martonosi, Wattch: a framework for architectural-level power analysis and optimizations, in: Proceedings of the 27th International Symposium on Computer Architecture, June 2000, 2000, pp. 83–94.

[19] P.S. Magnusson, M. Christensson, J. Eskilson, D. Forsgren, G. Hållberg, J. Högberg, F. Larsson, A. Moestedt, B. Werner, Simics: a full system simulation platform, Computer 35 (2002) 50–58.

[20] J. Dinan, E. Moss, Dsswattch: power estimations in dynamic simplescalar, Technical Report, 2004.

[21] N. Hardavellas, S. Somogyi, T.F. Wenisch, E. Wunderlich, S. Chen, J. Kim, B. Falsafi, J.C. Hoe, A.G. Nowatzyk, Simflex: a fast, accurate, flexible full-system simulation framework for performance evaluation of server architecture, SIGMETRICS Perform. Eval. Rev. 31 (2004) 31–35.

[22] W. Ye, N. Vijaykrishnan, M. Kandemir, M.J. Irwin, The Design and Use of SimplePower: A Cycle-Accurate Energy Estimation Tool, ACM, California, USA, 2000, pp. 340–345.

[23] Flexus 4.1.0, http://parsa.epfl.ch/simflex, 2005.
[24] D. Ponomarev, G. Kucuk, K. Ghose, AccuPower: an accurate power estimation tool for super-scalar microprocessors, in: Proceedings of the Conference on Design, Automation and Test in Europe Conference and Exhibition, 2002, pp. 124–129.
[25] R.E. Wunderlich, T.F. Wenisch, B. Falsafi, J.C. Hoe, SMARTS: accelerating microarchitecture simulation via rigorous statistical sampling, SIGARCH Comput. Archit. News 31 (2) (2003) 84–97.
[26] N. Binkert, B. Beckmann, G. Black, S.K. Reinhardt, A. Saidi, A. Basu, J. Hestness, D.R. Hower, T. Krishna, S. Sardashti, R. Sen, K. Sewell, M. Shoaib, N. Vaish, M.D. Hill, D.A. Wood, The gem5 simulator, SIGARCH Comput. Archit. News 39 (2011) 1–7.
[27] CGEN, The CPU Tools Generator, 2009, www.sourceware.org/cgen.
[28] M. Rosenblum, S.A. Herrod, E. Witchel, A. Gupta, Complete computer system simulation: the SimOS approach, IEEE Concurrency 3 (1995) 34–43.
[29] M. Vachharajani, N. Vachharajani, D.A. Penry, A. Blo Jason, S. Malik, D.I. August, The liberty simulation environment: a deliberate approach to high-level system modeling, ACM Trans. Comput. Syst. 24 (2006) 211–249.
[30] R. Lantz, Parallel SimOS: Scalability and performance for large system simulation, Ph.D. Thesis, Stanford University, 2007.
[31] Red Hat Inc. Red hat's sid. http://sourceware.org/sid/sid-guide.pdf, 2001.
[32] M.T. Yourst, PTLsim: a cycle accurate full system x86-64 microarchitectural simulator, in: ISPASS, IEEE Computer Society, San Jose, CA, 2007, pp. 23–34.
[33] H. Zeng, M. Yourst, K. Ghose, D. Ponomarev, MPTLsim: a cycle-accurate, full-system simulator for x86-64 multicore architectures with coherent caches, SIGARCH Comput. Archit. News 37 (2) (2009) 2–9.
[34] C.J. Mauer, M.D. Hill, D.A. Wood, Full-system timing-first simulation, SIGMETRICS Perform. Eval. Rev. 30 (1) (2002) 108–116.
[35] T.F. Wenisch, R.E. Wunderlich, B. Falsafi, J.C. Hoe. TurboSMARTS: accurate microarchitecture simulation sampling in minutes, Technical Report, SIGMETRICS Performance Evaluation Review, 2005.
[36] P.J. Mucci, S. Browne, C. Deane, G. Ho, PAPI: a portable interface to hardware performance counters, in: Proceedings of the Department of Defense HPCMP Users Group Conference, 1999, pp. 7–10.
[37] S.L. Graham, P.B. Kessler, M.K. McKusick, gprof: a call graph execution profiler (with retrospective), in: Best of PLDI, 1982, pp. 49–57.
[38] J. Levon, P. Elie, OProfile. http://oprofile.sourceforge.net, 2003.
[39] Z. Aral, Ilya Gertner, Parasight: a high-level debugger/profiler architecture for shared-memory multiprocessor, in: Proceedings of the 2nd International Conference on Supercomputing, ICS '88, ACM, New York, NY, 1988, pp. 131–139.
[40] Advance Micro Devices, AMD CodeAnalyst Performance Analyzer. http://developer.amd.com/tools/CodeAnalyst, April, 2012.
[41] S. Jarp, R. Jurga, A. Nowak, Perfmon2: a leap forward in performance monitoring, J. Phys. Conf. Ser. 119 (4) (2008) 042017.
[42] T.E. Anderson, E.D. Lazowska, Quartz: a tool for tuning parallel program performance, SIGMETRICS Perform. Eval. Rev. 18 (1990) 115–125.
[43] Intel, Intel VTune. http://software.intel.com/en-us/intel-vtune-amplifier-xe, 2013.
[44] A. Srivastava, A. Eustace, Atom: A System for Building Customized Program Analysis Tools, ACM, New York, NY, 1994, pp. 196–205.
[45] N. Tallent, J. Mellor-Crummey, L. Adhianto, M. Fagan, M. Krentel, HPCToolkit: performance tools for scientific computing, J. Phys. Conf. Ser. 125 (1) (2008) 012088.
[46] C.-K. Luk, R. Cohn, R. Muth, H. Patil, A. Klauser, G. Lowney, S. Wallace, V.J. Reddi, K. Hazelwood, Pin: building customized program analysis tools with

dynamic instrumentation, in: Programming Language Design and Implementation, ACM Press, New York, USA, 2005, pp. 190–200.

[47] S.S. Shende, A.D. Malony, The Tau parallel performance system, Int. J. High Perform. Comput. Appl. 20 (2006) 287–311.

[48] GDB, GDB: the GNU project debugger. http://www.sourceware.org/gdb.com, 2013.

[49] B. Buck, J.K. Hollingsworth, An API for runtime code patching, Int. J. High Perform. Comput. Appl. 14 (2000) 317–329.

[50] M. Schulz, J. Galarowicz, W. Hachfeld, Open SpeedShop: open source performance analysis for Linux clusters, in: Proceedings of the 2006 ACM/IEEE Conference on Supercomputing, SC '06, ACM, New York, NY, 2006.

[51] Allinea, Allinea DDT. http://www.allinea.com/products/ddt, 2002.

[52] T. Romer, G. Voelker, D. Lee, A. Wolman, W. Wong, H. Levy, B. Bershad, B. Chen, Instrumentation and optimization of Win32/Intel executables using etch, in: Proceedings of the USENIX Windows NT Workshop, 1997, pp. 1–7.

[53] ZIH TU Dresden, VampirTrace. http://www.tu-dresden.de/die_tu_dresden/ zentrale_einrichtungen/zih/forschung/software_werkzeuge_zur_unterstuetzung_von_ programmierung_und_optimierung/vampirtrace, 2007.

[54] J.R. Larus, E. Schnarr, EEL: machine-independent executable editing, in: Proceedings of the ACM SIGPLAN 1995 Conference on Programming Language Design and Implementation, PLDI '95, ACM, New York, NY, 1995, pp. 291–300.

[55] N. Nethercote, J. Seward, Valgrind: a framework for heavyweight dynamic binary instrumentation, SIGPLAN Not. 42 (2007) 89–100.

[56] D.L. Bruening, Efficient, transparent and comprehensive runtime code manipulation, Technical Report, 2004.

[57] D. Bruening, T. Garnett, S. Amarasinghe, An infrastructure for adaptive dynamic optimization, in: Proceedings of the International Symposium on Code Generation and Optimization: Feedback-Directed and Runtime Optimization, CGO '03, IEEE Computer Society, Washington, DC, 2003, pp. 265–275.

[58] C. Cifuentes, M. Van Emmerik, UQBT: adaptable binary translation at low cost, Computer 33 (3) (2000) 60–66.

[59] M. Fernández, R. Espasa, Dixie: a retargetable binary instrumentation tool, in: Proceedings of the Workshop on Binary Translation, 1999.

[60] J. Souloglou, A, Rawsthorne, Dynamite: a framework for dynamic retargetable binary translation. Technical Report, The University of Manchester, March 1997.

[61] T. Janjusic, K. Kavi, B. Potter, International Conference on Computational Science, ICCS 2011 Gleipnir: A Memory Analysis Tool, Procedia Computer Science, vol. 4, 2011, pp. 2058–2067.

[62] W. Cheng, Q. Zhao, B. Yu, S. Hiroshige, Tainttrace: efficient flow tracing with dynamic binary rewriting, in: Proceedings of the 11th IEEE Symposium on Computers and Communications, ISCC '06, IEEE Computer Society, Washington, DC, 2006, pp. 749–754.

[63] D. Bruening, Q. Zhao, Practical memory checking with Dr. Memory, in: Proceedings of the 9th Annual IEEE/ACM International Symposium on Code Generation and Optimization, CGO '11, IEEE Computer Society, Washington, DC, 2011, pp. 213–223.

[64] Q. Zhao, J.E. Sim, W.F. Wong, L. Rudolph, DEP: detailed execution profile, in: PACT '06: Proceedings of the 15th International Conference on Parallel Architectures and Compilation Techniques, ACM Press, Seattle, Washington, USA, 2006, pp. 154–163.

[65] J. Hollingsworth, B.P. Miller, J. Cargille, Dynamic Program Instrumentation for Scalable Performance Tools, IEEE Computer Society, Los Alamitos, CA, USA, 1994, pp. 841–850.

[66] W. Korn, P.J. Teller, G. Castillo, Just how accurate are performance counters? in: IEEE International Conference on Performance, Computing, and Communications, April 2001, 2001, pp. 303–310.

[67] B. Nikolic, Z. Radivojevic, J. Djordjevic, V. Milutinovic, A survey and evaluation of simulators suitable for teaching courses in computer architecture and organization, IEEE Trans. Educ. 52 (4) (2009) 449–458.

[68] M.M.K. Martin, D.J. Sorin, B.M. Beckmann, M.R. Marty, M. Xu, A.R. Alameldeen, K.E. Moore, M.D. Hill, D.A. Wood, Multifacet's general execution-driven multiprocessor simulator (gems) toolset, SIGARCH Comput. Archit. News 33 (2005) 92–99.

[69] V. Puente, J.A. Gregorio, R. Beivide, Sicosys: an integrated framework for studying interconnection network performance in multiprocessor systems, in: Proceedings of the 10th Euromicro Workshop on Parallel, Distributed and Network-Based Processing, 2002, pp. 15–22.

[70] K. Skadron, M.R. Stan, W. Huang, S. Velusamy, K. Sankaranarayanan, D. Tarjan, Temperature-aware microarchitecture, in: Proceedings of the 30th Annual International Symposium on Computer Architecture, June, 2003, pp. 2–13.

[71] T. Wada, S. Rajan, S.A. Przybylski, An analytical access time model for on-chip cache memories, IEEE J. Solid-State Circuits 27 (8) (1992) 1147–1156.

ABOUT THE AUTHORS

Dr. Tomislav Janjusic received his Bachelor of Science in Computer Science from Henderson State University in 2006 and a Ph.D. in Computer Science and Engineering in 2013 from the University of North Texas. Dr. Janjusic joined Oak Ridge National Laboratory in Oak Ridge Tennessee as a postdoctoral research associate in July 2013. His main focus is on application performance analysis and communication library development. Dr. Janjusic's research area is in computer systems with emphasis on computer architecture, memory allocation techniques, cache system performance, and parallel computing.

Dr. Krishna Kavi is currently a Professor of Computer Science and Engineering and the Director of the NSF Industry/University Cooperative Research Center for Net-Centric Software and Systems at the University of North Texas. During 2001–2009, he served as the Chair of the department. Previously, he was on the faculty of University of Alabama in Huntsville and the University of Texas at Arlington. His research is primarily on Computer Systems Architecture including multithreaded and multicore processors, cache memories, and hardware-assisted memory managers. He also conducted research in the area of formal methods, parallel processing, and real-time systems. He published more than 150 technical papers in these areas. He received his Ph.D. from Southern Methodist University in Dallas Texas and a BS in EE from the Indian Institute of Science in Bangalore, India.

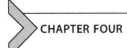

CHAPTER FOUR

Model Transformation Using Multiobjective Optimization

Mohamed Wiem Mkaouer, Marouane Kessentini
SBSE Laboratory, CIS Department, University of Michigan, Michigan, USA

Contents

Abstract

The evolution of languages and software architectures provides a strong motivation to migrate/transform existing software systems. Thus, more attention is paid to the transformation aspects in model-driven engineering (MDE) along with the growing importance of modeling in software development. However, a major concern in MDE is how to ensure the quality of the model transformation mechanisms. Most of existing work in model transformation has relied on defining languages to express transformation rules. The main goal of existing transformation approaches is to provide rules generating target models, from source models, without errors. However, other important objective is how to minimize the complexity of transformation rules (e.g., the number of rules and number of matching in the same rule) while maximizing the quality of target models. In fact, reducing rule complexity and improving target model quality are important to (1) make rules and target models easy to understand and evolve, (2) find transformation errors easily, and (3) generate optimal target models. In this chapter, we consider the transformation mechanism as a multiobjective problem where the goal is to find the best rules maximizing target model quality and minimizing rule complexity. Our approach starts by randomly generating a set of rules, executing them to generate some target models. Of course, only solutions ensuring full correctness are considered during the optimization process. Then, the quality of the proposed solution (rules) is evaluated by (1) calculating the number of rules and matching metamodels in each rule and (2) assessing the quality of generated target models using a set of quality metrics. To this end, we use the nondominated sorting genetic algorithm (NSGA-II) to automatically generate the best transformation rules satisfying the two conflicting criteria. We report the results of our validation using three different transformation mechanisms. The best solutions provided well-designed target models with a minimal set of rules.

1. INTRODUCTION

Model transformation plays an important role in model-driven engineering (MDE) [1]. The research efforts by the MDE community have produced various languages and tools [2–5] for automating transformations between different formalisms using mapping rules. These transformation rules can be implemented using general programming languages such as Java or C#, graph transformation languages like AGG [2] and the VIsual Automated model TRAnsformations (VIATRA) [3], or specific languages such as ATLAS Transformation Language (ATL) [4, 5] and the Query/View/Transformation (QVT) [6]. Sometimes, transformations are based on invariants (preconditions and postconditions specified in languages such as the Object Constraint Language (OCL) [7]).

One major challenge is to automate transformations while preserving the quality of the produced models [1]. Thus, the main goal is to reduce the number of possible errors when defining transformation rules. These transformation errors have different causes such as transformation logic (rules) or source/target metamodels. Existing approaches and techniques have been successfully applied to transformation problems with a minimum number of errors. Especially at the model level, correctness is the gold standard characteristic of models: it is essential that the user understands exactly how the target model deviates from fidelity to the source model in order to be able to rely on any results. However, other important objectives are how to minimize the complexity of transformation rules (e.g., the number of rules and number of matching in the same rule) while maximizing the quality of target models to obtain well-designed ones. In fact, reducing rule complexity and improving target model quality are important to (1) make rules and target models easy to understand and evolve, (2) find transformation errors easily, and (3) generate optimal target models.

The majority of existing approaches [1, 2, 5] formulate the transformation problem as a single-objective problem that maximizes rule correctness. In this case, the proposed transformation rules produce target models without errors. However, these rules are sometimes complex (e.g., size) and applying them may generate very large target model, for example, complex transformation rules in mapping from dynamic Unified Modeling Language (UML) models to colored Petri nets (CPN); their systematic application will generally results in large PNs [8]. This could compromise the subsequent analysis tasks, which are generally limited by the number of the PN states. Obtaining large PNs is not usually related to the size of the source models but to the rule complexity [9]. In addition, it is important to take into consideration the quality of produced target models (e.g., maximizing good design practices by reducing the number of bad smells [10] in a generated class diagram (CLD) from a relational schema (RS)). Another category of approaches [11, 12] proposes an additional step to minimize complexity, using refactoring operations [13, 14], after generating transformation rules. However, it is a difficult and fastidious task to modify, evolve, and improve quality of already generated complex rules.

In this chapter, to overcome some of the previously mentioned limitations, we propose to alternatively view transformation rule generation as a multiobjective problem. We generate solutions matching the source metamodel elements to their equivalent target ones, taking into consideration two objectives: (1) minimizing rule complexity and (2) maximizing target model quality. We start by randomly generating a set of rules, executing them on different source models to generate some target models, and then evaluate the quality of the proposed solution (rules). Of course, during the optimization process, we select only solutions ensuring full correctness (generating correct target models/rules). Correctness is the gold standard characteristic of models: it is essential that the user understand exactly how the target model deviates from fidelity to the source model in order to be able to rely on any results. To ensure the transformation correctness, we used a list of constraints to satisfy when generating target models. For the first objective, it calculates the number of rules and number of matching metamodels in each rule (one-to-one, many-to-one, etc.). For the second objective, we use a set of software quality metrics [15] to evaluate the quality of generated target models. To search for solutions, we selected and adapted, from the existing multiobjective evolutionary algorithms [16], the nondominated sorting genetic algorithm (NSGA-II) [17]. NSGA-II aims to find a set of representative Pareto-optimal solutions in a single run. In our case, the evaluation of these solutions is based on the two mentioned conflicting criteria.

The primary contributions of the chapter can be summarized as follows:

1. We introduce a new approach for model transformation using multi-objective techniques. Our proposal does not require to define rules manually, but only to input a set of source models and equivalent target models (without traceability links); it generates well-designed target models/rules without the need to refactor them; it takes into consideration the complexity of the generated rules; and it can be applied to any source or target metamodels (independent from source and target languages). However, different limitations are discussed in Section 6.3.

2. We report the results of an evaluation of our approach; we used three different transformation mechanisms to evaluate our proposal: CLDs to RS and vice versa and sequence diagrams (SDs) to CPN. The generated rules for both mechanisms achieved high-quality scores with a minimal set of rules.

The rest of this chapter is organized as follows. Section 2 is dedicated to the related work, while Section 3 describes the problem statement. The overview of our multiobjective proposal is described in Section 4. Section 5 explains the experimental method, the results of which are discussed in Section 6. The chapter concludes with Section 7.

2. STATE OF THE ART

2.1. Model Transformation Languages

Kleppe *et al.* [18] provide the following definition of model transformation, as illustrated in Fig. 4.1: a transformation is the automatic generation of a target model from a source model, according to a transformation definition. A transformation definition is a set of transformation rules that describe together how a model in the source language can be transformed into a model in the target language. A transformation rule is a description of how one or more constructs in the source language can be transformed into one or more constructs in the target language.

In the following, a classification of endogenous transformation (model-to-model) approaches is briefly reported. Then, some of the available

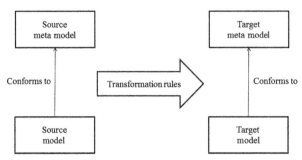

Figure 4.1 Model transformation process.

endogenous transformation languages are separately described. The classification is mainly based upon [18, 19]. Several endogenous transformation approaches have been proposed in the literature. In the following, classifications of model-to-model endogenous transformation approaches discussed by Czarnecki and Helsen [18, 19] are described.

2.1.1 Direct Manipulation Approach

It offers an internal model representation and some Application Programming interfaces (API) to manipulate it. It is usually implemented as an object-oriented framework, which may also provide some minimal infrastructure. Users have to implement transformation rules, scheduling, tracing, and other facilities in a programming language.

An example of used tools in direct manipulation approaches is Builder Object Network (BON), a framework that is relatively easy to use and is still powerful enough for most applications. BON provides a network of C++ objects. It provides navigation and update capabilities for models using C++ for direct manipulation.

2.1.2 Operational Approach

It is similar to direct manipulation but offers more dedicated support for model transformation. A typical solution in this category is to extend the utilized metamodeling formalism with facilities for expressing computations. An example would be to extend a query language such as OCL with imperative constructs. Examples of systems in this category are Embedded Constraint Language [20], QVT Operational Mappings [21], XMF [22], MTL [23], and Kermeta [24].

2.1.3 Relational Approach

It groups declarative approaches in which the main concept is mathematical relations. In general, relational approaches [25] can be seen as a form of constraint solving. The basic idea is to specify the relations among source and target element types using constraints that, in general, are nonexecutable. However, the declarative constraints can be given executable semantics, such as in logic programming where predicates can describe the relations. All of the relational approaches are side effect-free and, in contrast to the imperative direct manipulation approaches, create target elements implicitly. Relational approaches can naturally support multidirectional rules. They sometimes also provide backtracking. Most relational approaches require strict separation between source and target models, that is, they do not allow in-place update. Examples of relational approaches are QVT Relations and ATL [26]. Moreover, in Ref. [3], the application of logic programming has been explored for the purpose.

2.1.4 Graph Transformation-Based Approach

They exploit theoretical work on graph transformations and require that the source and target models be given as graphs [27]. Performing model transformation by graph transformation means to take the abstract syntax graph of a model and to transform it according to certain transformation rules. The result is the syntax graph of the target model. More precisely, graph transformation rules have an LHS and an RHS graph pattern. The LHS pattern is matched in the model being transformed and replaced by the RHS pattern in place. In particular, LHS represents the preconditions of the given rule, while RHS describes the postconditions. $LHS \cap RHS$ defines a part that has to exist to apply the rule, but that is not changed. $LHS - LHS \cap RHS$ defines the part that shall be deleted, and $RHS - LHS \cap RHS$ defines the part to be created. The LHS often contains conditions in addition to the LHS pattern, for example, negative conditions. Some additional logic is needed to compute target attribute values such as element names. Graph Rewriting and Transformation Language (GReAT) [28] and AToM3 [29] are systems directly implementing the theoretical approach to attributed graphs and transformations on such graphs. They have built-in fixed-point scheduling with nondeterministic rule selection and concurrent application to all matching locations.

Mens and Van Gorp [30] provide a taxonomy of model transformations. One of the main differences with the previous taxonomy is that Czarnecki and Helsen propose a hierarchical classification based on feature diagrams, while the Mens *et al.* taxonomy is essentially multidimensional. Another important difference is that Czarnecki *et al.* classify the specification of model transformations, whereas Mens *et al.* taxonomy is more targeted toward tools, techniques, and formalisms supporting the activity of model transformation.

For these different categories, many languages and tools have been proposed to specify and execute exogenous transformation programs. In 2002, the Object Management Group (OMG) issued the Query/View/Transformation request for proposal [21] to define a standard transformation language. Even though a final specification was adopted at the end of 2008, the area of model transformation continues to be a subject of intense research. Over the last years, in parallel to the OMG effort, several model transformation approaches have been proposed from both academia and industry. They can be distinguished by the used paradigms, constructs, modeling approaches, tool support, and suitability for given problems. We briefly describe next some well-known languages and tools.

ATL [5] is a hybrid model transformation language that contains a mixture of declarative and imperative constructs. The former allows dealing with simple model transformations, while the imperative part helps in coping with transformations of higher complexity. ATL transformations are unidirectional, operating on read-only source models and producing write-only target models. During the execution of a transformation, source models may be navigated through, but changes are not allowed. Transformation definitions in ATL form modules. A module contains a mandatory header section, import section, and a number of helpers and transformation rules. There is an associated ATL Development Toolkit available as open source from the GMT Eclipse Modeling Project [31]. A large library of transformations is available at Ref. [4].

GReAT [32] is a metamodel-based graph transformation language that supports the high-level specification of complex model transformation programs. In this language, one describes the transformations as sequenced graph rewriting rules that operate on the input models and construct an output model. The rules specify complex rewriting operations in the form of a matching pattern and a subgraph to be created as the result of the application of a rule. The rules (1) always operate in a context that is a specific subgraph of the input and (2) are explicitly sequenced for efficient execution. The rules are specified visually using a graphical model builder tool called the Generic Modeling Environment (GME) [33].

AGG is a development environment for attributed graph transformation systems that support an algebraic approach to graph transformation. It aims at specifying and rapid prototyping applications with complex, graph-structured data. AGG supports typed graph transformations including type inheritance and multiplicities. It may be used (implicitly in "code") as a general-purpose graph transformation engine in high-level Java applications employing graph transformation methods.

The source, target, and common metamodels are represented by type graphs. Graphs may additionally be attributed using Java code. Model transformations are specified by graph rewriting rules that are applied non-deterministically until none of them can be applied anymore. If an explicit application order is required, rules can be grouped in ordered layers. AGG features rules with negative application conditions to specify patterns that prevent rule executions. Finally, AGG offers validation support that is consistency checking of graphs and graph transformation systems according to graph constraints, critical pair analysis to find conflicts between rules (that could lead to a nondeterministic result), and checking of termination criteria for graph transformation systems. An available tool support provides graphical editors for graphs and rules and an integrated textual editor for Java expressions. Moreover, visual interpretation and validation are supported.

VIATRA2 [3] is an eclipse-based general-purpose model transformation engineering framework intended to support the entire life cycle for the specification, design, execution, validation, and maintenance of transformations within and between various modeling languages and domains. Its rule specification language is a unidirectional transformation language based mainly on graph transformation techniques. More precisely, the basic concept in defining model transformations within VIATRA2 is the (graph) pattern. A pattern is a collection of model elements arranged into a certain structure fulfilling additional constraints (as defined by attribute conditions or other patterns). Patterns can be matched on certain model instances, and upon successful pattern matching, elementary model manipulation is specified by graph transformation rules. There is no predefined order of execution of the transformation rules. Graph transformation rules are assembled into complex model transformations by abstract state machine rules, which provide a set of commonly used imperative control structures with precise semantics.

VIATRA2 is a hybrid language since the transformation rule language is declarative, but the rules cannot be executed without an execution strategy that should be specified in an imperative manner. Important specification features of VIATRA2 include recursive (graph) patterns, negative patterns with arbitrary depth of negation, and generic and meta-transformations (type parameters and rules manipulating other rules) for providing reuse of transformations.

A conclusion to be drawn from studying the existing endogenous transformation approaches, tools, and techniques is that they are often based on empirically obtained rules [34]. In fact, the traditional and common approach toward implementing model transformations is to specify the transformation rules and automate the transformation process by using an executable model transformation language. Although most of these languages are already powerful enough to implement large-scale and complex model transformation tasks, they may present challenges to users, particularly to those who are unfamiliar with a specific transformation language. Firstly, even though declarative expressions are supported in most model transformation languages, they may not be at the proper level of abstraction for an end user and may result in a steep learning curve and high training cost. Moreover, the transformation rules are usually defined at the metamodel level that requires a clear and deep understanding about the abstract syntax and semantic interrelationships between the source and target models. In some cases, domain concepts may be hidden in the metamodel and difficult to unveil (e.g., some concepts are hidden in attributes or association ends, rather than being represented as first-class entities). These implicit concepts make writing transformation rules challenging. Thus, the difficulty of specifying transformation rules at the metamodel level and the associated learning curve may prevent some domain experts from building model transformations for which they have extensive domain experience.

To address these challenges inherited from using model transformation languages, an innovative approach called model transformation by example (MTBE) is proposed that will be described in the Section 2.2.

2.2. Model Transformation by Example

Examples play a key role in the human learning process. There are numerous theories on learning styles in which examples are used. For a description of today's popular learning style theories, see Refs. [35, 36].

Our work is based on using past transformation examples. Various "by-example" approaches have been proposed in the software engineering literature [37].

What does by example really mean? What do all by-example approaches have in common? The main idea, as the name already suggests, is to give the software examples of how things are done or what the user expects and let it do the work automatically. In fact, this idea is closely related to fields such as machine learning or speech recognition. Common to all by-example approaches is the strong emphasis on user-friendliness and a "short" learning curve. According to Baudry *et al.* [38], the by-example paradigm dates back to 1970—see "Learning Structure Descriptions from Examples" in Ref. [39].

Programming by example [36] is the best-known by-example approach. It is a technique for teaching the computer a new behavior by demonstrating actions on concrete examples. The system records user actions and generalizes a program that can be used for new examples. The generalization process is mainly based on user responses to queries about user intentions. Another well-known approach is query by example (QBE) [40]. It is a query language for relational databases that are constructed from filled sample tables with examples: rows and constraints. QBE is especially suited for queries that are not too complex and can be expressed in terms of a few tables. In web engineering, Lechner and Schrefl [41] present the language TBE (XML transformers by example) that allows defining transformers for WebML schemes by example, that is, stating what is desired instead of specifying the operations to get it. Advanced XSLT tools are also capable of generating XSLT scripts using examples from schema levels (like MapForce from Altova) or document (instance)-level mappings (such as the pioneering XSLerator from IBM Alphaworks or the more recent Stylis Studio).

The problems addressed by the previously mentioned approaches are different from ours in both the nature and the objectives.

The commonalities of the by-example approaches for transformation can be summarized as follows: All approaches define an example as a triple consisting of an input model and its equivalent output model and trace between the input and output model elements. These examples have to be established by the user, preferably in a concrete syntax. Then, generalization techniques such as hard-coded reasoning rules, inductive logic, or relational concept analysis are used to derive model transformation rules from the examples, in a deterministic way that is applicable for all possible input models that have a high similarity with the predefined examples.

Varro and Balogh [42, 43] propose a semiautomated process for MTBE using inductive logic programming. The principle of their approach is to derive transformation rules semiautomatically from an initial prototypical set of interrelated source and target models. Another similar work is that of Wimmer *et al.* [44] that derives ATL transformation rules from examples of business process models. Both contributions use semantic correspondences between models to derive rules. Their differences include the fact that [44] presents an object-based approach that finally derives ATL rules for model transformation, while [45] derives graph transformation rules. Another difference is that they, respectively, use an abstract versus a concrete syntax: Varro uses IPL when Wimmer relies on an *ad hoc* technique. Both models are heavily dependent on the source and target formalisms. Another similar approach is that of Dolques *et al.* [46] that aims to alleviate the writing of transformations and where engineers only need to handle models in their usual (concrete) syntax and to describe the main cases of a transformation, namely, the examples. A transformation example includes the source model, the target model, and trace links that make explicit how elements from the source model are transformed into elements of the target model. The transformation rules are generated from the transformation traces, using formal concept analysis extended by relations, and they are classified through a lattice that helps navigation and choice. This approach requires the examples to cover all the transformation possibilities and it is only applicable for one-to-one transformations.

Recently, a similar approach to MTBE, called model transformation by demonstration (MTBD), was proposed [47]. Instead of the MTBE idea of inferring the rules from a prototypical set of mappings, users are asked to demonstrate how the MT should be done, through direct editing (e.g., add, delete, connect, and update) of the source model, so as to simulate the transformation process. A recording and inference engine was developed, as part of a prototype called MT-Scribe, to capture user operations and infer a user's intention during an MT task. A transformation pattern is then generated from the inference, specifying the preconditions of the transformation and the sequence of operations needed to realize the transformation. This pattern can be reused by automatically matching the preconditions in a new model instance and replaying the necessary operations to simulate the MT process. However, this approach needs a large number of simulated patterns to be efficient, and it requires a high level of user intervention. In fact, the user must choose the suitable transformation pattern. Finally, the authors do not show how MTBD can be useful to transform an entire source model and only provide examples of transforming model fragments. On the other hand, the MTBD approach, in contradiction with other by-example approaches, is applied to endogenous transformations.

Another very similar by demonstration approach was proposed by Langer *et al.* [48]. The difference from Sun *et al.*'s work, which uses the recorded fragments directly, is that Langer *et al.* use them to generate ATL rules. Another difference is that the Langer approach is related to exogenous transformation.

Brosch *et al.* [49] introduced a tool for defining composite operations, such as refactorings, for software models in a user-friendly way. This by-example approach prevents modelers from acquiring deep knowledge about the metamodel and dedicated model transformation languages. However, this tool is only able to apply refactoring operations and does not detect automatically refactoring operations.

The commonalities of the by-example approaches for the exogenous transformation can be summarized as follows: All approaches define an example as a triple consisting of an input model and its equivalent output model and trace between the input and output model elements. The examples have to be established by the user, preferably in a concrete syntax. Then, generalization techniques such as hard-coded reasoning rules, inductive logic, or relational concept analysis are used to derive model transformation rules from the examples, in a deterministic way that is applicable to all possible input models that have a high similarity with the predefined examples.

None of the mentioned approaches claims that the generation of the model transformation rules is correct or complete. In particular, all approaches explicitly state that some complex parts of the transformation involving complex queries, attribute calculations such as aggregation of values, nondeterministic transformations, and counting of elements have to be developed by the user, by changing the generated model transformations. Furthermore, the approaches recommend developing the model transformations using an iterative methodology. This means that, after generating the transformations from initial examples, these examples can be adjusted or the transformation rules should be changed if the user is not satisfied with the outcome. However, in most cases, deciding that the examples or the transformation rules need changing is not an obvious process to the user.

2.3. Traceability-Based Model Transformation

Some other metamodel matching works can also be considered as variants of by-example approaches. Garcia-Magarino *et al.* [11] propose an approach to generate transformation rules between two metamodels that satisfy some manually introduced constraints by the developer. In Ref. [50], the authors propose to automatically capture some transformation patterns in order to generate matching rules at the metamodel level. This approach is similar to MTBD, but it is used at the metamodel level.

Most current transformation languages [11, 51, 52] build an internal traceability model that can be interrogated at execution time, for example, to check if a target element was already created for a given source element. This approach is specific to each transformation language and sometimes to the individual transformation specification. The language determines the traceability metamodel, and the transformation specification determines the label of the traces (in case of QVT/relational, the traceability metamodel is deduced from the transformation specification). The approach taken only provides an access to the traces produced within the scope of the current transformation. Marvie describes a transformation composition framework [53] that allows manual creation of linkings (traces). These linkings can then be accessed by subsequent transformation, although this is limited to searching specific traces by name, introducing tight coupling between subtransformations.

In order to transform models, they need to be expressed in some modeling language (e.g., UML for design models and programming languages for source code models). The syntax and semantics of the modeling language itself are expressed by a metamodel (e.g., the UML metamodel). Based on the language in which the source and target models of a transformation are expressed, a distinction can be made between endogenous and exogenous transformations.

2.4. Search-Based Software Engineering

Our approach is largely inspired by contributions in search-based software engineering (SBSE). SBSE is defined as the application of search-based approaches to solve optimization problems in software engineering [54]. Once a software engineering task is framed as a search problem, there are numerous approaches that can be applied to cope with that problem, from local searches such as exhaustive search and hill climbing to metaheuristic searches such as genetic algorithms (GAs) and ant colony optimization [55].

Many contributions have been proposed for various problems, mainly in cost estimation, testing, and maintenance [40, 56]. Module clustering, for example, has been addressed using exhaustive search [55], GAs [56], and simulated annealing (SA) [57]. In those studies that compared search techniques, hill climbing was perhaps surprisingly found to produce better results than metaheuristic GA searches. Model verification has also been addressed using search-based techniques. Shousha *et al.* [58] propose an approach to detect deadlocks in UML models, but the generation of a new quality predictive model, starting from a set of existing ones by using SA, is probably the problem that is the most similar to MT by examples. In that work, the model is also decomposed into fine-grained pieces of expertise that can be combined and adapted to generate a better prediction model. To the best of our knowledge, inspired among others by the road map paper of Harman [56], the idea of treating model transformation as a combinatorial optimization problem to be solved by a search-based approach was not studied before our proposal.

2.5. Summary

This section has introduced the existing work in different domains related to our work. The closest work to our proposal is MTBE. Once the examples have been established, generalization techniques, such as hard-coded reasoning rules, inductive logic [43], or relational concept analysis or pattern, are used to derive model transformation rules from the examples, in a deterministic way that is applicable for all possible input models that have a high similarity with the predefined examples.

Table 4.1 summarizes an existing transformation by-example approaches according to given criteria. The majority of these approaches are specific to exogenous transformation and based on the use of traceability.

One conclusion to be drawn from studying the existing by-example approaches is that they use semiautomated rule generation, with the

Table 4.1 By-Example Approaches

By-Example Approaches	Exogenous Transformation	Endogenous Transformation	Traceability	Rule Generation
[43]	X		X	X
[44]	X		X	X
[47]		X	X	
[46]	X		X	X
[48]	X		X	X
[49]		X	X	

generated rules further refined by the user. In practice, this may be a lengthy process and require a large number of transformation examples to assure the quality of the inferred rules. In this context, the use of search-based optimization techniques can be a more preferable transformation approach since it directly generates the target model from the existing examples, without using the rule step. This also leads to a higher degree of automation than existing by-example approaches.

As shown in Section 2.4, like many other domains of software engineering, MDE is concerned with finding exact solutions to these problems or those that fall within a specified acceptance margin. Search-based optimization techniques are well suited for the purpose. For example, when testing model transformations, the use of deterministic techniques can be unfeasible due to the number of possibilities to explore for test case generation, in order to cover all source metamodel elements. However, the complex nature of MDE problems sometimes requires the definition of complex fitness functions [59]. Furthermore, the definition is specific to the problem to solve and necessitate expertise in both search-based and MDE fields. It is thus desirable to define a generic fitness function, evaluating a quality of a solution that can be applied to various MDE problems with low adaptation effort and expertise.

To tackle these challenges, our contribution combines search-based and by-example techniques. The difference with case-based reasoning approaches is that many subcases can be combined to derive a solution, not just the most adequate case. In addition, if a large number of combinations have to be investigated, the use of search-based techniques becomes beneficial in terms of search speed to find the best combination.

3. MOTIVATIONS AND PROBLEM STATEMENT

In this section, we emphasize the motivations of our work and the specific problems that are addressed by our multiobjective approach.

3.1. Defining Transformation Rules

Although there is a consensus about the necessity of defining transformation rules, our experience with industrial partners showed that there are many open issues that need to be addressed when defining a transformation mechanism. Sometimes, the transformation may not be obvious to realize, due to different reasons [9]. The process of defining rules manually for model transformation is complex, time-consuming, and error-prone. Thus, we need to define an automated solution to generate rules automatically instead of the manual process. One solution is to propose a semiautomated approach for a rule generation in order to help the designer. In the majority of existing approaches, the rules are generated from traceability links interrelating different source and target model examples. However, defining traces is a fastidious task because they are manually defined. Generating transformation rules can be difficult since the source and target languages may have elements with different semantics; therefore, one-to-one mappings are not often sufficient to express the semantic equivalence between metamodel elements. Indeed, in addition, to ensure structural (static) coherence, the transformation should guarantee a behavioral coherence in terms of time constraints and weak sequencing. In addition, various rule combination possibilities may be used to transform between the same source and target languages: how to choose between different possible rule combinations having the same correctness.

3.2. Reducing Transformation Complexity

In general, the majority of existing transformation approaches generates transformation rules without taking into consideration complexity (but only correctness). In such situations, applying these rules could generate large target models, it is difficult to test complex rules and detect/correct transformation errors, and it is a fastidious task to evolve complex rules (modifying the transformation mechanism) when the source or target metamodels are modified. Some transformation approaches [12, 60, 61] propose to refactor the rules after defining them. However, it is difficult to manipulate and modify complex rules. For this reason, it is better to optimize the complexity when generating the rules.

3.3. Improving Transformation Quality

The majority of model maintenance work [10, 12, 62, 63] is concerned with the detection and correction of bad design fragments, called design defects or bad smells, after the generation of target models [8]. Design defects refer to design situations that adversely affect the development of models [2]. In Ref. [62], Beck defines 22 sets of symptoms of common defects. For UML CLDs, these include large classes, feature envy, long parameter lists, and lazy classes. In most of the existing model transformation work, the main goal is to generate correct target models. The quality of target models is not considered when generating transformation rules. However, it is important to ensure that generated transformation rules provide well-designed target models with a minimum number of bad smells. Otherwise, each target model should be revised to improve its design quality, which can be a fastidious task. In fact, detecting and fixing design defects is, to some extent, a difficult, time-consuming, and manual process [8].

4. APPROACH OVERVIEW

This section shows how the previously mentioned issues can be addressed using our proposal. This section starts by presenting an illustration of an example of the transformation mechanism. Then, we provide an overview of the approach and we discuss the computational complexity of our problem.

A model transformation mechanism takes as input a model to transform, the source model, and produces as output another model, the target model. The source and target models must conform to specific metamodels and, usually, relatively complex transformation rules are defined to ensure this.

We can illustrate this definition of the model transformation mechanism with the case of CLD-to-RS transformation. Our choice of CLD-to-RS transformation is motivated by the fact that it is well known and reasonably complex; this allows us to focus on describing the technical aspects of our approach. In Section 6, we show that our approach can also be applied to more complex transformations such as SDs to CPNs [64].

Figure 4.2A shows a simplified metamodel of the UML CLD, containing concepts like class, attribute, and relationship between classes. Figure 4.2B shows a partial view of the RS metamodel, composed of table, column, attribute, etc. The transformation mechanism, based on rules, will then specify how the persistent classes, their attributes, and their associations should be transformed into tables, columns, and keys.

Figure 4.3 shows the example of a source model, as CLD containing four classes and two association links, and its related target model.

The associated target model is expressed as an RS. Four classes are mapped to tables (Client, Order, Order details, and Product). The two association links become foreign keys. Finally, attributes in subclasses are mapped into columns of the derived table from the parent class. The CLD-to-RS transformation is used to illustrate our approach described in the rest of this chapter.

The general structure of our approach is introduced in Fig. 4.4. The following two sections give more details about our proposals.

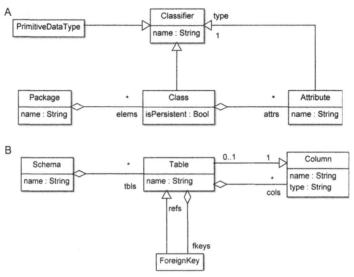

Figure 4.2 Class diagram and relational schema metamodels. (A) Class diagram metamodel. (B) Relational schema metamodel.

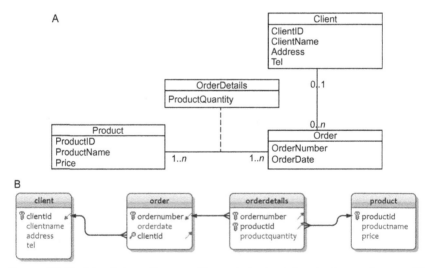

Figure 4.3 Models of class diagram with equivalent relational schema diagram. (A) Class diagram example. (B) Relational schema diagram example. (For color version of this figure, the reader is referred to the online version of this chapter.)

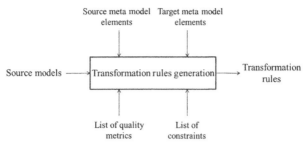

Figure 4.4 Overview of the approach: General architecture.

As described in Fig. 4.4, the number of source models and the expected target ones is used to generate the transformation rules. In fact, our approach takes as inputs a set of source models with their equivalent target models, a list of quality metrics, and another list of constraints (to ensure transformation correctness) and takes as controlling parameters a list of source and target metamodel elements. Our approach generates a set of rules as output.

The rule generation process combines source and target metamodel elements within rule expressions. Some logical expressions (union OR and intersection AND) can be used to combine between metamodel elements. Consequently, a solution to the transformation problem is a set of rules that transforms well the source models to target models within the satisfaction of the list of all transformation constraints. For example, the following rule states that a class is transformed to a table with the same name having a primary key:

> R1: IF Class(A) THEN Table(A) AND Column(idA, A, pk).

In this example of a rule, a class, a table, and a primary key column correspond to some extracted elements from the source and target metamodels. The first part of the rule contains only elements from the source metamodel. Consequently, the second part of the rule contains only elements from the target metamodel.

To ensure the transformation correctness when generating transformation rules, the idea is that the transformation of source models into target models is coupled with a contract consisting of pre- and postconditions. Hence, the transformation is tested with a range of source models that satisfy the preconditions to ensure that it always yields target models that satisfy the postconditions. If the transformation produces an output model that violates a postcondition, then the contract is not satisfied and the transformation needs to be corrected. The contract is defined at the metamodel level and conditions are generally expressed in OCL. We used these constraints as input in our approach.

After ensuring the transformation correctness, our multiobjective optimization process uses two criteria to evaluate the generated solutions. The first criterion consists of minimizing the rule complexity by reducing the number of rules and the number of matching metamodels in each rule. The second criterion consists of maximizing the quality of generated target models, based on different quality metrics. Quality metrics provide useful information that helps in assessing the level of conformance of a software system to a desired quality such as *evolvability* and *reusability*. For instance, Ehrig *et al.* and Marinescu [12, 63] propose different metrics to evaluate the quality of RSs such as depth of relational tree of a table T that is defined as the longest referential path between tables, from the table T to any other table in the schema database; referential degree of a table T (RD(T)) consisting of the number of foreign keys in the table T; percentage of complex columns metric of a table T; and size of a schema (SS) defined as the sum of the tables size (TS) in the schema.

We selected also a set of quality metrics that can be applied on CLDs as target models. These metrics include number of associations (Naccoc), the total number of associations; number of aggregations (Nagg), the total number of aggregation relationships; number of dependencies (Ndep), the total number of dependency relationships; number of generalizations (Ngen), the total number of generalization relationships (each parent–child pair in a generalization relationship); number of aggregations hierarchies, the total number of aggregation hierarchies; number of generalization hierarchies, the total number of generalization hierarchies; and maximum DIT, the maximum of the DIT (depth of inheritance tree) values for each class in a CLD. The DIT value for a class within a generalization hierarchy is the longest path from the class to the root of the hierarchy; number of attributes (NA), the total number of attributes; number of methods (LOCMETHOD), the total number of methods; and number of private attributes (NPRIVFIELD), number of private attributes in a specific class.

During the multiobjective optimization process, our approach combines randomly source and target metamodel elements within logical expressions (union OR and intersection AND) to create rules. In this case, the number n of possible combinations is very large. The rule generation process consists of finding the best combination between m source metamodel elements and k target metamodel elements. In addition, a huge number of possibilities to execute the transformation rules exist (rule execution sequence). In this context, the number NR of possible combinations that have to be explored is given by $NR = ((n + k)!)^m$.

This value quickly becomes huge. Consequently, the rule generation process is a combinatorial optimization problem. Since any solution must satisfy two criteria (complexity and quality), we propose to consider the search as a multiobjective optimization problem instead of a single-objective one. To this end, we propose an adaptation of the NSGA-II proposed in Ref. [17]. This algorithm and its adaptation are described in Section 5.

5. MULTIOBJECTIVE MODEL TRANSFORMATION

In this section, we describe the NSGA-II that is used to generate model transformation rules. After ensuring transformation correctness, this algorithm takes into consideration two objectives: (1) minimizing rule complexity (number of rules and number of matching metamodels in each rule) and (2) maximizing target model quality using quality metrics.

5.1. NSGA-II Overview

The NSGA-II is a powerful search method. It is stimulated by natural selection that is inspired from the theory of Darwin. Hence, the basic idea is to make a population of candidate solutions evolving toward the best solution in order to solve a multiobjective optimization problem. NSGA-II was designed to be applied to an exhaustive list of candidate solutions, which creates a large search space.

The main idea of the Pareto NSGA-II is to calculate the Pareto front that corresponds to a set of optimal solutions, so-called nondominated solutions, or also Pareto set. A nondominated solution is the one that provides a suitable compromise between all objectives without degrading any of them. Indeed, the concept of Pareto dominance consists of comparing each solution x with every other solution in the population until it is dominated by one of them. If any solution does not dominate it, the solution x will be considered nondominated and will be selected by the NSGA-II to be one of the set of Pareto front. If we consider a set of objectives f_i, $i \in 1, \ldots, n$, to maximize, a solution x dominates x' if $\forall i, f_i(x') \leq f_i(x)$ and $\exists j \mid f_j(x') < f_j(x)$.

The first step in NSGA-II is to create randomly the initial population P_0 of individuals encoded using a specific representation. Then, a child population Q_0 is generated from the population of parents P_0 using genetic operators such as crossover and mutation. Both populations are merged and a subset of individuals is selected basely on the dominance principle to create the next generation. This process will be repeated until it reaches the last iteration according to stop criteria.

To be applied, NSGA-II needs to specify some elements that have to be considered in its implementation: (1) the representation of individuals used to create a population, (2) a fitness function according to each objective to evaluate the candidate solutions, and (3) the crossover and mutation operators that have to be designed according to the individual's representation. In addition, a method to select the best individuals has to be implemented to create the next generation of individuals. The result of NSGA-II is the best individuals (with highest fitness scores), produced along all generations. In the following sections, we show how we adapted all of these concepts to guide our search-based transformation approach.

5.2. NSGA-II Adaptation

We adapted NSGA-II to the problem of generating transformation rules, taking into consideration both complexity and model quality dimensions. We consider each one of these criteria as a separate objective for NSGA-II. The algorithm's pseudocode is given in Fig. 4.5.

As Fig. 4.5 has shown, the algorithm takes as input a set of source and target metamodel elements and a set of source models and its equivalent target ones. Lines 1–5 construct an initial based population on a specific representation, using the list of metamodel elements, given at the inputs. Thus, the initial population stands for a set of possible transformation rule solutions that represents a set of source and target metamodel elements, selected and combined randomly. Lines 6–30 encode the main NSGA-II loop whose goal is to make a population of candidate solutions that evolve toward the best rule combination, that is, the one that minimizes as much as possible the number of rules and matching metamodels in the same rule and maximizes the target model quality by improving quality metric values. During each iteration t, a child population Q_t is generated from a parent generation P_t (line 7) using genetic operators. Then, Q_t and P_t are assembled in order to create a global population R_t (line 8). After that, each solution S_i in the population R_t is evaluated using the two fitness functions, complexity and quality (lines 11–18):

- Complexity function (line 13) calculates the number of rules and matching metamodels in each rule.
- Quality function (line 14) represents the quality score of based target models on a combination of quality metrics.

Input : Source metamodel elements SMM

Input : Target metamodel elements TMM

Input : source models SM

Input: Correctness constraints CC

Input: Quality metrics QM

Output : Near-optimal transformation rules

1: initialize_population(P, Max_population)

2: P_0:= set_of(S)

3: S:= set_of(Rules:SMM:TMM)

4: SM:= Source_Models

5: iteration:=0

6: repeat

7:    Q_t:= Gen_Operators(P_t)

8:    R_t:=P_t U Q_t

9:    for all $S_i \in R_t$ do

10:       TM:= execute_rules(Rules, SM);

11:        Correctness(S_i) := calculate_constraints_coverage(SM, TM, CC);

12:        if (Correctness(S_i) ==1) then

13:            Complexity(S_i) := calculate_complexity(Rules);

14:            QualityModels(S_i) := calculate_qualityModels(TM, QM);

15:        else

16:            Complexity(Si) == 0;

17:            QualityModels(Si) == 0;

18:        End if

19:    end for

20:    F:=fast-non-dominated-sorting(R_t)

21:    P_{t+1} :=Ø

22:    while |P_{t+1}|<Max_size

23:        F_i := crowding_distance_assignment(F_i)

24:        P_{t+1} := P_{t+1}+F_i

25:    end while

26:    P_{t+1} :=P_{t+1}[0:Max_size]

27:    iteration:= iteration +1;

28: until (iteration ==max_iterations)

29: best_solutions = Pareto_front(R_t)

30: return best_solutions

Figure 4.5 High-level pseudocode for NSGA-II adaptation to our problem.

These two functions take the value 0 if the transformation correctness is not ensured. The correctness function (line 11) represents the percentage of source/target metamodel constraints that are satisfied by the proposed solution S_i. We consider during the optimization process only solutions that satisfy all correctness constraints.

Once quality and complexity are calculated, solutions are sorted in order to return a list of nondominated fronts F (line 20). When the whole current population is sorted, the next population P_{t+1} will be created using solutions that are selected from sorted fronts F (lines 21–26). When two solutions are in the same front, that is, same dominance, they are sorted by the crowding distance, a measure of density in the neighborhood of a solution. The algorithm terminates (line 28) when it achieves the termination criterion (maximum iteration number). The algorithm returns the best solutions that are extracted from the first front of the last iteration (line 29).

We give more details in the following subsections about the representation of solutions, genetic operators, and fitness functions.

5.2.1 Solution Representation

An individual is a set of declarative IF–THEN rules. To ease the manipulation of the source and target metamodels and their transformation, the metamodels are described using a set of predicates that corresponds to the included element. For example, Fig. 4.6 shows the rule interpretation of an individual containing two rules. So, the mapping between predicates *Class* (A) and *Table* (A) indicates that the class A is transformed to a table with the same name.

Similarly, the mapping between *Association(1,n,1,n,N,A, B)* and *Table(N)* *AND Column(idA, N,pfk)* *AND Column(idB, N,pfk)* indicates that the association link N is transformed to a table with the same name containing two primary foreign keys *pfk*, *idA* and *idB* that are primary keys, respectively, in tables A and B.

Consequently, a transformation rule has the following structure:

```
IF "Combination of source metamodel elements" THEN "Combination of
target metamodel elements"
```

> Rule 1 : Class(A) THEN Table(A)
>
> Rule 2 : Association(1,n,1,n,N,A, B). THEN Table(N) AND Column(idA, N,pfk)
>
> AND Column(idB, N,pfk).

Figure 4.6 Rule interpretation of an individual.

As shown in Fig. 4.6, the IF clause contains a combination of source metamodel elements. These elements are combined using logic operators (AND and OR). Consequently, THEN clauses highlight the equivalent target metamodel elements. Some other additional rules determine the sequence of applying transformation rules.

One of the most suitable computer representations of rules is based on the use of trees. In our case, the rule interpretation of an individual will be handled by a tree representation, which is composed of two types of nodes: terminals and functions. The terminals (leaf nodes of a tree) correspond to source or target metamodel elements. The functions that can be used between these elements correspond to logical operators, which are union (OR) and intersection (AND).

Consequently, the rule interpretation of the individual of Fig. 4.6 has the following tree representation of Fig. 4.7. The sequence of applying the rules is determined randomly.

5.2.2 Generation of an Initial Population

To generate an initial population, we start by defining the maximum tree length including the number of nodes and levels. Because the individuals

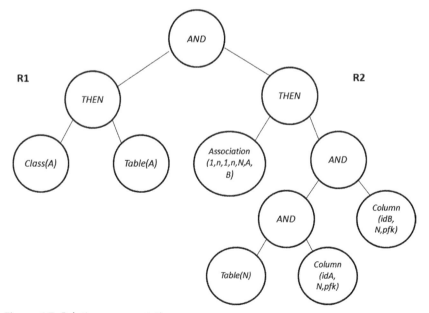

Figure 4.7 Solution representation.

will evolve with different tree lengths (structures), we randomly assign for each one:
- One source or target metamodel element to each terminal node
- A logic operator (AND or OR) to each function node

5.2.3 Selection and Genetic Operations

5.2.3.1 Selection

There are many selection strategies where fittest individuals are allocated more copies in the next generations than the other ones. Thus, to guide the selection process, NSGA-II uses a comparison operator, based on a calculation of the crowding distance, to select potential individuals to construct a new population P_{t+1}. Furthermore, for our initial prototype, we used stochastic universal sampling (SUS) to derive a child population Q_t from a parent population P_t, in which each individual's probability of selection is directly proportional to its relative overall fitness value (average score of the two fitness values) in the population. We use SUS to select elements from P_t that represents the best elements to be reproduced in the child population Q_t using genetic operators such as mutation and crossover.

5.2.3.2 Crossover

Two parent individuals are selected, and a subtree is picked on each one. Then, the crossover operator swaps the nodes and their relative subtrees from one parent to the other. Each child thus combines information from both parents.

Figure 4.8 shows an example of the crossover process. In fact, the rule R1 and a rule R2 are combined to generate two new rules. The right subtree of R1 is swapped with the left subtree of R2.

As result, after applying the cross operator, the new rule R1 will be:

`Rule 1: Class(A) THEN Table(A).`

`Rule 2: Association (1,n,1,n,N,A, B). THEN Table(N) AND Column(idA, N,pfk) AND Column(idB, N,pfk).`

5.2.3.3 Mutation

The mutation operator can be applied to either function or terminal nodes. This operator can modify one or many nodes. Given a selected individual, the mutation operator first randomly selects a node in the tree representation of the individual. Then, if the selected node is a terminal (source or target metamodel element), it is replaced by another terminal (another metamodel element).

If the selected node is a function (e.g., AND operator), it is replaced by a new function (i.e., AND becomes OR). If a tree mutation is to be carried out, the node and its subtrees are replaced by a new randomly generated subtree.

To illustrate the mutation process, consider again the example that corresponds to a candidate rule. Figure 4.9 illustrates the effect of a mutation to

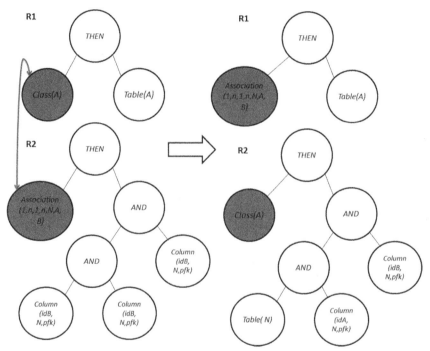

Figure 4.8 Crossover operator. (For color version of this figure, the reader is referred to the online version of this chapter.)

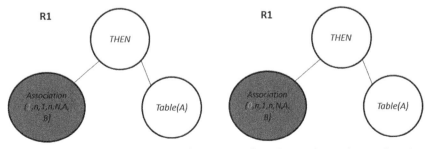

Figure 4.9 Mutation operator. (For color version of this figure, the reader is referred to the online version of this chapter.)

modify the metamodel element association link in the rule R1. Thus, after applying the mutation operator, the new rule R1 will be:

```
Rule 1: Association (0,n,0,n,N,A, B). THEN Table(A).
```

When the crossover and mutation operators are executed, many pre- and postconditions should be satisfied to ensure that the rule modifications are valid. We specified these conditions for each metamodel element.

5.2.4 Multicriteria Evaluation

In the majority of existing work, the fitness function evaluates a generated solution by verifying its ability to ensure transformation correctness. In our case, in addition to ensuring transformation correctness, we define two new fitness functions in our NSGA-II adaptation: (1) rule complexity and (2) target model quality.

To ensure transformation correctness, different constraints are defined manually including two parts: pre- and postconditions. The preconditions constrain the set of valid models and the postconditions declare a set of properties that can be expected on the output model. For example, a table should contain at least one primary key or a foreign key should be a primary key in another table. As described in Fig. 4.4, the transformation correctness constraints are verified before evaluating the rule complexity and model quality. If the proposed solution generates correct transformation rules, then complexity and quality criterion can be evaluated. Thus, the correctness C parameter takes 1 if all constraints are satisfied otherwise 0:

$$C = \begin{cases} 1, & \text{if all transformation correctness constraints are satisfied} \\ 0, & \text{otherwise} \end{cases}$$

5.2.4.1 Complexity Criterion

In our approach, we define the complexity function, to minimize, as the sum of number of generated rules and number of metamodel elements in each rule:

$$f_1 = c^*(n+m) \tag{4.1}$$

where n is the number of rules to define and m is the number of metamodel elements in the same rule. Of course, the complexity function takes 0 if the transformation correctness is not ensured $(c=0)$.

5.2.4.2 Quality Criterion

The quality criterion is evaluated using the fitness function given in Eq. (4.2). The quality value increases when the metric values (m_i) are in the range of well-designed model thresholds ($m_{i,\text{best\_minOrmax}}$). This function, to minimize, returns a real value that represents the difference between good metric values (expected) and those extracted from the generated target models. The choice of good metric thresholds is based on our previous works in model quality improvements:

$$f_2 = \sum_{i=0}^{\text{nbMetrics}} \text{Min}\left(\left|m_{i,\min} - m_i\right|, \left|m_{i,\max} - m_i\right|\right) \qquad (4.2)$$

In this case, the quality of generated target models is maximized when f_2 is minimized. To illustrate the fitness function, we consider that a solution generated contains these four rules:

R1: IF Class(A) THEN Table(A) AND Column(idA,A,pk).

R2: IF Attribute(a,A) THEN Column(a,A,_).

R3: IF Association(0,1,0,n,N,A,B) THEN Column(idA,B,fk).

R4: IF Association(1,n,1,n,N,A, B) THEN Table(N) AND Column(idA,idB, N,pfk).

To evaluate this solution, let us consider the CLD source model of Fig. 4.3A. After executing this set of four rules, we obtain the RS target model of Fig. 4.3B. We consider, for example, that the correctness is ensured based on two constraints: (C1) each table should contain, at least, one primary key; and (C2) a foreign key in a table A should be a primary key in another table B. To evaluate the design quality of target models, we use two quality metrics:

- RD(T) consists of the number of foreign keys in the schema: $m_{1,\text{best}} = (\min = 1; \max = 3)$.
- SS defined as the sum of the TS in the schema: $m_{2,\text{best}} = (\min = 3; \max = 5)$.

In such scenario, the parameters of the complexity fitness function take the following values: $c = 1$ since both correctness constraints are satisfied by the target model; $n = 4$, which corresponds to the number of rules; and $m = 3 + 2 + 2 + 3 = 10$ (*number of matching metamodels*). Thus, the complexity score of the generated solution is

$$f_1 = 1^*(4 + 10) = 14$$

Regarding the quality dimension, based on Fig. 4.3B, RD and SS take, respectively, the values 3 $(0 + 1 + 2 + 0)$ and 4. Thus, the quality fitness function is defined as follows:

$$f_2 = \text{Min}(|1 - 3|, |3 - 3|) + \text{Min}(|3 - 4|, |5 - 4|) = 0 + 1 = 1$$

6. VALIDATION

To evaluate the feasibility of our approach, we conducted an experiment with three transformation mechanisms. We start by presenting our research questions. Then, we describe and discuss the obtained results.

6.1. Research Questions

Our study addresses two research questions, which are defined here. We also explain how our experiments are designed to address them. The goal of the study is to evaluate the efficiency of our approach for generating correct transformation rules while minimizing rule complexity and maximizing the quality of generated target models. The three research questions are then:

- RQ1: To what extent can the proposed approach minimize rule complexity?
- RQ2: To what extent can the proposed approach maximize the quality of generated target models?
- RQ3: To what extent can the proposed multiobjective approach perform compared to mono-objective search algorithms?

To answer RQ1, we compared the complexity of the generated rules with expected ones that are defined manually: number of rules and number of elements in each rule.

To answer RQ2, the transformation result is checked for quality using two methods: (1) we calculate the dissimilarity between reference metric threshold and those related to generated target models and (2) we evaluate the variation in terms of size between generated target models using NSGA-II and those provided manually by experts.

To answer RQ3, we implemented a mono-objective GA where the goal is to generate a minimal set of correct transformation rules (one objective is used, which is the complexity). Then, we compared the results to those generated by our NSGA-II approach; the comparison is based on complexity and quality criteria.

6.2. Settings

To evaluate the feasibility of our approach, we conducted an experiment on generating rules for CLD to RS and vice versa (RS to CLD) and SD to CPN. We used 12 large class diagrams with their equivalent RSs. The examples were provided by an industrial partner. The size of the CLDs varied from 28 to 92 model elements, with an average of 58. In addition, we collected the transformations of 10 SDs to SDs from the Internet and textbooks. We ensured by manual inspection that all the transformations are valid. The size of the SDs varied from 16 to 57 constructs, with an average of 36. The 10 SDs contained many complex fragments: loop, alt, opt, par, region, neg, and ref.

As described in Section 2, we selected a set of 12 quality metrics for CLD, 9 for RS, and 2 for CPN (number of places and transitions). Based on our previous work, we define the threshold range for each of those metrics. As described previously, we implemented a set of constraints to ensure the correctness of generated target models during the optimization process.

6.3. Results and Discussions

In this section, we present the answer to each research question in turn, indicating how the results answer each. Figure 4.10 shows the rule complexity and target model quality for all the three transformation mechanisms, based on the two fitness function values. These two fitness functions, to minimize, correspond to (1) complexity, the number of rules and matching metamodels in each rule and (2) dissimilarity, the difference between the solution-calculated metric values and the reference metric values; so, decreasing the dissimilarity will increase the solution's quality. For all the transformation mechanisms, different solutions generate well-designed target models with a minimal set of rules.

As shown in Fig. 4.10, NSGA-II converges to Pareto-optimal solutions that are considered as good compromises between quality and complexity. In this figure, each point is a solution with the complexity score represented in the x-axis and the dissimilarity score (deviation from reference metric threshold) in the y-axis. The best solutions exist in the middle representing the Pareto front that minimizes dissimilarity with reference metric threshold and the rule complexity. The user can choose a solution from this front depending on his preferences in terms of compromise. However, at least for our validation, we need to have only one best solution that will be suggested by our approach. To this end and in order to fully automate

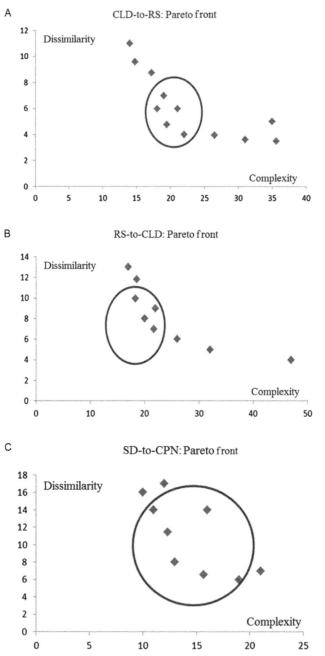

Figure 4.10 Pareto front optimal solutions. (A) CLD-to-RS transformation results. (B) RS-to-CLD transformation results. (C) SD-to-CPN transformation results. (For color version of this figure, the reader is referred to the online version of this chapter.)

our approach, we propose to extract and suggest only one best solution from the returned set of solutions. Equation (4.3) is used to choose the solution that corresponds of the best compromise between quality and complexity. Hence, we select the nearest solution to the ideal one in terms of Euclidian distance:

$$\text{bestSol} = \operatorname*{Min}_{i=0}^{n} \left(\sqrt{(\text{Dissimilarity } [i])^2 + (\text{Complexity } [i])^2} \right) \qquad (4.3)$$

where n is the number of solutions in the Pareto front returned by NSGA-II.

Since the two objectives of quality and complexity are conflicting/contradicting, the results of Fig. 4.10 confirm that a solution that scores better in complexity is better than any other solution that is of lower quality.

As described in Figs. 4.10 and 4.11, the majority of proposed transformation rules generate good quality of target models with minimal complexity compared to those provided manually by experts or a mono-objective GA. For all the three transformation mechanisms, the dissimilarity of generated target models using NSGA-II is lower than those generated by the manual and GA methods, which means that NSGA-II quality is much better than the other transformation mechanisms. In fact, when experts write rules manually, they did not take into consideration, in general, the quality of produced models but only the correctness. Since the mono-objective algorithm has considered only correctness when generating transformation rules, then, it is evident that NSGA-II performs better in terms of target model quality. The generated rules using NSGA-II are less complex than those generated by an expert for all the three transformation mechanisms. In fact, experts ensure that the rules are correct as a main goal. However, GA provides less complex rules for CLD to RS and RS to CLD than our NSGA-II algorithm. This can be explained by the reason that these two transformation mechanisms are not complex. However, with more complex transformation mechanisms, such as SD to CPN, it is difficult to obtain a minimal set of rules without specifying complexity as a separate objective in addition to correctness. In addition, based on NSGA-II algorithm, we can sacrifice a small complexity decrease to improve the quality of generated target models.

Figure 4.11 shows that, in general, we generate, approximately, the same number of rules for all transformation mechanisms. The number of generated rules is comparable to those provided by our expert in terms of number of matching metamodels. The different generated rules are verified manually and we did not find any errors.

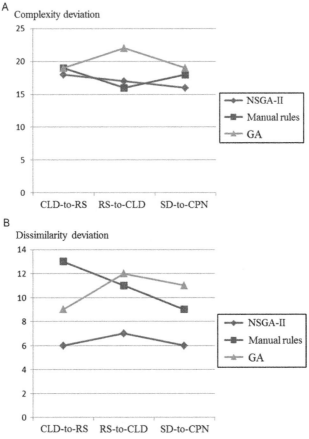

Figure 4.11 Comparison between NSGA-II, manually defined rules and GA. (For color version of this figure, the reader is referred to the online version of this chapter.)

As described in Figs. 4.10 and 4.11, the average of quality deviation, from reference metric values, for all transformed source models is low. This is confirming the good quality of generated target models. After a manual investigation of the results, we found that most of quality deviation is due to the bad quality of source models to transform. In conclusion, our approach produces good refactoring suggestions, both from the point of views of complexity and target model quality. The generated rules might vary depending on search space exploration, since solutions are randomly generated, though guided by a metaheuristic. To ensure that our results are relatively stable, we compared the results of multiple executions for NSGA-II as shown in Fig. 4.12; we, consequently, believe that our technique is stable, since the quality and complexity scores are approximately the same for different executions (each fold).

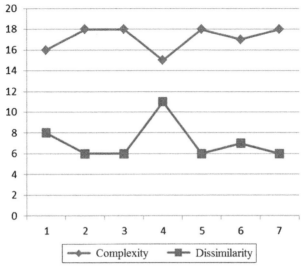

Figure 4.12 An example of seven executions on CLD-to-RS (best solutions). (For color version of this figure, the reader is referred to the online version of this chapter.)

Since we viewed the maintainability defects correction problem as a combinatorial problem addressed with heuristic search, it is important to contrast the results with the execution time. We executed our algorithm on a standard desktop computer (i7 CPU running at 4 GHz with 4 GB of RAM). The execution time for finding the optimal rules with a number of iterations (stopping criteria) fixed to 1000 was <1 h. This indicates that our approach is reasonably scalable from the performance standpoint. However, the execution time depends on the source and target metamodels.

As described in Table 4.2, we used the CPN-SD transformation mechanism to compare between the quality of the generated CPNs using mono–objective GA (minimizing only rule complexity) and multiobjective approach.

When developing our approach, we conjectured that the multiobjective approach produces CPNs less complex/better quality (e.g., in size) than the one obtained by a mono-objective approach. Table 4.2 compares the obtained CPN sizes by using both approaches for the 10 source models to transform.

The size of a CPN is defined by the number of elements. In all cases, a reduction in size occurs when using our multiobjective approach, with an average reduction of 13% in comparison with mono-objective. The obtained results confirm our assumption that systematic application of rules using a mono-objective approach results in larger CPNs.

Table 4.2 Complexity Comparison

CPN Size (Mono-objective)	CPN Size (Multiobjective)	Variation (%)
13	11	15
22	19	14
24	24	0
31	26	17
36	33	9
39	29	25
44	37	16
52	43	18
54	46	15
Average variation		13

7. CONCLUSION

In this chapter, we introduced a new multiobjective approach for generating model transformation rules. Our algorithm starts by randomly generating a set of rules, executing them to generate some target models, and then evaluates the complexity by reducing the number of generated rules and the quality of generated target models, based on some quality metric thresholds. Our approach differs from rule-based transformation approaches as it does not require writing rules. To our best knowledge, our proposal represents the first work that uses multiobjective techniques to automated model transformations. It also differs from existing by-example approaches by the fact that no traceability links are needed in the examples.

We have evaluated our approach on three transformation mechanisms. The experimental results indicate that the quality of derived target models is comparable and sometimes better than those defined by experts in the base of examples in terms of correctness with a minimal set of rules.

Finally, we discussed some limitations and open research directions that were related to our proposal. First, all our performance contribution depends on the availability of examples, which could be difficult to collect. However, as we have shown in the experiments, only few examples are needed to obtain good results. Second, due to the nature of our solution, that is, an optimization technique, the process could be time-consuming for large models. Furthermore, as we use heuristic algorithms, different executions for the same input could lead to different outputs. This can be a disadvantage for some MDE applications, for example, when a model transformation is required to be a deterministic process and the generated target model is unique. Nevertheless, having different and equivalent output models is close to what happens in the real world where different experts may propose different target models.

Different future work directions can be explored. The application of new search-based techniques like artificial immune system to model evolution or model refactoring is challenging. We are working on an extension of our first contribution about exogenous transformation by example. The idea is to generate transformation rules from examples using heuristic search. Our approach starts by randomly generating a set of rules, executing them to generate some target models. Then, it evaluates the quality of the proposed solution (rules) by comparing the generated target models to the expected ones in the base of examples. In this case, the search space is large and a heuristic search is needed.

We are actually working to extend our proposal to other problems. A new technique for predicting "buggy" changes, when modifying an existing version of a model, can be proposed. The idea is to classify the changes as clean or not. The change classification determines whether a new model change is more similar to prior "buggy" or clean changes in the base of examples. In this manner, a change classification can predict the existence of "bugs" in model changes.

Furthermore, we are working on a transformation composition using examples. We propose a solution based on a music-inspired approach. We draw an analogy between the transformation composition process and finding the best harmony when composing music. Say, for example, that we have a transformation mechanism M1 that transforms formalism T1 into T2, but the metamodel of T2 evolved into T3, after deleting or adding elements. We want to generate new transformation rules that transform T1 into T3. The idea is to compose two transformation mechanisms T1 to T2 and T2 to T3. To this end, we propose to view the transformation rule generation as an optimization problem where rules are automatically derived from available examples. Each example corresponds to a source model and its corresponding target model, without transformation traces from T1 to T3. Our approach starts by composing a set of rules (T1 to T2 and T2 to T3), executing them to generate some target models, and then evaluating the quality of the proposed solution (rules) by comparing the generated target models and the expected ones in the base of examples.

REFERENCES

[1] R. France, B. Rumpe, Model-driven development of complex software: a research roadmap, in: L. Briand, A. Wolf (Eds.), International Conference on Software Engineering: Future of Software Engineering, IEEE Computer Society Press, Los Alamitos, 2007.

[2] G. Taentzer, AGG: a graph transformation environment for modeling and validation of software, applications of graph transformations with industrial relevance, Springer, Berlin, Heidelberg, vol. 3062, 2004, pp. 446–453.

[3] D. Varro, A. Pataricza, Generic and meta-transformations for model transformation engineering, The Unified Modeling Language. Modelling Languages and Applications, in: T. Baar, A. Strohmeier, A. Moreira, S.J. Mellor (Eds.), vol. 3273, 2004, pp. 290–304.

[4] ATLAS Group, The ATLAS Transformation Language. http://www.eclipse.org/gmt, 2000.

[5] F. Jouault, I. Kurter, Transforming models with ATL, in: Proceedings of the International Conference on Satellite Events at the MoDELS (MoDELS), Jean-Michel Bruel (Ed.), Springer-Verlag, Berlin, Heidelberg, 2005, pp. 128–138.

[6] Compuware, SUN. MOF 2.0 Query/Views/Transformations RFP, Revised Submission. OMG Document ad/2003-08-07. http://www.omg.org/cgi-bin/doc?ad/2003-08-07, 2003.

[7] T. Clark, J. Warmer, Object modeling with the OCL, in: The Rationale Behind the Object Constraint Language, vol. 2263, Springer, London, 2002.

[8] O. Ribeiro, J. Fernandes, Some rules to transform sequence diagrams into coloured Petri nets, in: K. Jensen (Ed.), Workshop and Tutorial on Practical Use of Coloured Petri Nets and the CPN Tools, Aarhus, 2006, pp. 237–256.

[9] A. Ouardani, P. Esteban, M. Paludetto, J. Pascal, A meta-modeling approach for sequence diagrams to Petri nets transformation, in: The European Simulation and Modeling Conference, 2006, pp. 345–349.

[10] A. Ouni, M. Kessentini, H.A. Sahraoui, M. Boukadoum, Maintainability defects detection and correction: a multi-objective approach, Journal of Automated Software Engineering (JASE), Springer, US, vol. 20, 2013, pp. 47–79.

[11] I. Garcia-Magarino, J.J. Gomez-Sanz, R.F. Ferandez, Model transformation by-example: an algorithm for generating many-to-many transformation rules in several model transformation languages, in: International Conference on Theory and Practice of Model Transformations, Berlin, 2009, pp. 52–66.

[12] H. Ehrig, K. Ehrig, C. Ermel, Refactoring of model transformations, in: Graph Transformation and Visual Modeling Techniques, 2009.

[13] K. Dhambri, H.A. Sahraoui, P. Poulin, Visual detection of design anomalies, in: IEEE European Conference on Software Maintenance and Reengineering, 2008, pp. 279–283.

[14] S. Forrest, A.S. Perelson, L. Allen, R. Cherukuri, Self-nonself discrimination in a computer, in: IEEE Symposium on Security and Privacy, Washington, 1994, pp. 202–212.

[15] M. Harman, J.A. Clark, Metrics are fitness functions too, in: IEEE Metrics, 2004, pp. 58–69.

[16] E. Zitzler, L. Thiele, Multiobjective optimization using evolutionary algorithms: a comparative case study, IEEE Transactions on Evolutionary Computation, vol. 3(4), 1999, pp. 257–271

[17] K. Deb, A. Pratap, S. Agarwal, T. Meyarivan, A fast and elitist multiobjective genetic algorithm: NSGA-II, IEEE Trans. Evol. Comput. 6 (2002) 182–197.

[18] G. Kleppe, J. Warmer, W. Bast, MDA Explained: The Model Driven Architecture: Practice and Promise, Addison-Wesley, Boston, 2003.

[19] K. Czarnecki, S. Helsen, Classification of model transformation approaches, in: OOSPLA Workshop on Generative Techniques in the Context of Model-Driven Architecture, Anaheim, 2003.

[20] J. Gray, Aspect-Oriented Domain-Specific Modeling: A Generative Approach Using a Meta-weaver Framework, (Ph.D. thesis), Vanderbilt University, 2002.

[21] OMG, MOF 2.0 Query/Views/Transformation RFP, 2002.

[22] Xactium. Xmf-mosaic. http://xactium.com.

[23] D. Vojtisek, J. Jézéquel, MTL and Umlaut NG: engine and framework for model transformation, in: INRIA Technical Report, 2004.

[24] J. Falleri, M. Huchard, C. Nebut, Towards a traceability framework for model transformations in Kermeta, in: The European Conference on MDA Traceability Workshop, Bilbao, 2006.

[25] D.H. Akehurst, S. Kent, A relational approach to defining transformations in a metamodel, in: J.M. Jézéquel, H. Hussmann, S. Cook (Eds.), The Unified Modeling Language 5th International Conference, Dresden, vol. 2460, 2002, pp. 243–258.

[26] F. Jouault, F. Allilaire, J. Bézivin, I. Kurtev, ATL: a model transformation tool, Science of Computer Programming, vol. 72, 2008, pp. 31–39.

[27] M. Andries, G. Engels, A. Habel, B. Hoffmann, H.J. Kreowski, S. Kuske, D. Kuske, D. Plump, A. Schürr, G. Taentzer, Graph transformation for specification and programming, in: Technical Report 7/96, Universität Bremen, 1996.

[28] G. Karsai, Lessons learned from building a graph transformation system, in: Graph Transformations and Model-Driven Engineering, 2010, pp. 202–223.

[29] J. De Lara, H. Vangheluwe, AToM3: a tool for multi-formalism and meta-modelling, Fundamental Approaches to Software Engineering, Springer, Berlin, Heidelberg, vol. 2306, 2002, pp. 174–188.

[30] T. Mens, P. Van Gorp, A taxonomy of model transformation, Electronic Notes in Theoretical Computer Science, vol. 152, 2006, pp. 125–142.

[31] Eclipse. Generative Modeling Technologies (GMT) Project, 2006.

[32] A. Agrawal, G. Karsai, S. Neema, F. Shi, A. Vizhanyo, The design of a language for model transformations, Software & Systems Modeling, Springer-Verlag, vol. 5, 2006, pp. 261–288.

[33] A. Lédeczi, A. Bakay, M. Maroti, P. Völgyesi, G. Nordstrom, J. Sprinkle, G. Karsai, Composing domain-specific design environments, IEEE Computer Society Press, Los Alamitos, vol. 34, 2001, pp. 44–51.

[34] A.F. Egyed, Heterogeneous View Integration and Its Automation, (Ph.D. Dissertation) University of Southern California, Los Angeles, 2000.

[35] P. Baker, M. Harman, K. Steinhofel, A. Skaliotis, Search based approaches to component selection and prioritization for the next release problem, in: IEEE International Conference on Software Maintenance, Washington, 2006, pp. 176–185.

[36] A. Repenning, C. Perrone, Programming by example: programming by analogous examples, Commun. ACM 43 (2000) 90–97.

[37] M. Kessentini, H.A. Sahraoui, M. Boukadoum, Example-based model-transformation testing, Automat. Softw. Eng. 2 (2011) 199–224.

[38] B. Baudry, F. Fleurey, J. Jézéquel, Y. Le Traon, Automatic test cases optimization using a bacteriological adaptation model: application to NET components, in: IEEE International Conference on Automated Software Engineering, Washington, 2006, pp. 253–256.

[39] O. Cinnéide, P. Nixon, Automated software evolution towards design patterns, in: International Workshop on Principles of Software Evolution, New York, 2001, pp. 162–165.

[40] R. Krishnamurthy, S.P. Morgan, M. Zloof, Query-by-example: operations on piecewise continuous data (extended abstract), in: Proceedings of the 9th International Conference on Very Large Data Bases (VLDB '83), Mario Schkolnick and Costantino Thanos (Eds.), Morgan Kaufmann Publishers Inc., San Francisco, CA, USA, 1983, pp. 305–308.

[41] S. Lechner, M. Schrefl, By-example schema transformers for supporting the process of conceptual web application modelling, in: Technical Report TR0301, University of Linz, Austria, 2003.

[42] D. Varro, Model transformation by example, in: Model Driven Engineering Languages and Systemsvol. 4199, 2006, pp. 410–424.

[43] D. Varro, Z. Balogh, Automating model transformation by example using inductive logic programming, in: ACM Symposium on Applied Computing | Model Transformation Track, 2007.

[44] M. Wimmer, M. Strommer, H. Kargl, G. Kramler, Towards model transformation generation by-example, in: Proceedings of HICSS-40 Hawaii International Conference on System Sciences, Hawaii, 2007.

[45] H. Alikacem, H. Sahraoui, Détection d'anomalies utilisant un langage de description de règle de qualité, in: actes du 12e colloque LMO, 2006.

[46] X. Dolques, M. Huchard, C. Nebut, P. Reitz, Learning transformation rules from transformation examples: an approach based on relational concept analysis, in: IEEE EDOC Workshops and Short Papers, 2010.

[47] Y. Sun, J. White, J. Gray, Model transformation by demonstration, in: Model Driven Engineering Languages and Systems, vol. 5795, Springer, Berlin, Heidelberg, 2009, pp. 712–726.

[48] P. Langer, M. Wimmer, G. Kappel, Model-to-model transformations by demonstration, in: L. Tratt, M. Gogolla (Eds.), International Conference on Theory and Practice of Model Transformations, Berlin, 2010, pp. 153–167.

[49] P. Brosch, P. Langer, M. Seidl, K. Wieland, M. Wimmer, G. Kappel, W. Retschitzegger, W. Schwinger, An example is worth a thousand words: composite operation modeling by-example, in: International Conference on Model Driven Engineering Languages and Systems, 2009, pp. 271–285.

[50] M.D. Del Fabro, P. Valduriez, Towards the efficient development of model transformations using model weaving and matching transformations, Software & Systems Modeling, Springer-Verlag, vol. 8, 2009, pp. 305–324.

[51] K. Erni, C. Lewerentz, Applying design metrics to object-oriented frameworks, in: IEEE Symposium in Software Metrics: From Measurement to Empirical Results, IEEE Computer Society, Washington DC, 1996, pp. 64–74.

[52] F. Jouault, Loosely coupled traceability for ATL, in: The European Conference on Model Driven Architecture Workshop on Traceability, 2005, pp. 29–37.

[53] R. Marvie, A transformation composition framework for model driven engineering, in: Technical Report, LIFL, 2004.

[54] M. Kessentini, H. Sahraoui, M. Boukadoum, Model transformation as an optimization problem, in: Proceedings of the 11th International Conference on Model Driven Engineering Languages and Systems (MoDELS), vol. 5301, Springer, Toulouse, 2008, pp. 159–173.

[55] M. Harman, L. Tratt, Pareto optimal search based refactoring at the design level, in: Conference on Genetic and Evolutionary Computation, New York, 2007, pp. 1106–1113.

[56] M. Harman, The current state and future of search based software engineering, in: International Conference on Software Engineering, Minneapolis, 2007, pp. 20–26.

[57] S. Kirkpatrick, C.D. Gelatt, M.P. Vecchi, Optimization by simulated annealing, Journal of Science, vol. 220, 1983, pp. 671–680.

[58] M. Shousha, L. Briand, Y. Labiche, A UML/SPT model analysis methodology for concurrent systems based on genetic algorithms, in: Proceedings of the 11th International Conference on Model Driven Engineering Languages and Systems (MoDELS), vol. 5301, Springer, Toulouse, 2008, pp. 475–489.

[59] M. O'Keeffe, M. Cinnéide, Search-based refactoring: an empirical study, Journal of Software Maintenance, vol. 20, 2008, pp. 345–364.

[60] Y. Kataoka, M.D. Ernst, W.G. Griswold, D. Notkin, Automated support for program refactoring using invariants, in: IEEE International Conference on Software Maintenance, 2001, pp. 736–743.

[61] W.F. Opdyke, Refactoring, A Program Restructuring Aid in Designing Object-Oriented Application Frameworks, (Ph.D. thesis), University of Illinois at Urbana-Champaign, 1992.

[62] M. Fowler, K. Beck, J. Brant, W. Opdyke, D. Roberts (Eds.), Refactoring—Improving the Design of Existing Code, Addison-Wesley Professional, 1999, p. 431.

[63] R. Marinescu, Detection strategies: metrics-based rules for detecting design flaws, in: International Conference on Mechatronics, 2004, pp. 350–359.

[64] M. Kessentini, A. Bouchoucha, H.A. Sahraoui, M. Boukadoum, Example-based sequence diagrams to colored Petri nets transformation using heuristic search, in: ECMFA, 2010, pp. 156–172.

ABOUT THE AUTHORS

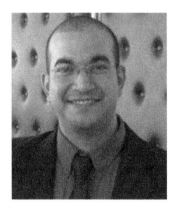

Mohamed Wiem Mkaouer received his MS degree in Computer Science from the University of Tunis in 2010, Tunisia. He is currently a Ph.D. student in Software Engineering at University of Michigan-D, USA, under the supervision of Dr. Marouane Kessentini. His research interests include software quality, software testing, model-driven engineering, and search-based software engineering. He is a member of the Search-based Software Engineering@Michigan research group, and he is also a student member of the IEEE and the IEEE Computer Society.

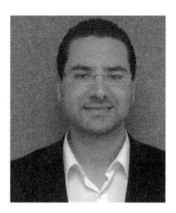

Marouane Kessentini is a Tenure-Track Assistant Professor at the University of Michigan-D. He is the founder of the research group: Search-based Software Engineering@Michigan. He holds a Ph.D. in Computer Science, University of Montreal (Canada), 2011. His research interests include the application of artificial intelligence techniques to software engineering (search-based software engineering), model-driven engineering, software quality, and reengineering. He has published around 50 papers in conferences, workshops, books, and journals. He has served as a program committee/organization member in several conferences and journals.

CHAPTER FIVE

Manual Parallelization Versus State-of-the-Art Parallelization Techniques: The SPEC CPU2006 as a Case Study

Aleksandar Vitorović[*], Milo V. Tomašević[†], Veljko M. Milutinović[†]

[*]EPFL, Lausanne, Switzerland
[†]School of Electrical Engineering, University of Belgrade, Belgrade, Serbia

Contents

Advances in Computers, Volume 92
ISSN 0065-2458
http://dx.doi.org/10.1016/B978-0-12-420232-0.00005-2

Abstract

Being multiprocessors (both on-chip and/or off-chip), modern computer systems can automatically exploit the benefits of parallel programs, but their resources remain underutilized in executing still-prevailing sequential applications. An obvious solution is in the parallelization of such applications. The first part overviews the broad issues in parallelization. Various parallelization approaches and contemporary software and hardware tools for extracting parallelism from sequential applications are studied. It also attempts to identify typical code patterns amenable for parallelization. The second part represents a case study where the SPEC CPU2006 suite is considered as a representative collection of typical sequential applications. Following that, it discusses the possibilities and potentials of automatic parallelization and vectorization of the sequential C++ applications from the CPU2006 suite. Since these potentials are generally limited, it explores the issues in manual parallelization of these applications. After previously identified patterns are applied by source-to-source code modifications, the effects of parallelization are evaluated by profiling and executing on two representative parallel machines. Finally, the presented results are carefully discussed.

1. INTRODUCTION

There is an everlasting strive for an increasing power and speed of computer systems. Parallel systems have long been considered as a promising solution for both throughput-oriented and speedup-oriented computing. Parallel processing has been used predominantly for demanding scientific applications and for large-scale systems over the years, but the architecture, technology, and application trends have been forcing it rapidly towards the commercial computing in medium-scale and even small-scale systems [1].

The importance of parallel processing has been boosted in the last decade by current trends in processor architecture and technology. Until recently, the performance of the processors grew steadily following Moore's law primarily as a consequence of an ever-increasing number of progressively faster transistors. However, inability to obtain further benefits of instruction-level parallelism (ILP), the problems with power dissipation, technology constraints, and design and verification difficulties in complex superscalars gave rise to chip multiprocessors (CMP) [2]. Since a CMP includes multiple simple superscalar cores on a chip, in addition to having the benefits of ILP, a multicore processor can issue multiple instructions per cycle from instruction streams (threads) [3]. Hence, parallel processing is brought further down to the laptop and embedded-system level. While parallelism in superscalars is extracted on the instruction level transparently to a software designer, an increasing level of parallelism in multicores (thread-level parallelism) requires the more intensive involvement of a programmer.

The first part of this chapter represents a survey on parallelization issues and approaches. It reviews some important issues in solving data dependences by loop transformations in order to improve the parallelization abilities. Then, a broad spectrum of parallelization approaches and contemporary tools is explored in order to provide the state-of-the-art in the field. A special attention is devoted to typical parallelization patterns found within sequential applications. Speedups obtained by applying these simple yet powerful patterns are significant, as we show later in our case study.

In a situation where all contemporary processors are multicores, the benefits of multithreaded, parallel workloads are easily exploited. However, the real challenge nowadays is to fully utilize the resources of multicore processors to improve the performance of a considerable amount of existing general-purpose sequential applications. Since the nature of such applications is best reflected in benchmark suites, the second part of this chapter is a case study on parallelization of the SPEC CPU2006 benchmark suite [4,5] as one of the most representative and widely used suites for uniprocessors. It examines the potentials of autoparallelization and vectorization of the SPEC CPU2006 benchmarks in the state-of-the-art compilers and the efforts to parallelize its applications outside this suite. In order to achieve an additional level of parallelism, this study is oriented towards making manual source-to-source code modifications based on profiling information. To this end, the SPEC CPU2006 benchmarks are carefully examined for places where typical parallelization patterns can be efficiently applied. Finally, the resulting speedups are evaluated on two large parallel machines. The evaluation environment and methodology are also described in order to illustrate the details of entire process. Based on this experience, some general indications on where to find the parallelization potential are discussed.

2. PARALLELIZATION THEORY

The main goal of parallelization is to decrease the application execution time as much as possible. The success in parallelization is mainly reflected in a performance indicator referred to as speedup, which shows how much a parallel program is faster than a corresponding sequential program. Amdahl's law determines the maximum speedup when only part of the program can be parallelized. This law tells that speedup of a program is limited by the time spent in the nonparallelized section. Typically, speedup increases almost linearly with the increasing number of processors and saturates at some level, which is less than N, where N is the number of processors. Exceptionally, speedup can be higher than N (superlinear). That happens when all working data sets fit into caches in a multiprocessor but not in single-processor execution. Speedup can be obtained in conditions of weak or strong scaling. As the number of processors increases, with weak scaling, the problem size per processor is kept constant. Ideally, the performance should increase linearly with respect to the number of processors. Strong scaling implies that the total problem size remains the same, and it is uniformly distributed among the increasing number of processors. Ideally, the performance should be constant as more processors are polled in.

2.1. Data Dependences

The major obstacle for parallelization is the presence of data dependences in the code. Correctness problems arise whenever it is possible for two statements to read or write the same memory location at the same time, and at least one of the statements writes to this location, as it was illustrated in [6]. Consequently, these statements cannot be executed in parallel.

Classification of dependences is crucial from the aspect of parallelization. It is based on the dataflow relation between the two dependent statements and it concerns whether or not the two statements communicate the values through the memory location. Let us take a look at the following example (Fig. 5.1): S1 and S2 are statements performed in a sequential execution of a loop, and S1 is executed before S2. The most important and difficult kind of dependences to handle is when S1 writes the memory location and S2 reads the location. Due to the fact that the result of a computation produced by S1 communicates, or "flows," to S2, this kind of dependences is denoted as *flow dependence*. Since S1 must execute first to produce the value that is consumed by S2, in general, this dependence cannot be removed and S1 and S2 cannot

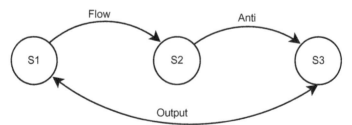

Figure 5.1 Flow, anti-, and output dependences. Statements S1, S2, and S3 appear in sequential execution in the specified order. S1: A = 1; S2: B = A; S3: A = 3.

be executed in parallel. Hence, it is sometimes referred as a "true" dependence.

There are two other kinds of dependences that can always be removed since they do not incur the communication of data between S1 and S2. Instead, they actually represent the reuse of the memory location with the same name for different purposes at different points in the program. They are also known as name dependences and can be removed by renaming. In the first one, S1 reads the location, and then S2 writes to it. Because this memory access pattern is the opposite of the flow dependence, this case is referred to as *antidependence*. We can parallelize a loop that contains an antidependence by giving each iteration a private copy of the location and initializing the copy related to S1 with the value S1 would have read from the location during a sequential execution.

In another name dependence, both S1 and S2 write to the same location. Because only the writing occurs, this is denoted as *output dependence*. Parallelization in the presence of an output dependence is possible if the memory location is made private for both statements. In addition, if the location is live after the loop, the value produced by S2 has to be copied back to the shared copy of the location at the end of the loop. The process of copying back the location written in the last iteration is called finalization. Fortunately, in OpenMP, there is `lastprivate` pragma, which ensures that the output of the private value from last iteration is copied to the main thread. Figure 5.1 illustrates these dependences.

When a program is modified in order to remove a dependence in a parallel loop, it is critical that any other present dependences are not violated. In addition, if some new loop-carried dependences are introduced by renaming the locations, they must be removed as well.

2.2. Loop Transformations

The most of the potential for parallelization is commonly found in loops when their iterations can be executed concurrently. There are two different types of loops according to their parallelization abilities. *DoAcross* loops cannot be generally executed in parallel, while *DoAll* loops can be safely executed in parallel. *DoAcross* loops are sometimes classified in the literature as those with loop-carried dependences, while the others are classified as *DoAll*. However, a programmer can write a loop in a form that contains loop-carried dependences, which can be removed with some loop transformations. Such a loop is amenable for parallelization, so we denote it as *DoAll*.

Thus, the distinction between *DoAll* and *DoAcross* refers to essence of the loop itself and not to its actual code representation. Hurson et al. did a thorough study on *DoAll* and *DoAcross* loops [7]. They parallelized both *DoAcross* and *DoAll* loops by using different strategies for allocation of the processors to the loop iterations.

The rest of this subsection is adapted from Ref. [6] and it contains the loop transformation examples, which translate the loop-carried dependences form to the dependence-free form. *Loop skewing* is one such loop transformation. In the example from Table 5.1,[1] there is a loop-carried flow dependence between two consecutive iterations, that is, from write to *a[i]* to the read of *a[i-1]* in the next iteration. We can move the read of *a[i-1]* to the previous iteration ("skew" the loop) such that all the dependences are within an iteration.

There are some other situations in which loop-carried dependences can be removed. A *reduction* is a collective operation in which a single process collects data from other processes in a group and performs an operation on them, resulting in a single data item [6]. The following form in sequential code yields the possibility for reduction:

```
s = s op f(loopIndex)
```

An example is shown in Table 5.2.[2] Such a code segment implies loop-carried dependences, as *x* is updated based on the value from the previous iteration. We can parallelize the code segment by marking *x* as the reduction variable, which allows each machine to keep its own copy of *x*. These copies are eventually combined in a single value. To be able to compute copies independently, constraints are that *s* is not allowed to appear in f(loopIndex) or anywhere else in the loop body.

Table 5.1 Loop Skewing Removes the Loop-Carried Dependences

```for(int i = 2; i<=N; i++){ b[i] = b[i] + a[i - 1]; a[i] = a[i] + c[i]; }``` ⇨	```b[2] = b[2] + a[1]; #pragma omp parallel for \ shared(a, b, c) for (i = 2; i<=N-1; i++){ a[i] = a[i] + c[i]; b[i + 1] = b[i + 1] + a[i]; } a[N] = a[N] + c[N];```

---

[1] Adapted from Example 3.21 from Ref. [6], with permission from Elsevier, 2001.
[2] Adapted from Example 3.19 from Ref. [6], with permission from Elsevier, 2001.

Table 5.2 Sequential and Parallel Code of the Reduction Example

```
x = 0;                          x=0;
for(i = 0; i<N; i++)  ⟹  #pragma omp parallel for reduction
    x = x + a[i];                                        (+: x)
                                for (i=0; i<N; i++)
                                    x = x + a[i];
```

Table 5.3 Sequential and Parallel Code of the Induction Example

```
idx = N/2 + 1;
i_sum = 1;
pow2 = 2;                               #pragma omp parallel for \
                                        shared(a, b, c)
for[i = 1 i<N/2; i++]{  ⟹  for[i=1; i<N/2; i++] {
    a[i] = a[i] + a[idx];                   a[i] = a[i] + a[i + N/2];
    b[i] = i_sum;                           b[i] = i * (i + 1)/2;
    c[i] = pow2;                            c[i] = exp(2, i);
    idx = idx + 1;                      }
    i_sum = i_sum + i;
    pow2 = pow2 * 2;
}
```

In certain cases, we can relax the constraints, that is, although f ($loopIndex$) may depend on s, these dependences sometimes could be removed by expressing $f(loopIndex)$ differently. This code transformation is denoted as *induction variable elimination*[6], and it is demonstrated in Table 5.3.[3] The sequential code has the loop-carried flow dependences on idx, i_sum, and $pow2$. The parallel version of the code removes all these dependences by computing variables using a simple expression containing the loop index. For example, the expression for i_sum takes advantage of the equality:

$$\sum_{i=1}^{N} N = \frac{N(N+1)}{2}$$

These code patterns appear frequently in real-world applications, as the programmer usually tends to break a long expression into more short ones.

Other loop transformations include fissioning the loop into serial and parallel portions and eliminating dependences in a serial part of the loop

---

[3] Adapted from Example 3.20 from Ref. [6], with permission from Elsevier, 2001.

by expanding a scalar into an array [6]. An extensive study of code transformations and optimizations for parallel architectures was performed in Refs. [8,9].

2.3. Speculative Loop Execution

Due to the code complexity, compile-time techniques for loop transformations do not recognize all the parallelizable loops. To improve the situation, a combination of static and run-time techniques was proposed [10]. The loops that were not marked as parallelizable at compile-time are attempted to be speculatively executed as *DoAll* loops. The framework monitors dependences during the speculative execution using LRPD (Lazy Reduction and Privatization Doall) parallelization test. At run-time, the test detects reduction and antidependences (for the latter, the framework performs privatization). If the test finds any other loop-carried dependence or an exception is encountered, the loop reexecutes sequentially. This requires saving the state prior to speculative execution, which is done through checkpointing or privatizing shared variables.

The framework does not attempt speculative execution for all the loops. Rather, it considers the probability that the loop is parallelizable and the expected speedup (slowdown) if the execution succeeds (restarts).

3. PARALLELIZATION TECHNIQUES AND TOOLS

Some sequential programs can be easily transformed into their parallel counterparts consisting of tasks that can run independently. These parallel programs, known as *embarrassingly parallel*[1], can be executed very efficiently, and they scale perfectly, since there is no communication among the tasks. Some examples are genetic algorithms and brute-force searches in cryptography. For such programs, parallel paradigms, models, and languages are presented. For sequential programs that cannot be trivially parallelized, there are parallelization techniques and tools that can automatically generate the code ready for parallel execution. They are further classified as compiler or hardware techniques/tools. Compiler techniques are based on source-to-source transformations a compiler can do, usually with no human intervention. Hardware techniques imply running programs on specific platforms. Usually, these techniques require some level of code adaptation.

3.1. Levels of Parallelism

Domain decomposition or "data parallelism" implies partitioning data to processes (or parallel computing nodes), such that a single portion of data is assigned to a single process. The portions of data are of approximately equal size. If the portions require rather different amounts of time to be processed, the performance is limited by the speed of the slowest process. In that case, the problem can be mitigated by partitioning the data into a large number of smaller portions. Then, a process takes another portion once it finishes with the previous one, and a faster process is assigned more portions. Single-program-multiple-data (SPMD) paradigm is an example of data parallelism, as the processes share the same code but operate on different data. Another example is parallelization of a loop with no loop-carried dependences in which the processes execute the same loop body, but for different loop indices, and consequently, for different data.

In functional decomposition or "task parallelism," processes are assigned pieces of code. Each piece of code works on the same data and is assigned to exactly one process. An example of task parallelism is computing the average and standard deviation on the same data. These two tasks can be executed by separate processes. Another example is parallelization of a loop with an *if–then–else* construct inside, such that different code is executed in different iterations.

In the development of application software for parallel machines, the parallelism can be specified and extracted either implicitly or explicitly by applying an appropriate parallel programming model.

3.2. Parallel Programming Models

A parallel programming model is a set of program abstractions for fitting parallel activities from the application to the underlying parallel hardware. It spans over different layers: applications, programming languages, compilers, libraries, network communication, and I/O systems. Two widely known parallel programming models are *shared memory* and *message passing*, but there are also different combinations of both. *Data-parallel* programming model is also among the most important ones as it was revived again with increasing popularity of MapReduce [11] and GPGPU (General-Purpose computing on Graphics Processing Units) [12].

In the shared-memory programming model, tasks share a common address space, which they read and write in an asynchronous manner. The communication between tasks is implicit. If more than one task accesses the same variable, the semaphores or locks can be used for synchronization. By keeping data local to the processor and making private copies, expensive memory accesses are avoided, but some mechanism of coherence maintenance is needed when multiple processors share the same data with the possibility of writing.

In the message-passing programming model, tasks have private memories, and they communicate explicitly via message exchange. To exchange a message, each sends operation needs to have a corresponding receive operation. Tasks are not constrained to exist on the same physical machine.

A suitable combination of two previous models is sometimes appropriate. Processors can directly access memory on another processor. This is achieved via message passing, but what the programmer actually sees is shared-memory model.

Mainstream parallel programming environments are based on augmenting traditional sequential programming languages with low-level parallel constructs (library function calls and/or compiler directives).

The MPI is a library of routines with the bindings in Fortran, C, and C++ and it is an example of an explicitly parallel API that implements the message-passing model via library function calls [13]. The set of processes with separate address spaces coordinate the computation by explicitly sending and receiving messages. Each process has a separate address space, its own program counter, and its own call stack.

However, high-level constructs such as synchronization, communication, and mapping data to processes are left to a programmer to implement. MPI supports point-to-point communication between any two processes. It also enables the collective communication operations where a group of processes perform global/collective operations, such as gather, scatter, reduce, and scan.

In a heterogeneous environment, in order to optimize the performance, an MPI implementation may map processes to processors in a particular way. Similarly, an MPI implementation may optimize the way processes communicate during a global operation. For example, in case of MPI_Reduce, the communicating nodes do not have to form a tree structure, if an alternative structure brings better performance for the underlying parallel machine.

On the other side, OpenMP is an example of mainly implicit parallel API intended for shared-memory multiprocessors [14]. It exploits parallelism through compiler directives and the library function calls. Unlike MPI, where all threads are spawned at the beginning of the execution and are active until the program terminates, in OpenMP, a single master thread starts

Table 5.4 The `Sections` Construct

```
#pragma omp parallel{
        #pragma omp sections{
                #pragma omp section
                        block1
                #pragma omp section
                        block2
        }
}
```

Table 5.5 The `For` Construct

```
#pragma omp parallel for
for(i=0; i<n; i++)
    a[i] = b[i] + c[i];
```

execution, and additional threads are active only during the execution of a parallel region. To reduce the overheads, these threads are spawned when the program enters a parallel region for the first time, and they are blocked while the program is executing a nonparallel region.

`Sections` work-sharing construct breaks work into multiple distinct sections, such that each section is entirely executed by a single thread. It is an example of task parallelism paradigm. Its general form is presented in Table 5.4.

`For` work-sharing construct splits iterations of a loop among different threads, such that each iteration is entirely executed by a single thread. It is an example of data-parallelism paradigm. Its general form is shown in Table 5.5.

Cilk [15] is a language extension for C programming language with parallel constructs, resembling to OpenMP. Both OpenMP and Cilk can automatically choose parallelism to achieve good performance. Cilk++ [16] brings the same for C++ language.

3.3. Parallel Languages

A few fully implicit parallel programming languages exist, either as spanking ones (SISAL and Occam) or as parallel extensions of existing languages (HPF, C*, IntelTBB, and STAPL). SISAL is a general-purpose single assignment functional programming language with strict semantics and efficient array handling, which avoids data hazards, mainly by privatizing every write into a variable [17]. However, for large contemporary programs, it may be inefficient since the memory overhead is enormous.

Unified Parallel C (UPC) [18] is a programming language from partitioned global address space group of languages offering multiple-data layouts by combining shared-memory and message-passing paradigms in a fine-grained fashion. Depending on a specific user trade-off between latency of acquiring data and amount of data, it offers private, shared-local, and shared-remote data layouts.

Intel TBB is an approach for expressing parallelism in C++ programs [19]. It exploits a higher-level, task-based parallelism that abstracts the platform details and threading mechanisms for scalability and performance. A similar noncommercial product is STAPL [20]. Both approaches rely on manual code interventions to exploit the benefits of parallel execution.

Algorithmic skeletons [21] strictly separate parallelization details (communication and synchronization patterns) from sequential building blocks. Starting from a basic set of patterns (skeletons), a user can build more complex patterns via nesting. Then, these patterns can be instantiated by parameterization with number of nodes used, data distribution, etc., so a user can concentrate on and write only the sequential part of the application (denoted as muscle functions). In addition to algorithmic abstraction, this approach offers the platform independence. Although these models are restricted, they drastically reduce the burden on a programmer.

According to Ref. [22], there are three main skeleton constructs:
1. *Data-parallel*: It operates on data structures (e.g., map, scan, and reduce).
2. *Task-parallel*: It operates on task level (e.g., sequential, if, and loop).
3. *Resolution family of problems*: (e.g., divide-and-conquer, branch-and-bound, and dynamic programming).

Nowadays, numerous skeleton libraries based on these paradigms are available. Algorithmic skeletons for Java parallel programming on multicore machines are proposed in Ref. [23], while in Ref. [24], a generic set of skeletons is provided as a C library on top of MPI.

As presented in Ref. [25], in an append-only system where no previously written data are revoked, the application is order-insensitive, which allows the parallel execution. If code segments do not fulfill these conditions, we have to exit order-insensitive mode and do some synchronization among threads.

MapReduce [11] and Dryad [26] are programming models for distributed processing on a cluster. Both of them exploit data parallelism and

Table 5.6 The Characteristics of Some Parallel Languages

Language	Implementation	Data Parallelism	Task Parallelism/ Parallel Algorithms
SISAL	Stand-alone	Yes	No
UPC	C extension	Yes	No
STAPL	C++ extension	Yes	Yes
Intel TBB	C++ extension	Yes	Yes
Skeletons	Various languages	Yes	Yes
MapReduce	Various languages	Yes	No
Dryad	Various languages	Yes	No
MATLAB	Stand-alone	Yes	Yes

provide great scalability accompanied with a fault-tolerance support. MapReduce programs are built as a sequence of map and reduce operations. These operations are executed one after another, but an operation can be scaled out on many processors. MapReduce is extremely popular nowadays due to an open-source implementation [27]. Dryad offers user-specified dataflow direct acyclic graphs. It supports all connection relationships (one-to-one, one-to-many, and many-to-one) and different communication channels (TCP, files, etc.).

MATLAB has Parallel Computing Toolbox and Distributed Computing Server, which allow for parallel/distributed execution [28]. This environment has

- a possibility for specifying task parallelism through `parfor` (parallel for loops) and data parallelism through `spmd` annotations
- high-level constructs such as distributed collections (i.e., arrays)
- many parallel algorithms

The key issues of mentioned parallel languages are summarized in Table 5.6.

3.4. Compiler Techniques

Although the explicit expression of parallelism enables the absolute control over the parallel execution and offers the advantages for achieving the best performance, it often requires a tedious involvement of a programmer. Therefore, an automatic parallelization provided by parallelizing compilers is highly desirable. Unfortunately, compiler possibilities for automatic parallelization are usually limited, especially for general-purpose applications with complex control flows and a substantial use of pointers. The major problem in these conditions is that a compiler cannot statically prove that parallelization is safe and most conversions have to be done manually. Even if the compiler can recognize that some construction is possibly parallel, it can hardly detect whether the parallelization is worthwhile. Namely, due to the overheads of spawning threads, a parallelization of a loop with a small iteration count can even result in a slowdown. This is why the compiler usually behaves conservatively and surrenders parallelization of a loop if it does not know the iteration count in advance.

Model-based parallelization was proposed for automatic parallelization. Each loop transformation is mathematically modeled as a sequence (schedule) of parallelization steps. The compiler frameworks for dependence analysis and loop transformations based on these models are denoted as polyhedral frameworks. A constraint is that loops have only array accesses inside. Representative frameworks are Refs. [29–31].

Vectorization is a standard feature in most of the compilers. It refers to an automatic transformation of the sequential code to the code suitable for execution on a processor with vector instructions, where a vector instruction can simultaneously be performed on multiple pairs of vector operands.

Some compilers follow a special approach for program speedup using profile-guided optimizations even without parallelization. It consists of three phases: program instrumentation, trial run with test data input, and final run. First, a program is instrumented for profiling during compilation. Information collected in this phase can be used for basic block optimizations, conditional branch optimizations, inlining, and function splitting/grouping. In the second phase, the instrumented program is executed with representative test input and all necessary statistics for running the code are collected. These statistics are used for code optimizations. Finally, the program can be run with arbitrary input data. Besides the need for two program runs, the main problem with this approach is the sensitivity to the input data. If the current data impose that the program control flow goes around the optimized blocks, no speedup is obtained.

Kremlin [32] is a profiler of serial programs, helping a user to parallelize them. It analyzes code regions that are amenable for parallelization and reports those with the highest potential speedup. A user can do manual parallelization based on the profiler's output.

Some compilers have implemented quite advanced optimizations. The SUIF compiler is roughly based on the C semantics and can deal with both C and Fortran programs. SUIF can automatically parallelize and optimize the sequential programs for shared-memory multiprocessors [33]. It performs symbolic execution, and using that information, it exploits coarse-grain parallelism and interprocedural optimizations. In order to maximize parallelism from different calling contexts, the compiler may decide to instantiate multiple clones of a single procedure, by replacing some the formal parameters with their actual counterparts.

Another example is Polaris compiler [34]. Unfortunately, it targets only Fortran programs. At the top of this compiler, new frameworks can be built, such as the one for improving program parallelism by finding induction variables in a loop consisting of complex index functions (i.e., those with indirection) or complex control flow [35]. This framework employs a novel data structure, called Value Evolution Graph, for representing the value flow of induction variables.

Cetus [36] and ROSE [37] are source-to-source translators that automatically parallelize loops by augmenting the original sequential code with OpenMP pragmas. Cetus [36] supports C language and performs optimizations such as array privatization and parallelization of code with induction and reduction variables. An interesting project based on Cetus is a translation from OpenMP to MPI programs [38]. The ROSE [37] supports Fortran, C, and C++ and automatically performs loop transformations (loop fusion, fission, interchange, unrolling, and blocking). It also provides a user with tools for an extensive analysis of the call graph, class hierarchy, and data dependences. Both Cetus [36] and ROSE [37] allow writing user-specified code analysis and optimizations.

There are also other tools that allow a user to specify a custom optimization or analysis. Semantic Designs developed DMS Software Reengineering Toolkit [39], which automatically recognizes specified patterns in the code and applies user-specified transformations on them. Mercurium [40], developed at UPC, is specialized for OpenMP source-to-source transformations, allowing for fast testing of new OpenMP constructs. A user specifies desired transformations using templates.

Recently, a framework for automatic distribution of computation across heterogeneous cores was proposed [41]. It contains a compiler and run-time for their language, which uses the MapReduce pattern, akin to Ref. [11]. In Ref. [42], a framework for running MapReduce-like applications in heterogeneous environments (consisting of both CPUs and GPUs) is presented.

Performance gain can also be obtained by transforming data structures under certain conditions. Harmen et al. [43] transform accesses to a linked list in a loop to array-based accesses, so that all loop transformations become applicable.

The parallelism detection went beyond usual exploiting parallelism on arrays within a loop. Kulkarni et al. [44] presented a novel amorphous data parallelism. By using run-time detection mechanisms, they observed that certain applications exploit a noticeable level of data parallelism on complex data structures (trees and graphs). The authors studied the commutation properties of these data structures in order to parallelize the programs. An example is a parallelization of the Kruskal minimum spanning tree (MST) algorithm [45]. A sufficient condition for adding multiple edges to the tree at the same time is that these edges are lighter than any unprocessed edge and that no cycles are formed in MST. In terms of the final result, adding multiple MST edges to the MST is commutative. In a similar manner, a user can specify complex commutativity conditions for other applications as well. An effort in Ref. [46] offers commutation for collections, but the authors of Ref. [44] expand this analysis on more complex data structures (including even union-find).

Using similar ideas, Liao et al. presented exploiting parallelism on C++ STL collections in [47]. The authors use ROSE to specify source-to-source transformations. In Ref. [48], the authors attempted to perform automatic parallelization of recursive data structures.

The knowledge-based (machine learning) systems have also been proposed. A problem with those techniques is that formal proof of correctness can still be missing or they can be applied for programs with some domain constraints. A system combining machine learning techniques with profiling was presented in Ref. [49]. They obtained the results close to those conceivable by the best-effort manual parallelization.

3.5. Hardware Techniques

Multicore processors with 32 and 64 cores are already widely available and such hardware performs very well with the inherent data-parallel software. An example is Tilera Tile64 chip [50], particularly suitable for digital video processing. Still, executing a program containing a lot of data dependences remains a challenge.

However, general-purpose solutions are generally more important. ILP is supported on superscalar processors for a long time, but performance gain can be only two to three times in average and it does not scale beyond this level because of the control and data dependences between the adjacent instructions.

An approach to mitigate the impact of branch misprediction on performance is to apply *branch predication* mechanisms. Predication [51] is a technique opposite to the classical branch prediction; instead of predicting a single path and executing it, all possible paths are executed in parallel. After realizing which path is the correct one, the effects of all other paths are undone. Trade-offs of applying predication in different settings were studied in Refs. [52,53]. Predication combined with out-of-order execution is presented in Ref. [54], whereas an integration of control and data dependence speculation and predication is shown in Ref. [55].

The TLS (thread-level speculation) technique is characterized by an aggressive parallelization, even if there are possible data dependences between threads [56,57]. Dedicated hardware monitors the execution and, if these dependences really occur, mispredicted speculation is squashed and the execution rolled back to the correct state. This can bring some speedup, but the overhead in case of incorrect speculation can be high.

There are several proposed approaches for controlling TLS performance trade-offs. The mechanism for control of the speculation can be integrated with the coherence protocol. The heuristics for deciding where to use TLS (TLS task selection) in Java programs by monitoring dynamic speculation profiles is investigated in Ref. [58].

A cost model for TLS task selection was proposed in Ref. [59]. The authors also developed DProf, a tool for profiling dependences at run-time and mapping them to the corresponding source code. They examined their model on some SPEC CPU2006 benchmarks by estimating the percentage rate of successful speculations using DProf. In Ref. [60], by utilizing the information obtained from DProf, the authors manually parallelized (using OpenMP) some SPEC CPU2006 benchmarks and obtained up to 2.6 times speedup on a 4-core machine.

DSWP [61] allows parallelizing loops with loop-carried dependences by splitting the loop body in multiple threads, which are executed in a pipeline. The assignment is performed in such a way that critical path dependences are within a thread. In SpecDSWP [62], DSWP is applied speculatively to allow for more parallelism within a loop. In Ref. [63], a combination of TLS and SpecDSWP techniques was pursued on the SPEC CPU2000 integer-intensive benchmarks. On a 32-core machine, it resulted in an average speedup of 4.5 times. The programs were parallelized manually, using code annotations.

The Bulk Multicore [64] automatically parallelizes programs on shared-memory multiprocessors, transparently to the programming language used and without user intervention. It groups the instructions into blocks, which are denoted as chunks. A chunk is executed on a single processor, and processors execute their chunks in parallel. The Bulk Multicore executes the chunks atomically and in isolation with respect to each other using hardware address signatures. This allows for aggressive optimizations (such as reordering) within a chunk.

The transactional memory model [65] is a relatively novel approach that relieves the problems of explicit low-level synchronization. However, TM model works well only if the transactions are relatively small and if shared data items are rarely accessed concurrently, that is, in integer and client/server workloads, as explained in Ref. [56]. In Ref. [66], TLS and transaction memory were combined. This approach brought a geometric mean 15.5 times speedup on 24-core machine on five SPEC CPU benchmarks.

The GPGPU is an increasingly widespread approach that supports the execution of general-purpose applications on graphical processing units. NVIDIA CUDA is such a platform, which makes data-parallel computing on GPUs convenient and efficient by using an extension of C language [12]. NVIDIA GPUs consist of a number of multiprocessors, each of them having one or more groups of cores. The cores in the same group concurrently execute the same instruction. On the programming side, a program consists of sequentially executed kernels. A kernel contains blocks, each of which is assigned to a single multiprocessor, allowing for data sharing and synchronization within a block. Each block has multiple threads, each of which is assigned to a single core.

As explained in Ref. [67], memory access latencies can be hidden by a technique called hardware multithreading, based on the fact that context switches in GPGPUs are very cheap. Namely, cores are provided with multiple thread contexts, such that when a thread stalls, a context switch is performed. This results in almost 100% utilization. The main drawback of CUDA is the lack of support for recursion and function pointers.

4. ABOUT MANUAL PARALLELIZATION

The automatic parallelization is quite attractive since it relieves the programmer of a great burden; however, this approach has its disadvantages. It is limited in detecting data dependences and thus inappropriate for complex code. As we will see, it can even induce performance degradation. In these conditions, manual parallelization approach where the programmer is directly involved in identifying and implementing parallelism is preferred.

This section discusses the issues in manual parallelization. The ideas presented here can be used to improve the compiler's ability for automatic parallelization.

4.1. Problems and Pitfalls

The loops are commonly recognized as the program constructs where parallelism is primarily searched for. The analysis of data dependences is aggravated by aliasing of variables, overriding and operator functions, and especially by templatized inheritance and recursion. In addition, mutable variables and register-allocated variables inhibit any level of parallelism.

Optimization of loops can indeed provide speedup if that code segment is executed often enough for longer periods of time. However, the parallelization of loops can even lead to slowdown when the iteration count is insufficient to amortize the parallelization overhead. This is why existing compilers conservatively decide to parallelize a code segment, and as we will see, even in that case, they can introduce slowdowns.

To avoid the slowdown effect, in manual parallelization, we insert a guard in front of the parallelized *for* loop that compares its iteration count against some predefined threshold value. If the iteration count is above this threshold, parallel execution is enabled. Otherwise, the loop iterations are performed sequentially. A more formal method for measuring the performance benefits from loop parallelization is elaborated in Section 5.5.

Even comparing the performance of the sequential and manually parallelized version of a program is not trivial. Namely, to avoid inaccurate speedup results, we have to make sure that compiler optimizations (e.g., inlining and autoparallelization) are performed in the same way in both versions.

Interestingly, a parallel version of the program can yield slightly different results when run multiple times. This is due to the fact that the order of operations is run-time-dependent (e.g., consider a reduction) and floating-point operations are not associative [68]. However, CPU2006 validation passes successfully if the results are within a certain absolute or relative error margin.

As noticed in Ref. [69], library calls, such as *malloc*, are usually not thread-safe, since they might cause some interthread data dependences. A safe solution is to always use parallel libraries instead.

4.2. General Ideas for Parallelization

In trying to parallelize programs, a few things should be kept in mind. The first and most important issue is that the source code has to be thoroughly understood. All implementation issues are not so important, but an ability to establish the precise mapping between algorithm steps and code segments is essential. Using the domain knowledge, one can infer which code segments are inherently parallel.

Also, an experience from some existing parallel versions, which is usually an algorithm replacement, may offer some hints about parallel sections of a program. Still, the induced ideas have to be applied with extreme caution, as the goal is not to rewrite the program, but to discover code transformations, which, in principle, could be implemented in a compiler.

An educated guess about some code sections based on variable names can also help. For example, a variable named temp most probably can be privatized. On the other hand, if a time variable is a counter in a *for* loop, the loop-carried dependences are quite probable.

Profiling is a very helpful technique for identifying and localizing the places in a program with a potential for performance improvements. Profiling data can point out the code segments that are relatively small yet consume relatively huge amount of processor time. These code segments are denoted as hot spots. According to the Amdahl's law, if parallelizable, hot spots can lead to significant speedups. We devote special attention to loops that are hot spots and profile them additionally to extract the number of times a loop is entered, the number of the loop iterations executed, and the average time spent in a single iteration.

Cutting-edge compilers can recognize code segments feasible for automatic parallelization. As already mentioned, in most cases, the compiler is too conservative and it is not able to parallelize the code segments with complex data dependences. Still, reading compiler reports along with manually analyzing the code might lead to a good parallelization idea.

Inlining of function calls within loops is generally considered as a good idea, since it would most probably provide enough work for parallelization. However, this is not always feasible due to data dependences that are not known at compile time or eventual side effects of the function. One can infer whether a method has side effects by looking at const modifiers within its signature. System calls cannot be parallelized.

If a function is fairly long and if it is invoked frequently enough, one should consider parallelizing within a function. Task parallelism may be available immediately. If not, one should attempt to split the function into multiple function calls and merge their results.

There is an interesting phenomenon with nested loops. It is typical to search for parallelism at the innermost level. Even if found, that parallelism can sometimes lead to a very limited speedup. Moreover, it is possible that the innermost loop exhibits loop-carried dependences, while some outer loop is dependence-free. Parallelism on that level can be significant. The execution of the inner loop will not be affected, since the inner loop inside parallelized outer loop is executed sequentially.

4.3. Examples of Typical Parallelization Patterns

As previously mentioned, parallelism is looked for at the loops first. Parallelization of a loop with even one simple instruction may bring speedup if the loop has a large number of iterations, as illustrated for PARALLEL_RESET pattern in Table 5.7.

Operations on vectors are also indicative for parallelization. The PARALLEL_VECTOR pattern is shown in Table 5.8.

For both PARALLEL_RESET and PARALLEL_VECTOR, we still need to check if output dependences exist, that is, if any two elements of g(i) accessed within a loop have the same value. The loop can be executed speculatively and data dependences checked with a run-time test, for example, LRPD [10]. In PARALLEL_VECTOR, even if there are loop-carried dependences, they are actually reductions on different elements of vector. Consequently, this pattern is always parallelizable with LRPD test [10], as the test detects reductions at run-time.

Even a *for* loop with a single operation but with a large number of iterations can be indicative for parallelization, as in the PARALLEL_RESET pattern. This is especially the case when an operator is overloaded and implemented with a rather long operator function.

Also, the sequential search of an unordered large data collection is amenable for parallel processing by searching across distinct data sets (the PARALLEL_SEARCH pattern).

Table 5.7 PARALLEL_RESET Pattern

```
for(i = ...)
  vector[g(i)]=0;
```

Table 5.8 PARALLEL_VECTOR Pattern

```
for (i =...)
  vector[g(i)] += y * x(i);
```

Table 5.9 REPEAT_SET_CALC_WRITE Pattern

```
for ( i = 0; i < iteration_count; ++i ) {
    SET
      CALC
      WRITE
    SET
      CALC
      WRITE
      ...
}
```

If a loop contains loop-carried dependences, the loop can still be amenable for task-level parallelism within an iteration. This particularly holds when an iteration takes considerable amount of time, as in iterative algorithms. The parallelism can be extracted by partitioning the code within an iteration into distinct segments, which have no data dependences, or they can be easily eliminated. We observed a pattern that consists of repetitively setting some initial conditions and calculating and writing the results. This pattern is referred to as REPEAT_SET_CALC_WRITE and its general form can be found in Table 5.9.

5. CASE STUDY: PARALLELIZATION OF SPEC CPU2006

In situation where all contemporary processors are multicores, the benefits of multithreaded, parallel workloads are easily exploited. However, the real challenge nowadays is to fully utilize resources of multicore processors to improve the performance of a bunch of existing general-purpose sequential applications. Since the nature of such applications is best reflected in uniprocessor benchmark suites, the focus of this case study is parallelization of SPEC CPU2006 [4,5] as one of the most representative and widely used suites for uniprocessors.

5.1. Parallelization of Benchmark Suites

Benchmark programs are very useful since they represent the important and typical details of applications. There is a variety of parallel benchmark suites, too. The ParBenCCh suite is a collection of small C and C++ applications designed to characterize the compiler optimization capabilities and machine performance [70]. It consists of five benchmarks, which include parallel tests implemented using MPI and OpenMP. The SPLASH-2 suite consists of multiprocessor benchmarks written in C both of kernel and application type [71]. The SPEC MPI2007 is benchmark suite for evaluating MPI-parallel, floating-point, compute-intensive performance across a wide range of cluster and SMP hardware. The SPEC OMP2001 suite measures performance using applications based on the OpenMP standard for shared-memory parallel processing. These suites are written in a parallel fashion and they are mostly used for measuring characteristics of some particular parallel environments.

SPEC CPU2006 is a collection of programs written in Fortran, C, and C++ that provides a comparative measure of the compute-intensive performance using workloads developed from typical sequential real-world applications, rather than using artificial loop kernels or synthetic benchmarks. Every SPEC CPU2006 benchmark represents a class of problems, having in mind that solving some problems from different areas is quite similar (e.g., computing the forces between atoms is very similar to computing the forces between planets).

The SPEC CPU suite was the target of some earlier parallelization efforts. Autoparallelization of CPU2000FP was pursued in Ref. [72]. The authors reported speedup (up to 40%) in 4 out of 14 benchmarks, when 2 threads were used. In Ref. [73], in three out of eight SPEC CPU2000FP benchmarks, the authors managed to achieve almost linear speedup for four and eight cores. TLS was attempted for both CPU2000 [74] and CPU2006 [57,75] benchmarks. SPEC CPU2006 benchmarks have been generally found hard to parallelize. The authors of [75] showed that this suite has a very limited potential for TLS (less than 1%). However, a recent study based on a more advanced profile-driven compiler succeeded in extracting more TLS parallelism by extending speculation on multiple loop levels [57]. When eight cores were used, the geometric mean of achieved speedup for three SPEC CPU2006 C++ benchmarks examined was 153%.

There are other benchmark suites besides CPU2006 written in a sequential manner, which can also be parallelized. BioBench suite targets the biological applications, but it already has a parallel version—BioParallel [76] where predominantly integer applications are written mostly in C. The NAS Parallel Benchmarks are a set of computations, five kernels and three pseudoapplications [77]. They are focused on some important aspects of highly parallel computations in aerophysics applications. The NAS benchmarks do not provide parallel implementations, but they specify into details the problems to be solved and the high-level method to be used (e.g., multigrid or conjugate gradient method). The user is free to choose the language constructs (though the language must be an extension of Fortran or C), data structures, communication abstractions, etc.

Since SPEC CPU2006 contains representative sequential applications from broad range of domains, it was chosen in this case study for leveraging manual parallelization techniques. This study is focused on C++ benchmarks since the use of C++ is prevalent nowadays and Fortran programs are already highly parallelized. Some interesting details about C++ benchmarks in the SPEC CPU2006 are described in Ref. [78].

5.2. Description of the SPEC Benchmarks

Out of 29 benchmarks from CPU2006, 7 are written in C++. For each benchmark, its nature is described first. Then, its known existing parallel version outside CPU2006, or potential for parallelization, is elaborated upon. Finally, the results of autoparallelization and vectorization obtained using the Intel compiler are presented (details about the evaluation environment can be found in Section 5.4).

5.2.1 Namd

This benchmark represents the classical molecular dynamics simulation. It adapts an extract of the code from the homonymous parallel program.

There is also a manually parallelized version outside CPU2006 based on CHARM++ parallel objects [79,80]. It spatially decomposes the 3-D space into cubes. These cubes, along with interactions between pairs of cubes, are spread over available processors.

Compiler did not recognize any section in the sequential namd that can be parallelized. Vectorization introduces 12.5% speedup obtained from the code segment presented in Table 5.10.

An occurrence of REPEAT_SET_CALC_WRITE pattern can be found in the top-level loop in main function in spec_namd.C. Due to the fact that calculations of forces between two atoms do not depend on other calculations, code segments within an iteration can be executed in parallel. Macrodefinitions for three phases of the pattern are presented in Table 5.A5, while the original and transformed codes are presented in

Table 5.10 Vectorization in namd

```
for ( j = i + 1; j < j_hgroup; ++j ) {
    pairlist[pairlistindex++] = j;
}
```

Table 5.A6. The time spent in the pattern code (and its descendants) is around 99% of the total benchmark execution time, clearly identifying this code segment as a hot spot. Since the template method takes almost all the execution time, parallelizing the six sections has almost 600% speedup potential. In order to preserve correctness, privatization of `patchList` variable, as well as merging output files from six parallel sections, is required.

5.2.2 Dealii

This benchmark is a partial differential equation solver based on the adaptive finite element method. It uses the homonymous C++ library [81], which provides support for adaptivity through the appropriate complex data structures and algorithms. This benchmark extensively uses modern C++ features and libraries, such as Boost.

Within this CPU2006 benchmark, parallelization is specified for some code segments by using the Adaptive Communication Environment, a cross-platform communication library. Parallel segments were specified manually by experts, who knew their potential for parallelization (by profiling their execution times and inspecting data dependences). In some cases, they aided parallelization by using synchronization through mutexes. Consequently, not much space is left for further optimizations and improvements.

Autoparallelization is done nowhere. Vectorization is applied in a few places, for example, in the standard library vector method call, but produces 4.16% slowdown.

5.2.3 Soplex

This benchmark represents Simplex Linear Program Solver. It is based on SoPlex 1.2.1. The Linear Program (LP) consists of a sparse matrix A, vector b, and the coefficient vector c, which represents the objective function. SoPlex takes the advantage of the fact that the matrix is sparse and extensively uses sparse linear algebra algorithms, such as a sparse LU factorization.

This is an iterative problem (each iteration depends on the results of the previous iteration). Outside CPU2006, there is a version for shared-memory systems (SMoPlex) and a version for distributed-memory systems (DoPlex) [82]. SMoPlex exploits parallelism both within iteration and on the level of multiple consecutive iterations. The former is attained by parallelizing pricing and ratio tests (task parallelism) and by parallelizing within linear algebra routines. The latter is achieved using a technique called block pivoting.

The compiler did not recognize any sections that can be autoparallelized, yet vectorization of the benchmark brings 5.3% speedup.

5.2.4 Povray

This benchmark represents computer visualization/ray tracing. It is based on POV-Ray, a popular ray tracer (renderer) [83]. Ray tracing is a rendering technique that generates a realistic image by simulating the light ray paths in the real world of objects that the image represents.

There are third-party parallel patches for POV-Ray, such as MPIPOV and PVM patch. The PVM patch for POV-Ray is based on message passing in which the master partitions the image into small blocks and distributes them among the slaves [84]. The slaves return the rendered blocks to the master. Finally, the master merges them into the final image. The main problem with these patches is huge memory consumption. Namely, memory is proportional to the number of processors.

The new POV-Ray 3.7 beta [83] allows for parallel execution without substantial increase in memory requirements. This is achieved by redesigning the algorithm and restructuring the code to make it aware of parallelism.

The compiler applied autoparallelization with 1.9% slowdown and vectorization with 1.3% slowdown.

5.2.5 Omnetpp

This benchmark represents discrete-event simulation. It is based on OMNeT++ [85]. This benchmark simulates a large Ethernet network and it models CSMA/CD protocol of Ethernet and the Ethernet frame in detail. The generated traffic is following a generic request–response protocol.

Outside CPU2006, OMNeT++ [85] supports parallel simulation using MPI. The Ethernet model is partitioned into logical processes, which are assigned to available processors. As LPs execute independently from each other, the causality of events could be violated, that is, events could be processed out of timestamp order. To preserve correctness of the simulation, LPs need to synchronize when exchanging messages.

The compiler did not apply any parallelization, while vectorization achieved 13% speedup.

5.2.6 Astar

This benchmark implements the algorithms of pathfinding. It is derived from a 2-D pathfinding library. The library implements classical A* algorithm and its two modifications: one for supporting different motion speeds and another for graphs. There are two input files for this benchmark and we use `rivers.cfg` input for performance measurements.

Outside CPU2006, there exist parallel counterparts of `astar`, but they are based on parallel versions of the `astar` algorithm [86]. These versions are totally different from the sequential version found in CPU2006.

As in the previous benchmark, the compiler did not succeed in autoparallelization, but it embedded some vectorization, which yielded 4.7% speedup.

5.2.7 Xalancbmk

This benchmark represents an XSLT processor. It is a modified version of Xalan-C++, an XSLT processor for converting XML documents into other document types, such as HTML text.

`Xalancbmk` expresses an SPMD type of parallelism. Parallel execution can be employed only when more documents are manipulated at once. Traditionally, dealing with a single XML file is considered inherently sequential. However, Berkeley Parallel Browser Project [87] attempts to parallelize processing within a single file.

The benchmark is nowhere automatically parallelized, but vectorization gives 3% speedup.

The functional description and parallelization possibilities of the benchmarks are summarized in Table 5.11.

5.3. Details of Parallelization

Some real-life programs exhibit bad performance due to subroutines that are written in a suboptimal way. These routines are sometimes denoted as *"low-hanging fruit"*[88], and the performance can easily be improved by optimizing them. Such subroutines do not exist within CPU2006, as the benchmarks were written by the domain experts, and usual sequential optimizations such as loop interchange, padding, and data alignment were consistently applied wherever possible and beneficial. Therefore, CPU2006 cannot be easily optimized. Very careful and deep analysis of a program is needed to reveal the code sections that are feasible for parallelization.

Table 5.11 Description of the SPEC CPU2006 Benchmarks

Program	Function	Parallelization Possibilities
namd	Molecular dynamics simulation	Outside the benchmark, the algorithm totally rewritten
dealII	Solving partial differential equations using adaptive finite elements method	Inside the benchmark
soplex	Simplex Linear Program Solver	Outside the benchmark, a slightly changed algorithm
povray	Ray tracer renderer	Outside the benchmark, the algorithm totally rewritten
omnetpp	Discrete-event simulation on Ethernet	Outside the benchmark, a slightly changed algorithm
astar	Pathfinding algorithm	Outside the benchmark, the algorithm totally rewritten
xalancbmk	Transformation of XML documents into HTML	Outside the benchmark, for more input files

Our primary goal was to find the parallelization patterns at the interprocedural level for obtaining coarse-grain parallelism in these benchmarks and, if possible, apply them and estimate their speedup potentials. Some examples along with the evaluations are discussed in Section 5.5.

Since each program from the suite represents a class of problems, this analysis in a long run could lead to some conclusions for parallelization of an entire program class rather than for a particular program only. Also, if some parallelization pattern is recognized as quite general and decently frequent in the code, it could deserve to be considered for implementation as a plug-in, which enhances the compiler's ability for automatic parallelization.

5.4. Evaluation Environment and Methodology

In this study, the benchmarks are prepared and executed on two machines, Hydra and BigSpring, using a number of software tools. This section presents the details of hardware platforms and describes the software tools used and the methodology of evaluation.

5.4.1 Hardware and Software Platforms

Hydra is a 640-processor "IBM Cluster 1600" system. The processors are IBM's 1.9GHz Power5+ physically packaged and organized into nodes.

A p575 node is a symmetrical multiprocessor system with 16 Power5+ processors (8 dual-cores) and 32 GB DDR2 shared memory. The 40 nodes are further organized and housed into four physical racks and interconnected by a high-performance switch. Hydra runs the 64-bit version of AIX 5L (5.3) as a single-system image.

BigSpring consists of 24 "x335 Type 8676 server Model 6EX" nodes connected with the gigabit Ethernet switch. Each node has two Intel Xeon 2.4 GHz dual-core processors, which gives a total of 96 processors, and 4 GB DDR shared memory. BigSpring runs the 32-bit version of Linux CentOS release 5 (Final) on 2.6.18 kernel.

In both systems, no more than eight processors were used for all the experiments. Experimenting with larger number of processors is left for future work.

5.4.2 Compilers

Since Intel's and IBM's compilers are among the best, they are employed in this study in order to obtain a deeper insight into parallelization possibilities of the state-of-the-art compilers. Intel compiler on BigSpring is used for measuring the execution time of the autoparallelized and vectorized code. The IBM compiler on Hydra is used for measuring the execution time of the manually parallelized benchmarks.

When comparing sequential and manually parallelized versions of the benchmarks, we must guarantee fairness, that is, the sequential optimizations applied by the compiler must be the same for both versions. To ensure this, the optimization level on xlC was set conservatively (no interprocedural analysis) to -O2 -qnoinline. However, -qnoinline is not used for dealII benchmark since it takes too long and, therefore, does not represent the benchmark correctly. When running a manually parallelized version of the benchmark, -qsmp=noauto:omp option was added. This option specifies that the compiler should not parallelize segments of code that are not explicitly marked with OpenMP directives. The intention was to measure only speedup provided by modifying the desired code segments. Table 5.12 summarizes the compiler options.

5.4.3 Profilers

The profiler is an inevitable software tool in measuring run-time characteristics and resource utilization of a program. Profiling results can vary as they are dependent on the hardware and the software platform details [88].

Table 5.12 Compiler Options

Mode	Machine	Compiler	Options
Profiling	BigSpring	Intel C++ 9.1.042	–O1 –p
Autoparallelization	BigSpring	Intel C++ 9.1.042	–O3 –openmp
Vectorization	BigSpring	Intel C++ 9.1.042	–O3 –xN
Profiling	Hydra	xlC 8.0	–O2 –q64 –qnoinline –pg
Sequential version	Hydra	xlC 8.0	–O2 –q64 –qnoinline
Manual parallelization	Hydra	xlC 8.0	–O2 –q64 –qnoinline –qsmp=noauto:omp

To avoid the platform-specific bias, both machines were used for gathering the statistics.

We used `gprof` for profiling. It gives CPU time instead of the real wall time. Disk delays and eventual thrashing due to input/output are not accounted.

Although the sampling is the principal method, there is also some instrumentation during compile time, since the correct number of calls for each method was needed. The tick period is OS-dependent, yet it is 0.01 s on both machines. This is obviously not enough, since some methods take only a few nanoseconds. As stated in Ref. [89], the expected time measurement error in this case is

$$\text{TICK\_PERIOD} * \sqrt{\frac{\text{PROGRAM\_EXECUTION\_TIME}}{\text{TICK\_PERIOD}}}$$

5.4.4 General Methodology

The basic procedure for running CPU2006 benchmarks is described in Ref. [90]. Benchmarks can be run in the interactive mode or in the batch mode. The interactive mode provides for direct benchmark execution on a limited number of processors that are usually front ends shared among all users. This mode is used to test the benchmark and to check the environment. After that, in order to acquire the accurate results of the execution, the benchmark is run in the batch mode where one processor can be dedicated to only one user process.

A benchmark has to be copied on the fastest hard drive available, since the goal is not to measure the memory access time, but speedups in general. During benchmark execution, its status (running, dispatched, or finished) can be seen using a platform-dependent tool. The operating system schedules processes across the network. Selecting particular processors where OpenMP instances should be executed is better to leave to the OS and environment, since they are more aware of available resources and their collaboration. Also, there is no process migration if the hardware operates correctly.

After the source codes had been modified, a procedure of preparation for execution was carried out using as many CPU2006 tools as possible. Firstly, CPU2006 configuration files were adjusted according to the processor, OS, and compiler type, as well as the compiler optimization flags and various test settings. After the benchmarks had been compiled, the job files were submitted to the batch queue. The job files may contain information about the number of processors, memory resources for each particular process, the upper limit for wall clock time execution, and environment variables, such as the benchmark name and location.

When the job successfully passed the queue, output/error files from the benchmark and queue facility had to be checked. `Specdiff` was used to compare the obtained and expected results. Some slight differences in the compared results are allowed and even expected due to compiler optimizations and operation reordering in the parallel environment.

As for the scalability, the strong scaling is followed in this study, since data size was the same for the sequential and parallel benchmark versions.

5.5. Evaluation Results

The optimizations elaborated upon in this section tend to be general since only source-to-source code transformations are used. The profiling information was collected on both machines, so that platform-dependent extremes were eliminated. To account for slight variations in run-time conditions, all the profiling measurements were run at least twice on each machine. The biggest difference observed in a function profile was 1.34% within `astar` on Hydra.

In order to anticipate if the OpenMP parallelization of a code segment brings a performance improvement, without the actual running of the modified program, we introduce an estimation model. The model leverages the parallelization benefits (or penalties) by predicting parallelization overhead. It is generic enough to work on any platform by measuring the execution time of a small parallel program with different number of processors. We illustrate the model and perform the measurements on Hydra, as we run manually parallelized benchmarks on that machine. The program consists of an outer sequential loop and an inner OpenMP loop (Table 5.13). To measure only the overheads, the program does no useful work. To prevent the compiler from performing dead code elimination, the inner loop invokes an empty method. The optimization was indeed prevented, as the measured execution time grows with the number of processors and iterations.

The execution time of this segment is measured in systems with different processor counts (2 and 16) and for a different number of the inner loop iterations (from 100 up to 100,000). Table 5.14 presents the execution times of the inner loop in microseconds averaged over BIGLOOP = 10,000 outer iterations. Since the threads are spawned only in the first iteration of the outer loop, the thread creation time can be neglected. We are actually measuring the overheads of blocking/unblocking parallel threads.

It is obvious from the results that the overhead for thread creation prevails for smaller iteration counts (100, 1000) and the execution time on 16 processors is even longer than on 2 processors. For higher iteration counts (10,000 and more), this overhead is amortized over a higher number of

Table 5.13 Code Segment for Measuring Parallelization Overhead

```
for(int i=0; i<BIGLOOP; i++){
#pragma omp parallel for \
private(j) shared(PARLOOP) schedule(static)
    for(j=0; j<PARLOOP; j++){
        empty();
    }
}
```

Table 5.14 Execution Time of the Inner Loop for 2 and 16 Processors

PARLOOP/Number of Processors	2	16
100	2.63 µs	9.58 µs
1000	4.74 µs	9.09 µs
10,000	26.27 µs	18.36 µs
100,000	239.85 µs	50.39 µs

Table 5.15 Calculated Overhead of Parallelization

PARLOOP/Overhead	Overhead (2)	Overhead (16)
100	2.4 μs	9.54 μs
1000	2.34 μs	8.78 μs
10,000	2.73 μs	15.35 μs

iterations and the benefit of more processors is evident in the decreased execution time.

The execution times in Table 5.14 contain both the parallelization overheads and the time to execute the loop in parallel. We can estimate the overhead in the following way. Since each of two processors runs a half of the iteration count due to the static scheduling, two equations follow from the results from Table 5.14.

$$\text{Overhead(2)} + 50*\texttt{iter} = 2.63\mu s$$
$$\text{Overhead(2)} + 50000*\texttt{iter} = 239.85\mu s$$

Considering that `Overhead(2)` can be neglected in the second equation, the iteration time (`iter`) is estimated to 4.8 ns. By substituting the value of `iter` in the first equation, we can compute `Overhead(2)`. In the same way, the values `Overhead(2)` and `Overhead(16)` are calculated for other iteration counts. The calculated values are presented in Table 5.15.

Since a node of Hydra has 16 processors, an upper bound for the parallelization overhead can be estimated to 20 μs. With this value, the benefit of parallelizing a code segment on N processors could be easily foreseen. If `seq_time` is the execution time of the segment on a single machine, the execution time of the parallelized segment is `par_time=overhead (N) + seq_time/N`. If `par_time < seq_time`, the parallelization brings speedup. The total speedup is determined from Amdahl's law. Namely, the total execution time of the parallelized program is a sum of the time spent in a nonparallelized portion of the code and the `par_time`.

In the following sections, the specific findings about possible parallelization and its effects (either speedup or slowdown) are discussed for particular C++ applications from CPU2006.

5.5.1 Namd

In the `main` function of `namd`, a parallelization of the computation within each time step is extremely beneficial, as shown in Section 5.2.1. Here, we examine the effects of some lower-level parallelizations.

As a straightforward approach, parallelization of the inner loops was firstly attempted. An example is the *for* loop in `ComputeNonboundedBase.h` with two instructions and a *switch* command with three cases, each of them having one instruction (Table 5.A1). It was parallelized by using three OpenMP sections containing an *if* clause for each case. The *for* loop stayed in all three sections, but the computation of the variables used in the loop body was moved in front of this code, in a separate parallel *for*, and here, they only read from memory. The number of loop iterations was less than 60, and the time spent in one entry of this *for* loop was insignificant. We set the iteration count threshold for parallel execution to 40. The effect was a slowdown of 1.2% with four processors.

Another example is the *while* loop in `ComputeNonboundedBase.h`. It was transformed into a *for* loop and the three statements for the computation of some constants were put inside the loop (Table 5.A2). The transformed loop contains 10 statements and up to 286 iterations were executed. We set the iteration number threshold to 100. The purpose of the original *while* loop was to compute the prefix sum. This is a well-known problem for which parallel algorithms exist [91]. Due to the small number of iterations, employing the parallel prefix sum resulted in the 47% slowdown on four processors. To find out the number of iterations that brings benefits in the parallel execution, we compared the parallel prefix sum against its sequential counterpart outside the benchmark. The parallel version was faster if the number of iterations was at least 5500 for two processors and at least 11,000 for four processors.

5.5.2 Dealii

`ConstraintMatrix::add_line` is the routine that consumes most of the execution time in this benchmark. It adds an element at the end of the collection, so the parallel structures and algorithms can help. It is called from `DoFTools::make_hanging_node_constraints` in average 15,750 times in the loop. Average time spent in `add_line` is around $105\mu s$ due to checking whether the line structure already exists in the collection. `DoFTools::make_hanging_node_constraints` also calls `ConstraintMatrix::add_entry` in loop for 121,000 times on average, but rather a small amount of time is spent in `add_entry` in the entire benchmark. In addition, one call of this method lasts for about $2\,\mu s$. Table 5.A3 presents the `ConstraintMatrix::add_line` method, while Table 5.A4 shows the `DoFTools::make_hanging_node_constraints` method.

The `MappingQ1::compute_fill` method in `compute_fill.cc` is also a hot spot. Although four nested *for* loops found in some summations in this method look promising, their parallelization was not possible.

5.5.3 Soplex

The PARALLEL_RESET pattern is recognized in the `SSVector::clear` method (see Table 5.16). There were no loop-carried dependences due to the semantics of benchmark. The *for* loop inside this method has up to almost 800,000 iterations, but it takes only 1.15% of the total benchmark execution time. Setting the threshold for parallel execution to 4000 iterations resulted in a 2% slowdown with eight processors. Increasing the threshold did not help. The justification for these results is that most of the time the actual iteration count was rather low.

A single invocation of `SSVector::assign2productFull` in `ssvector.cc` takes in average 16.7 ms (see Table 5.17). The method is invoked 1950 times on Hydra and 2200 times on BigSpring. These facts clearly

Table 5.16 The PARALLEL_RESET Pattern in `soplex`

```
                                    int i;
                                    if(num>THRESHOLD) {
                                      #pragma omp parallel for \
                                      shared(num,val,idx) \
                                        private(i)
for(int i = 0; i<num; ++i)            for(i = 0; i < num; ++i)
    val[idx[i]] = 0.0;      ⟹           val[idx[i]] = 0.0;
                                    }else{
                                        for(i = 0; i < num; ++i)
                                            val[idx[i]] = 0.0;
                                        }
                                    }
```

Table 5.17 The PARALLEL_VECTOR Pattern in `soplex`

```
                                    for (i=x.size(); i-->0; ++xi)
                                    {
for(i = x.size(); i-->0;++xi)         svec = const_cast<SVector*>
{                                                     ( & A[*xi] );
 svec = const_cast<SVector*>         y = vl[*xi];
               ( & A[*xi] );         #pragma omp parallel for \
 elem = &(svec->element(0));           shared(y,v,svec)
 last = elem + svec->size();  ⟹        private(j,elem)
 y = vl[*xi];                          for (j=0;j<svec->size();j++)
 for (; elem < last; ++elem)           {
  v[elem->idx]+=y *elem->val;            elem = &(svec->element(j));
}                                        v[elem->idx]+=y*elem->val;
                                         }
                                    }
```

identify the method as a candidate for parallelization within the method. The inner *for* loop in this method has more inherent potential since the iteration count goes from 1 up to 47,500, while the outer loop iteration count goes up to 1500. Thus, the PARALLEL_VECTOR pattern was applied for the inner loop. Due to the benchmark semantics, there were no loop-carried dependences in the inner loop. With no threshold specified, the achieved speedup was 4% on an 8-processor system. Interestingly, setting the threshold degrades the performance, as most of the time the iteration count was large enough, and adding the *if* condition comes with a nonzero cost.

The `updateTest` method from `soplex::SoPlex` was promising for consideration since it calls `test` method in a loop and the `test` method does not have side effects. The PARALLEL_VECTOR pattern is clearly recognized in the updateTest (see Table 5.18). In a single invocation of `updateTest`, `test` method is in average invoked 395,000 times. A single invocation of `test` takes 10ns on average. Therefore, in one *for* loop of updateTest, the average accumulated time spent in `test` is about 4 ms. In the 8-processor system, the execution time of the parallelized code segment is

$$20\mu s + 4ms/8 \text{ processors} = 520\mu s \ll 4ms.$$

Since the `updateTest` method takes about 5% time of the entire program, a speedup of 4% could theoretically be obtained. Due to the

Table 5.18 Potential for PARALLEL_VECTOR in `soplex`

```
void SoPlex::updateTest()
{
    METHOD( "SoPlex::updateTest()" );
    thePvec->delta().setup();
    const IdxSet& idx = thePvec->idx();
    const SPxBasis::Desc& ds = desc();

    int i;
    for (i = idx.size() - 1; i >= 0; --i)
    {
        int j = idx.index(i);
        SPxBasis::Desc::Status stat = ds.status(j);
        if (!isBasic(stat))
            theTest[j] = test(j, stat);
        else
            theTest[j] = 0;
    }
}
```

parallelization test that is required to check for loop-carried dependences, the expected speedup is slightly smaller.

5.5.4 Astar

In this benchmark, the PARALLEL_RESET pattern can be found in the `regmngobj::getregfillnum` method (see Table 5.19). This method takes 11.2% (about 112 s) of the execution time and it is invoked 93,000 times in total. *For* loop within the method contains a single statement; it has up to 41,000 iterations, but in average, a single-loop execution takes 1200 μs. Due to the semantics of the benchmark, the loop has no loop-carried dependences. We parallelized the loop and obtained 6% speedup using eight processors.

Now we compare the measured speedup against the one computed from the estimation model. The total execution time can be computed from the formula.

`88.8% total_seq_time + 11.2% total_seq_time/N + number_of_calls*overhead`

---

where `total_seq_time` is the execution time of the entire sequential program (1120 s in our case), N is the number of processors (eight in our case), `overhead` is estimated to 20 μs, and the `number_of_calls` is the number of times the method is invoked (93,000 in our case). By substituting all the variables, it can be computed that the theoretically estimated speedup is around 8%. This is close to the measured speedup. These results validate our estimation model.

A potential for parallelization was also considered in the `regwayobj::makebound2` method, but the execution time of an entire outer loop is less than 20 μs on average. This method is not an extreme hot spot, so a significant speedup cannot be obtained anyway. In addition, the synchronization of the parallel structures would be necessary, since in the `regwayobj::addtobound` method, the elements are added into the same collection.

Table 5.20 summarizes the speedup for each particular benchmark (negative values mean slowdown). The first two rows refer to the measured

Table 5.19 The PARALLEL_RESET Pattern in `astar`

`for (i=0; i<rarp.elemqu; i++)`
`    rarp[i]->fillnum=0;` ⟹
	`#pragma omp parallel for \`
	`    shared(rarp) \`
	`    private(i)`
	`    for (i=0; i<rarp.elemqu; i++)`
	`        rarp[i]->fillnum=0;`

Table 5.20 The Application Speedups for Different Parallelization Methods

Method/Program	namd	dealll	soplex	povray	omnetpp	astar	xalancbmk
Autoparallelization	n/a	n/a	n/a	−1.9%	n/a	n/a	n/a
Vectorization	12.5%	−4.16%	5.3%	−1.3%	13%	4.7%	3%
Manual interventions	n/a	n/a	4%	n/a	n/a	6%	n/a
Estimated potential with manual changes	600%	n/a	7%	n/a	n/a	6%	n/a

effects of autoparallelization and vectorization, respectively. The third row (manual interventions) gives the measured speedups, while the fourth row (full potential with manual changes) presents the sum of the measured and estimated speedup when all the considered optimizations for a particular benchmark are applied.

6. CONCLUSION

Rapidly growing acceptance of parallel systems and multicore processors emphasizes the importance of more efficient use of their resources in case of execution of the sequential programs. Therefore, the problem of their parallelization is imminent. The chapter first explores theoretical background in the field and overviews various parallelization approaches and tools. As a case study, the chapter also examines the manual parallelization of the standard SPEC CPU2006 benchmark suite. Automatic parallelization of these benchmarks by the compiler was not shown to be very effective and even slowdown was occasionally incurred, while vectorization can bring some speedup. Therefore, the approach of manual parallelization based on the profiling information was pursued in this study.

Although more thorough evaluation is needed, the experience gained in this study has confirmed that the potential for speedup by manual parallelization can be found even in highly optimized sequential applications such as those from the SPEC CPU2006. Profiling data can help in setting threshold iteration counts for conditional parallelization of the loops according to useful performance prediction models (as a simple one from this study) and can provide valuable information to identify hot spots. Speedups obtained by manual parallelization of these hotspots are significant, keeping in mind that they are incurred by applying parallelization on a single code segment. Up to 600% speedup was predicted by applying a single parallelization pattern.

Much more effort in parallelization of the SPEC CPU2006 and other sequential applications is needed to build up strong conclusions and provide the experience that can lead to implementation of some techniques in compilers to enhance their abilities of autoparallelization.

ACKNOWLEDGMENTS

A. V. would like to thank Prof. Lawrence Rauchwerger, who accepted him for an internship, for many very helpful suggestions, and also to the entire Parasol Laboratory faculty and staff at Texas A&M University, who helped him a lot in configuring machines and starting jobs on them.

 APPENDIX

Table 5.A1 Transformed *switch* in namd

```
                                        int startk = k;
                                        int* excl_flag_val =
                                            new int[npair2-startk];

                                            for (; k<npair2; ++k ) {
                                                int j = pairlist2[k];
                                                int atom2 = p_1[j].id;
                                                excl_flag_val[k-startk]=
                                                    excl_flags[atom2];
                                            }
                                        #pragma omp parallel
                                        {

                                        #pragma omp sections private(k)
                                        {
                                        #pragma omp section
                                        {
for (; k < npair2; ++k ) {              for (k=startk; k<npair2; ++k) {
    int j = pairlist2[k];                int j = pairlist2[k];
    int atom2 = p_1[j].id;               if (excl_flag_val[k-startk]==0)
    int excl_flag =                        {
        excl_flags[atom2];                   *(plin++) = j;
    switch ( excl_flag ) {                 }
        case 0:                          }
*(plin++) = j;  break;                   }
        case 1:                          #pragma omp section
*(plix++) = j;  break;                   {
```

```
      case 2:                        for (k=startk; k<npair2; ++k ){
 *(plim++) = j;   break;              int j = pairlist2[k];
   }                                  if (excl_flag_val[k-startk]==1)
}                                         {
                                            *(plix++) = j;
                                          }
                                      }
                                    }
                                    #pragma omp section
                                    {
                                    for (k=startk; k<npair2; ++k ) {
                                     int j = pairlist2[k];
                                     if (excl_flag_val[k-startk]==2)
                                        {
                                          *(plim++) = j;
                                        }
                                      }
                                     }
                                    }
                                    }

                                    delete [] excl_flag_val;
```

Table 5.A2 Transformed *while* in namd

```
if ( g < gu ) {
      int j2 = glist[g];
      BigReal p_j_x = p_1[j2].position.x;
      BigReal p_j_y = p_1[j2].position.y;
      BigReal p_j_z = p_1[j2].position.z;
      while ( g < gu ) {
      j = j2;
      j2 = glist[++g];
        BigReal r2 = p_i_x - p_j_x;
        r2 *= r2;
      p_j_x = p_1[j2].position.x;
        BigReal t2 = p_i_y - p_j_y;
        r2 += t2 * t2;
      p_j_y = p_1[j2].position.y;
        t2 = p_i_z - p_j_z;
        r2 += t2 * t2;
      p_j_z = p_1[j2].position.z;
        // use a slightly large cutoff to include hydrogens
        if ( r2 <= groupcutoff2 )
        { *gli = j; ++gli; }
      }
}
```

⇩

```
if ( g < gu ) {
     const int THRESHOLD=100;
     int start_g=g;
     int sizearr= gu - start_g;
     if (sizearr>THRESHOLD){
          /****************************************
          optimized way if data size is critical
          ****************************************/
        /*forming data input for prefix*/
        int* r2arr = new int[sizearr];

        #pragma omp parallel for \
        shared(start_g, gu, r2arr,groupcutoff2) \
        private(g, j)
           for(g=start_g; g<gu; g++){
               j=glist[g];
               BigReal p_j_x = p_1[j].position.x;
               BigReal p_j_y = p_1[j].position.y;
               BigReal p_j_z = p_1[j].position.z;

               BigReal r2 = p_i_x - p_j_x;
               r2 *= r2;
               BigReal t2 = p_i_y - p_j_y;
               r2 += t2 * t2;
               t2 = p_i_z - p_j_z;
               r2 += t2 * t2;

               r2arr[g-start_g]=0;
               if ( r2 <= groupcutoff2 ) {
                   r2arr[g-start_g]=1;
               }
           }

        long* prefix =
               parallelPrefixSum(r2arr, sizearr);

        #pragma omp parallel for \
        shared(start_g, gu, r2arr, glist, gli,prefix) \
        private(g, j)
           for(g=start_g; g<gu; g++){
               int index = g-start_g;
               if(r2arr[index]!=0){
               j=glist[g];
```

```
            gli[prefix[index]-1]=j;
                    //  -1 since first element
                    // (with prefix sum 1)
                    // to put in zero slot
        }
      gli+=prefix[sizearr-1];

      //cleaning data on heap
      delete [] prefix;
      delete [] r2arr;
    }else{
       // original sequential version
    }
}
```

Table 5.A3 ConstraintMatrix::add_line in dealll

```
void ConstraintMatrix::add_line (const unsigned int line)
{
  Assert (sorted==false, ExcMatrixIsClosed());

   // check whether line already exists;
   // it may, but then we need to quit

   for (unsigned int i=0; i!=lines.size(); ++i)
     if (lines[i].line == line)
       return;

     // push a new line to the end of the
     // list
   lines.push_back (ConstraintLine());
   lines.back().line = line;
}
```

Table 5.A4 DoFTools::make_hanging_node_constraints in dealll

```
for (unsigned int row=0; row!=dofs_on_children.size(); ++row){
    constraints.add_line (dofs_on_children[row]);
    for (unsigned int i=0; i!=dofs_on_mother.size(); ++i)
        constraints.add_entry (dofs_on_children[row],
                               dofs_on_mother[i],
                               fe.constraints()(row,i));
}
```

Table 5.A5 Macro Definitions in namd

```
#define RUN_AND_CHECKSUM \
    patchList.zeroresults(); \
    computeList.runComputes(&patchList); \
    if ( patchList.reductionData[exclChecksumIndex] != \
                      molecule.numCalcExclusions ) { \
      printf("exclusion checksum failure!\n"); \
      exit(-8); }
```

```
#define SET_MODE(E,F,M) \
    patchList.doEnergy = E; patchList.doFull = F; \
    patchList.doMerge = M; \
    printf("iteration %d: %d %d %d\n",i,E,F,M);
```

```
#define WRITE(R) \
    patchList.setresults(&R); \
    if ( output ) R.writefile(output_file); \
    if ( standard ) { \
      comp.readfile(standard_file); \
      R.samemode(comp); R.compare(comp); }
```

Table 5.A6 Original and Transformed Code in namd

```
for(i=0; i<iterations; ++i) {          for(i=0; i<iterations; ++i){
    SET_MODE(1,0,0)                    #pragma omp parallel
    RUN_AND_CHECKSUM                     {
    WRITE(r100)                           #pragma omp sections
    SET_MODE(1,1,0)                        {
    RUN_AND_CHECKSUM                        #pragma omp section
    WRITE(r110)                             SET_MODE(1,0,0)
    SET_MODE(1,1,1)                         RUN_AND_CHECKSUM
    RUN_AND_CHECKSUM                        WRITE(r100)
    WRITE(r111)
    SET_MODE(0,0,0)                         #pragma omp section
    RUN_AND_CHECKSUM                        SET_MODE(1,1,0)
    WRITE(r000)                             RUN_AND_CHECKSUM
    SET_MODE(0,1,0)                         WRITE(r110)
    RUN_AND_CHECKSUM
    WRITE(r010)                           #pragma omp section
    SET_MODE(0,1,1)                         SET_MODE(1,1,1)
    RUN_AND_CHECKSUM                        RUN_AND_CHECKSUM
    WRITE(r011)                             WRITE(r111)

    r100.compare(r110);        ⟹        #pragma omp section
    r100.compare(r111);                    SET_MODE(0,0,0)
```

```
r100.compare(r000);              RUN_AND_CHECKSUM
r100.compare(r010);              WRITE(r000)
r100.compare(r011);
                                 #pragma omp section
r110.compare(r111);              SET_MODE(0,1,0)
r110.compare(r000);              RUN_AND_CHECKSUM
r110.compare(r010);              WRITE(r010)
r110.compare(r011);
r111.compare(r000);              #pragma omp section
r111.compare(r010);              SET_MODE(0,1,1)
r111.compare(r011);              RUN_AND_CHECKSUM
r000.compare(r010);              WRITE(r011)
r000.compare(r011);              } /* end of sections */
r010.compare(r011);             } /* end of parallel */
                                } /* end of for loop
patchList.moveatoms();
}
```

REFERENCES

[1] D. Culler, J. Singh, A. Gupta, Parallel Computer Architecture: A Hardware/Software Approach, Morgan Kaufmann Publishers Inc., Burlington, Massachusetts, 1998.

[2] K. Olukotun, L. Hammond, J. Laudon, Chip Multiprocessor Architecture Techniques to Improve Throughput and Latency, Morgan & Claypool Publishers, San Rafael, CA, USA, 2007.

[3] K. Asanovic, et al., The Landscape of Parallel Computing Research: A View from BerkeleyTechnical report UCB/EECS-2006-183, EECS Department, University of California, Berkeley, 2006.

[4] SPEC CPU2006. http://www.spec.org/cpu2006/ (accessed 23 July 2013).

[5] J.L. Henning, SPEC CPU2006 benchmark descriptions, SIGARCH Comput. Archit. News 34 (4) (2006) 1–17.

[6] R. Chandra, R. Menon, L. Dagum, et al., Parallel Programming in OpenMP, first ed., Morgan Kaufmann, San Francisco, USA, 2001.

[7] A.R. Hurson, J.T. Lim, K.M. Kavi, et al., Parallelization of DOALL and DOACROSS loops—a survey, in: Advances in Computers, 45 Elsevier, 1997, pp. 53–103.

[8] R. Allen, K. Kennedy, Optimizing Compilers for Modern Architectures: A Dependence-Based Approach, first ed., Morgan Kaufmann, San Francisco, USA, 2001.

[9] A.V. Aho, R. Sethi, J.D. Ullman, Compilers: Principles, Techniques, and Tools Used, Addison Wesley, Boston, USA, 1986.

[10] L. Rauchwerger, D. Padua, The LRPD test: speculative run-time parallelization of loops with privatization and reduction parallelization, IEEE Trans. Parallel Distrib. Syst. 10 (2) (1999) 160–180.

[11] J. Dean, S. Ghemawat, MapReduce: simplified data processing on large clusters, in: OSDI, San Francisco, CA, USA, 2004.

[12] M. Wolfe, Understanding the CUDA data parallel threading model. http://www.pgroup.com/lit/articles/insider/v2n1a5.htm (accessed 23 July 2013).

[13] Message Passing Interface (MPI) tutorial. https://computing.llnl.gov/tutorials/mpi/ (accessed 23 July 2013).

[14] OpenMP tutorial. https://computing.llnl.gov/tutorials/openMP/ (accessed 23 July 2013).

[15] M. Frigo, C.E. Leiserson, K.H. Randall, The implementation of the Cilk-5 multi-threaded language, in: PLDI, 1998, pp. 212–223.

[16] C.E. Leiserson, The Cilk++ concurrency platform, in: Proceedings of the 46th Annual Design Automation Conference, 2009, pp. 522–527.

[17] J.-L. Gaudiot, W. Bohm, W. Najjar, et al., The Sisal model of functional programming and its implementation, in: Proceedings of the 2nd AIZU International Symposium on Parallel Algorithms/Architecture Synthesis, 1997, pp. 112–123.

[18] W.W. Carlson, J.M. Draper, D.E. Culler, et al., Introduction to UPC and Language SpecificationTechnical report CCS-TR-99-157, IDA Center for Computing Sciences, 1999.

[19] J. Reinders, Intel Threading Building Blocks: Outfitting C++ for Multicore Processor Parallelism, O'Reilly Media, Sebastopol, CA, USA, 2007.

[20] P. An, A. Jula, S. Rus, et al., STAPL: an adaptive, generic parallel C++ library, in: Languages and Compilers for Parallel Computing, Springer, Berlin, Heidelberg, 2001, pp. 193–208.

[21] M. Cole, Algorithmic Skeletons: Structured Management of Parallel Computation, MIT Press, Cambridge, MA, USA, 1991.

[22] H. González-Vélez, M. Leyton, A survey of algorithmic skeleton frameworks: high-level structured parallel programming enablers, Softw. Pract. Exp. 40 (12) (2010) 1135–1160.

[23] M. Leyton, J.M. Piquer, Skandium: multi-core programming with algorithmic skeletons, in: 18th Euromicro International Conference on Parallel, Distributed and Network-Based Processing, 2010, pp. 289–296.

[24] A. Benoit, M. Cole, Two fundamental concepts in skeletal parallel programming, in: Proceedings of the 5th International Conference on Computational Science, vol. Part II, 2005, pp. 764–771.

[25] P. Alvaro, N. Conway, J.M. Hellerstein, et al., Consistency analysis in bloom: a CALM and collected approach, in: Proceedings of the 5th Conference on Innovative Data Systems Research, 2011.

[26] M. Isard, M. Budiu, Y. Yu, et al., Dryad: distributed data-parallel programs from sequential building blocks, in: EuroSys, 2007.

[27] Apache™ Hadoop®. http://hadoop.apache.org/ (accessed 23 July 2013).

[28] MathWorks MATLAB. http://www.mathworks.com/products/matlab/ (accessed 23 July 2013).

[29] M. Griebl, Automatic parallelization of loop programs for distributed memory architectures, habilitation thesis, University of Passau, 2004.

[30] C. Bastoul, Efficient code generation for automatic parallelization and optimization, in: Proceedings of the Second International Symposium on Parallel and, Distributed Computing, 2003, pp. 23–30.

[31] C. Chen, J. Chame, M. Hall, CHiLL: A Framework for Composing High-Level Loop Transformations, Technical report 08-897, University of Southern California, 2008.

[32] S. Garcia, D. Jeon, C.M. Louie, et al., Kremlin: rethinking and rebooting gprof for the multicore age, in: PLDI, 2011, pp. 458–469.

[33] M.W. Hall, J.M. Anderson, S.P. Amarasinghe, et al., Maximizing multiprocessor performance with the SUIF compiler, Computer 29 (12) (1996) 84–89.

[34] D. Padua, Polaris: An Optimizing Compiler for Parallel Workstations and Scalable MultiprocessorsTechnical report 1475, Center for Supercomputing Research & Development, University of Illinois, Urbana-Champaign, 1996.

[35] S. Rus, D. Zhang, L. Rauchwerger, The value evolution graph and its use in memory reference analysis, in: Proceedings of the 13th International Conference on Parallel Architectures and Compilation Techniques, Washington, D.C., USA, 2004, pp. 243–254.

[36] C. Dave, H. Bae, S.-J. Min, et al., Cetus: a source-to-source compiler infrastructure for multicores, Computer 42 (12) (2009) 36–42.

[37] D. Quinlan, et al., ROSE user manual: a tool for building source-to-source translators. http://rosecompiler.org/ (accessed 23 July 2013).

[38] A. Basumallik, R. Eigenmann, Towards automatic translation of OpenMP to MPI, in: Proceedings of the 19th Annual International Conference on Supercomputing, New York, USA, 2005, pp. 189–198.

[39] DMS Software Reengineering Toolkit. http://www.semdesigns.com/products/DMS/DMSToolkit.html (accessed 23 July 2013).

[40] M. Gonzàlez, et al., Nanos mercurium: a research compiler for OpenMP, in: Proceedings of the European Workshop on OpenMP, 2004, pp. 103–109.

[41] M.D. Linderman, J.D. Collins, H. Wang, et al., Merge: a programming model for heterogeneous multi-core systems abstract, in: Proceedings of the 13th International Conference on Architectural Support for Programming Languages and Operating Systems, 2008, pp. 287–296.

[42] V.T. Ravi, W. Ma, D. Chiu, et al., Compiler and runtime support for enabling generalized reduction computations on heterogeneous parallel configurations, in: Proceedings of the 24th ACM International Conference on Supercomputing, New York, USA, 2010, pp. 137–146.

[43] H.L.A. van der Spek, S. Groot, E.M. Bakker, et al., A compile/run-time environment for the automatic transformation of linked list data structures, Int. J. Parallel Prog. 36 (6) (2008) 592–623.

[44] M. Kulkarni, D. Prountzos, D. Nguyen, et al., Defining and Implementing Commutativity Conditions for Parallel ExecutionTechnical report, ECE Department, Purdue University, 2009.

[45] T.H. Cormen, C.E. Leiserson, R.L. Rivest, et al., Introduction to Algorithms, MIT Press, Cambridge, Massachusetts, 2003.

[46] Y. Ni, V.S. Menon, A.-R. Adl-Tabatabai, et al., Open nesting in software transactional memory, in: Proceedings of the 12th ACM SIGPLAN Symposium on Principles and Practice of Parallel Programming, 2007, pp. 68–78.

[47] C. Liao, D.J. Quinlan, J.J. Willcock, et al., Semantic-aware automatic parallelization of modern applications using high-level abstractions, Int. J. Parallel Prog. 38 (5–6) (2010) 361–378.

[48] R. Asenjo, R. Castillo, F. Corbera, et al., Parallelizing irregular C codes assisted by interprocedural shape analysis, in: IEEE International Symposium on Parallel and Distributed Processing, 2008, pp. 1–12.

[49] G. Tournavitis, Z. Wang, B. Franke, et al., Towards a holistic approach to auto-parallelization: integrating profile-driven parallelism detection and machine-learning based mapping, in: PLDI, 2009.

[50] TILE64 Processor. http://www.tilera.com/products/processors/TILE64 (accessed 23 July 2013).

[51] A. Klauser, T. Austin, D. Grunwald, et al., Dynamic hammock predication for non-predicated instruction set architectures, in: PACT, 1998, pp. 278–285.

[52] D.I. August, W.W. Hwu, S.A. Mahlke, A framework for balancing control flow and predication, in: MICRO, 1997, pp. 92–103.

[53] Hyesoon Kim, J.A. Joao, O. Mutlu, et al., Profile-assisted compiler support for dynamic predication in diverge-merge processors, in: International Symposium on Code Generation and Optimization, 2007, pp. 367–378.

[54] M. Stephenson, Lixin Zhang, R. Rangan, Lightweight predication support for out of order processors, in: HPCA, 2009, pp. 201–212.

[55] D.I. August, D.A. Connors, S.A. Mahlke, et al., Integrated predicated and speculative execution in the IMPACT EPIC architecture, in: Proceedings of the 25th International Symposium on Computer, Architecture, 1998, pp. 227–237.

[56] R. Ramaseshan, F. Mueller, Toward thread-level speculation for coarse-grained parallelism with regular access patterns, in: MULTIPROG, 2008.

[57] V. Packirisamy, A. Zhai, Wei-Chung Hsu, et al., Exploring speculative parallelism in SPEC2006, in: IEEE International Symposium on Performance Analysis of Systems and Software, 2009, pp. 77–88.

[58] J. Whaley, C. Kozyrakis, Heuristics for profile-driven method-level speculative parallelization, in: International Conference on Parallel Processing, 2005, pp. 147–156.

[59] P. Wu, A. Kejariwal, C. Caşcaval, Compiler-driven dependence profiling to guide program parallelization, in: J.N. Amaral (Ed.), Languages and Compilers for Parallel Computing, Springer-Verlag, Edmonton, Canada, 2008, pp. 232–248.

[60] D. Das, Peng Wu, Experiences of using a dependence profiler to assist parallelization for multi-cores, in: IEEE International Parallel & Distributed Processing Symposium, 2010, pp. 1–8.

[61] G. Ottoni, R. Rangan, A. Stoler, et al., Automatic thread extraction with decoupled software pipelining, in: MICRO, 2005, pp. 105–118.

[62] N. Vachharajani, R. Rangan, E. Raman, et al., Speculative decoupled software pipelining, in: PACT, Washington, D.C., USA, 2007, pp. 49–59.

[63] M. Bridges, N. Vachharajani, Y. Zhang, et al., Revisiting the sequential programming model for multi-core, in: MICRO, Washington, D.C., USA, 2007, pp. 69–84.

[64] J. Torrellas, L. Ceze, J. Tuck, et al., The Bulk Multicore architecture for improved programmability, Commun. ACM 52 (12) (2009) 58.

[65] J.R. Larus, R. Rajwar, Transactional memory, Synth. Lect. Comput. Archit. 1 (1) (2006) 1–226.

[66] A. Raman, H. Kim, T.R. Mason, et al., Speculative parallelization using software multi-threaded transactions, in: Proceedings of the Fifteenth edition of Architectural Support for Programming Languages and Operating Systems, 2010, pp. 65–76.

[67] K. Fatahalian, M. Houston, A closer look at GPUs, Commun. ACM 51 (10) (2008) 50–57.

[68] Tuning MPI programs for peak performance. http://www.mcs.anl.gov/research/projects/mpi/tutorial/perf/mpiperf/index.htm (accessed 23 July 2013).

[69] V. Packirisamy, Efficient architecture support for thread-level speculation, University of Minnesota, PhD Thesis, April 2009.

[70] ParBenCCh 1.0 Parallel C++ Benchmarking Suite. https://asc.llnl.gov/computing_resources/purple/archive/benchmarks/parbencch/ (accessed 23 July 2013).

[71] S.C. Woo, M. Ohara, E. Torrie, et al., The SPLASH-2 programs: characterization and methodological considerations, in: International Symposium on Computer, Architecture, 1995, pp. 24–36.

[72] G. Zhang, P. Unnikrishnan, J. Ren, Experiments with auto-parallelizing SPEC2000FP benchmarks, in: Languages and Compilers for High Performance Computing, vol. 3602, Springer, Berlin, Heidelberg, 2005, pp. 348–362.

[73] H. Zhong, M. Mehrara, S. Lieberman, et al., Uncovering hidden loop level parallelism in sequential applications, in: HPCA, 2008.

[74] M.K. Prabhu, K. Olukotun, Exposing speculative thread parallelism in SPEC2000, in: Proceedings of the Tenth ACM SIGPLAN Symposium on Principles and Practice of Parallel Programming, 2005, pp. 142–152.

[75] A. Kejariwal, X. Tian, M. Girkar, et al., Tight analysis of the performance potential of thread speculation using spec CPU 2006, in: Proceedings of the 12th ACM SIGPLAN Symposium on Principles and Practice of Parallel Programming, 2007, pp. 215–225.

[76] BioBench and BioParallel: a benchmark suite for bioinformatics applications. http://www.ece.umd.edu/biobench/ (accessed 23 July 2013).

[77] NASA Supercomputing Benchmarks. https://www.nas.nasa.gov/cgi-bin/software/start (accessed 23 July 2013).

[78] M. Wong, C++ benchmarks in SPEC CPU2006, SIGARCH Comput. Archit. News 35 (1) (2007) 77.

[79] J.C. Phillips, R. Braun, W. Wang, et al., Scalable molecular dynamics with NAMD, J. Comput. Chem. 26 (16) (2005) 1781–1802.

[80] J. Phillips, NAMD serial and parallel performance. http://www.ks.uiuc.edu/Research/namd/tutorial/PSC2001/pdf/performance.pdf (accessed 23 July 2013).

[81] deal.II Homepage. http://www.dealii.org/ (accessed 23 July 2013).

[82] SoPlex, SMoPlex and DoPlex: parallel and object-oriented simplex algorithms. http://typo.zib.de/vis-long_projects/par/simplex.html (accessed 23 July 2013).

[83] POV-Ray—the persistence of vision raytracer. http://www.povray.org/ (accessed 23 July 2013).

[84] PVM patch for POV-Ray. http://pvmpov.sourceforge.net/ (accessed 23 July 2013).

[85] OMNeT++ Network Simulation Framework. http://omnetpp.org/ (accessed 23 July 2013).

[86] Z. Cvetanovic, C. Nofsinger, Parallel Astar search on message-passing architectures, in: Proceedings of the Twenty-Third Annual Hawaii International Conference on System Sciencesvol. 1, 1990, pp. 82–90.

[87] Berkeley Parallel Browser Project. http://parallelbrowser.blogspot.ch/ (accessed 23 July 2013).

[88] R.P. Weicker, J.L. Henning, Subroutine profiling results for the CPU2006 benchmarks, SIGARCH Comput. Archit. News 35 (1) (2007) 102.

[89] GNU gprof. http://www.cs.utah.edu/dept/old/texinfo/as/gprof.html (accessed 23 July 2013).

[90] C.D. Spradling, SPEC CPU2006 benchmark tools, SIGARCH Comput. Archit. News 35 (1) (2007) 130–134.

[91] J. JaJa, An Introduction to Parallel Algorithms, first ed., Addison-Wesley Professional, Boston, USA, 1992.

ABOUT THE AUTHORS

Aleksandar Vitorović received a Bachelor degree in Computer Science in 2008 and a Master degree in Computer Science in 2010 by the School of Electrical Engineering, University of Belgrade. In 2010, he started a Ph.D. program at EPFL, Lausanne, Switzerland. His main research interests are program parallelization and distributed systems.

Milo Tomašević was born in Nikšić, Montenegro. He received his B.Sc. in Electrical engineering and M.Sc. and Ph.D. in Computer Engineering from the University of Belgrade, Serbia, in 1980, 1984, and 1992, respectively. He is currently an Associate Professor and Head of Department of Computer Engineering, School of Electrical Engineering, University of Belgrade, Serbia. He was previously with the Pupin Institute, Belgrade, for over a decade where he was involved in many research and development projects. His current research interests are mainly in computer architecture (especially multiprocessor systems), parallel programming, cryptography, and algorithms and data structures. In these areas, he published almost 100 papers in international scientific journals, books, and proceedings of international and domestic conferences. He served as a reviewer for several journals and conferences and delivered tutorials at major conferences from the field of computer architecture and companies.

Veljko Milutinović received his Ph.D. in Electrical Engineering from University of Belgrade in 1982. During the 1980s, for about a decade, he was on the faculty of Purdue University, West Lafayette, Indiana, USA, where he coauthored the architecture and design of the world's first DARPA GaAs microprocessor. Since the 1990s, after returning to Serbia, he is on the faculty of the School of Electrical Engineering, University of Belgrade, where he is teaching courses related to computer engineering, sensor networks, and data mining. During the 1990s, he also took part in teaching at the University of Purdue, Stanford and MIT. After the year 2000, he participated in several FP6 and FP7 projects through collaboration with leading universities and industries in the EU/US, including Microsoft, Intel, IBM, Ericsson, especially Maxeler. He has lectured by invitation to over 100 European universities. He published about 50 papers in SCI journals and about 20 books with major publishers in the United States. Professor Milutinović is a Fellow of the IEEE and a Member of Academia Europaea.

AUTHOR INDEX

Note: Page numbers followed by "*f*" indicate figures, "*t*" indicate tables and "*np*" indicate footnotes.

SUBJECT INDEX

Note: Page numbers followed by "*f*" indicate figures and "*t*" indicate tables.

CONTENTS OF VOLUMES IN THIS SERIES

Volume 82

Volume 83

Volume 84

Printed and bound by CPI Group (UK) Ltd, Croydon, CR0 4YY

03/10/2024

01040425-0007

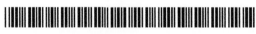